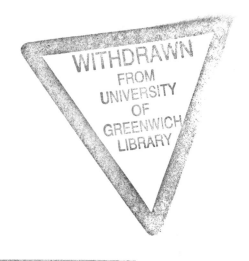

Operative Hip Arthroscopy

J.W. Thomas Byrd

Editor

Operative Hip Arthroscopy

Third Edition

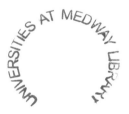

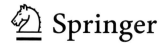 Springer

Editor
J.W. Thomas Byrd, M.D.
Nashville Sports Medicine Foundation
Nashville, TN
USA

ISBN 978-1-4419-7924-7   ISBN 978-1-4419-7925-4   (eBook)
DOI 10.1007/978-1-4419-7925-4
Springer New York Heidelberg Dordrecht London

Library of Congress Control Number: 2012940854

Printed on acid-free paper

Springer is part of Springer Science+Business Media (www.springer.com)

This third edition remains dedicated to my family, Donna, Allison, and Ellen, and to the two finest surgeons that I have known, the late Benjamin Franklin Byrd, Jr., and James Reuben Andrews.

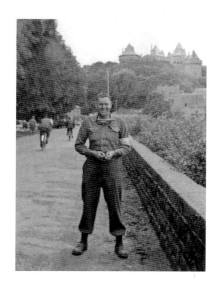

My father, B.F. Byrd, Jr., dedicated his entire life to fighting cancer, a much more admirable pursuit than anything that I will do. He detoured only briefly from this battle to champion another cause, as a highly decorated medical officer overseeing the care of wounded from Normandy Beach through the fields of Europe. Through his lifelong example, he showed me what being a physician is all about. As he put it, "A surgeon is just a regular doctor, with a few special skills."

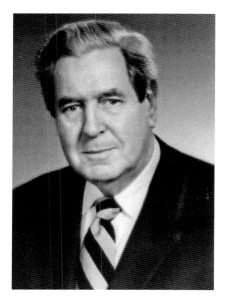

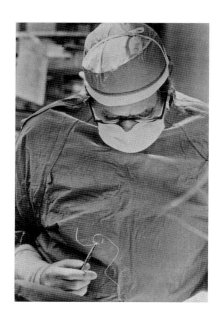

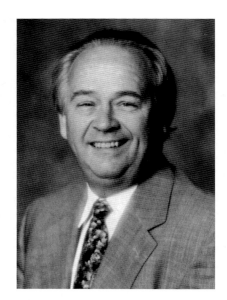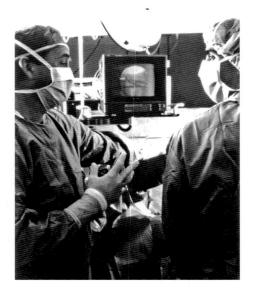

Dr. Andrews taught me the art and the philosophy of sports medicine. He also taught me much about how to treat patients as people and, fortunately, he shared with me a few of his remarkable surgical skills. Perhaps more importantly, through his example, he instilled in me the burning desire to make the most of my abilities.

Foreword to the Third Edition

One may be surprised to find a foreword from an orthopedic surgeon who is not an expert in arthroscopy. However, the motivation comes from the mutual interest in joint preserving surgery of the hip.

Dr. Byrd merits to be one of the first to describe the different technical aspects of hip arthroscopy in a textbook and editions one and two were well received by the orthopedic community. The third edition is urgently awaited because it merges the latest technical progress with the pathophysiological concept of hip impingement, yet enhancing hip arthroscopy to a larger basis of raison d'etre and vice versa, offering an additional approach to the surgical treatment of hip impingement.

The book covers all technical aspects of today's hip arthroscopy, and Dr. Byrd's arthroscopic technique is safe, efficient, and reproducible. The reader, however, should take into consideration that it pertains especially for the anterior impingement and it is very successful when this is the only localization. The more complex deformities, particularly when extra-articular components are hidden behind the intra-articular ones, may be better treated with open surgery; such complex deformities are less seen in a sports medicine practice but rather frequent in general and pediatric orthopedics.

It is foreseeable that ongoing progress of hip arthroscopy will necessitate in a few years time a further edition. The reader may then additionally wish to get information about the relevance of this treatment beyond the revival of athletic activities.

Switzerland   Reinhold Ganz, M.D.

Foreword to the Second Edition

Dr. Byrd's textbook, *Operative Hip Arthroscopy*, is a must-have for every physician and surgeon who cares for patients with hip problems. Dr. Byrd is to be complimented for advancing the art and science of medicine with this comprehensive dissertation that not only illustrates what is possible in the diagnosis and treatment of hip pathology but teaches a procedure that was thought to be impossible in the not too distant past.

This second edition is another major step forward in the application of minimally invasive procedures that, until recently, would only have been undertaken with great hesitation because of the magnitude of the surgical exposure. This text includes a comprehensive review of the pertinent anatomy and pathological processes that are potentially amenable to the ever widening application of arthroscopy as well as the critical aspects of the physical examination and postoperative care.

Physicians and surgeons face the challenge of bringing these diagnostic tools and surgical treatments into the real world of everyday practice. This is no easy task, but this text goes a long way in helping to prepare them for this adventure. It continues the revolution in orthopedic hip surgery that has been advanced by Dr. Byrd and his colleagues. It provides the best opportunity for learning these techniques outside of a personal visit and observation and will undoubtedly encourage others to join Dr. Byrd in advancing the techniques of arthroscopy in the hip.

Lanny L. Johnson, M.D.

Foreword to the First Edition

The hip is a site of pathology ranging from degenerative disorders to work- and sports-related injuries. The hip is also one of the final frontiers for arthroscopic intervention.

Unique anatomic considerations challenge the hip arthroscopist and have slowed the advancement of hip arthroscopy. The dense soft tissue encasing the joint, the relatively non-compliant capsule, and the ball-and-socket architecture constrain both access and maneuverability of instrumentation.

The evolution of hip arthroscopy has followed a different course from other joints. In the knee, for example, standard practice for recognized pathology evolved from open techniques to less invasive arthroscopic procedures. Conversely, in the hip, standard practice evolved from no treatment at all because of the failure to recognize the existence of these lesions. Arthroscopic assessment defined the presence of symptomatic hip pathology amenable to something other than a total hip replacement, which is the major surgical procedure for patients with hip disease.

Rarely has arthrotomy been an accepted practice for elusive sources of hip pathology. However, arthroscopy for certain causes of hip pain offers an alternative where previously the only option was living within the constraints of the symptoms.

There are several merits to hip arthroscopy. First, arthroscopic assessment has identified previously unrecognized disorders. Second, arthroscopy is a less invasive alternative to arthrotomy for certain pathologies. Third, for such elusive causes of hip pain as labral or chondral injuries, arthroscopy offers a definitive treatment where none existed before. Fourth, it has a role as a staging procedure for osteotomy candidates and patients with avascular necrosis. Finally, arthroscopy may have a role as a palliative and temporizing procedure for select patients with degenerative hip disease.

The authors have prepared a comprehensive text covering all facets of hip arthroscopy. I believe the reader will find this work informative and helpful in the care of patients and in the understanding of the principles of arthroscopic surgery of the hip. I congratulate the authors on their excellent work and wish the reader success in the challenging and rewarding endeavor of hip arthroscopy.

James R. Andrews, M.D.

Preface

Seven years elapsed between the first and second editions of *Operative Hip Arthroscopy*. That period signaled a wave of growing attention to the hip. It has been another 7 years to the publication of the third edition. During this time, there has been an explosion of interest in hip arthroscopy with exponential growth in the understanding of hip disorders and technology available for treatment. All of these latest advancements are contained within the pages of this third edition.

The earlier editions set the foundation for the proven fundamentals that have facilitated continuing intellectual and technological revolution. These many arthroscopic innovations have been garnered by a legion of brilliant young clinical scientists with a passion for hip arthroscopy, as well as insight from surgeons who perform open techniques. The revolution of less invasive arthroscopic and endoscopic methods is far from complete, but this third edition of *Operative Hip Arthroscopy* covers all the latest technology available for our patients.

This edition contains the newest advancements in atraumatic access to the joint and provides an understanding of the numerous disorders to be encountered, ranging from FAI and beyond and the current treatments for preservation, restoration, and reconstruction. Management of problems in the central and peripheral compartments is detailed, and we have long been dealing with issues outside the joint such as the iliopsoas tendon. These less invasive methods have now expanded into the surrounding soft tissue regions of the hip. Arthroscopy has evolved into endoscopic techniques for the peritrochanteric space and subgluteal region and even hamstring disorders. We have redefined some disorders such as greater trochanteric pain syndrome, abductor tendinopathies, and subgluteal syndrome previously described with open technology and have newly defined some previously unrecognized problems.

There are unique challenges to hip arthroscopy that should discourage casual consideration of this procedure without clear indication and purpose. The dos and don'ts are clearly emphasized in this text. If you prepare to embark on a case of arthroscopic surgery of the hip, be sure of your indications, be versed in the technique, but read about the complications twice. As my father's chief, Barney Brooks, M.D., chief of surgery at Vanderbilt University, 1925–1952, was quoted as saying to one of his residents "Son, you don't have to learn all the complications for yourself, you can read about a few of them."

In summary, this textbook details the clinical assessment including examination and imaging that is necessary for patient selection in the decision making process for arthroscopy. The numerous forms of pathology and their treatment are detailed including expectations of outcomes and results. Of equal importance, efforts have been made to discern the underlying etiology and how to address this with the goal of genuinely improving the natural history and progression of many of these disorders.

Acknowledgment

Sharon Simmons and Kay Jones have been involved since the beginning. They along with every member of the Nashville Sports Medicine team have been an essential element of everything that we have accomplished. Sharon has deftly orchestrated every manuscript and educational endeavor, while Kay has tirelessly cared for and followed all the patients. Lisa Donnelly, fueled by her passion and drive, has reached iconic status within industry through her contributions. Encouraged and supported by her mentors at Smith & Nephew, Lisa has raised the bar on industry commitment to hip arthroscopy. A legion of talented individuals have contributed to everything that we have done in surgery, including Jim who has assisted in more hip arthroscopy cases than any other known person. This just scratches the surface of those who have touched the lives of our patients and influenced the treatment of patients worldwide. It takes a village.

J.W. Thomas Byrd

Contents

Contributors

Oscar Fariñas Barberá, M.D. Transplant Services Foundation, Musculoskeletal Tissue Unit, Sant Boi de Llobregat, Barcelona, Spain

Ray Barile, M.S. St. Louis Blues Hockey Club, Scottrade Center, St. Louis, MO, USA

Asheesh Bedi, M.D. Sports Medicine and Shoulder Surgery, Department of Orthopaedic Surgery, Hospital for Special Surgery, Ann Arbor, MI, USA

MedSport, Ann Arbor, MI, USA

Luise Berger, M.D. Department of Plastic Surgery and Hand Surgery, Klinikum rechts der Isar, Munich, Bavaria, Germany

Itamar Botser, M.D. Hinsdale Orthopaedics Associates, Westmont, IL, USA

Loyola Stritch School of Medicine, Chicago, IL, USA

Michael Brunt, M.D. Section of Minimally Invasive Surgery, Barnes-Jewish Hospital, Washington University School of Medicine, St. Louis, MO, USA

J.W. Thomas Byrd, M.D. Nashville Sports Medicine Foundation, Nashville, TN, USA

Javier Camacho-Galindo, M.D. Adult Joint Reconstruction Service, Hip and Knee, National Rehabilitation Institute of Mexico, Mexico City, DF, Mexico

Department of Hip and Knee Surgery, Universidad Nacional Autónoma de México, Mexico City, DF, Mexico

Erica M. Coplen, DPT Department of Physical Therapy, Nashville Sports Medicine Physical Therapy, Nashville, TN, USA

Benjamin Domb, M.D. Hinsdale Orthopaedics Associates, Westmont, IL, USA

Loyola Stritch School of Medicine, Chicago, IL, USA

Roy E. Erb, M.D. Department of Medical Imaging, St. Mary's Hospital, Grand Junction, CO, USA

Trevor R. Gaskill, M.D. Bone and Joint Sports Medicine Institute, Naval Medical Center Portsmouth, Portsmouth, VA, USA

Steadman Philippon Research Institute, The Steadman Clinic, Vail, CO, USA

Carlos A. Guanche, M.D. Southern California Orthopedic Institute, Los Angeles, Van Nuys, CA, USA

Sommer Hammoud, M.D. Department of Sports Medicine, Massachusetts General Hospital, Boston, MA, USA

Marcia Horner, B.A. Vincera Core Physicians, Philadelphia, PA, USA

Victor M. Ilizaliturri, Jr. M.D. Adult Joint Reconstruction Service, Hip and Knee, National Rehabilitation Institute of Mexico, Mexico City, DF, Mexico

Department of Hip and Knee Surgery, Universidad Nacional Autónoma de México, Mexico City, DF, Mexico

Kay S. Jones, MSN, RN Nashville Sports Medicine Foundation, Nashville, TN, USA

Tina Joseph, M.D. Department of Surgery, Drexel University, College of Medicine/Hahnemann Hospital, Philadelphia, PA, USA

Patrick Jost, M.D. Milwaukee Orthopedic Group, Milwaukee, WI, USA

Bryan T. Kelly, M.D. Center for Hip Preservation, Hospital for Special Surgery, New York, NY, USA

Michael Knesek, M.D. Department of Orthopaedic Surgery, University of Michigan, Ann Arbor, MI, USA

Mininder S. Kocher, M.D., MPH Department of Orthopaedic Surgery, Harvard Medical School, Boston, MA, USA

Division of Sports Medicine, Department of Orthopaedic Surgery, Children's Hospital Boston, Boston, MA, USA

Christopher M. Larson, M.D. Minnesota Orthopedic Sports Medicine Institute, Twin Cities Orthopedics, Edina, MN, USA

Erin Magennis, B.A. Center for Hip Preservation, Hospital for Special Surgery, New York, NY, USA

G. Peter Maiers II M.D. Methodist Sports Medicine – The Orthopedic Specialists, Indianapolis, IN, USA

Department of Orthopaedic Surgery, Indiana University, Indianapolis, **IN, USA**

Hal David Martin, DO The Hip Clinic, Oklahoma Sport Science and Orthopaedics, Oklahoma City, OK, USA

Phillip Mason, M.D. Department of Orthopaedic Surgery, Wake Forest University, Winston-Salem, NC, USA

Richard C. Mather III M.D. Department of Orthopaedic Surgery, Duke University Medical Center, Durham, NC, USA

William C. Meyers, M.D. Departments of Surgery, Drexel University College of Medicine and Thomas Jefferson University, Philadelphia, PA, USA

Duke University Health System, Durham, NC, USA

Core Performance Physicians, Philadelphia, PA, USA

Ulrike Muschaweck, M.D., Ph.D. Hernienzentrum Dr. Muschaweck, Munich, Bavaria, Germany

Ivan Sáenz Navarro, M.D. Department of Human anatomy and Embriology, Facultat de Medicina, Barcelona, Spain

Shane J. Nho, M.D., M.S. Department of Orthopedic Surgery, Rush University Medical Center, Midwest Orthopaedics at Rush, Chicago, IL, USA

Marc J. Philippon, M.D. Department of Hip Arthroscopy, Steadman Philippon Research Institute and Steadman Clinic, Vail, CO, USA

Elizabeth A. Potts, MSN, APN, ACNP-BC Nashville Sports Medicine Foundation, Nashville, TN, USA

Avinish Reddy, B.S. Department of Orthopedic Surgery, Rush University Medical Center, Chicago, IL, USA

Thomas G. Sampson, M.D. Department of Hip Arthroscopy, Post Street Surgery, San Francisco, CA, USA

Jack G. Skendzel, M.D. Department of Orthopaedic Surgery, University of Michigan, Ann Arbor, MI, USA

Austin V. Stone, M.D. Department of Orthopaedic Surgery, Wake Forest University, Winston-Salem, NC, USA

Rebecca M. Stone, M.S., ATC Minnesota Orthopedic Sports Medicine Institute, Twin Cities Orthopedics, Edina, MN, USA

Allston J. Stubbs, M.D. Department of Orthopaedic Surgery, Wake Forest University, Winston-Salem, NC, USA

Humberto Gonzalez Ugalde, M.D. Adult Joint Reconstruction Service, Hip and Knee, National Rehabilitation Institute of Mexico, Mexico City, DF, Mexico

Department of Hip and Knee Surgery, Universidad Nacional Autónoma de México, Mexico City, DF, Mexico

Michael L. Voight, DHSc, PT, OCS, SCS, ATC, FAPTA School of Physical Therapy, Belmont University, Nashville, TN, USA

James E. Voos, M.D. Department of Orthopaedic Surgery, Orthopaedic and Sports Medicine Clinic of Kansas City, Leawood, KS, USA

Christopher Walsh, M.D. Department of Orthopaedic Surgery, University of Michigan Health System, Ann Arbor, MI, USA

Corey A. Wulf, M.D. Department of Orthopedics, CNOS, Dakota Dunes, SD, USA

Yi-Meng Yen, M.D., Ph.D. Division of Sports Medicine, Department of Orthopaedic Surgery, Children's Hospital Boston, Harvard Medical School, Boston, MA, USA

Adam Zoga, M.D. Department of Radiology, Thomas Jefferson University, Philadelphia, PA, USA

Overview and History of Hip Arthroscopy

J.W. Thomas Byrd

The first recorded attempt at arthroscopic visualization of the hip is attributed to Michael S. Burman in 1931 (Figs. 1.1 and 1.2) [1]. For his purposes, an arthroscope was constructed by Reinhold Wappler with a diameter of 4 mm, not dissimilar to the dimensions of our current arthroscopes (Fig. 1.3). Burman used fluid distension for visualization, examining the interior of more than 90 various joints in cadaver specimens, correlating the arthroscopic anatomy with the gross anatomy on subsequent dissection. Twenty of these were hip joints. Dr. Burman practiced at the Hospital for Joint Diseases in New York City, but according to Ejnar Eriksson, he performed his landmark cadaver work at a lab in Germany.

Burman made several pertinent and prudent observations that still hold true today, more than over 80 years later. His examination of the hip did not use distraction, and the structures that he successfully visualized correspond with the structures that currently are discernible via arthroscopy without distraction (Fig. 1.4). These aspects include much of the articular surface of the femoral head, seen by placing the hip through range of motion, and the intracapsular portion of the femoral neck. With this approach, the acetabulum, fossa, and ligamentum teres could not be visualized.

Burman noted that "visualization of the hip joint is limited to the intracapsular part of the joint." This statement still has much bearing in current applications of hip arthroscopy. Although arthroscopy has been used for release of a snapping iliopsoas tendon and for extracapsular bone fragments that impinge on the joint, intra-articular sources of pathology are most amenable to arthroscopic intervention.

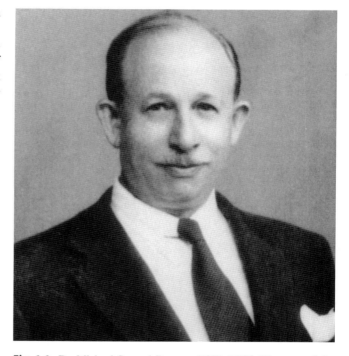

Fig. 1.1 Dr. Michael Samuel Burman (1901–1975) (Courtesy of the New York Academy of Medicine Library)

Burman further stated:

We experimented with a number of punctures and the anterior paratrochanteric puncture proved the best… The anterior paratrochanteric puncture is undoubtedly the best and is made slightly anterior to the greater trochanter along the course of the neck of the femur… The puncture is not hard to do and one can visualize the hip with it in almost every case. Originally we were skeptical as to whether anything could be seen in the hip joint, but we have had unusual success with this puncture.

The anterior paratrochanteric (or anterolateral) portal is clearly the workhorse portal for modern arthroscopy. Although there is some variation of the other portals described by numerous authors, this is the one position common to all, and according to an anatomic study, it is the safest [3].

J.W.T. Byrd, M.D.
Nashville Sports Medicine Foundation,
2011 Church Street, Suite 100, Nashville, TN 37203, USA
e-mail: byrd@nsmfoundation.org

J.W.T. Byrd (ed.), *Operative Hip Arthroscopy*,
DOI 10.1007/978-1-4419-7925-4_1, © Springer Science+Business Media New York 2013

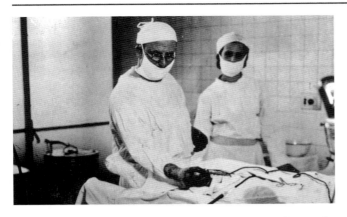

Fig. 1.2 Dr. Burman performing an arthroscopic procedure at the Hospital for Joint Diseases in 1935 (Reprinted from: Parisien and Present [2]. With permission)

Burman continued:

We have been careful to choose cadavers of slender build since our trochar is not long enough to puncture the hip of a well mus-cled person… A special long trochar with a correspondingly long telescope should thus be used for the hip joint. The line of the femoral artery and the position of the head of the femur should be marked beforehand to avoid possible damage to the vessels. This should only be a theoretical accident.

For the surgeon who only occasionally is challenged by the role of arthroscopic surgery of the hip, size may be a rela-tive contraindication, and even for an experienced arthrosco-pist, it may preclude the ability to enter the hip joint. Indeed, as recommended by Burman, extra-length cannulas and instruments are used, but in some cases, even these may not be adequate. Also, a careful appreciation of the orientation of

Fig. 1.3 Photograph reprinted from Burman's article illustrates the arthroscopic instruments devised by Reinhold Wappler and used by Dr. Burman in his investigative studies. The *upper portion* is the telescope (measuring 3 mm in diameter), the *lower portion* is the trochar sheath (measuring 4 mm in diameter) (Reprinted by permission, Burman [2])

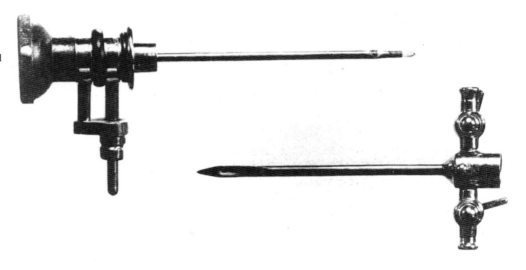

Fig. 1.4 Burman's illustration of the arthroscopic view of a hip visualizing the ridging of the neck of the femur, the junction of the neck and the femoral head, and a portion of the articular surface of the femoral head (Reprinted by permission, Burman [2])

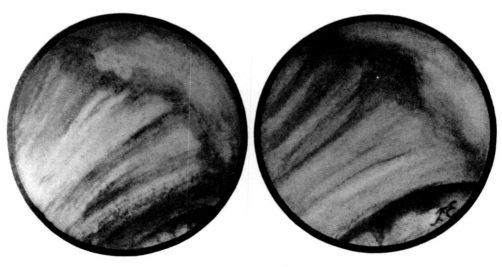

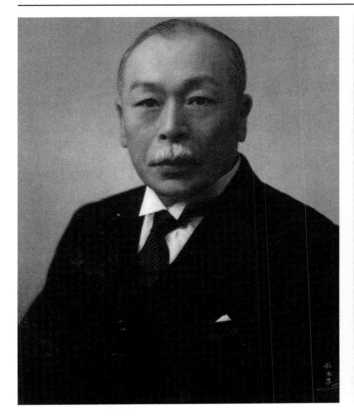

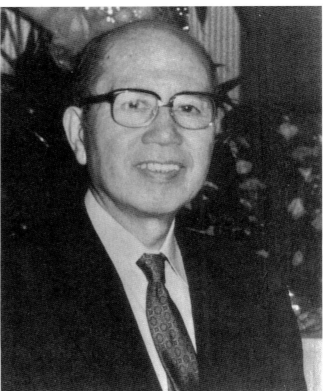

Fig. 1.5 Dr. Kenji Takagi (1888–1963) (Courtesy, Tokyo Teishin Hospital)

Fig. 1.6 Dr. Masaki Watanabe (1911–1994) (Courtesy, Tokyo Teishin Hospital)

the major neurovascular structures is always critical. There are anecdotal accounts such as a case of irreparable damage to the femoral nerve. This type of catastrophic scenario should be unlikely with basic understanding and orientation of the extra-articular anatomy.

The first clinical application of the arthroscope in the hip of a patient was reported by Takagi in 1939 (Fig. 1.5) [4]. This report consisted of four hips, including two cases of Charcot's joints, one tuberculous arthritis, and one suppurative arthritis.

The clinical implications of arthroscopic techniques, especially about the knee, began to flourish following the publication of the second edition of *Atlas of Arthroscopy* by Masaki Watanabe et al. [5] in 1965 (Fig. 1.6). Watanabe was a student of Takagi. He also visited with Michael Burman in the evolution of his techniques.

However, following Takagi's report in 1939, the clinical applications of arthroscopy about the hip went unmentioned until the 1970s with Aignan's [6] report of attempted diagnostic arthroscopy and biopsy of 51 hips. This study was presented at the 1975 meeting of the International Arthroscopy Association in Copenhagen. In 1977, Richard Gross described 32 diagnostic arthroscopic procedures in 27 children for a variety of pediatric hip disorders including congenital dislocation, Legg-Calve-Perthes disease, neuropathic

subluxation, prior sepsis, and slipped capital femoral epiphysis [7]. A second clinical series appeared in the pediatric literature in 1981 when Svante Holgersson et al. [8] from Sweden reported on the role of arthroscopy in assessing 15 hips in 13 children with juvenile chronic arthritis. Between these two series, there were two case reports on removal of entrapped cement fragments following total hip arthroplasty, one from the New York City Hospital for Special Surgery and one from Israel [9, 10].

The 1980s brought several important advancements that contributed to the applications of operative hip arthroscopy. In 1981, Lanny Johnson [11] addressed the role of arthroscopy of the hip joint in the second edition of his textbook, *Diagnostic and Surgical Arthroscopy* (Fig. 1.7). In 1985, Watanabe [12] also described the technique for carrying out the procedure in *Arthroscopy of Small Joints*. In 1986, Ejnar Eriksson et al. [13] from Sweden described the forces necessary for adequate hip distraction (Fig. 1.8). This was an in vivo study of patients undergoing arthroscopy as well as a study of unanesthetized volunteers, which included Professor Eriksson himself.

James Glick from San Francisco has been recognized as the single greatest influence on the development of hip arthroscopy in North America (Fig. 1.9). Motivated by the creative ideas of Lanny Johnson, Glick began performing the

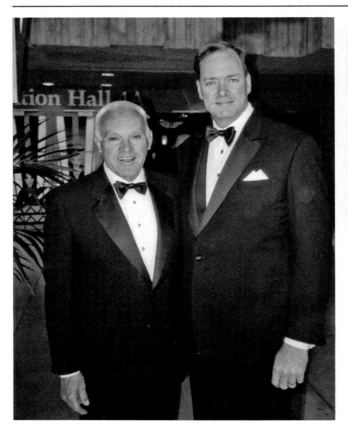

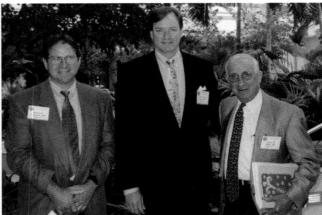

Fig. 1.9 The author with James Glick (*right*) and Thomas Sampson (*left*). Jim Glick, the single greatest figure in modern hip arthroscopy, was motivated by Lanny Johnson and influenced in his techniques by his younger partner, Tom Sampson (Courtesy of J.W. Thomas Byrd, M.D., Nashville, TN)

Fig. 1.7 The author (*right*) with Lanny Johnson (*left*), a pioneer of arthroscopy as a clinician, scientist, and inventor (Courtesy of J.W. Thomas Byrd, M.D., Nashville, TN)

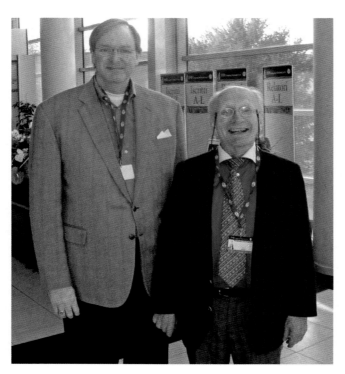

Fig. 1.8 The author with Professor Eriksson (*right*), a pioneer in arthroscopy and modern techniques in surgical reconstruction of the knee (Courtesy, Ejnar Eriksson, M.D.)

procedure in 1977. He recognized limitations of the technique in obese patients. Influenced by his partner, Thomas Sampson, in 1985 Glick modified the procedure and began placing the patient in the lateral decubitus position. Their preliminary experiences were reported in 1987 [14]. This and subsequent works became the cornerstones upon which other surgeons founded their approach [15, 16].

In the mid-1980s, Richard Villar from Cambridge, England, envisioned several useful roles for arthroscopy of the hip. He corresponded with James Glick and Richard Hawkins, who had published some of the few articles available on the topic at the time [14–17]. Villar subsequently pioneered the technique in England. He published the first textbook on the subject, and through his teachings, he has influenced many others to begin performing the procedure in the United Kingdom [18].

By the late 1980s, numerous authors contributed to the slowly growing knowledge base for hip arthroscopy [19–21]. Joe McCarthy from Boston has particularly remained active as a prolific author and educator [22]. There was a brief influx of reports from Japan, especially focusing on lesions of the acetabular labrum [23–26]. In Nashville, this author redefined the application of the supine position and has nurtured the field of hip arthroscopy through preparation of several textbooks and numerous scientific publications [27–29]. These efforts have been possible through a database diligently maintained over these last two decades by Kay Jones.

In the United States, little attention has been given to the prospect of performing hip arthroscopy without distraction [30]. However, Henri Dorfmann and Thierry Boyer, a pair of rheumatologists from Paris, France, have accumulated a large number of cases performed by this method [31, 32] (Fig. 1.10). Dr. Dorfmann learned the techniques of arthroscopy while training under Dr. Watanabe in Japan and pioneered his own

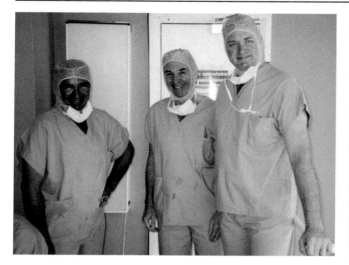

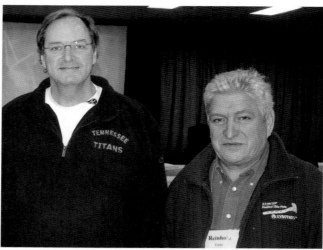

Fig. 1.10 The author on the occasion of a visit with Drs. Dorfmann (*center*) and Boyer (*left*) at their surgery center in Paris (Courtesy of J.W. Thomas Byrd, M.D., Nashville, TN)

Fig. 1.11 The author with Professor Ganz (*right*) at Jeffrey Mast's hip symposium at Mammoth Lakes (Courtesy of J.W. Thomas Byrd, M.D., Nashville, TN)

Fig. 1.12 The founding board members of the International Society for Hip Arthroscopy, Paris, 2008. From *left* to *right* are Thierry Boyer, Giancarlo Polesello, Robert Buly, Victor Ilizaliturri, Michael Dienst, Tom Sampson, Richard Villar, Marc Philippon, Joe McCarthy, John O'Donnell, Thomas Byrd, and Hassan Sadri (Courtesy of Robert Buly, M.D.)

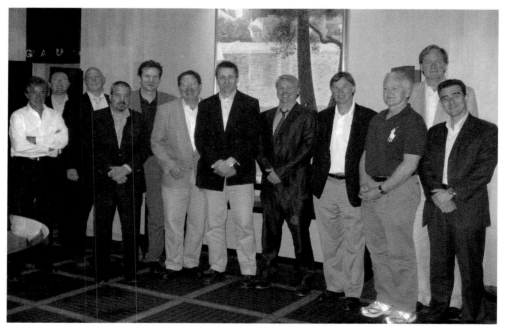

method of hip arthroscopy, especially important for viewing the peripheral compartment. However, it was a young orthopedic surgeon, Michael Dienst, who brought the Parisians' technique to the orthopedic world, successfully integrating arthroscopy of the intra-articular joint with that of the periphery [33]. Unbeknown at the time, this set the stage for arthroscopic access of femoroacetabular impingement lesions, which were soon to be described by Professor Reinhold Ganz and colleagues in Bern, Switzerland (Fig. 1.11) [34]. The most innovative contributor in the transition from resection to restorative reconstructive techniques has been Marc Philippon from Vail.

We have now seen exponential growth of interest in hip arthroscopy. There has been extensive work in the realms of both basic science and clinical research, with a steady stream of peer-reviewed scientific publications. A groundswell of participation of talented young surgeons with brilliant scientific minds has occurred. Some of these representative individuals are noted in the photograph (Fig. 1.12) of the founding board members of the International Society for Hip Arthroscopy (ISHA), which was the brainchild of Ricky Villar. This organization, with its popular science-packed annual meetings, best epitomizes the explosion of worldwide innovations and evidence-based medicine in the field of hip arthroscopy.

References

1. Burman M. Arthroscopy or the direct visualization of joints. J Bone Joint Surg. 1931;13(4):669–94.
2. Parisien JS, Present DA. Dr. Michael S. Burman, pioneer in the field of arthroscopy. Bull Hosp Jt Dis Orthop Inst. 1985;45(2):119–26.
3. Byrd JWT, Pappas JN, Pedley MJ. Hip arthroscopy: an anatomic study of portal placement and relationship to the extraarticular structures. Arthroscopy. 1994;11(4):418–23.
4. Takagi K. The arthroscope: the second report. J Jpn Orthop Assoc. 1939;14:441–66.
5. Watanabe M, Takeda S, Ikeuchi H. Atlas of arthroscopy. 2nd ed. Tokyo: Igaku-Shoin; 1970.
6. Aignan M. Arthroscopy of the hip. In: Proceedings of the International Association of Arthroscopy. Rev Int Rheumatol. 1976;33:458.
7. Gross R. Arthroscopy in hip disorders in children. Orthop Rev. 1977;6(9):43–9.
8. Holgersson S, Brattström H, Mogensen B, Lidgren L. Arthroscopy of the hip in juvenile chronic arthritis. J Pediatr Orthop. 1981;1(3):273–8.
9. Shifrin L, Reis N. Arthroscopy of a dislocated hip replacement: a case report. Clin Orthop. 1980;146:213–4.
10. Vakili F, Salvati EA, Warren RF. Entrapped foreign body within the acetabular cup in total hip replacement. Clin Orthop. 1980;150:159–62.
11. Johnson LL. Hip joint. In: Johnson LL, editor. Diagnostic and surgical arthroscopy, the knee and other joints. 2nd ed. St. Louis: CV Mosby; 1981. p. 405–11.
12. Watanabe M. Arthroscopy of small joints. Tokyo: Igaku-Shoin; 1985.
13. Eriksson E, Arvidsson I, Arvidsson H. Diagnostic and operative arthroscopy of the hip. Orthopaedics. 1986;9(2):169–76.
14. Glick JM, Sampson TG, Gordon BB, Behr JT, Schmidt E. Hip arthroscopy by the lateral approach. Arthroscopy. 1987;3(1):4–12.
15. Glick JM. Hip arthroscopy using the lateral approach. Instr Course Lect. 1988;37:223–31.
16. Glick JM, Sampson TG. Hip arthroscopy by the lateral approach. In: McGinty J, Caspari R, Jackson R, Poehling G, editors. Operative arthroscopy. 2nd ed. New York: Raven Press; 1995. p. 1079–90.
17. Hawkins RB. Arthroscopy of the hip. Clin Orthop. 1989;249:44–7.
18. Villar RN. Hip arthroscopy. Oxford: Butterworth-Heinemann; 1992.
19. Dvorak M, Duncan CP, Day B. Arthroscopic anatomy of the hip. Arthroscopy. 1990;6:264–73.
20. Parisien JS. Arthroscopy of the hip, present status. Bull Hosp Jt Dis Orthop Inst. 1985;45(2):127–32.
21. Parisien JS. Arthroscopy surgery of the hip. In: Parisien JS, editor. Arthroscopic surgery. New York: McGraw-Hill; 1988. p. 283–91.
22. McCarthy JC, Day B, Busconi B. Hip arthroscopy: applications and technique. J Am Acad Orthop Surg. 1995;3(3):115–22.
23. Ikeda T, Awaya G, Suzuki S, Okada Y, Tada H. Torn acetabular labrum in young patients. J Bone Joint Surg. 1988;70B:13–6.
24. Ueo T, Suzuki S, Iwasaki R, Yosikawa J. Rupture of the labra acetabularis as a cause of hip pain detected arthroscopically, and partial limbectomy for successful pain relief. Arthroscopy. 1990;6(1):48–51.
25. Suzuki S, Awaya G, Okada Y, Maekawa M, Ikeda T, Tada H. Arthroscopic diagnosis of ruptured acetabular labrum. Acta Orthop Scand. 1986;57:513–5.
26. Ide T, Akamatsu N, Nakajima I. Arthroscopic surgery of the hip joint. Arthroscopy. 1991;7(2):204–11.
27. Byrd JWT. Hip arthroscopy utilizing the supine position. Arthroscopy. 1994;10(3):275–80.
28. Byrd JWT. Operative hip arthroscopy. New York: Thieme; 1998.
29. Byrd JWT. Operative hip arthroscopy. 2nd ed. New York: Springer; 2004.
30. Klapper RC, Silver DM. Hip arthroscopy without distraction. Contemp Orthop. 1989;18(6):687–93.
31. Dorfmann H, Boyer T, Henry P, de Bie B. A simple approach to hip arthroscopy. Arthroscopy. 1988;4(2):141–2.
32. Dorfmann H, Boyer T. Arthroscopy of the hip: 12 years of experience. Arthroscopy. 1999;15(1):67–72.
33. Dienst M, Godde S, Seil R, Hammer D, Kohn D. Hip arthroscopy without traction: in vivo anatomy of the peripheral hip joint cavity. Arthroscopy. 2001;17(9):924–31.
34. Ganz R, Parvizi J, Beck M, et al. Femoroacetabular impingement. A cause for osteoarthritis of the hip. Clin Orthop Relat Res. 2003;7:112–20.

Patient Selection and Physical Examination

J.W. Thomas Byrd

The key to successful outcomes in hip arthroscopy lies most clearly in proper patient selection. The best operation will fail when performed for the wrong reasons. Selection revolves around imaging evidence or at least clinical findings of a problem potentially amenable to arthroscopic intervention. Another important selection factor is assuring that the patient has reasonable expectations of what may or may not be accomplished by the procedure. The success of the operation is gauged by the patient's function and subjective sense of satisfaction. If the patient has unreasonable expectations of what the procedure may accomplish, then it will be deemed a failure, even in the presence of a well-performed procedure.

Examination of the hip joint is succinct and requires only a few minutes. However, examination of the hip region can be complex and requires much more detail. Numerous disorders can mimic a hip joint problem. Generally, these are neurological, visceral or musculoskeletal. An upper lumbar disk problem causes anterior hip pain and minimal traction signs, which is different than the findings that would be more easily distinguished in association with more common lower lumbar disk problems. Major nerves include the sciatic, femoral, and obturator, but any nerves of the lumbosacral plexus can become entrapped with sometimes variable and overlapping pain patterns that may need to be deciphered [1]. Referred symptoms from a visceral origin include disorders of the gastrointestinal, urological, or gynecological systems. Other musculoskeletal problems such as mechanical back pain or pelvic dysfunction from the SI joint or symphysis pubis must be differentiated.

Additionally, not all hip problems are amenable to arthroscopic intervention. Stress fractures, avascular necrosis, and advanced degenerative disease are just a few examples. Also, keep in mind that the hip and pelvis are the sites of origin of approximately 10–15% of all primary musculoskeletal tumors, although metastatic disease is more common among older adults. Because of the joint's deeply situated anatomy, tumors can grow to considerable size before being clinically evident. Radiographs are important. These are helpful to rule out other problems in addition to assisting in the diagnosis of intra-articular disorders amenable to arthroscopy.

It is refreshing to evaluate a patient who has a simple isolated hip joint problem. Often there may be coexistent disease or secondary disorders where the patient has been compensating for the hip or simply other coexistent abnormalities.

It is not uncommon for an adult patient with early degenerative hip disease to perhaps have some concomitant degenerative problems of the lumbar spine. Differentiating the contribution of each can be a clinical challenge. Among athletes, hip and back problems often coexist, especially in sports where rotational velocity is a premium. Dysfunction of one results in reduced ability to compensate for the other. The physician may find himself alternately treating one or the other, but they actually require a comprehensive management strategy. There is ample data that hip disorders often go undetected for a protracted period of time [2]. As individuals compensate for their hip problem, secondary disorders develop such as gluteal symptoms or trochanteric bursitis. On examination, the secondary disorders may be more evident and obscure the underlying primary hip problem. Treatment of these secondary disorders fails when the primary problem is not addressed. Lastly, there may simply be other coexistent problems such as snapping of the iliopsoas tendon or iliotibial band. Since these have a recognized prevalence in a normal population and may be present in someone with a hip disorder, these can further challenge the clinical assessment [3].

Patient demographics provide useful tips in formulating a differential diagnosis. Age, gender, vocation, or avocation all provide useful clues. For example, femoroacetabular impingement (FAI) is a common source of problems in ice hockey. Dysplasia is more common in dancers where mobility

J.W.T. Byrd, M.D.
Nashville Sports Medicine Foundation,
2011 Church Street, Suite 100, Nashville, TN 37203, USA
e-mail: byrd@nsmfoundation.org

is more of a premium. Also in this group, even slight impingement can become problematic because of the super physiologic demands of motion. Older patients are more likely to have problems with arthritis. Advancing age is not an indicator of poor results with arthroscopy, but the amount of arthritis is [4].

History

There are various disorders that can result in a painful hip, and thus the history may be equally varied as far as onset, duration, and severity of symptoms. For example, acute labral tears associated with an injury have gone undiagnosed for decades, presenting as a chronic disorder. Conversely, patients with a degenerative labral tear may describe the acute onset of symptoms associated with a relatively innocuous episode and gradual progression of symptoms.

In general, a history of a significant traumatic event is a better prognostic indicator of a problem potentially correctable with arthroscopy [5]. Insidious onset of symptoms can be a less favorable prognostic indicator but not a contraindication to arthroscopy. This situation reflects the likely existence of underlying predisposition to injury. Patients may recount a specific precipitating episode such as a twisting injury, but even with these circumstances, there is a likelihood of some underlying susceptibility to joint damage.

Mechanical symptoms such as locking, catching, popping, or sharp stabbing in nature are better prognostic indicators of a problem correctable by arthroscopy [6]. Simply pain in absence of mechanical symptoms is a poorer predictor. However, the presence of a "pop" or "click" is an often overrated feature of the hip examination. This may indicate an unstable lesion inside the joint, but many painful intra-articular problems never demonstrate this finding, and popping and clicking can occur due to many extra-articular causes, most of which are normal. Constant intractable pain present even with inactivity presents a particular challenge and is often unlikely to be solved by arthroscopy.

There are characteristic features of the history that can indicate a mechanical hip problem (Table 2.1). These are helpful in localizing the hip as the source of trouble but are not specific for the type of pathology. As expected, the pain is worse with activities, although the degree is variable. Straight plane activities such as straight-ahead walking or even running are often well tolerated, while twisting maneuvers such as simply turning to change direction may produce sharp pain, especially turning toward the symptomatic side which places the hip in internal rotation. Sitting may be uncomfortable, especially if the hip is placed in excessive flexion. Rising from the seated position is especially painful,

Table 2.1 Characteristic hip symptoms

Symptoms worse with activities
Twisting, such as turning changing directions
Seated position may be uncomfortable, especially with hip flexion
Rising from seated position often painful (catching)
Difficulty ascending and descending stairs
Symptoms with entering/exiting an automobile
Dyspareunia
Difficulty with shoes, socks, hose, etc.

and the patient may experience an accompanying catch or sharp stabbing sensation. Also, after a period of sitting, the first few steps upon rising may be painful. Symptoms are worse with ascending or descending stairs or other inclines. Entering and exiting an automobile is often difficult with accompanying pain. This loads the hip in a flexed position along with twisting maneuvers. Dyspareunia is almost uniformly present and a problem for sexually active individuals, although often patients may be reluctant to share this bit of information. Difficulty with shoes, socks, or hose may simply be due to pain or may reflect restricted rotational motion and more advanced hip joint involvement.

Based on the information obtained in the history, a preliminary differential diagnosis should be formulated. The history assists the examiner in performing an appropriately directed physical examination.

Physical Examination

The information obtained in the history is just a screening tool. It helps direct the examination, but it should not unduly prejudice the approach. The examiner must be systematic and thorough to avoid potential pitfalls and missed diagnoses (Fig. 2.1). In reference to examination of the hip, Otto Aufranc [7] noted that "more is missed by not looking than by not knowing."

Inspection

The most important aspect of inspection is stance and gait. The patient's posture is observed in both the standing and seated position. Any splinting or protective maneuvers used to alleviate stresses on the hip joint are noted. While standing, a slightly flexed position of the involved hip and concomitantly the ipsilateral knee is common (Fig. 2.2). In the seated position, slouching or listing to the uninvolved side avoids extremes of flexion (Fig. 2.3).

An antalgic gait is often present but dependent on the severity of symptoms. Typically, the stance phase is

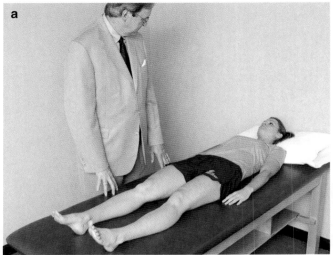

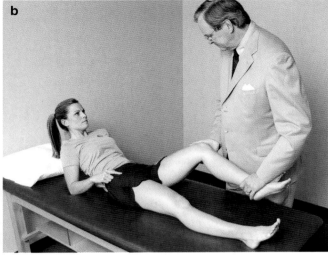

Fig. 2.1 (**a**) It is important that both hips be examined. This necessitates that the examination table be positioned so that the examiner can approach the patient from both sides. (**b**) Always begin the examination with the uninvolved extremity. This can gain the patient's confidence and provide potentially useful information for comparison when examining the involved hip. Failure to do so can result in possibly missing useful information. (All rights are retained by Dr. Byrd)

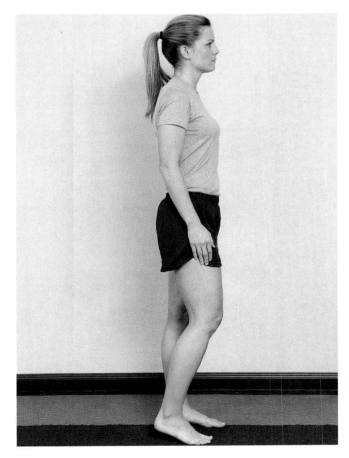

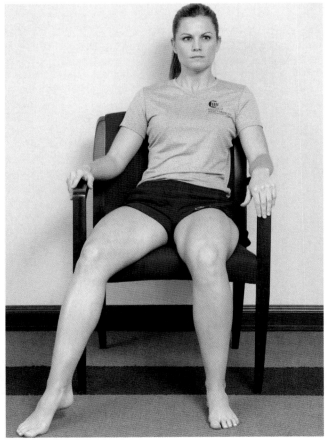

Fig. 2.2 During stance, the patient with an irritated hip will tend to stand with the joint slightly flexed. Consequently, the knee will be slightly flexed as well. This combined position of slight flexion creates an effective leg length discrepancy. To avoid dropping the pelvis on the affected side, the patient will tend to rise slightly on his or her toes. (All rights are retained by Dr. Byrd)

Fig. 2.3 In the seated position, slouching and listing to the uninvolved side allow the hip to seek a slightly less flexed position. This is usually combined with slight abduction and external rotation, which relaxes the capsule. (All rights are retained by Dr. Byrd)

Fig. 2.4 Normal phases of gait.
(All rights are retained by
Dr. Byrd)

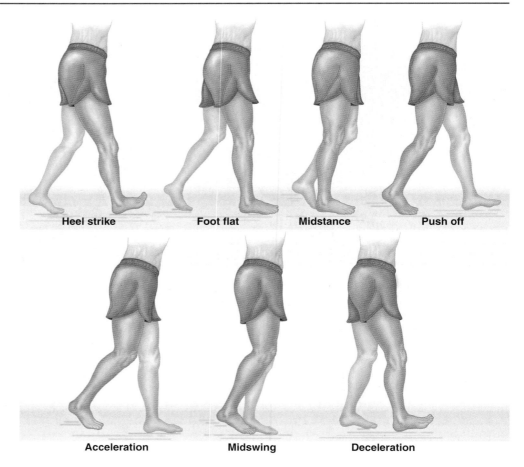

Heel strike   Foot flat   Midstance   Push off

Acceleration   Midswing   Deceleration

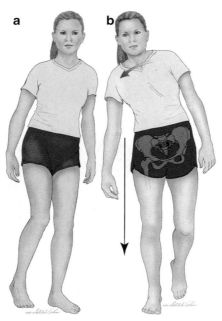

Fig. 2.5 (**a**) During ambulation, the stance phase of gait is shortened. Hip extension is avoided by keeping the joint in a slightly flexed position. This slight flexion creates a functional leg length discrepancy with shortening on the involved side and partially creates a lurch. (**b**) Further abductor lurch may occur as a compensatory mechanism to reduce the forces across the joint. Shifting the torso over the involved hip moves the center of gravity closer to the axis of the hip, shortens the lever arm moment, and reduces compressive joint force. (All rights are retained by Dr. Byrd)

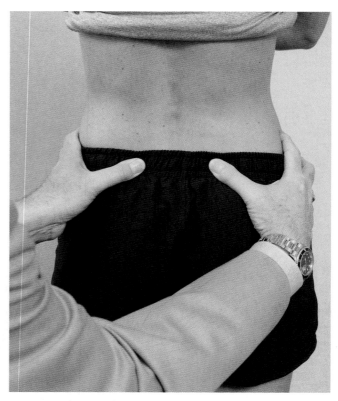

Fig. 2.6 Assessment is made of spinal alignment, pelvic obliquity, or asymmetry. (All rights are retained by Dr. Byrd)

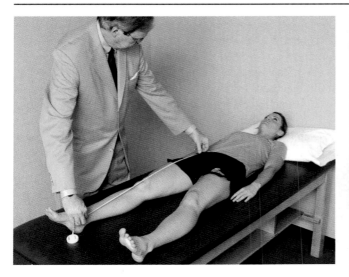

Fig. 2.7 Leg lengths are measured from the anterior superior iliac spine to the medial malleolus. (All rights are retained by Dr. Byrd)

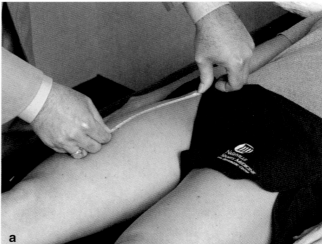

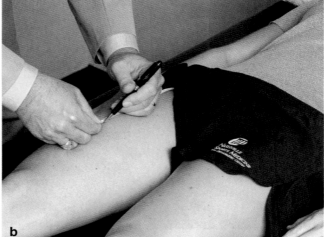

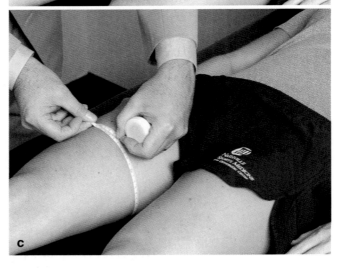

shortened, and hip flexion appears accentuated as extension is avoided during this phase (Fig. 2.4). Varying degrees of abductor lurch may be present as the patient attempts to place the center of gravity over the hip, reducing the forces on the joint (Fig. 2.5).

Observation is made for any asymmetry, gross atrophy, spinal alignment, or pelvic obliquity that may be fixed or associated with a gross leg length discrepancy (Fig. 2.6).

Measurements

Certain measurements should be recorded as a routine part of the assessment. Leg lengths should be measured from the anterior superior iliac spine to the medial malleolus (Fig. 2.7). Significant leg length discrepancies (greater than 1.5 cm) may be associated with a variety of chronic conditions. Typically, if this appears to be a contributing factor, we try to correct for half of the recorded discrepancy in the course of conservative treatment, preferably with an insert that is cosmetically more acceptable than a built-up shoe.

Thigh circumference, although a crude measurement, may reflect chronic conditions and muscle atrophy (Fig. 2.8). The involved leg is compared to the uninvolved side. Sequential measurement on subsequent examination can be an indicator of response to therapy. This only indirectly reflects hip function, but hip disease affects the entire lower extremity.

Range of motion of the hip must be recorded in a consistent and reproducible fashion. This is important for comparing sides and also chronicling the response to treatment on

Fig. 2.8 Thigh circumference should be measured at a fixed position, both for consistency of measurement of the affected and unaffected limbs and for consistency of measurement on subsequent examinations. (**a**) A tape measure is placed from the anterior superior iliac spine (ASIS) toward the center of the patella. (**b**) A selected distance below the anterior superior iliac spine is marked (typically 18 cm). (**c**) Thigh circumference is then recorded at this fixed position. (All rights are retained by Dr. Byrd)

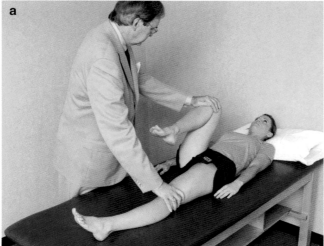

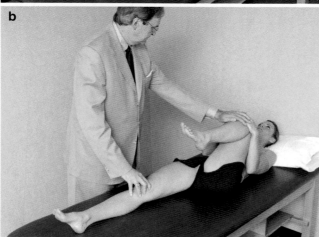

Fig. 2.9 (a) In the supine position, the uninvolved hip is kept in maximal extension. This stabilizes the pelvis and avoids contribution of pelvic tilt to hip flexion. The affected hip is then maximally flexed and motion recorded. (b) To check extension or presence of a flexion contracture, the unaffected hip is brought into maximal flexion and held by the patient, locking the pelvis. The affected hip is then brought out toward extension and motion recorded. (All rights are retained by Dr. Byrd)

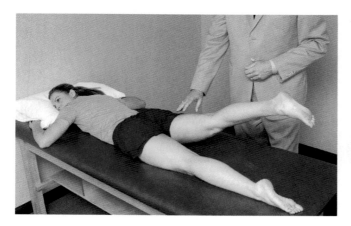

Fig. 2.10 In the prone position, extension can also be quantitated. (All rights are retained by Dr. Byrd)

subsequent examinations. The degree of flexion and the presence of a flexion contracture are determined by using the Thomas test (Fig. 2.9). Extension is recorded with the patient in the prone position, raising the leg (Fig. 2.10). There are several methods for recording rotational motion of the hip. It is important to select one and be consistent. Flexing the hip 90° and then internally and externally rotating the joint are easy and reproducible means for recording rotational motion (Fig. 2.11). Abduction and adduction are recorded as well (Fig. 2.12).

People with limited range of motion of the hip become adept at compensating by increased pelvic motion. Thus, when assessing motion, the examiner must be vigilant that the pelvis remains stable.

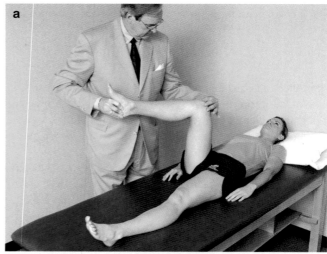

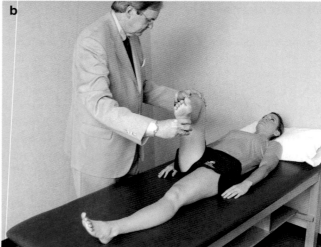

Fig. 2.11 (a, b) Supine, with the hip flexed 90°, the hip is maximally rotated internally and externally with motions recorded. This method is simple quick and reproducible. (c, d) Alternatively, rotational motion can be recorded with the hip extended in the prone position. Whatever method is chosen, it is important to be consistent on sequential examinations. (All rights are retained by Dr. Byrd)

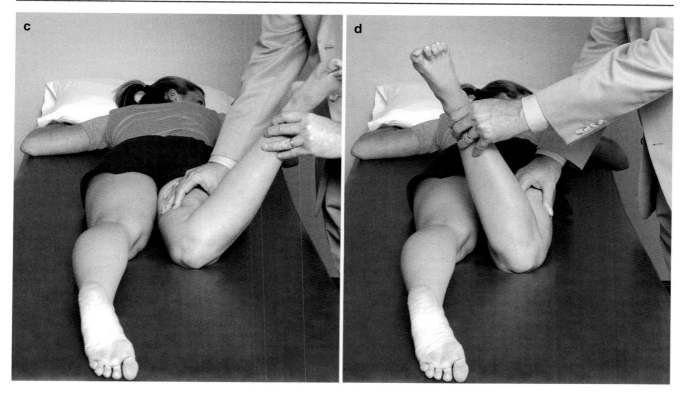

Fig. 2.11 (continued)

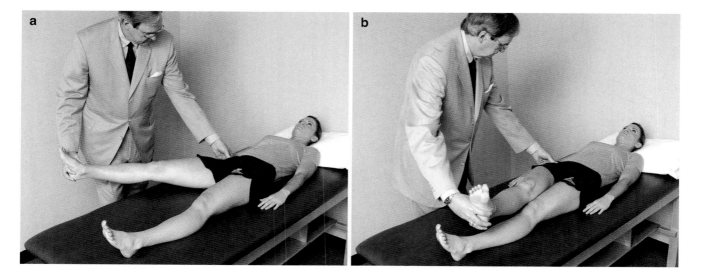

Fig. 2.12 (**a**, **b**) The hip is abducted and adducted and range of motion recorded relative to the midline. (All rights are retained by Dr. Byrd)

Symptom Localization

The One Finger Rule

Although this is less well applied to the hip than to other joints, such as the knee, it is still important to ask the patient to use one finger and point to the spot that hurts the worst

(Fig. 2.13). This provides much useful information before beginning palpation. It allows the examiner to discern the point of maximal tenderness. Consequently, this area is reserved until last when performing the examination. This forces the examiner to be more systematic, exploring uninvolved areas first, and enhances the patient's trust by not stimulating pain at the beginning of the examination (Fig. 2.14).

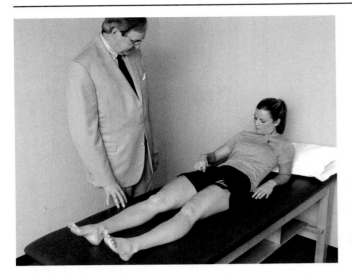

Fig. 2.13 Often the patient will wave over a large area of involvement. However, the patient is asked, with encouragement and instruction, to point with one finger to the area of maximal involvement. (All rights are retained by Dr. Byrd)

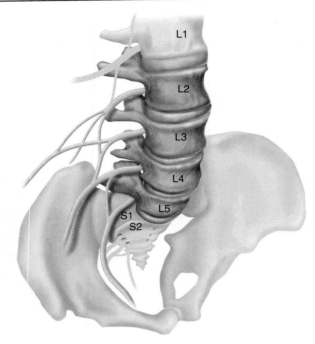

Fig. 2.15 The hip joint receives innervation from branches of *L2* to *S1* of the lumbosacral plexus but predominantly from the *L3* nerve root. (All rights are retained by Dr. Byrd)

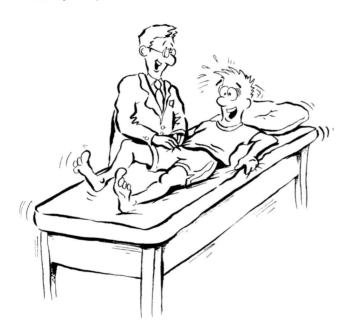

Fig. 2.14 "This is where it hurts?". (All rights are retained by Dr. Byrd)

Hilton's law states that "the same trunks of nerves whose branches supply the groups of muscles moving a joint furnish also a distribution of nerves to the skin over the insertion of the same muscles, and the interior of the joint receives its nerves from the same source" [8]. While this may ensure physiological harmony among the various structures, it also explains why muscle spasms and cutaneous sensations may accompany joint irritation.

Classic mechanical hip pain is described as being anterior, typically emanating from the groin area. The hip joint receives

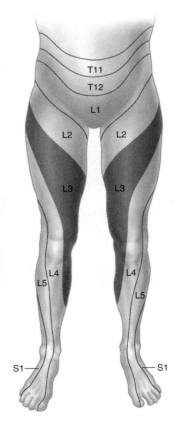

Fig. 2.16 The *L3* dermatome crosses the anterior thigh and extends distally along the medial thigh to the level of the knee. (All rights are retained by Dr. Byrd)

innervation from branches of L2 to S1 of the lumbosacral plexus, predominantly L3 (Fig. 2.15). Consequently, hip symptoms may be referred to the L3 dermatome, explaining the presence of symptoms referred to the anterior and medial thigh, distally to the level of the knee (Fig. 2.16).

Intracapsular hip pathology usually has a component of anterior hip pain. Occasionally, there may be more deep lateral discomfort but only rarely posterior pain.

The C Sign

The classic complaint of patients with hip pathology is "groin pain." However, the author has identified a very common characteristic sign of patients presenting with hip disorders. The patient will cup their hand above the greater trochanter when describing deep interior hip pain. The hand forms a C, and thus, this has been termed the "C sign" (Fig. 2.17). Because of the position of the hand, this can be misinterpreted as indicating lateral pathology such as the iliotibial band or trochanteric bursitis, but quite characteristically, the patient is describing deep interior hip pain.

Palpation

Deep palpation over the anterior hip capsule may create slight discomfort with an irritable hip. Palpation is otherwise more useful for distinguishing various extra-articular problems. The examiner must be systematic and familiar with the topographic and deep anatomy in order to correlate the structures being palpated. Aufranc noted in reference to examination that "a continuing study of anatomy marks the difference between good and expert ability" [7]. Palpation is generally broken down into anterior, lateral, and posterior regions. These are detailed in Figs. 2.18, 2.19, and 2.20.

Manual muscle testing is a crude measure of hip function but may elicit useful information (Fig. 2.21). If injury to a specific muscle group is suspected, resisted contraction should reproduce localized symptoms.

Active range of motion and resisted active range of motion may also reproduce joint symptoms. However, when carefully interpreted, a distinction can be made between symptoms of a muscle strain and hip pain. This differentiation may be least clear with a strain of the hip flexors. In this setting, active hip flexion reproduces pain while passive flexion should not.

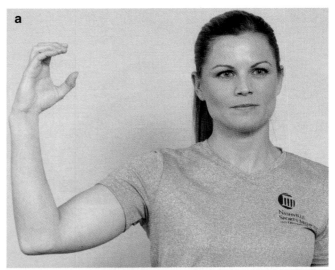

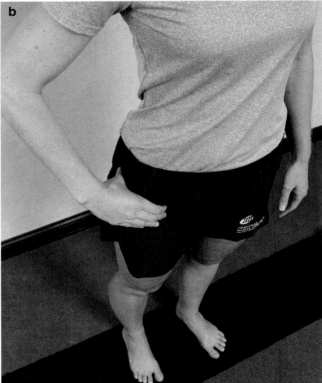

Fig. 2.17 (**a**, **b**) The C sign. This term reflects the shape of the hand when a patient describes deep interior hip pain. The hand is cupped above the greater trochanter with the thumb posterior and the fingers gripping deep into the anterior groin. (All rights are retained by Dr. Byrd)

Special Tests

There are various specific examination maneuvers for evaluating the hip joint as well as assessing the surrounding extra-articular structures. These are helpful to distinguish different disorders that may have similar presentations as well as coexistent problems that may occur either coincidentally or as a compensatory disorder. Keep in mind that none of these tests are 100% reliable in every circumstance. Also, as part of the clinical reality of evaluating patients, the

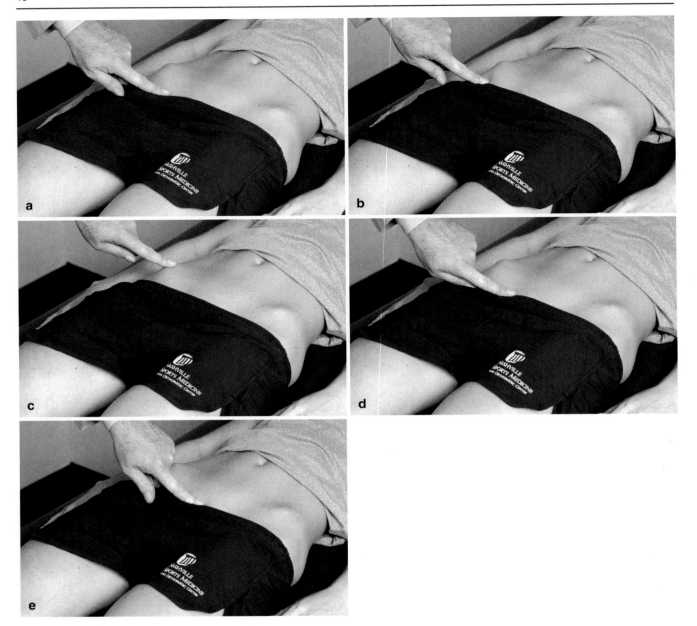

Fig. 2.18 Anterior palpation includes the following structures. (**a**) Anterior hip and hip flexor region. (**b**) Sartorius. (**c**) Anterior superior iliac spine. (**d**) Pubic ramus. (**e**) Symphysis pubis. (All rights are retained by Dr. Byrd)

examiner may be confronted with conflicting examination findings that will require prioritizing the importance of the observations encountered.

The single most specific test for hip pain is logrolling of the hip back and forth (Fig. 2.22). This moves only the femoral head in relation to the acetabulum and the surrounding capsule. There is no significant excursion or stress on myotendinous structures or nerves. Absence of a positive logroll test does not preclude the hip as a source of symptoms, but its presence greatly raises the suspicion.

Forced flexion, adduction and internal rotation is a one manuever. That may elicit symptoms associated with even subtle hip pathology (Fig. 2.23). This is often referred to as an "impingement test" in reference to testing for FAI [9]. However, we have found that this test is not specific for impingement as most irritable hips will be painful with this maneuver regardless of the etiology of the intra-articular pathology. This maneuver may normally be uncomfortable, so it is important to compare the response on the symptomatic and asymptomatic sides.

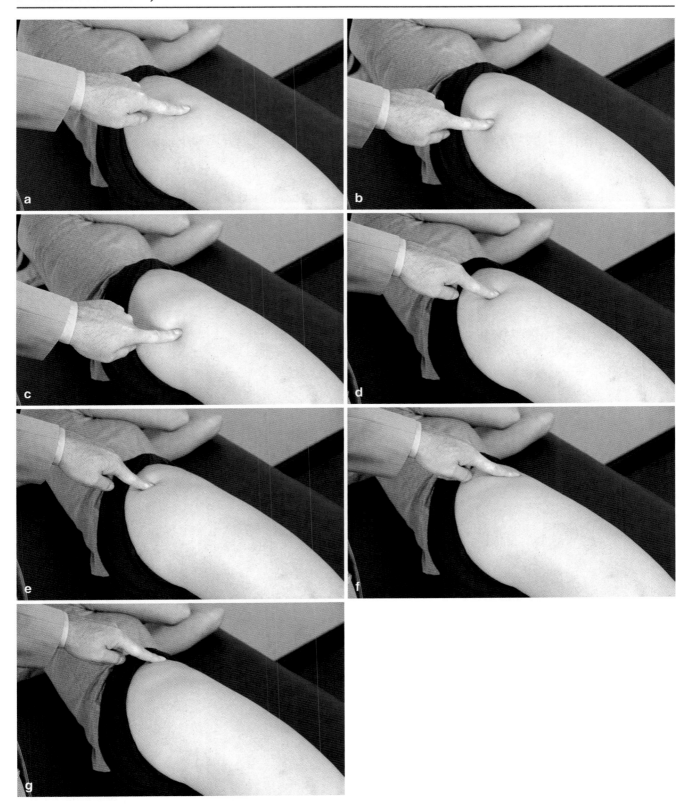

Fig. 2.19 Lateral palpation includes the following structures. (**a**) Greater trochanter and trochanteric bursa. (**b**) Posterior trochanter and trochanteric bursa. (**c**) Insertion site of the gluteus maximus. (**d**) Proximal tip of the trochanter and insertion of the gluteus medius. (**e**) Muscle belly of the gluteus medius. (**f**) Tensor fascia lata originating from the anterior margin of the iliac crest. (**g**) Iliac crest. (All rights are retained by Dr. Byrd)

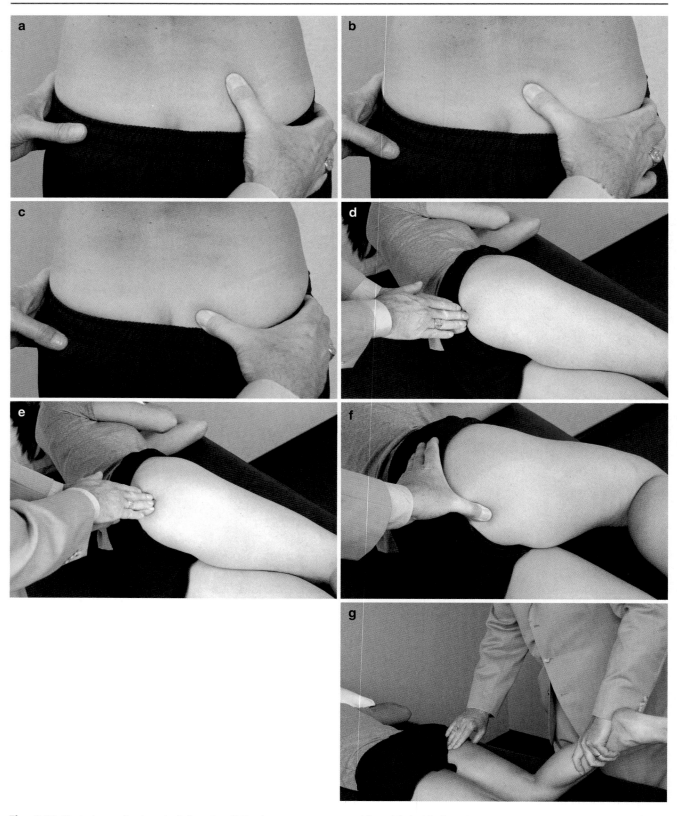

Fig. 2.20 Posterior palpation includes the following structures. (**a**) Posterior iliac crest. (**b**) Posterior superior iliac spine. (**c**) Sacroiliac joint. (**d**) Sciatic notch. (**e**) Region of the piriformis and overlying gluteus maximus. (**f**) The ischium is best palpated in the lateral decubitus position with the hip flexed. (**g**) The origin of the hamstrings is palpated prone with resisted contraction of the hamstring muscle group. (All rights are retained by Dr. Byrd)

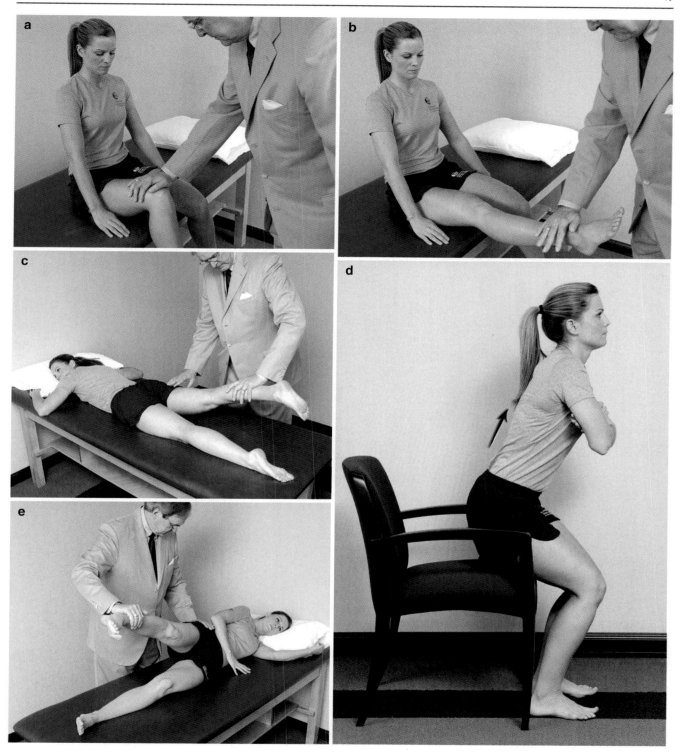

Fig. 2.21 (**a**) Resisted hip flexion with the knee flexed isolates the iliopsoas tendon. Contribution from the sartorius is minimal as this is a very weak muscle. (**b**) Resisted hip flexion combined with knee extension recruits the rectus femoris, which crosses both joints as a hip flexor and knee extensor. (**c**) Resisted hip extension can be tested with the patient prone. (**d**) Another useful test for extensor weakness is to simply have the patient rise from the seated position with the arms crossed. This is difficult when significant extensor muscle weakness is present. (**e**) Manual testing of abductor strength is most easily performed in the lateral position. Resistance testing across the extended knee recruits the tensor fascia lata. (**f**) Resistance testing with the knee flexed isolates the gluteus medius. (**g**) The Trendelenburg test is another dynamic method for assessing abductor strength. Lifting the unaffected leg off of the ground, with normal abductor strength, the patient should be able to maintain a level pelvis. (**h**) If the abductors are weak, the patient is unable to maintain a level pelvis, and it drops toward the unaffected side with the raised leg. (**i**) Manual testing of adductor strength can similarly be tested but with the patient supine. (All rights are retained by Dr. Byrd)

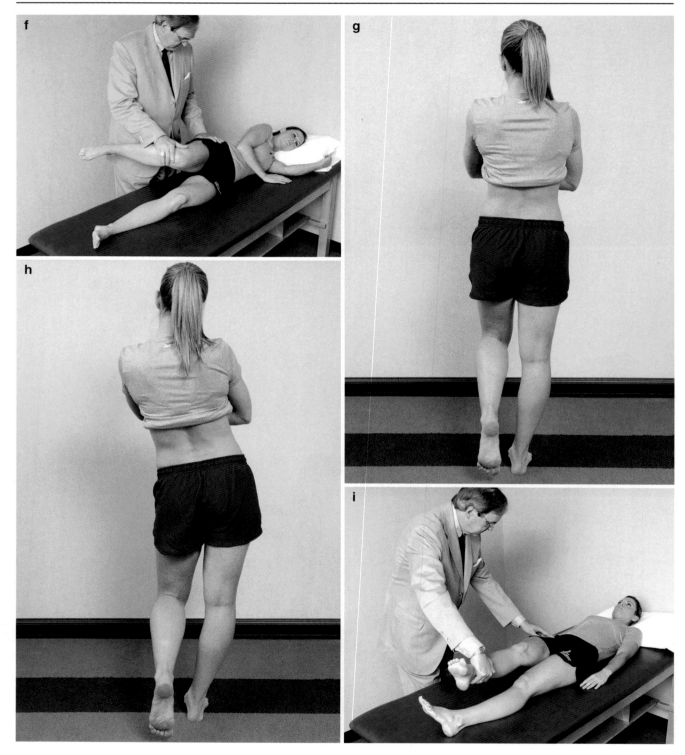

Fig. 2.21 (continued)

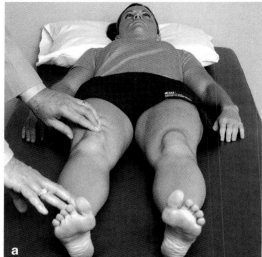

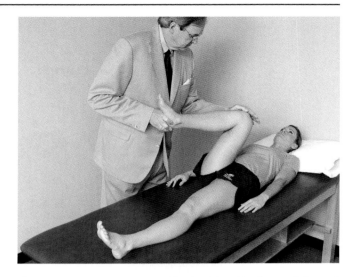

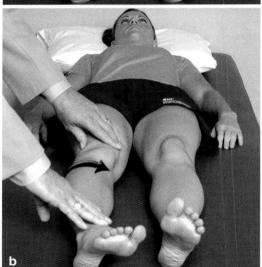

Fig. 2.23 Forced flexion combined with adduction and internal rotation is often very uncomfortable and usually elicits symptoms associated with even subtle degrees of hip pathology. (All rights are retained by Dr. Byrd)

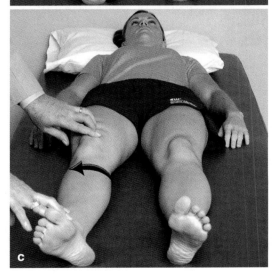

Fig. 2.22 The logroll test is the single most specific test for hip pathology. With the patient supine (a), gently rolling the thigh internally (b) and externally (c) moves the articular surface of the femoral head in relation to the acetabulum but does not stress any of the surrounding extra-articular structures. (All rights are retained by Dr. Byrd)

Forced abduction with external rotation may also create symptoms with a hip joint problem (Fig. 2.24a–c). The fist test is a useful method for quantitating the amount of restriction in abduction and external rotation [10]. This is usually present to a lesser extent than pain with flexion and internal rotation in cases of degenerative disease or severe impingement. Isolated tightness and pain with abduction and external rotation occur in the presence of posterior impingement or adhesive capsulitis [11, 12]. Global over coverage of the acetabulum can occur due to an ossified labrum resulting in painful restricted motion in all planes and what has been termed as a "captured hip." With adhesive capsulitis, external rotation is more restricted and painful than internal rotation. Both of these conditions find their highest prevalence among middle-aged females. Isolated posterior impingement is not common. It can be checked by forcing the extended hip into external rotation eliciting painful posterior impingement symptoms (Fig. 2.25). This same maneuver can be used testing for anterior instability as the femoral head can translate anteriorly with forced external rotation.

An active straight leg raise or straight leg raise against resistance tests the hip flexors but can also elicit joint symptoms (Fig. 2.26). This maneuver generates a force of several times body weight across the articular surfaces and is more than the normal forces of walking [13].

A conventional straight leg raise test is important for assessing signs of lumbar nerve root irritation (Fig. 2.27). The Patrick or Faber test (flexion, abduction, external rotation) has been described for stressing the SI joint looking for symptoms localized to this area and for isolating symptoms to the hip (Fig. 2.28). Differentiation between pain localized to the SI joint in the hip is usually easy. Occasionally, this may also elicit symptoms referable to the symphysis pubis.

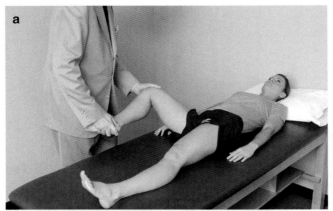

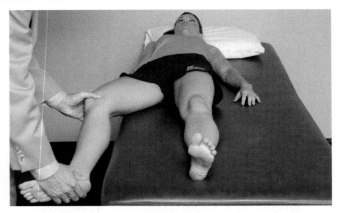

Fig. 2.25 Supine, the patient is positioned close to the edge of the table so the hip can be extended along with maximal external rotation. This can elicit symptoms of painful posterior impingement. However, anterior translation of the femoral head in this position may also evoke symptoms of anterior instability or possibly elicit pain trapping an anterior labral tear. Thus, the maneuver may be positive for various forms of hip joint pathology. (All rights are retained by Dr. Byrd)

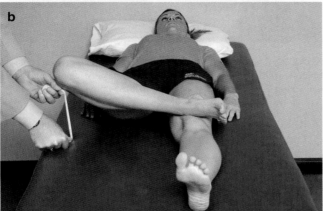

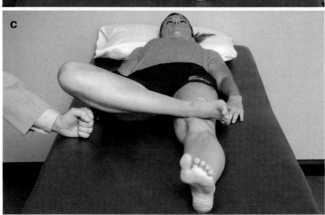

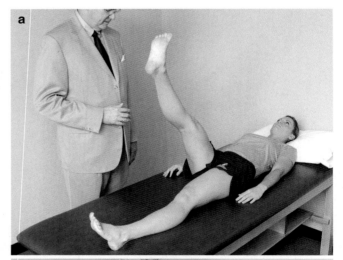

Fig. 2.24 (**a**) Flexion combined with abduction and external rotation may be uncomfortable and can produce catching-type sensations associated with labral and chondral lesions. (**b**) Restriction in abduction and external rotation is quantitated by measuring knee elevation off of the examination table. (**c**) Estimating the number of fist widths provides a quick method of assessment. (All rights are retained by Dr. Byrd)

The Dial test has been described as an assessment of anterior capsular laxity and possible instability (Fig. 2.29) [14]. It is characterized by increased external rotation of the affected limb when resting in extension. Also, subjectively, there is loss of the normal springy endpoint with external rotation which can be indicative of compromise of the

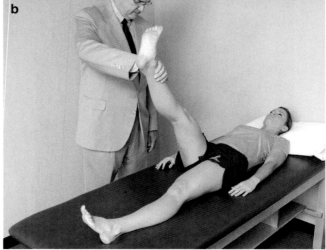

Fig. 2.26 (**a**, **b**) An active straight leg raise, or especially a leg raise against resistance, generates compressive forces of multiple times body weight across the hip joint. Consequently, this is often painful, especially when there is even a mild degree of underlying degenerative disease. (All rights are retained by Dr. Byrd)

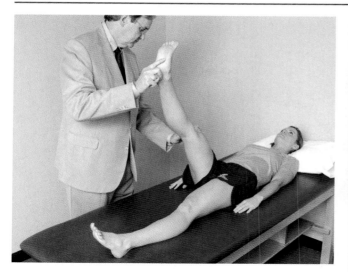

Fig. 2.27 The classic straight leg raise (SLR) test is performed to assess tension signs of lumbar nerve root irritation. A positive interpretation is characterized by reproduction of radiating pain along a dermatomal distribution of the lower extremity. It may also re-create discomfort from stretching of the hamstring tendons. (All rights are retained by Dr. Byrd)

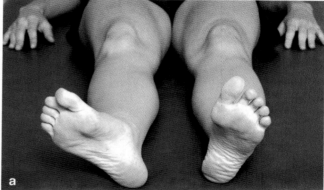

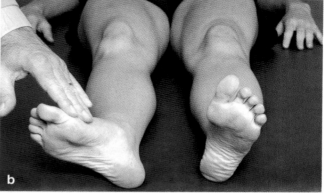

Fig. 2.29 A positive Dial test is ascribed to anterior capsular laxity. (**a**) In the resting position, the affected hip tends to lie in excessive external rotation. (**b**) Passively externally rotating the limb, a soft end point is encountered. (All rights are retained by Dr. Byrd)

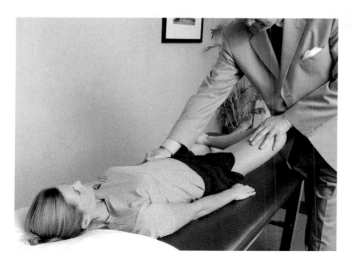

Fig. 2.28 With the patient supine, the Patrick of Faber test is performed by crossing the ankle over the front of the contralateral knee and then forcing the knee of the involved extremity down on the table while applying counterforce to the contralateral iliac crest. This combination of flexion, abduction, and external rotation stresses the sacroiliac (SI) joint, and when injury or inflammation is present, this movement may exacerbate symptoms localized to the SI area. This same maneuver can irritate the hip joint as well but with distinctly different localization of symptoms. Occasionally, it may also elicit symptoms emanating from the symphysis pubis. (All rights are retained by Dr. Byrd)

structural integrity of the anterior capsule. Forced external rotation of the extended hip translates the femoral head anteriorly and may evoke symptoms of anterior instability (Fig. 2.25). Assessing for pathological laxity in the hip is aided by looking for generalized signs of excessive laxity (Fig. 2.30) [15].

Athletic pubalgia ("sports hernia") can mimic or coexist with a hip joint problem [16, 17]. Groin tenderness to palpation is elicited over the pubis at the tendinous confluence of the insertion of the rectus abdominis and origin of the adductors (Fig. 2.18c). Hip flexor soreness may be present (Fig. 2.31a). Tenderness is isolated by palpating the adductor origin during resisted contraction (Fig. 2.31b). Similarly, tenderness is localized palpating the insertion of the rectus abdominis during resisted sit-ups (Fig. 2.31c). These maneuvers are normally not painful with isolated joint pathology. Conversely, passive flexion with internal rotation should exacerbate a hip joint problem and not be painful with athletic pubalgia. Keep in mind that various elements of both problems may coexist. Symptoms of osteitis pubis, characterized by point tenderness over the symphysis, may occur as an isolated entity or in conjunction with athletic pubalgia caused by excessive micromotion that can occur with compromise of the pelvic stabilizers.

Snapping of the iliopsoas tendon is a common condition [3]. The examination findings and symptoms when painful can be challenging to differentiate from an intra-articular problem. The snapping occurs as the iliopsoas transiently lodges on the anterior aspect of the hip capsule or pectineal eminence (Fig. 2.32). It may be audible and sometimes palpable. The characteristic maneuver for creating this type of

Fig. 2.30 Beighton described five examination features of generalized laxity. (**a**) Fifth finger hyperextension greater than 90°. (**b**) Ability to approximate the thumb against the proximal forearm. (**c**) Elbow hyperextension greater than 10°. (**d**) Knee hyperextension greater than 10°. (**e**) Ability to place palms flat on the floor with knees extended. (All rights are retained by Dr. Byrd)

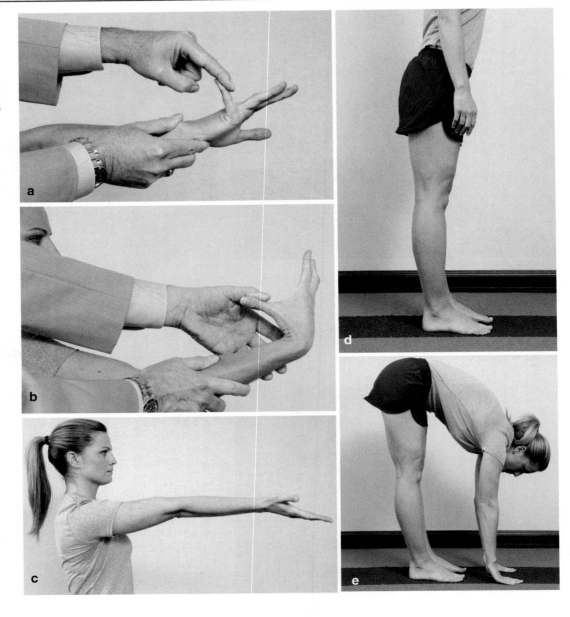

snap is bringing the hip from a flexed, abducted, externally rotated position into extension with internal rotation (Fig. 2.33). Applying direct pressure over the front of the hip may block the snapping. Often the snapping phenomenon is better demonstrated by the patient than can be detected on examination. This may variously be shown standing, sitting, or lying, but a consistent feature is the snapping almost always occurs going from flexion to extension. With close questioning, the patient can usually tell you whether the snapping is the cause of their pain or just a coincidental finding.

Snapping of the iliotibial band is not likely to be confused with a joint problem since the findings are located laterally [3]. However, these are patients who frequently present with a sense that their hip is subluxing. They can dynamically per-

form a maneuver that suggests hip instability. This visual appearance is uniformly created by the tensor fascia lata flipping back and forth across the greater trochanter (Fig. 2.34). The patient is examined on their side, flexing and extending and rotating the hip to assess the snapping (Fig. 2.35). Ober testing is also performed as a routine assessment for tightness of the iliotibial band (Fig. 2.36). However, this snapping phenomenon is again better demonstrated by the patient than elicited by the examiner. Typically, the patient will stand internally and externally rotating the hip creating the visual snapping. Radiographs will demonstrate that the hip remains concentrically reduced regardless of the visual positional alterations.

Piriformis syndrome is uncommon but is likely one of the most common causes of non-spinal origin sciatica [18]. This

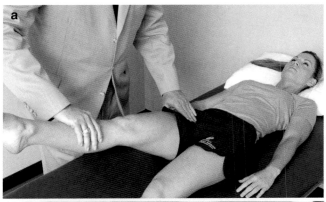

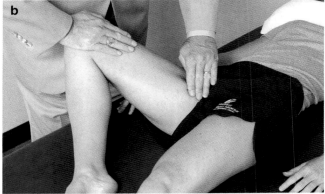

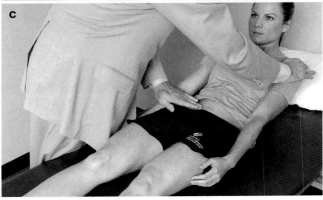

Fig. 2.31 Findings associated with athletic pubalgia. (**a**) Hip flexor soreness is elicited by palpation during resisted contraction. (**b**) Tenderness is elicited at the origin of the adductors by palpation during resisted contraction. (**c**) The insertion of the rectus abdominis is palpated for tenderness during resisted contraction. Counter pressure is applied to the contralateral shoulder causing selective recruitment and contraction on the involved side. (All rights are retained by Dr. Byrd)

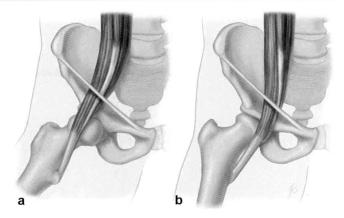

Fig. 2.32 Illustration of the iliopsoas tendon flipping back and forth across the anterior hip capsule and pectineal eminence. (**a**) With flexion of the hip, the iliopsoas tendon lies lateral to the center of the femoral head. (**b**) With extension of the hip, the iliopsoas shifts medial to the center of the femoral head. (All rights are retained by Dr. Byrd)

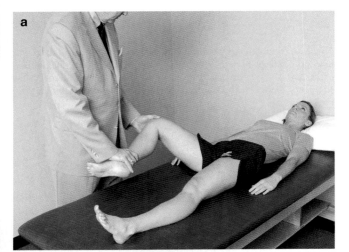

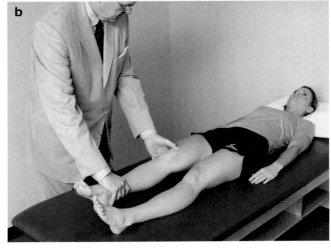

Fig. 2.33 The characteristic examination maneuver for snapping of the iliopsoas is performed with the patient lying supine. The hip is placed in a position of flexion, abduction, and external rotation (**a**) and then rotated down into extension with internal rotation (**b**) creating the snap. (All rights are retained by Dr. Byrd)

condition is probably overlooked and overdiagnosed in equal proportions. Piriformis function changes with hip position. Provocative exam maneuvers include passive internal (Freiberg's test) and resisted external rotation of the extended hip, resisted abduction of the flexed hip (Pace's sign), and stretching in flexion, adduction, and internal rotation (Fig. 2.37). Posterior tenderness to palpation is present, but the piriformis is obscured by the overlying mass of the

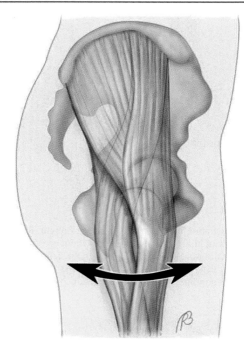

Fig. 2.34 Snapping of the iliotibial band can occur either as the tendinous portion flips back and forth across the trochanter with flexion and extension, or the trochanter may move back and forth underneath the stationary tendon with internal and external rotation. (All rights are retained by Dr. Byrd)

gluteus maximus (Fig. 2.20); and for recalcitrant cases, the most specific examination maneuver is rectal or vaginal palpation of the piriformis from inside the pelvis. There are also other less well-defined causes of extraspinal sciatica.

Radiology

In the past, with the emergence of advanced imaging such as magnetic resonance studies, the importance of plain radiography in the assessment of hip problems has been overlooked. Fortunately, the interest in FAI and other morphological conditions has led to a resurgence in appreciation for what plain x-rays offer [19]. A well-centered AP pelvis x-ray is important for assessing various radiographic indices as well as simply looking at closely related surrounding structures and providing a comparison view of the contralateral hip that can help in assessing subtle variations (Figs. 2.38 and 2.39). A lateral view of the affected hip is also needed. A frog lateral is not a true lateral of the hip but provides a perpendicular view of the proximal femoral anatomy (Fig. 2.40). It has good utility and is easily obtained in a consistent fashion [20]. There is much discussion about other optimal lateral radiographs for assessing FAI, but none of these are predictably reliable in all cases [21]. A false profile view can be

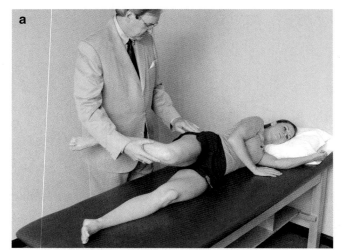

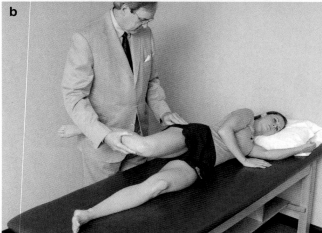

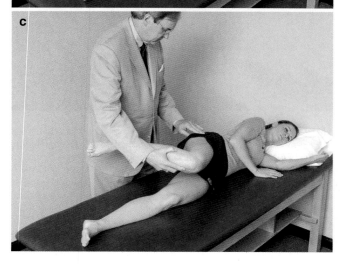

Fig. 2.35 With the patient on the side, the limb is supported (**a**) as it is moved back (**b**) and forth (**c**) in order to elicit snapping of the iliotibial band. (All rights are retained by Dr. Byrd)

helpful looking for deficiencies of the anterior acetabulum as well as assessing the anterior contour of the proximal femur.

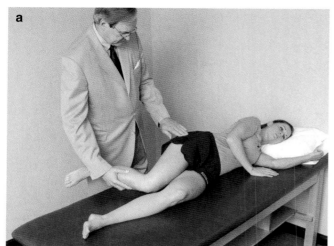

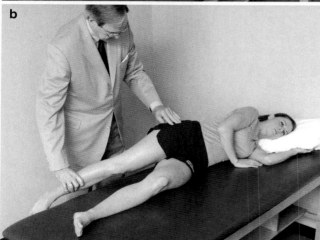

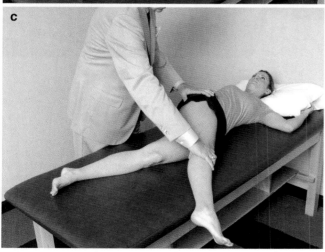

Fig. 2.36 The patient is in the lateral decubitus position with the affected side up. (**a**) Classic Ober testing is described, lowering the knee toward the table assessing for tightness of the iliotibial band. (**b**) The tensor fascia lata and iliotibial band are isolated checking for tightness in adduction with the hip and knee extended. (**c**) Tightness of the gluteus maximus is checked in adduction with the hip flexed and the shoulders squared on the examination table. (All rights are retained by Dr. Byrd)

Numerous measurements can be obtained to quantitate the variations of hip morphology that exist on a spectrum from dysplasia to impingement [19]. Many of these variations may exist among asymptomatic individuals. Thus, it is important not to base a treatment strategy solely on radiographic abnormalities. However, it is equally important to interpret the contribution of hip morphology with joint damage. This has great implication in the strategy of arthroscopic management and also knowing when arthroscopy may not be appropriate.

Two important considerations regarding plain radiography are offered. First, the damage inside the joint must be advanced before starting to notice any radiographic changes (Fig. 2.41). Thus, subtle radiographic abnormalities may have great significance regarding the severity of intra-articular pathology. Second, x-ray changes may occur in a short period of time (Fig. 2.42). Thus, in the course of treating patients with a hip joint problem, when the symptoms do not subside, repeat plain films before embarking on surgical intervention. Especially among middle-aged and older patients, degenerative changes may start to occur at an accelerated rate. You may be initiating treatment on the beginning of a steep downhill slope that cannot be reversed. Progressive radiographic changes with joint space loss may explain the severity of symptoms and avoid potentially recommending an unsuccessful arthroscopic procedure.

Lastly are a few comments regarding magnetic resonance imaging (MRI) and MRI with gadolinium arthrography (MRA) [22]. Not all MRIs are the same. Low-resolution studies (small magnets and open scanners) are unreliable at assessing hip joint pathology. High-resolution studies with small-field-of-view images and dedicated surface coils are better but still imperfect. Gadolinium arthrography can provide more sensitivity but is not always necessary, and there are caveats. Any magnetic resonance study should include a minimum of the following: coronal and axial large-field-of-view images of the pelvis showing both hips, and small-field-of-view axial, coronal, sagittal, and oblique axial images of the affected hip. Anything less is an incomplete study.

The literature will support high reliability of MRIs and MRAs in sensitivity and specificity [23, 24]. However, in clinical practice, it is best not to put too much faith solely in these studies. They are pretty good at showing labral pathology but will usually underestimate the severity of accompanying articular damage that is present. You must simply anticipate that it is likely that the articular damage encountered at the time of arthroscopy will be more extensive, and prepare your patients with this possibility in mind since this can influence the success of arthroscopy.

Contrasted images obscure whether an effusion may have been present, which is a valuable indicator of clinically relevant hip pathology (Fig. 2.43). Also, contrasted images can obscure edema in the subchondral bone and surrounding

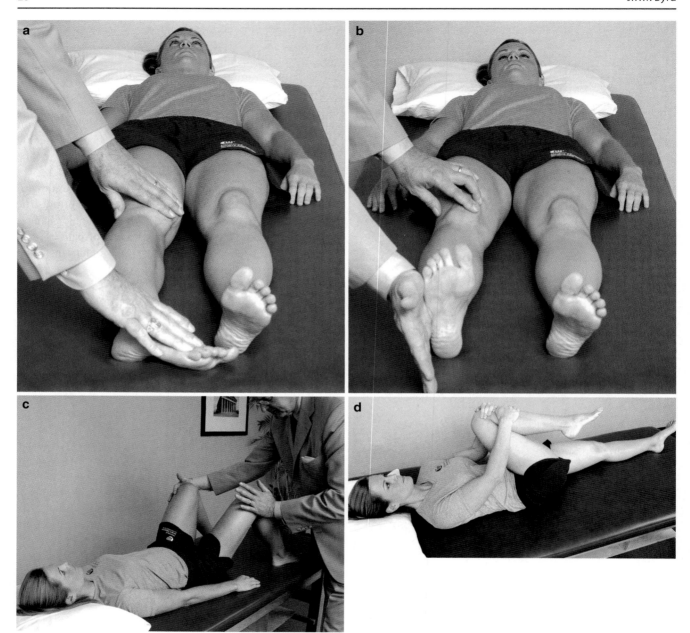

Fig. 2.37 Tests for piriformis syndrome. (**a**) Passive internal rotation of the extended hip placing tension on the piriformis is referred to as Freiberg's test. (**b**) Resisted external rotation of the extended hip with contraction of the piriformis may also re-create symptoms. (**c**) Resisted abduction of the flexed hip causes contraction of the piriformis in a different hip position and is referred to as Pace's sign. (**d**) The piriformis stretch test is performed with passive flexion, adduction, and internal rotation. This may stretch the piriformis provoking posterior symptoms but can also create anterior discomfort if the hip joint is irritable. (All rights are retained by Dr. Byrd)

soft tissues (Fig. 2.44). Thus, our strategy has been to perform a limited series of pre-contrast MRI followed by a more detailed post-contrast study.

Historically, we have relied mostly simply on the response to a fluoroscopically guided intra-articular injection of anesthetic to determine whether the hip was the principal pain generator [22]. As contrasted images became more popular,

we simply injected the anesthetic along with the contrast. For clinical relevance, we rely more on the response to the injection than simply findings on the images. However, there has been anecdotal experience by numerous experienced hip specialists that the contrast may somehow negate some of the anesthetic effect causing a false-negative interpretation. Presently, we have transitioned more to ultrasound-guided

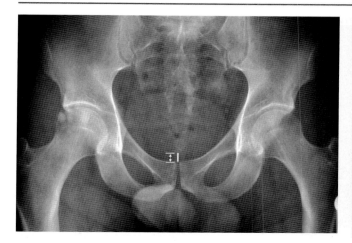

Fig. 2.38 A properly centered AP radiograph must be controlled for rotation and tilt. Proper rotation is confirmed by alignment of the coccyx over the symphysis pubis (*vertical line*). Proper tilt is controlled by maintaining the distance between the tip of the coccyx and the superior border of the symphysis pubis at 1–2 cm. (All rights are retained by Dr. Byrd)

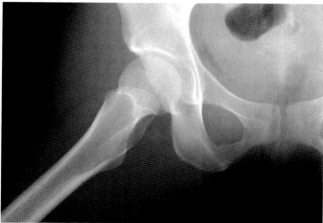

Fig. 2.40 A frog lateral radiograph is useful as a routine screening film. It is easy to obtain in a reproducible fashion. (All rights are retained by Dr. Byrd)

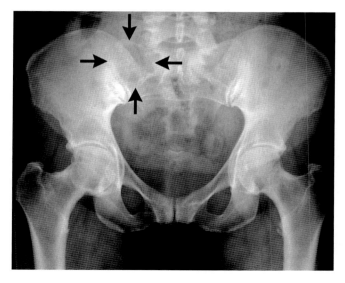

Fig. 2.39 AP pelvis radiograph of a 50-year-old woman with a chief complaint of "right hip pain." Chronic bony changes are apparent around both hips, but an aggressive lytic lesion is identified in the right sacrum (*arrows*). (All rights are retained by Dr. Byrd)

diagnostic injections which can be conveniently performed for the patient in the office setting. It also allows real-time assessment of the patient's response, testing the hip both pre- and postinjection to determine the level of pain relief. Office-based ultrasonography now offers many new diagnostic and interventional options for patients and these are detailed in chapter 34. With the advantage and patient convenience of ultrasound-guided injections, we usually obtain only a high-resolution conventional MRI.

It is important to keep in mind that some of the greatest value of the MRI is in assessing disorders that would not be evident during arthroscopy such as stress fractures, AVN, transient regional osteoporosis, tumors, and various extra-articular soft tissue disorders. The indication for arthroscopy is most often determined by the presence of recalcitrant hip joint pain that has failed conservative treatment, which may or may not be supported by obvious imaging findings of the nature of the pathology.

Summary

This chapter has detailed a practical approach to the assessment of patients presenting with a complaint of hip pain. The evaluation includes the history and examination and how to interpret the clinical relevance of various imaging studies. This strategy evolved as a direct consequence of arthroscopy, which began mainly with the removal of loose bodies then gradually the treatment of other previously unrecognized sources of hip pain such as labral tears. This evolution has included recognizing the existence of treatable hip disorders, learning how to interpret the history and symptoms, developing examination skills, and subsequently understanding the value and limitations of imaging studies. It is hoped that this practical approach can be useful for all clinicians challenged with the evaluation of hip problems. Others have attempted to address this in an evidence-based fashion, which may complement the practical experiences expressed here [25].

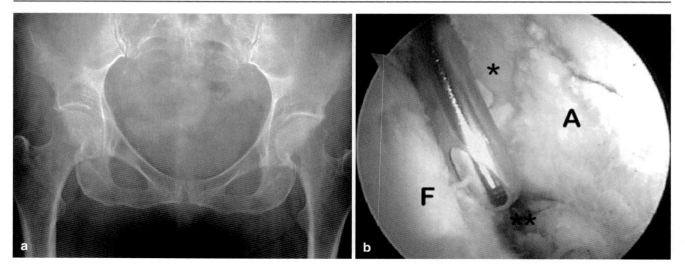

Fig. 2.41 (**a**) AP pelvis radiograph of a 74-year-old woman with chronic rheumatoid arthritis who presented with recent onset of intractable mechanical hip pain. Radiographs were reported as superficially normal with only modest evidence of inflammatory degenerative changes, insufficient to solely explain the magnitude of her symptoms. (**b**) Arthroscopic view of the left hip from the anterolateral portal revealing extensive articular surface erosion of both the femoral head (*F*) and acetabulum (*A*) with areas of exposed bone (*) and extensive synovial disease (**). (All rights are retained by Dr. Byrd)

Fig. 2.42 A 54-year-old orthopedic surgeon's wife experiences spontaneous onset of worsening mechanical right hip pain. (**a**) An AP radiograph demonstrates joint space preservation, and she was scheduled for arthroscopic surgery with MRI evidence of labral damage. (**b**) A repeat AP radiograph the day prior to surgery and only 1 month since her previous film demonstrates complete joint space loss. Arthroscopic surgery was canceled as this patient demonstrated rapidly progressive degenerative disease warranting a total hip arthroplasty. (All rights are retained by Dr. Byrd)

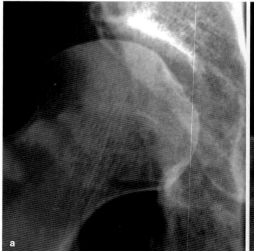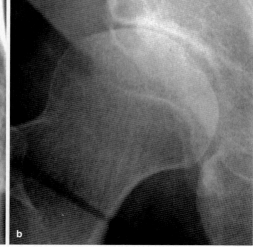

Fig. 2.43 (**a**) A coronal MRA image demonstrates contrast separating the lateral labrum (*arrow*), which could be indicative of a pathological tear or normal labral cleft. (**b**) Pre-contrast coronal T2-weighted large-field-of-view pelvis image demonstrates an effusion (*arrows*) of the right hip which is significant indirect evidence of joint pathology. (All rights are retained by Dr. Byrd)

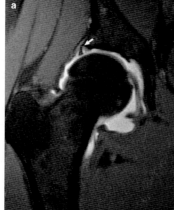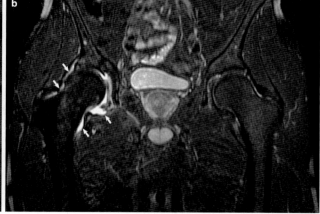

Fig. 2.44 Pre-contrast coronal (**a**) and sagittal (**b**) MRI images demonstrate subchondral signal changes of the femoral head (*arrows*). Post-contrast coronal (**c**) and sagittal (**d**) images substantially obscure the subchondral changes. (All rights are retained by Dr. Byrd)

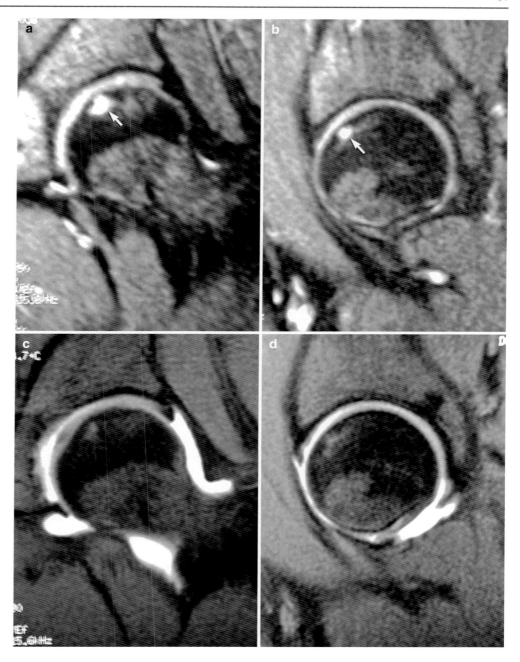

References

1. McCrory P, Bell S. Nerve entrapment syndromes as a cause of pain in the hip, groin and buttock. Sports Med. 1999;27(4):261–74.
2. Byrd JWT, Jones KS. Hip arthroscopy in athletes. Clin Sports Med. 2001;20(4):749–62.
3. Byrd JWT. Snapping hip. Oper Tech Sports Med. 2005;13(1): 46–54.
4. Byrd JWT, Jones KS. Prospective analysis of hip arthroscopy with 10-year follow up. Clin Orthop Relat Res. 2010;468(3):741.
5. Byrd JWT, Jones KS. Prospective analysis of hip arthroscopy with two year follow up. Arthroscopy. 2000;16(6):578–87.
6. O'Leary JA, Berend K, Vail TP. The relationship between diagnosis and outcome in arthroscopy of the hip. Arthroscopy. 2001;17(2): 181–8.
7. Aufranc OE. The patient with a hip problem. In: Aufranc OE, editor. Constructive surgery of the hip. St. Louis: CV Mosby; 1962. p. 15–49.
8. Hilton J. Rest and pain. London: Bell; 1863.
9. Ganz R, Parvizi J, Beck M, Leunig M, Notzli H, Siebenrock KA. Femoroacetabular impingement: a cause for osteoarthritis in the hip. Clin Orthop. 2003;417:112–20.

10. Philippon MJ. New frontiers in hip arthroscopy: the role of arthroscopic repair and capsulorrhaphy in the treatment of hip disorders. Instr Course Lect. 2006;55:309–16.

11. Sierra RJ, Trousdale RT, Ganz R, Leunig M. Hip disease in the young, active patient: evaluation and nonarthroplasty surgical options. J Am Acad Orthop Surg. 2008;16:689–703.

12. Byrd JWT. Adhesive capsulitis of the hip. Arthroscopy. 2006;22(1):89–94.

13. Rydell NW. Forces acting on the femoral head-prosthesis. Department of Orthop Surgery, University of Goteborg, Sweden, Munksgaard, Copenhagen. 1966. p. 77.

14. Philippon MJ, Schenker ML. Athletic hip injuries and capsular laxity. Oper Tech Orthop. 2005;15:261–6.

15. Beighton P, Horan F. Orthopaedic aspects of the Ehlers-Danlos syndrome. J Bone Joint Surg Br. 1969;51(3):444–53.

16. Tibor LM, Sekiya JK. Differential diagnosis of pain around the hip joint. Arthroscopy. 2008;24(12):1407–21.

17. Meyers WC, McKechnie A, Philippon MJ, Horner MA, et al. Experience with "sports hernia" spanning two decades. Ann Surg. 2008;248(4):656–64.

18. Byrd JWT. Piriformis syndrome. Oper Tech Sports Med. 2005;13(1):71–9.

19. Clohisy JC, Carlisle JC, Beaule PE, et al. A systematic approach to the plain radiographic evaluation of the young adult hip. J Bone Joint Surg Am. 2008;90:47–66.

20. Clohisy JC, Nunley RM, Otto RJ, Schoenecker PL. The frog-leg lateral radiograph accurately visualized hip cam impingement abnormalities. Clin Orthop. 2007;472:115–21.

21. Meyer DC, Beck M, Ellis T, et al. Comparison of six radiographic projections to assess femoral head/neck asphericity. Clin Orthop Relat Res. 2006;445:181–5.

22. Byrd JWT, Jones KS. Diagnostic accuracy of clinical assessment, MRI, gadolinium MRI, and intraarticular injection in hip arthroscopy patients. Am J Sports Med. 2004;32(7):1668–74.

23. Mintz DN, Hooper T, Connell D, et al. Magnetic resonance imaging of the hip: detection of labral and chondral abnormalities using noncontrast imaging. Arthroscopy. 2005;21(4):385–93.

24. Ziegert AL, et al. Comparison of standard hip MR arthrographic imaging planes and sequences for detection of arthroscopically proven labral tears. Am J Roentgenol. 2009;192(5):1397–400.

25. Martin HD, Kelly BT, Leunig M, et al. The pattern and technique in the clinical evaluation of the adult hip: the common physical examination tests of hip specialists. Arthroscopy. 2010;26(2):161–72.

Adult Hip Imaging for the Arthroscopist

3

Roy E. Erb

Imaging plays an important role in the evaluation of unexplained hip pain in the adult. Over the past decade, much has changed with the approach to diagnosing and treating labral pathology based on an increased understanding and awareness of the concept of femoroacetabular impingement (FAI) as a potential cause of idiopathic osteoarthritis [1]. Historically, MR arthrography has shown success with detecting labral pathology [2–10]. Recent studies have demonstrated characteristic MR arthrographic findings [11–14] associated with cam and pincer FAI that can offer a road map for the arthroscopist. The addition of 3T MRI has provided a significant improvement in image resolution, increasing our ability to visualize articular cartilage and labral abnormalities as well as other intra-articular and extra-articular causes of hip pain. This chapter focuses on the role of various imaging modalities used in the evaluation of adult hip pain with emphasis on the diagnosis of intra-articular hip pathology. Included in this overview are examples of intra-articular pathology demonstrated with 3T MR arthrography.

Diagnostic Imaging Modalities and Procedures

Plain Radiography

Plain radiography is the initial imaging exam obtained for suspected hip disease. Plain radiographs may demonstrate obvious causes of pain such as avascular necrosis, developmental dysplasia, degenerative joint disease, stress fracture, or tumor. Plain radiographs also can reveal more subtle abnormalities associated with femoroacetabular impingement [15] and mild cases of hip dysplasia. Plain radiographic series vary among institutions and orthopedic surgeons, but

standard hip radiographic series include an anteroposterior (AP) view of the pelvis and coned-down AP and frog leg lateral views of the symptomatic hip. This series may be augmented with 45° and 90° Dunn views, cross table lateral, and false profile views [15]. Oblique or Judet views are typically used in the setting of trauma to better depict acetabular fractures.

Common to the aforementioned projections of the hip (except the false profile view), the patient is lying supine on the exam table [15]. The AP view of the hip/pelvis is obtained with the x-ray beam directed in the AP plane with the patient's feet internally rotated 15° [16]. The frog leg lateral view is obtained with the hip abducted and the x-ray beam oriented in the AP plane [16]. Although less often included in hip series, the 90° and 45° Dunn views are taken with the hip flexed 90° and 45°, respectively, with 20° of abduction and the x-ray beam oriented in the AP direction [15]. Judet views of the hip are often obtained to evaluate acetabular fractures and are obtained with the patient supine with rotation of the pelvis 45° and the x-ray beam oriented in the AP plane [17].

Much recent attention has been given to the plain radiographic findings (Figs. 3.1, 3.2, and 3.3) associated with FAI [15, 18]. Plain radiographic findings suggestive of cam FAI include an aspherical femoral head (Fig. 3.1), focal prominence at the anterior femoral head-neck junction, pistol grip deformity of the proximal femur (Fig. 3.2), cystic change at the femoral head-neck junction, and abnormally increased alpha angle [15, 18]. Findings supportive of pincer-type FAI include a crossover sign (Fig. 3.3), posterior wall sign, and excessive acetabular coverage [15, 18]. Although these plain radiographic findings may be suggestive of FAI, considerable variability in measurements arises from variations in pelvic positioning [15]. A recent prospective assessment of the prevalence of plain radiographic findings associated with FAI in a group of healthy young adults revealed that these findings were common with approximately one-half demonstrating a crossover sign [18]. These findings support the fact that plain radiographic findings suggestive of FAI should

R.E. Erb, M.D.
Department of Medical Imaging,
St. Mary's Hospital, 2635 N, 7th St,
Grand Junction, CO 81502, USA
e-mail: roy.erb@stmarygj.org

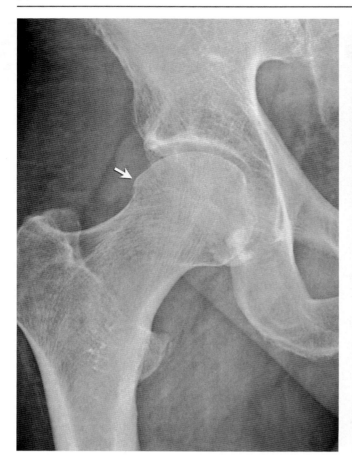 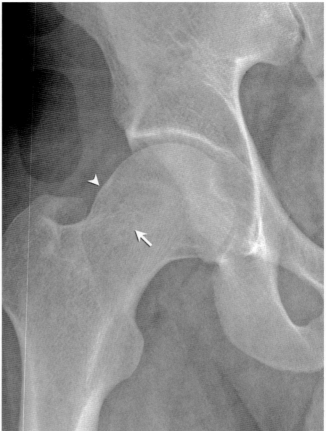

Fig. 3.1 Cam impingement seen on plain radiography. AP view demonstrates aspherical shape (*arrow*) of the femoral head

Fig. 3.2 Mixed impingement seen on plain radiography. AP view demonstrates mixed impingement with pistol grip deformity of the femoral head (*arrowhead*) and cystic change (*white arrow*) in the femoral neck indicative of cam impingement and crossover sign of pincer impingement

always be correlated with clinical findings [18]. Secondary imaging with conventional MR or MR arthrography should be considered to corroborate evidence for FAI and to help guide therapeutic intervention.

Computed Tomography

CT offers cross-sectional information of bony detail of the hip not available on plain radiographs and is typically used to further characterize acute fractures (Fig. 3.4), to assist with preoperative planning for prosthesis, to detect small particle disease, and to evaluate for nonunion [19]. Multislice helical CT has markedly improved our ability to rapidly acquire high-resolution images with multiplanar 2D and 3D reconstructions with the added benefits of shortened exam time, improved resolution, and lower radiation dose than conventional CT [20]. In our institution, CT is performed using multislice helical scanners, with images acquired in the axial plane from the anterior inferior iliac spine through the lesser trochanter with coronal and sagittal 2D reformations. 3D reconstructions (Fig. 3.4) are

constructed on request and may be helpful in aiding spatial orientation of complex fractures for surgical planning.

In the setting of trauma, CT is used to depict the spatial relationship of fractures and to aid in detection of articular surface fractures and intra-articular loose fragments (Fig. 3.4). CT has replaced conventional tomography in evaluating fractures for nonunion. Near isotropic imaging allows exquisite depiction of fracture healing in multiplanar display, and metallic artifact from hardware is not typically a hindrance, given the ability to adjust technique parameters and availability of metallic artifact suppression software [21]. CT offers a means for preoperative measurements and planning for patients undergoing hip arthroplasty, and protocols are typically recommended by the prosthesis manufacturers. CT can also be helpful in detecting and determining the extent of osteolysis associated with hip prosthesis [22]. Finally, although MRI is much better able to demonstrate bone marrow and soft tissue abnormalities, CT can be used in the

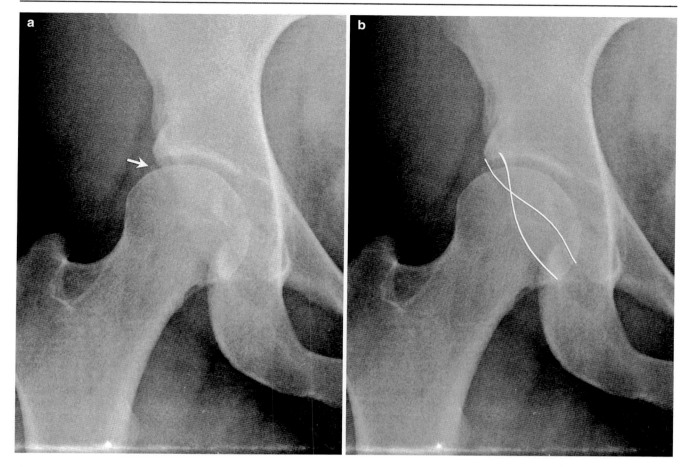

Fig. 3.3 Pincer impingement seen on plain radiography. (**a**) AP view reveals para-articular ossification (*arrow*) and crossover sign. (**b**) *Crossover sign* indicated by white tracing of the anterior rim crossing the posterior rim before reaching the edge of the lateral sourcil

setting of proximal femur or acetabular neoplasm to further characterize tumor matrix and to depict cortical destruction and breakthrough.

CT Arthrography

Due to recent attention given to the increased use [23] and potential risks [24] of radiation from CT, CT arthrography of the hip is unlikely to be employed widely but is an excellent alternative to MR arthrography in patients with a contraindication to MRI or in the presence of metallic hardware (Fig. 3.5). CT arthrography utilizing multislice helical CT can readily depict intra-articular abnormalities as contrast imbibes into sites of chondral, labral, or ligamentous injury and may outline loose bodies. At our institution, intra-articular injection is performed using a technique similar to MR arthrography (described later) but with approximately 10 cc of diluted mixture of iodinated contrast (10 cc contrast, 5 cc normal saline, 5 cc 0.25% bupivacaine). The inclusion of

anesthetic in the mixture is helpful in differentiating intra-articular from extra-articular sources of pain. Axial images are obtained from the anterior inferior iliac spine through the lesser trochanter with routine construction of coronal, sagittal, and oblique sagittal reformations.

Ultrasound

Ultrasound should be considered a complementary exam to MRI in the evaluation of hip pain, particularly suited for dynamic evaluation of the snapping hip syndrome (described later in this work) and image-guided intervention [25]. Sonography has several advantages over other imaging modalities in that it is noninvasive, lacks ionizing radiation, offers dynamic imaging of extremities in motion, allows concomitant evaluation of the contralateral joint, can depict tendon and other soft tissue abnormalities, and can be easily used as a guide for therapeutic injections and aspirations [25, 26]. Despite these advantages, MRI remains the

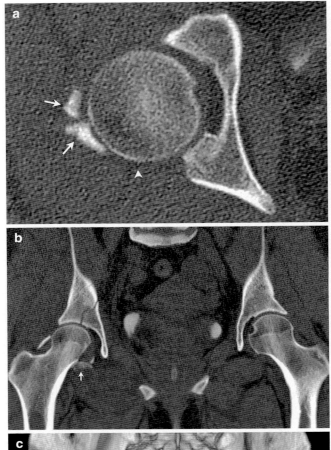

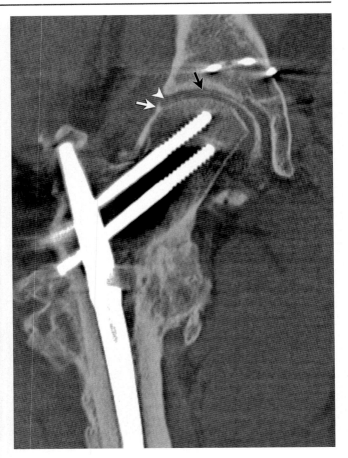

Fig. 3.5 CT arthrogram with metallic hardware. Coronal reformation demonstrates visualization of the labrum (*arrowhead*), perilabral sulcus (*white arrow*), and articular cartilage despite (*black arrow*) presence of metallic hardware in the proximal femur and acetabulum

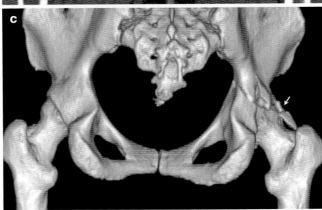

Fig. 3.4 Complex acetabular fracture seen on CT. (**a**) Axial CT reveals intra-articular fragments (*white arrows*) and large deficiency of the posterior wall (*arrowhead*). (**b**) Coronal reformation demonstrates complex Pipkin fracture pattern with fragment of femoral head (*arrow*) displaced caudally. (**c**) Posterior projection of 3D reformation reveals posterior wall deficiency and orientation of fracture fragments (*arrow*)

secondary imaging study of choice for most presentations of unexplained hip pain, as ultrasound is heavily operator dependent and does not provide the global overview and comprehensive information about the supporting soft tissues of the hip, intra-articular structures, and bone marrow available from MRI.

Ultrasound is well suited for image-guided interventional procedures including injection of the joint, tendon sheaths, or bursa; aspiration of ganglion cysts; drainage of para-articular fluid collections; and in the treatment of calcific tendinosis [25, 26]. The choice of ultrasound probe depends on the depth of the intervention. Most superficial interventional procedures can be accomplished with a linear array high-frequency probe. Deeper interventions may require a curved or sector array lower frequency probe. Both intra-articular and extra-articular injections are typically performed with small caliber needles using sterile technique and real-time sonographic guidance. Sterile technique can be maintained by using a sterile ultrasound probe cover and sterile gel. For real-time ultrasound guidance, the probe is held in one hand oriented typically parallel to the course of the needle, while the other hand is used to advance the needle [26]. Orientation of the needle parallel to the probe allows continuous visualization of the tip of the needle. Continuous imaging during injection or aspiration insures proper positioning of the needle tip during the procedure. Aspiration of ganglion cysts is typically performed with a larger gauge needle (18 gauge) as the contents are typically more viscous than serous fluid [26].

Conventional Magnetic Resonance Imaging

MRI is the established secondary imaging exam of choice in the evaluation of unexplained hip pain for most clinical presentations. MRI provides exquisite anatomical detail and unique information regarding soft tissue and marrow abnormalities not seen on plain radiographs, CT, or nuclear medicine exams. MRI is very effective in demonstrating intra-articular and extra-articular pathology, often identifying the source of pain and thus helping guide the appropriate management. MRI readily depicts many sources of extra-articular hip pathology including bursitis [27, 28], myotendinous injury [29], sacroiliitis, pubic osteitis, and occult pelvic neoplasms. Conventional MRI can also demonstrate intra-articular sources of hip pain including joint effusions [30], osteonecrosis [31], occult fractures [32–34], and inflammatory arthritis [35]. With some exceptions [36], conventional MRI at 1.5T has had relatively poor success with demonstrating labral [3, 37] and cartilaginous abnormalities [4], but this may improve with 3T MRI and newer imaging techniques. An early investigation by Magee [38] comparing conventional 3T MRI and 3T MR arthrography in detecting labral tears appears favorable for conventional 3T MRI.

Protocols for conventional MRI of the adult hip vary among institutions. The quality of the examination depends on the field strength of the scanner, coil selection, technical parameters used, and whether or not dedicated small-field-of-view images of the hip are acquired. Small-field-of-view high-resolution imaging of the affected hip is essential in the evaluation of labral and cartilaginous abnormalities. MRI protocols are tailored to the clinical presentation. For instance, at our institution, an MRI exam obtained to exclude an occult hip fracture in an elderly patient presenting with hip pain after a fall with normal plain radiographs is directed toward maximizing the conspicuity of fractures (heavily T2 weighted) and is completed with an abbreviated number (3) of sequences. The typical exam for an adult with unexplained hip pain includes seven sequences and is tailored toward evaluating intra-articular and extra-articular pathology. Our 3T MRI hip protocol utilizes a General Electric (Milwaukee) magnetic resonance scanner and an 8-channel phased array torso coil and includes coronal T1 (TR=600, TE=min, 3.0-mm slice thickness, 0.5-mm gap, 512×256 matrix, 2 NEX, 36 FOV) and T2 FSE fat-suppressed (TR=3,984, TE=68, 3.0-mm slice thickness, 0.5-mm gap, 512×320 matrix, 2 NEX, 36.0 FOV), and axial T2 FSE fat-suppressed (TR=2,717, TE=60, 4.0-mm slice thickness, 1.0-mm gap, 384×224 matrix, 2 NEX, 36.0 FOV) images of both hips. In addition, small-field-of-view coronal proton density (TR=2,217,

TE=min, 3.0-mm slice thickness, 1.0-mm gap, 448×224 matrix, 2 NEX, 20 FOV), coronal PD fat-suppressed (TR=2,434, TE=min, 3.0-mm slice thickness, 1.0-mm gap, 448×256 matrix, 2 NEX, 20 FOV), sagittal PD fat-suppressed (TR=2,600, TE=min, 3.0-mm slice thickness, 1.0-mm gap, 448×256 matrix, 2 NEX, 20 FOV), and oblique sagittal 3D spoiled gradient-recalled (SPGR) (flip angle=20,TI=auto, TE min, 3.0-mm slice thickness, 320×192 matrix, 3 NEX, FOV 20) images of the affected hip are obtained. The coronal T1-weighted images of both hips demonstrate anatomy and marrow-based abnormalities such as osteonecrosis, occult fractures, or marrow replacement from tumor. The T2-weighted fat-suppressed images of both hips reveal intra-articular and extra-articular fluid collections such as joint effusions and bursitis; highlight marrow-based abnormalities including occult fractures or stress fractures, subchondral cysts, osteonecrosis, and tumor; and depict para-articular myotendinous injuries. Small-field-of-view proton density images of the affected hip are most helpful in evaluating the acetabular labrum and the articular surface cartilage of the femoral head and acetabulum. The oblique sagittal SPGR sequence is used to measure for cam and pincer FAI and to assess for the characteristic osseous bump seen with cam FAI.

Magnetic Resonance Arthrography

Magnetic resonance arthrography of the hip has evolved into the exam of choice in the evaluation of an adult with suspected intra-articular hip pathology that may qualify as a candidate for hip arthroscopy. Since the initial reports of the success of MR arthrography in detecting labral pathology [2–10] increased, experience in the interpretation of these exams coupled with greater understanding of FAI has led to recognition of injury patterns [11–14] and pitfalls [39–42] in diagnosing cartilage and labral injuries. MR arthrography can depict abnormalities of the labrum, articular surface cartilage, ligamentum teres, and joint capsule and demonstrate the presence of loose bodies or proliferative changes of synovitis. The introduction of fluid into the joint displaces the joint capsule from the underlying bone and normal structures, thus allowing better visualization of intra-articular anatomy (Fig. 3.6) than conventional MRI. Extension of contrast into the labrum or cartilage yields direct evidence of pathology of these structures. The concomitant injection of anesthetic with the contrast solution provides a unique form of MR arthrography yielding both anatomic and clinical information and is the preferred technique of the author. Byrd and Jones [43] found in a series of patients that underwent MR arthrography with anesthetic injection and subsequent hip arthroscopy that symptomatic pain relief with anesthetic injection alone was 90% accurate in diagnosing intra-articular pathology. Symptomatic pain relief with MR arthrography

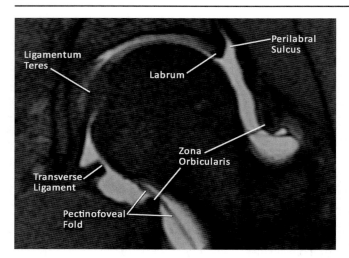

Fig. 3.6 Normal anatomy seen on magnetic resonance arthrography. Coronal T1-weighted fat-suppressed image of the left hip demonstrates the labrum, perilabral sulcus, transverse ligament, ligamentum teres, pectinofoveal fold, and zona orbicularis

with anesthetic injection provides strong clinical evidence of intra-articular pathology, and the MR images obtained can serve as a road map for the surgeon. Normal imaging in the setting of symptomatic pain relief with anesthetic injection may signify occult intra-articular pathology, most likely cartilaginous in nature in the author's experience.

MR arthrography technique varies among institutions but typically involves the intra-articular injection of dilute gadolinium solution (1–2 mmol). At our institution, gadolinium is diluted approximately 1:200 for the purposes of MR arthrography of any joint. The method to gain access to the hip is described later. A mixture of 0.05 cc of gadolinium (Magnevist, Bayer, Wayne, NJ) and 5 cc of iopamidol (Isovue, Bracco, Princeton, NJ) and 5 cc of anesthetic (1% lidocaine HCl or 0.25% bupivacaine HCl) is then injected into the hip. Following the injection, the patient is transferred to the MRI suite by foot or wheelchair, and MR imaging is typically performed within 45 min of the injection. In the author's experience, contrast extravasation from over exercise from the patient walking into the MR scanner has not been an issue.

MR arthrography of the hip at our institution is performed on a General Electric (Milwaukee) 3T MR scanner, and only the affected hip is scanned. An 8-channel torso coil is used yielding high-resolution small-field-of-view images of the hip. Triplane (coronal, sagittal, and axial) T1 fat-suppressed images (TR=617, TE=minimum, 2.5-mm slice thickness, 0 gap, 352×2,246 matrix, 2 NEX, FOV=18) are obtained and used as the primary sequences to detect labral pathology. Coronal PD images (TR=3,584, TE=minimum, 2.5-mm slice thickness, 0 gap, 448×224 matrix, 2 NEX, FOV=18) are acquired to assist in detection of cartilage and labral pathology, and T2 fat-suppressed images (TR=2,250, TE=65, 2.5-mm

slice thickness, 0 gap, 352×224 matrix, 3 NEX, FOV=18) are obtained to help indentify marrow-based findings (subchondral cysts, stress reactions, marrow edema, etc.) and para-articular soft tissue abnormalities such as gluteus tendon tears or bursitis. Oblique sagittal FSPGR images (TI=auto, TE=minimum, 3.0-mm slice thickness, 0 gap, 320×192 matrix, 3 NEX, FOV=18) are used to measure the alpha angle and acetabular overcoverage associated with FAI.

Nuclear Scintigraphy

With the advent of MRI, nuclear scintigraphy is seldom used in the workup of unexplained pain in the native hip. Today, bone scanning of the hip is most often used to assess for loosening or infection in a patient with a painful hip following arthroplasty. Although increased activity can normally be seen around hip arthroplasty components for up to 2 years following surgery, persistent activity at the tip of the femoral component or near the trochanters can indicate loosening, and more generalized activity around the femoral component can indicate infection [44]. Bone scanning employs the use of a radiopharmaceutical (typically technetium-99 methylene diphosphonate, MDP) injected into the patient with subsequent passive imaging with a gamma camera. Planar whole-body images or regional anatomic images are acquired typically 2–4 h (delayed) after the injection of radiopharmaceutical. Although not often used as a secondary examination in the workup of adult hip pain, the bone scan findings of FAI have been reported [45].

Hip Arthrography, Injection, Aspiration, and Bursography

Today, most arthrography of the hip is performed for MR arthrograms, therapeutic injections, and for aspiration in the setting of suspected septic arthritis. Traditionally, image guidance for arthrography of the hip has been with fluoroscopy, though sonographic guidance is a valid option and may become more increasingly popular given its increased usage in musculoskeletal applications and its lack of exposure to ionizing radiation. At our institution, fluoroscopy remains the preferred method of image guidance, and whether performed as an arthrogram, injection, or aspiration, similar technique is used to gain access to the hip joint. An anterior approach (Fig. 3.7) centered over the lateral aspect of the femoral neck is used. Informed written consent is obtained on all patients. With the patient supine on the fluoroscopic table, an ink mark is placed on the skin directly over the lateral aspect of the femoral neck near the head-neck junction (Fig. 3.7). The overlying skin is then prepped with betadine solution, and the skin and subcutaneous tissues are anesthetized with buffered 1% lido-

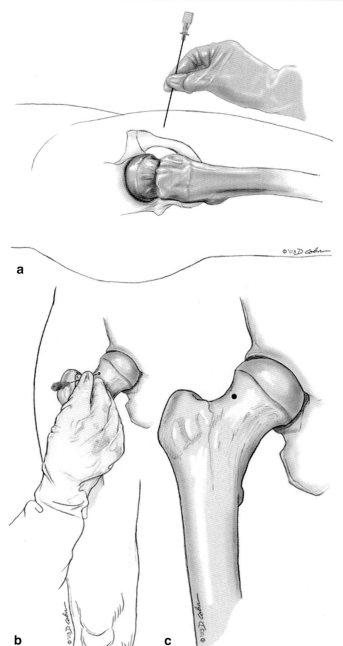

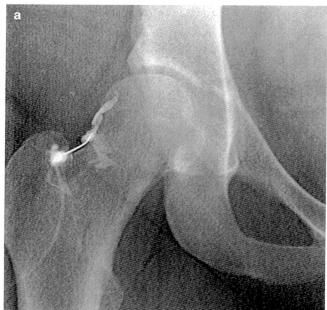

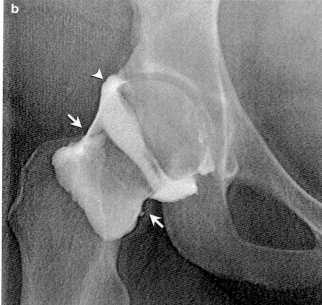

Fig. 3.7 Technique for fluoroscopic hip injection. Note anterior approach targeting the lateral aspect of the femoral neck. (**a**) direction of intra-articular needle placement from a lateral view. (**b**) direction of intra-articular needle placement from a frontal view. (**c**) dot over the lateral aspect of the femoral neck represents the target for intra-articular needle placement

Fig. 3.8 Intra-articular contrast injection and arthrogram. (**a**) Spinal needle coursing along the lateral femoral neck with early contrast filling the lateral joint confirming intra-articular needle position. (**b**) Completed arthrogram demonstrating the perilabral sulcus (*arrowhead*) and zona orbicularis (*white arrows*)

caine HCl. A 22-gauge spinal needle is then advanced to the cortex of the lateral femoral head-neck junction with the bevel of the needle oriented medially. Medial orientation of the bevel allows the needle to course laterally along the cortical surface of the femoral neck rather than to penetrate the cortex. Aspiration is then performed and allows gross evaluation for

infection as well as decompression of a joint effusion, if present, to allow space for mixtures used in injections. Approximately 1 cc of iodinated contrast is administered to confirm an intra-articular position of the needle (Fig. 3.8).

Diagnostic aspirations are performed in both native hips and in patients with hip prosthesis for suspected septic arthritis. For the native hip, the same approach is used as described above. For aspiration of a hip arthroplasty, the entry site is chosen lateral to the base of the neck of the femoral component allowing visualization of the needle as it is advanced to the surface of the junction of the neck and ball of the femoral component. For both native hips and in the setting of a hip arthroplasty, a 20-gauge spinal needle is typically used for aspiration as fluid associated with infection is often more viscous than simple joint fluid. If no fluid returns on aspiration (dry tap), a larger (18 gauge) needle can be used or injection with 10–15 cc of nonbacteriostatic water or saline can be injected and then reaspirated. A small amount of iodinated contrast is then injected to verify the position of the needle.

Diagnostic and therapeutic injections are often performed to distinguish intra-articular from extra-articular sources of pain and to alleviate pain and inflammation associated with arthritis. For both procedures, we routinely administer both long-acting anesthetic and corticosteroid. At our institution, we typically inject 80 mg of methylprednisolone acetate (Depo-Medrol) and 5–7 cc of 0.25% bupivacaine HCl, though the choice of steroid and anesthetic varies among orthopedic surgeons and radiologists. In these procedures, aspiration is first performed to exclude overt evidence of infection and to remove joint fluid to allow space for the anesthetic and steroid. If turbulent fluid is encountered, laboratory analysis of the fluid for infection is obtained, and injection of corticosteroid is deferred. The corticosteroid and long-acting anesthetic are injected as a mixture. Patient pain level before and after the procedure is documented, and the patient is given a pain log for follow-up with their referring physician. The injection technique for MR arthrography is similar to a therapeutic injection, and the contrast mixture administered has been described earlier in this work.

Historically, iliopsoas bursography has been used to diagnose iliopsoas snapping syndrome [46] and relies on fluoroscopic guidance to confirm an intrabursal location of contrast administration as well as fluoroscopic observation of the tendon, thus exposing the patient to ionizing radiation. Ultrasound has essentially replaced this exam as it is noninvasive, can be performed at the bedside, and can allow evaluation of both internal and external forms of snapping hip syndrome [25, 47–49]. Injection of the iliopsoas bursa for pain relief in cases of bursitis is occasionally performed and is similar to the technique used for diagnostic iliopsoas bursography. Injection of the bursa can be performed with either fluoroscopic or ultrasound guidance depending on the preference and experience of the operator. For injection of the bursa with fluoroscopic guidance, a 22-gauge spinal needle is advanced to the anterior acetabular rim directly over the upper portion of the femoral head using sterile technique and 1% lidocaine HCl as a local anesthetic. After contact with bone, a small volume of iodinated contrast is injected as the needle is gently retracted 2–3 mm. Upon entering the bursa, there should be a lack of resistance, and the tendon should be visualized as a longitudinally oriented filling defect positioned centrally in the bursa. For therapeutic injections of the bursa, we inject 40 mg of methylprednisolone acetate and 5 cc of 0.25% bupivacaine.

Use of fluoroscopic guidance can be more time consuming [25] and less accurate than ultrasound guidance. Sonographic guidance is easy and allows direct visualization of the location of the needle tip relative to the tendon and bursa and avoids patient exposure to ionizing radiation. An anterior approach can be used lateral to the vascular bundle. Doppler can be used to identify and avoid the femoral artery. Fluid within the bursa will appear anechoic or hypoechoic to the tendon. Observation of the needle tip during injection allows confirmation of an intrabursal position as the injected fluid will appear anechoic and should surround the tendon.

Normal Intra-articular Hip Anatomy and Pitfalls on MR Arthrography

MR arthrography of the hip allows excellent visualization of the acetabular labrum and intra-articular structures by displacing the joint capsule and outlining articular surfaces and the ligamentum teres. The labrum is a horseshoe-shaped fibrocartilaginous structure attached to the outer margin of the acetabulum that increases the depth of the joint [50] (Fig. 3.6). The inferior portion of the labrum is continuous with the transverse ligament that spans from the anterior margin to the posterior margin of the acetabulum inferiorly. The labrum typically demonstrates a triangular configuration in cross section and uniformly decreased signal relative to cartilage on all sequences, though variations in the shape and intrasubstance signal have been reported in earlier studies with conventional MR [51, 52]. In a group of asymptomatic patients, Lecouvet et al. [51] found that the presence of increased intrasubstance signal in the labrum on T1-weighted images and absence of the labrum increased in incidence with age. In a separate series of asymptomatic patients Cotten et al. [52] reported increased intrasubstance signal in the labrum on T1- and T2-weighted images and absence of the labrum occurred frequently. Note is made that these studies [51, 52] were based on conventional MRI and likely lacked distention of the perilabral sulcus that helps outline the labrum as seen on MR arthrography. In the author's experience, absence of the labrum is rare.

Since the initial report of the potential for a normal anterior sublabral sulcus by Byrd [53], several reports have documented the presence of normal sublabral sulci seen at MR arthrography and arthroscopy [39–41]. In a series of 121 patients, Saddik et al. [40] reported that 22% of patients who underwent hip arthroscopy and either conventional MR or MR arthrography were found to have normal sublabral sulci distributed as follows: 44% anterosuperior, 48% posteroinferior, 4% anteroinferior, and 4% posterosuperior. In their series [40], the accuracy of conventional MRI was 70%. Dinauer [39], in a series of 58 patients, noted 22.4% of patients without arthroscopic evidence of a labral tear had a normal posteroinferior sublabral sulcus on conventional MR or MR arthrography.

Differentiation of a sublabral sulcus from a labral tear can be challenging. Studler et al. [41] suggest that sublabral recesses occur most commonly anteroinferiorly (8 o'clock position) and can be distinguished from a labral tear by the linear shape of contrast between the labrum and acetabulum, partial separation of the labrum from the acetabulum (as opposed to complete separation), and absence of perilabral abnormalities. In this author's experience, normal sublabral sulci located posteroinferiorly are common. As tears of the posteroinferior labrum are uncommon, diagnosis of a posterior labral tear on MR arthrography should be reserved for cases where contrast extends the full thickness of the labrum or into the substance of the labrum (Fig. 3.9). Distinction of anterior sublabral sulci from labral detachment (Fig. 3.10) can be challenging, especially when the finding is small and not associated with adjacent acetabular chondral abnormality or paralabral cyst. In addition to the suggestions by Studler et al. [41], in distinguishing a normal sublabral sulcus from partial detachment or tear, clinical response to intra-articular anesthetic can be very helpful in the presence of equivocal MR findings.

The ligamentum teres is also well seen on MR arthrography as a low signal band-like structure with a broad-based attachment to the posteroinferior portion of the cotyloid fossa of the acetabulum and extending cephalad and laterally to attach to the fovea of the femoral head (Fig. 3.6). Low signal fat in the acetabular fossa can be mistaken for the ligamentum teres (Fig. 3.11). Ligamentum teres pathology is described later in this chapter. Another commonly seen normal variant on MR arthrography that could be confused with a pathologic plicae is the pectinofoveal fold (Fig. 3.6) [42]. The pectinofoveal fold is a thin band-like structure that is best seen on coronal images and extends caudally from the proximal medial femoral neck to attach to either the femoral neck or capsule and can be smooth or irregular in appearance, the latter of which is clinically insignificant [42].

Finally, the articular cartilage of the femoral head and acetabulum is seen as intermediate signal intensity (Fig. 3.6) and is the most difficult structure in the hip to evaluate on MR arthrography. Proton density with or without fat-suppression sequences can be helpful in demonstrating articular surface cartilage. Assessment of the articular cartilage in all three planes should be performed to maximize accuracy.

Imaging Features of Hip Pathology

Osteoarthritis, Femoroacetabular Impingement, and Labral Pathology

Osteoarthritis (OA) is the most commonly observed arthropathy in adults and can be subdivided into primary and secondary forms. Secondary OA occurs as a result of an insult to the hip such as trauma or infection, or in association with inflammatory arthropathies, crystal deposition disease, or hip dysplasia. The etiology of primary OA is less well understood. Initial plain radiographic findings of OA include nonuniform superolateral joint space narrowing indicative of cartilage loss (Fig. 3.12). As the disease progresses, reactive bone formation occurs (subchondral sclerosis, osteophytosis, medial buttressing) as a result of changes in mechanical stresses. Subchondral cyst formation in the superior acetabulum and femoral head is typically a late plain-film change of OA.

The recent proposal of FAI as a potential cause of primary or idiopathic OA in adults by Ganz et al. [1] has largely redirected our attention toward diagnosing causative structural abnormalities of the proximal femur and acetabulum rather than simply cartilage and labral abnormalities, thus directing surgical treatment toward correcting mechanical abnormalities and presumably delaying or slowing the progression of OA. Femoroacetabular impingement can be classified as cam, pincer, or mixed (both cam and pincer). Cam impingement most commonly occurs in males and results from premature impaction of a bony protuberance on the anterior femoral neck with the anterior acetabular rim [1]. Characteristically the anterosuperior acetabular cartilage is damaged and often associated with tearing or avulsion of the anterosuperior labrum [1]. Pincer impingement occurs more commonly in females from either retroversion or anteversion of the acetabular rim, or protrusio deformity of the acetabulum leading to premature impaction of the femoral neck on the acetabular rim due to acetabular overcoverage [1]. This mechanism results in a contrecoup injury to the posterior acetabulum and femoral head, and classically the labrum is thickened or enlarged and blunted and may demonstrate cystic change [1].

Assessment of the plain radiograph for FAI is well summarized in the work by Clohisy et al. [15]. Plain radiographic findings suggestive of cam FAI include a pistol grip deformity of the proximal femur (Fig. 3.3), focal prominence at the anterior femoral head-neck junction, aspherical femoral head (Fig. 3.1), cystic change at the femoral head-neck junction (Fig. 3.3), and abnormally increased alpha angle [15, 18]. MRI displays bony overgrowth on the anterior femoral neck best on oblique sagittal MRI sequences (Fig. 3.13). Measurement of the alpha angle is typically made from this MRI sequence according to the method outlined in the work of Notzli et al. (Fig. 3.13) [54]. In a comparison of a group of patients with symptoms of acetabular impingement and an asymptomatic group, they found a significant difference in the alpha angles of the two groups and proposed that an alpha angle greater than 55° was supportive of cam FAI [54]. In keeping with arthroscopic findings, classic distribution and appearance of acetabular labral and cartilage injuries seen on MR and MR arthrography in cam FAI have been established (Fig. 3.14) [11–14]. In a study of 50 patients who underwent MR arthrography of the hip and subsequent hip arthroscopy, Pfirmann et al. [11] noted large alpha angles, anterosuperior cartilage lesions, and osseous bump formation at the anterior

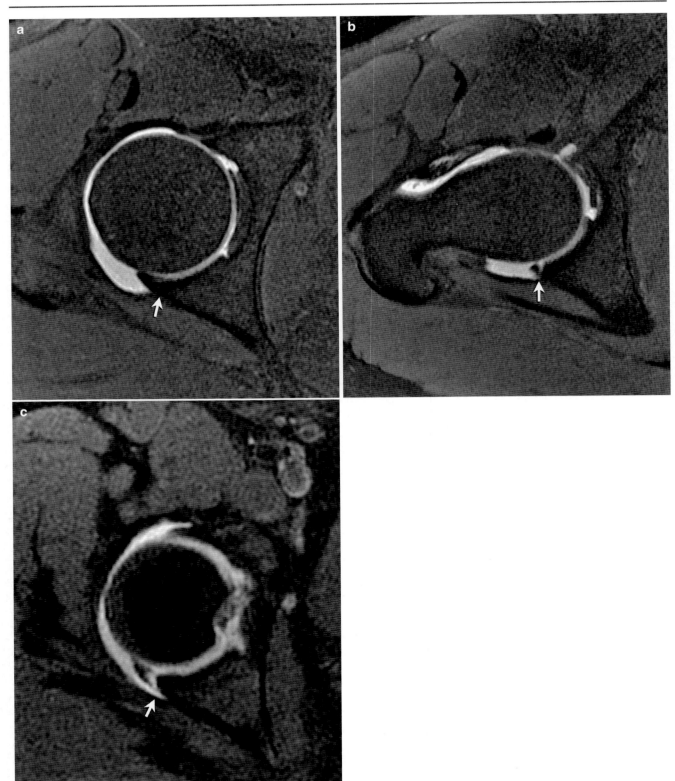

Fig. 3.9 Normal posterior labral acetabular interface, posterior sulcus, and posterior labral tear seen on MR arthrography. (**a**) Axial T1-weighted fat-suppressed image demonstrates lack of contrast between posterior labrum and acetabulum (*arrow*). (**b**) Axial T1-weighted fat- suppressed image reveals normal posterior sulcus with small amount of contrast extending between posterior labrum and acetabulum (*arrow*). (**c**) Axial T1-weighted fat-suppressed image demonstrates a posterior labral tear with contrast extending irregularly into the substance of the posterior labrum (*arrow*)

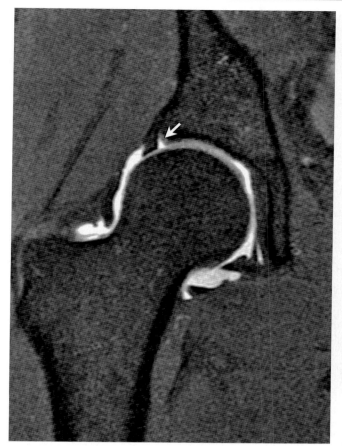

Fig. 3.10 Labral detachment. Coronal T1-weighted fat-suppressed 3T image of the right hip demonstrates contrast tracking between the labrum and acetabulum extending the full thickness of the labrum (*arrow*)

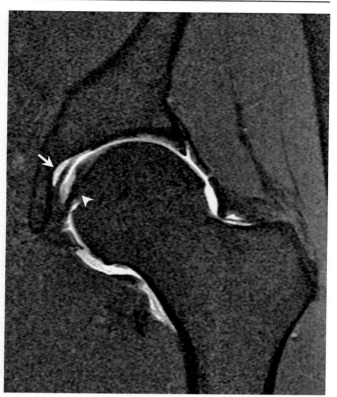

Fig. 3.11 Fat in the acetabular fossa mimicking the ligamentum teres. Coronal T1-weighted fat-suppressed 3T image from MR arthrogram reveals fat in the acetabular fossa (*white arrow*) appearing similar in morphology and coursing parallel to the ligamentum teres (*arrowhead*)

femoral head-neck junction in patients with cam FAI. Similarly, Kassarjian et al. [12] demonstrated a similar triad of findings on MR arthrography including abnormal head-neck morphology, anterosuperior cartilage, and anterosuperior labral abnormalities in the 88% of patients with clinical evidence of cam FAI.

Pincer FAI is less commonly seen and less well documented than cam FAI, thought to occur predominantly in females, and is associated with acetabular protrusion deformity or acetabular retroversion [1]. On plain radiographs, acetabular retroversion can be identified with the combination of a crossover sign (Fig. 3.2) and posterior wall sign [15, 18]. Measurement of acetabular overcoverage on MR and MR arthrography is less clearly documented in the literature than measurement of the alpha angle. Pfirmann et al. [11] proposed measuring the acetabular depth on the sagittal oblique sequence obtained through the center of the femoral neck (Fig. 3.15). Patients with pincer FAI demonstrated medial positioning of the center of the femoral head relative to a line connecting the anterior and posterior rim (averaging nearly 5 mm) as opposed to those patients with cam FAI that had neutral or lateral positioning of the femoral head relative to the anterior-posterior rim line [11]. In addition to potential

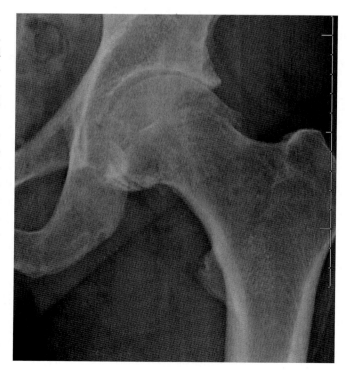

Fig. 3.12 Plain radiograph demonstrates superior joint space narrowing, subchondral sclerosis and osteophystosis associated with the femoral head

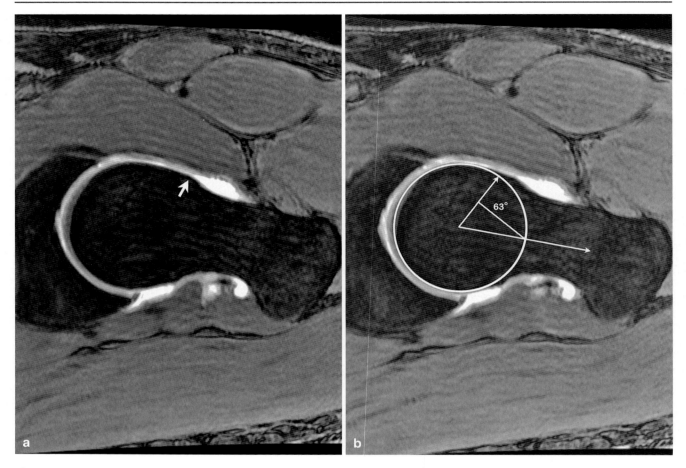

Fig. 3.13 Alpha angle measurement for cam impingement. (**a**) Oblique sagittal fast spoiled gradient recall (SPGR) 3T image at narrowest point of femoral neck demonstrates characteristic bump of anterior femoral head-neck junction (*arrow*). (**b**) A *circle* is made demarcating the margin of the femoral head. Measurement of the alpha angle is made by constructing the first ray of the angle parallel to the femoral neck from the center of the femoral neck to the center of femoral head (vertex of angle) and the second ray from center of the femoral head to the site at which the anterior femoral cortex extends beyond the circle

acetabular overcoverage, the authors found characteristic cartilage and labral lesions in the posteroinferior acetabulum in their series of 14 patients with pincer-type FAI [11].

As both forms of impingement are associated with labral pathology, knowledge of the MRI appearance of the normal and abnormal labrum is essential to proper diagnosis. Czerny et al. [2, 3] proposed the first MRI classification of labral pathology based on the morphology and intrinsic signal of the labrum, labrocapsular relationship, and presence of fluid tracking into the interface of the labrum and adjacent acetabular cartilage. One weakness to this classification is the established knowledge of normal sulci occurring at the junction of the labrum and adjacent acetabular cartilage. The most direct evidence for a labral tear is contrast or fluid tracking into the substance of the labrum (Fig. 3.16a, b). Detachment of the labrum is diagnosed when contrast extends the full thickness of the labrum between the labrum and acetabular cartilage (Fig. 3.10). As mentioned earlier, contrast extending between the labrum and acetabular

cartilage less than the full thickness of the labrum can represent a tear, partial detachment, or sublabral sulcus. The location of the finding and presence of neighboring chondral damage or a paralabral cyst should aid in distinguishing labral pathology from a sublabral sulcus. Labral hypertrophy with increased intrinsic signal is another abnormality observed on MR arthrography and implies chronic degeneration and degenerative tearing, most likely the result of pincer impingement [1].

Cartilage abnormalities adjacent to labral pathology in FAI are common, and identification of these changes is important as those patients with advanced chondral abnormalities have a poorer prognosis than those with limited or no chondral damage [55]. Identification of these chondral changes continues to be a weakness of conventional MRI and MR arthrography. Identification of cartilage abnormalities on MR and MR arthrography is likely limited by the curvature of the articular surfaces and the close apposition of the femoral head and acetabular cartilage. On

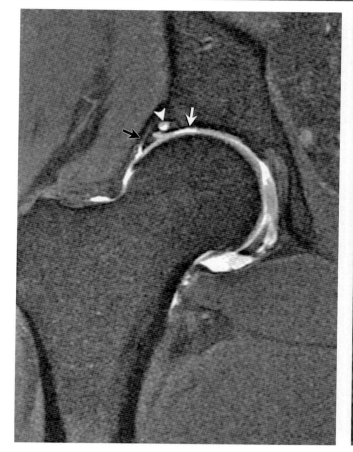

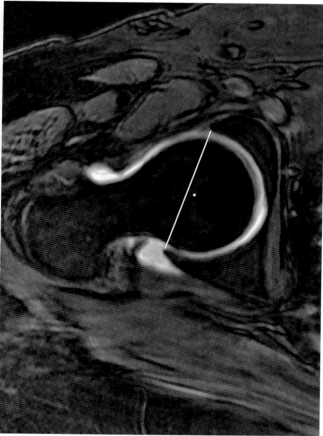

Fig. 3.14 Characteristic pattern of labral and cartilaginous abnormalities of cam impingement seen on MR arthrography. Coronal T1-weighted fat-suppressed 3T image of the right hip reveals a tear of the anterolateral labrum (*black arrow*), focal full thickness defect in adjacent acetabular cartilage (*white arrow*), and contrast filling a subjacent acetabular subchondral cyst (*arrowhead*)

Fig. 3.15 Measurement for pincer impingement on MR arthrography. Oblique sagittal SPGR 3T image reveals a *line* constructed from the anterior acetabular rim to the posterior acetabular rim is 5 mm lateral to the center of the femoral head (*dot*) indicating acetabular overcoverage

conventional MRI, focal cartilage is best seen on proton density fat-suppressed or proton density images as cartilage signal is less intense than fluid and higher than subjacent cortical bone. On MR arthrography, cartilage abnormalities can be seen as focal extension of contrast into cartilage (Fig. 3.16b) or contrast filling a focal cartilage defect (Fig. 3.16b). In a recent report by Pfirmann et al. [14] evidence of acetabular cartilage delamination associated with cam FAI can be seen as fluid undermining normal appearing cartilage or as a low signal intensity band or hypointense area in the acetabular cartilage on intermediate-weighted fat-suppressed or T1-weighted images. Unfortunately, MR arthrography was only moderately successful in demonstrating these findings [14]. Improvements in the diagnosis of cartilage abnormalities of the femoral head and acetabulum may be possible with greater awareness of their importance in treatment planning and new MR techniques and with 3T MRI (Fig. 3.17), but more investigation of this topic is needed.

Ligamentum Teres Pathology

The function of the ligamentum teres and its potential mechanical role remain problematic. It is unclear whether the ligament is a restraint and offers increased stability or is essentially an embryonic remnant with little or no function [56]. Injury to the ligament has been determined to be a mechanical source of hip pain that can be alleviated with arthroscopic debridement [57]. For this reason, evaluation of this structure on conventional MRI or MR arthrography of the hip is important, particularly in the setting of suspected intra-articular source of pain without evidence of labral or cartilaginous pathology. MR arthrography demonstrates this structure more consistently than conventional MRI by outlining ligament fibers with contrast, making fiber irregularity or disruption more conspicuous.

As described earlier, the ligamentum teres arises from the inferior portion of the acetabular or transverse ligament

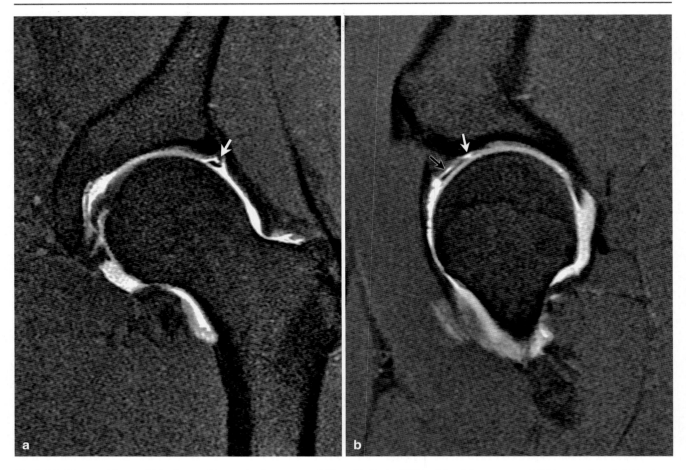

Fig. 3.16 Direct evidence of labral tear with cam impingement at MR arthrography. (**a**) Coronal T1-weighted fat-suppressed 3T image of the left hip reveals contrast tracking into labral tear anterolaterally (*arrow*).

(**b**) Sagittal T1-weighted fat-suppressed 3T image of the left hip demonstrates contrast tracking into the anterior labrum (*black arrow*) and adjacent cartilage (*white arrow*)

[56], attaches to the fovea of the femoral head, and contains a small artery. The ligament consists of two fascicles attached to the acetabular fossa [56], though distinction of such fascicles is not readily seen on MRI. Gray and Villar [58] proposed an arthroscopically based classification of abnormalities of the ligamentum teres that includes complete tears, partial tears, and degenerate ligamentum teres. Complete tear of the ligament accompanies dislocations of the hip and, depending on the timing of imaging after the injury, may appear on MRI as complete disruption of ligament fibers in the acute setting or absence of the ligament with remote injury. Partial tears or degeneration of the ligament may have similar appearances with focal enlargement of the ligament with increased intrasubstance signal. Partial thickness disruption of ligament fibers (Fig. 3.18) can also be seen with partial tears. As our awareness of ligamentum teres pathology has grown and utilization of 3T MRI has increased, preoperative detection of abnormalities of this ligament should improve.

Miscellaneous Hip Pathology

Osteonecrosis

Osteonecrosis of the femoral head is a commonly encountered source of hip pain and may be idiopathic or associated with underlying risk factors such as steroid use, sickle cell disease, trauma, alcohol use, or pancreatitis. MRI is the most sensitive imaging test for detecting osteonecrosis [31] and is particularly well suited to evaluate this disorder as it is sensitive to marrow-based pathology, allows concomitant evaluation of the contralateral hip that that is often affected, and can provide information that has prognostic and therapeutic implications [59–61]. The MRI appearance of osteonecrosis varies with temporal evolution of the disease. The MRI classification proposed by Mitchell et al. [31] is most commonly used and is believed to correlate with progression of osteonecrosis. A hallmark observation of osteonecrosis on MRI is the presence of a rim of low signal on T1-weighted images outlining the osteonecrotic area (Fig. 3.19). In the

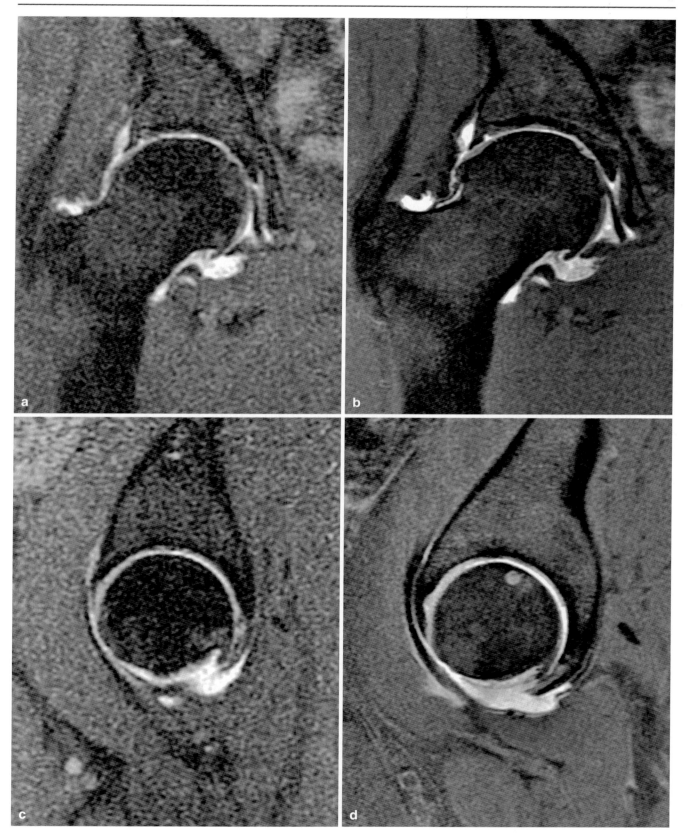

Fig. 3.17 Osteoarthritis at 1.5T and 3.0T MR arthrography. (**a, c**) Coronal and sagittal T1-weighted fat-suppressed 1.5T image of the right hip demonstrates joint space narrowing and irregularity of the articular cartilage and suggestion of a labral tear. (**b, d**) Coronal and sagittal T1-weighted fat-suppressed 3T image of same patient approximately 18 months later without interval surgery reveals similar findings with much better resolution and lesion conspicuity

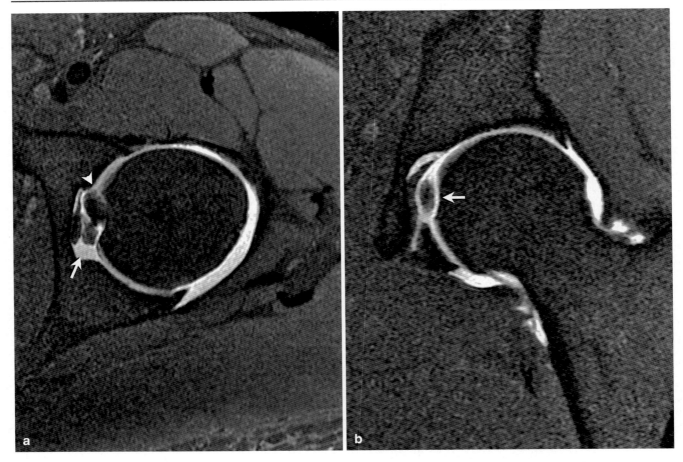

Fig. 3.18 Partial tear of the ligamentum teres as seen on MR arthrography. (**a**) Axial T1-weighted fat-suppressed 3T image reveals torn fibers of the ligamentum teres (*white arrow*) posterior and medial to intact foveal attachment fibers (*arrowhead*). (**b**) Coronal T1-weighted fat-suppressed 3T image demonstrates the unattached torn posterior fibers of the ligamentum teres (*arrow*)

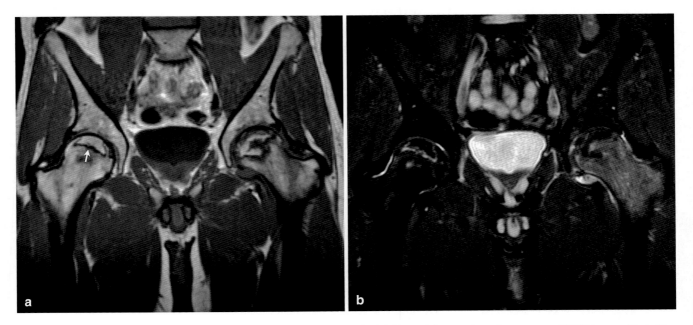

Fig. 3.19 Bilateral osteonecrosis. (**a**) Coronal noncontrasted T1-weighted images of both hips reveal characteristic rim of low signal (*arrow*) demarcating the zone of osteonecrosis (Class A) in the right hip. (**b**) Coronal short tau inversion recovery (STIR) image of both hips demonstrates an effusion and diffuse marrow edema in the femoral head and neck of the left hip

Mitchell classification system [31], the MR findings are subdivided into classes A–D depending on the signal of the central portion of the osteonecrotic focus as follows: Class A, signal analogous to fat; Class B, signal isointense to blood; Class C, signal isointense to fluid; and Class D, signal isointense to fibrous tissue. Another classic MRI observation of osteonecrosis on T2-weighted images is a *double line* composed of an inner band of high signal thought to correspond to granulation tissue and an outer band of low signal presumed to represent sclerosis from bone repair [31]. MRI can also show evidence of subchondral fracture, articular surface collapse, and evidence of secondary osteoarthritis associated with osteonecrosis. In addition, marrow edema in the femoral head and neck seen on MRI (Fig. 3.19) in association with osteonecrosis has been found to correlate with pain and subsequent collapse of the femoral head [61].

In addition to the detection and characterization of osteonecrosis, one of the most important contributions MRI provides is accurate depiction of the size of the lesion which strongly correlates with risk of future collapse [59, 60]. Beltran et al. [59] found, in a series of patients with osteonecrosis that underwent core decompression, 87% of cases involving greater than 50% of the weight-bearing surface area progressed to collapse. Forty-three percent of patients with 25–50% of the weight-bearing surface involved went on to collapse, and no patients with less than 25% of the weight-bearing surface area involved progressed to collapse [59]. Similarly, Shimizu et al. [60] found that 74% of patients with lesions greater than 25% of the femoral head diameter and involving 67% of the weight-bearing surface area demonstrated collapse. Collapse did not occur in patients with osteonecrosis involving less than 25% of the femoral head diameter in their study group [60].

Acute Trauma and Stress Injury

The radiographic evaluation of acute hip trauma is beyond the scope of this text. A brief review of imaging acute trauma to the hip and, in particular, in cases with high index of suspicion and normal plain radiographs is warranted. Plain radiographs remain the initial imaging exam in evaluating acute hip injury. Standard views may be augmented with Judet views for evaluation of acetabular fractures, and inlet and outlet views may be used to better assess displacement of pelvic ring fractures. CT is helpful in depicting the spatial relationship of fractures for surgical planning and for the detection of intra-articular bone fragments (Fig. 3.4). It is now established that MRI is the imaging modality of choice in the evaluation of the elderly patient with hip pain after a fall with normal radiographs and high clinical suspicion of fracture [32–34, 62]. MRI is very sensitive to marrow changes seen with an acute fracture and can readily demonstrate occult fractures of the femoral neck (Fig. 3.20), greater trochanter and intertrochanteric region (Fig. 3.20),

acetabulum, and superior and inferior pubic rami. MRI protocols used in the setting of acute trauma can be abbreviated and typically include T1-weighted and short tau inversion recovery (STIR) sequences. Acute fractures demonstrate decreased signal on T1-weighted images and increased signal on STIR sequences in the fracture site (Fig. 3.20). A common injury seen in the elderly is an incomplete fracture of the greater trochanter (Fig. 3.21) that extends caudally into the intertrochanteric region but without crossing to the lesser trochanter [63]. MRI can be helpful in delineating the extent of the fracture across the medullary canal that can aid in treatment planning [63]. In addition to detecting occult fractures in acute trauma, MRI can help identify and characterize the severity of extra-articular injuries to muscle and tendon (Fig. 3.22) [29, 64, 65].

Stress fractures occur as a result of insufficiency (as seen in the elderly or in patients with known risk factors) or overuse. As plain radiographs are often normal or show subtle changes, MRI is particularly suited to detect radiographically occult stress fractures as it is sensitive to marrow changes. Stress fractures of the hip can arise in the femoral neck (Fig. 3.23), femoral head, acetabulum, or pubic ring [66]. In a recent retrospective evaluation of MRI and CT exams of insufficiency fractures in elderly patients [66], 70% of patients had more than one fracture and 87% demonstrated marrow edema with fracture lines on MRI. A stress fracture of the femoral neck typically arises on the medial side, demonstrates a large area increased signal on T2-weighted images (marrow edema), and may have a linear focus of decreased signal at the epicenter of edema-oriented perpendicular to the trabecular pattern signifying the fracture line (Fig. 3.23). For follow-up of patients with femoral neck stress fractures, it is important to note that the MRI finding of marrow edema has been reported to resolve with appropriate therapy in 90% of patients by 6 months [67].

Septic Arthritis

Septic arthritis of the hip is an emergent condition that requires rapid diagnosis to prevent the sequela of delayed therapy. Plain radiographs are typically normal early in the clinical presentation. MRI should be considered if there is suspicion of a septic hip as it can suggest an intra-articular location of infection and help exclude a more superficial infection that would be a contraindication to an intra-articular needle aspiration. Septic arthritis often demonstrates a joint effusion with associated edema in the para-articular soft tissues and muscle (Fig. 3.24). Contrasted images can depict enhancement of the synovium and para-articular soft tissues. Marrow edema or bone enhancement with contrast may represent osteomyelitis but is nonspecific as these findings may be reactive [68].

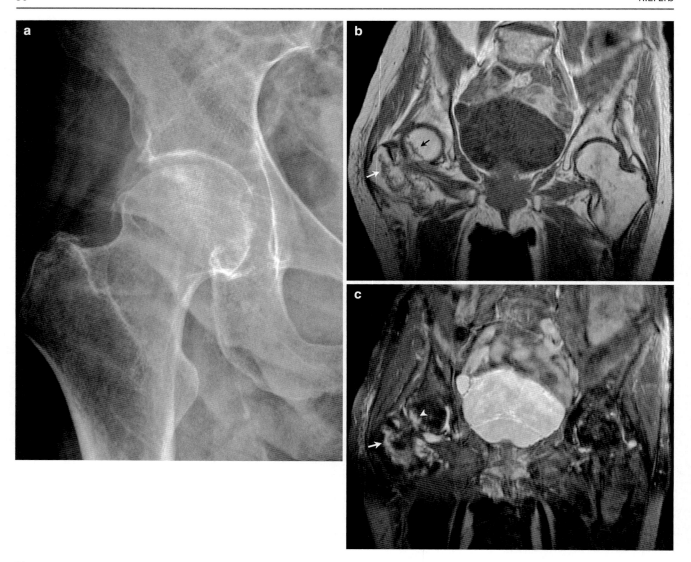

Fig. 3.20 Radiographically occult (or subtle) femoral neck and inter-trochanteric fractures depicted on MR. (**a**) Plain radiograph of the right hip is near normal with subtle linear band of sclerosis in the femoral neck and overlying artifact from skin folds. (**b**) Coronal T1-weighted 3T image of both hips demonstrates linear areas of decreased signal in the subcapital portion of the femoral neck (*black arrow*) and intertrochanteric region (*white arrow*). (**c**) Coronal STIR 3T image of both hips reveals marrow edema in the femoral neck (*arrowhead*) and intertrochanteric (*arrow*) fractures

Snapping Hip Syndrome

The snapping hip syndrome is a cause of hip pain associated with a snapping or popping sensation occurring with hip motion [69–71]. Ultrasound is well suited for the evaluation of extra-articular causes of the snapping hip syndrome [25, 47–49]. It offers a noninvasive means of dynamically evaluating the symptomatic hip and asymptomatic hip for comparison. The snapping hip syndrome can be designated as internal or external, or simply according to the structure that is snapping [69, 71]. Internal snapping syndrome has been theorized to occur as the iliopsoas tendon snaps or jerks as it crosses over the iliopectineal eminence, anterior joint capsule, or lesser trochanteric bony prominence [46]. A recent study by Deslandes et al. [48] challenges this assumption. In their review of dynamic ultrasound of 14 patients with extra-articular snapping hip syndrome, the most common finding was snapping of the iliopsoas tendon over the iliac muscle, occurring lateral to the iliopectineal eminence [48]. Other less common causes of snapping in their study included bifid iliopsoas tendons snapping over one another and snapping of the iliopsoas tendon over an anterior paralabral cyst [48]. Ultrasound for internal snapping syndrome is performed with the patient in the supine position with a

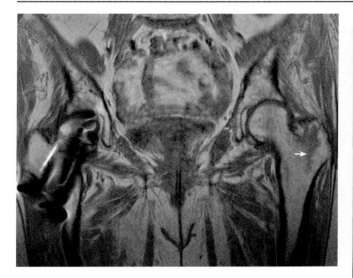

Fig. 3.21 Incomplete intertrochanteric fracture. Coronal T1-weighted image of both hips demonstrates a greater trochanteric fracture (*arrow*) extending longitudinally without crossing to medial femoral cortex

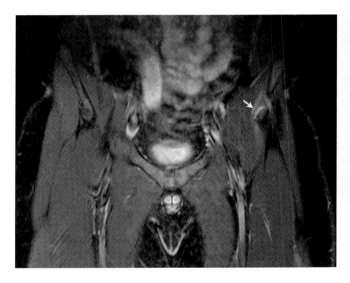

Fig. 3.22 Partial avulsion of the origin of the rectus femoris muscle. Coronal T2-weighted fat-suppressed image of both hips demonstrates partial avulsion of the rectus femoris from the anterior inferior iliac spine (*arrow*)

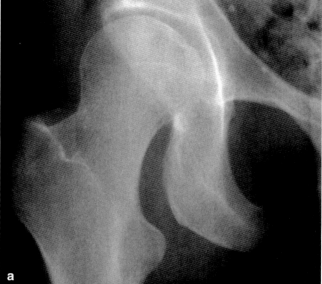

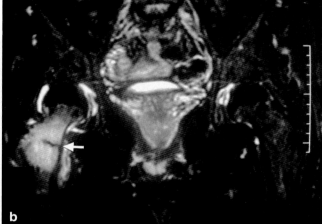

Fig. 3.23 Femoral neck stress fracture. (**a**) Plain radiograph is normal. (**b**) Coronal T2-weighted fat-suppressed image of both hips demonstrates a linear area of decreased signal (*arrow*) oriented perpendicular to the trabecular pattern surrounded by marrow edema

high-frequency linear or curved array transducer positioned directly over the hip in the transverse plane (Fig. 3.25). The iliopsoas is observed as the patient reproduces the snapping or clicking sensation typically extending the hip from the flexed, externally rotated, and abducted position. The abnormal snapping of the tendon with this maneuver can be seen in real time and can be captured with a cine clip for later review. External snapping syndrome is typically attributed to and has been sonographically visualized [49] as a jerking motion of the iliotibial band or gluteus maximus as it moves

over the greater trochanter. For this exam, the patient can be scanned in the lateral decubitus (symptomatic side up), supine, or standing position [25, 49]. The ultrasound probe is positioned in the transverse or longitudinal direction over the greater trochanter as the hip is extended from the flexed, internally or externally rotated position [25, 49].

Summary

Imaging plays a key role in the workup of unexplained hip pain. Plain radiographs remain the initial imaging exam obtained in the evaluation of hip pain and may be normal, reveal an obvious explanation of pain, or demonstrate more

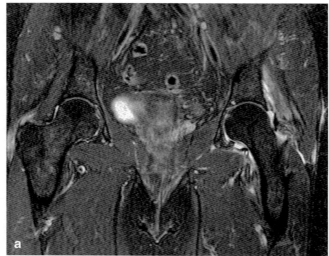

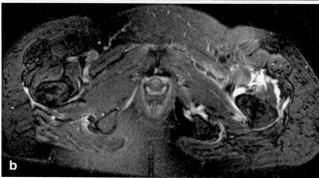

Fig. 3.24 Septic arthritis. (**a**) Coronal T2-weighted fat-suppressed image of both hips demonstrates a large left hip joint effusion with para-articular soft tissue edema. (**b**) Axial T2-weighted fat-suppressed image of the left hip reveals large joint effusion and edema in the para-articular soft tissues

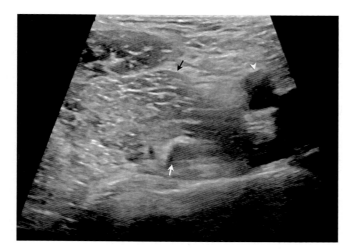

Fig. 3.25 Ultrasound of the right hip. Transverse image of the right hip at the level of the femoral head demonstrates the normal appearance of the iliopsoas tendon (*white arrow*), iliopsoas muscle (*black arrow*), and common femoral artery (*white arrowhead*)

subtle findings suggestive of FAI. Plain radiographic findings of FAI are common and should be carefully correlated with clinical findings and MR or MR arthrography as indicated. The selection of secondary imaging depends on the clinical setting and question to be answered. MRI of the hip is the secondary imaging exam for most presentations of unexplained hip pain. MR arthrography is especially helpful in the evaluation of the acetabular labrum and can reveal other intra-articular abnormalities including chondral damage, injury of the ligamentum teres, and loose bodies. Future advances in MRI technology and applications and greater experience with 3T MRI may improve our ability to visualize chondral damage associated with FAI, thus assisting the arthroscopist in selecting the most appropriate treatment and aiding surgical planning. Ultrasound plays a complimentary role to MRI in the evaluation and treatment of hip pain and currently is most helpful in the evaluation of snapping hip syndrome and therapeutic interventions.

References

1. Ganz R, Parvizi J, Beck M, et al. Femoroacetabular impingement: a cause for osteoarthritis of the hip. Clin Orthop Relat Res. 2003;417:112–20.
2. Czerny C, Hofmann S, Neuhold A, et al. Lesions of the acetabular labrum: accuracy of MR imaging and MR arthrography in detection and staging. Radiology. 1996;200:225–30.
3. Czerny C, Hofmann S, Urban M, et al. MR arthrography of the adult acetabular capsular-labral complex: correlation with surgery and anatomy. AJR Am J Roentgenol. 1999;173:345–9.
4. Haims A, Katz LD, Busconi B. MR arthrography of the hip. Radiol Clin North Am. 1998;36:691–702.
5. Hodler J, Yu JS, Goodwin D, et al. MR arthrography of the hip: improved imaging of the acetabular labrum with histologic correlation in cadavers. AJR Am J Roentgenol. 1995;165:887–91.
6. Leunig M, Werlen S, Ungersbrock A, et al. Evaluation of the acetabular labrum by MR arthrography. J Bone Joint Surg Br. 1997;79:230–4.
7. Palmer WE. MR arthrography of the hip. Semin Musculoskelet Radiol. 1998;12:349–61.
8. Petersilge CA, Haque MA, Petersilge WJ, et al. Acetabular labral tears: evaluation with MR arthrography. Radiology. 1996; 200:231–5.
9. Sadro C. Current concepts in magnetic resonance imaging of the adult hip and pelvis. Semin Roentgenol. 2000;35:231–48.
10. Petersilge CA. MR arthrography for evaluation of the acetabular labrum. Skeletal Radiol. 2001;30:423–30.
11. Pfirmann CWA, Mengiardi B, Dora C, et al. Cam and pincer Femoroacetabular impingement: characteristic MR arthrographic findings in 50 patients. Radiology. 2006;240:778–85.
12. Kassarjian A, Yoon LS, Belzile E, et al. Triad of MR arthrographic findings in patients with cam-type Femoroacetabular impingement. Radiology. 2005;236:588–92.
13. Filigenzi JM, Bredella MA. MR imaging of femoroacetabular impingement. Appl Radiol. 2008;37:12–9.
14. Pfirrmann CWA, Duc SR, Zanetti M, et al. MR arthrography of acetabular cartilage delamination in femoroacetabular cam impingement. Radiology. 2008;249:236–41.

15. Clohisy JC, Carlisle JC, Beaule PC, et al. A systematic approach to the plain radiographic evaluation of the young adult hip. J Bone Joint Surg Am. 2008;90:47–66.

16. Sartoris DJ, Resnick D. Plain film radiography: routine and specialized techniques and projections. In: Resnick D, Niwayana G, editors. Diagnosis of bone and joint disorders, vol. 1. 2nd ed. Philadelphia: Saunders; 1998. p. 38.

17. Judet R, Judet J, Letournel E. Fractures of the acetabulum: classification and surgical approaches to open reduction. J Bone Joint Surg. 1964;46A:1615–46.

18. Laborie LB, Lehmann TG, Engesaeter IO, et al. Prevalence of radiographic findings thought to be associated with femoroacetabular impingement in a population-based cohort of 2081 healthy young adults. Radiology. 2011;260:495–502.

19. Erb RE. Adult hip imaging. In: Byrd JWT, editor. Operative hip arthroscopy. 2nd ed. New York: Springer; 2005. p. 51.

20. Conway WF, Totty WG, McEnery KW. CT and MR imaging of the hip. Radiology. 1996;198:297–307.

21. Krestan CR, Noske H, Vasilevska V, et al. MDCT versus digital radiography in the evaluation of bone healing in orthopedic patients. AJR Am J Roentgenol. 2006;186:1754–60.

22. Park JS, Ryu KN, Hong HP, et al. Focal osteolysis in total hip replacement: CT findings. Skeletal Radiol. 2004;33:632–40.

23. Brenner DJ, Hall EJ. Computed tomography – an increasing source of radiation exposure. N Engl J Med. 2007;357:2277–84.

24. Smith-Bindman R, Lipson J, Marcus R, et al. Radiation dose associated with common computed tomography examinations and the associated lifetime attributable risk of cancer. Arch Intern Med. 2009;169:2078–86.

25. Miller TT. Abnormalities in and around the hip: MR imaging versus sonography. Magn Reson Imaging Clin N Am. 2005;13:799–809.

26. Joines MM, Motamedi K, Seeger LL, et al. Musculoskeletal interventional ultrasound. Semin Musculoskelet Radiol. 2007;11:192–8.

27. Kozlov DB, Sonin AH. Iliopsoas bursitis: diagnosis by MRI. J Comput Assist Tomogr. 1998;22:625–8.

28. Pritchard RS, Shah HR, Nelson CL, et al. MR and CT appearance of iliopsoas bursal distention secondary to diseased hips. J Comput Assist Tomogr. 1990;14:797–800.

29. Kneeland JB. MR imaging of sports injuries of the hip. Magn Reson Imaging Clin N Am. 1999;7:105–15.

30. Moss SG, Schweitzer ME, Jacobson JA, et al. Hip joint fluid: detection and distribution at MR imaging and US with cadaveric correlation. Radiology. 1998;208:43–8.

31. Mitchell DG, Rao VM, Dalinka MK, et al. Femoral head avascular necrosis: correlation of MR imaging, radiographic staging, radionuclide imaging, and clinical findings. Radiology. 1987;162:709–15.

32. Bogost GA, Lizerbram EK, Crues III JV. MR imaging in evaluation of suspected hip fracture: frequency of unsuspected bone and soft tissue injury. Radiology. 1995;197:263–7.

33. May DA, Purins JL, Smith DK. MR imaging of occult traumatic fractures and muscular injuries of the hip and pelvis in elderly patients. AJR Am J Roentgenol. 1996;166:1075–8.

34. Pandey R, McNally E, Ali A, et al. The role of MRI in the diagnosis of occult hip fractures. Injury. 1998;29:61–3.

35. Beltran J, Caudill JL, Herman LA, et al. Rheumatoid arthritis: MR imaging manifestations. Radiology. 1987;165:153–7.

36. Mintz DN, Hooper T, Connell D, et al. Magnetic resonance imaging of the hip: detection of labral and chondral abnormalities using noncontrast imaging. Arthroscopy. 2005;21:385–93.

37. Toomayan GA, Holman WR, Major NM, et al. Sensitivity of MR arthrography in the evaluation of acetabular tears. AJR Am J Roentgenol. 2006;186:449–53.

38. Magee T. Comparison of 3 Tesla MR versus 3 Tesla MR arthrography of the hip for detection of acetabular labral tears in the same patient population. AJR Am J Roentgenol. 2010;194:A91–5.

39. Dinauer PA, Murphy KP, Carroll JF. Sublabral sulcus at the posteroinferior acetabulum: a potential pitfall in MR arthrography diagnosis of acetabular labral tears. AJR Am J Roentgenol. 2004;183:1745–53.

40. Saddik D, Troupis J, Tirman P, et al. Prevalence and location of acetabular sublabral sulci at hip arthroscopy with retrospective MRI review. AJR Am J Roentgenol. 2006;187:507–11.

41. Studler U, Kalberer F, Leunig M, et al. MR arthrography of the hip: differentiation between an anterior sublabral recess as a normal variant and a labral tear. Radiology. 2008;249:947–54.

42. Blankenbaker DG, Davis KW, De Smet AA, et al. MRI appearance of the pectinofoveal fold. AJR Am J Roentgenol. 2009;192:93–5.

43. Byrd JWT, Jones KS. Diagnostic accuracy of clinical assessment, magnetic resonance imaging, magnetic resonance arthrography, and intra-articular injection in hip arthroscopy patients. Am J Sports Med. 2004;32:1668–74.

44. Mettler FA, Guibeerteau MJ. Skeletal system. In: Mettler FA, Guiberteau MJ, editors. Essentials of nuclear medicine imaging. 5th ed. Philadelphia: Saunders; 2006. p. 276–8.

45. Banks KP, Song WS. Acetabular impingement on planar and spect bone scintigraphy. Clin Nucl Med. 2008;33:916–9.

46. Harper MC, Schaberg JE, Allen WC. Primary iliopsoas bursography in the diagnosis of disorders of the hip. Clin Orthop Relat Res. 1987;221:238–41.

47. Cardinal E, Buckwalter KA, Capello WN, et al. US of the snapping iliopsoas tendon. Radiology. 1996;198:521–2.

48. Deslandes M, Guillin R, Cardinal E, et al. The snapping iliopsoas tendon: new mechanisms using dynamic sonography. AJR Am J Roentgenol. 2008;190:576–81.

49. Choi YS, Lee SM, Song BY, et al. Dynamic sonography of external snapping hip syndrome. J Ultrasound Med. 2002;21:753–8.

50. Santori N, Villar RN. Arthroscopic anatomy of the hip. In: Byrd JWT, editor. Operative hip arthroscopy. New York: Thieme; 1998. p. 93–104.

51. Lecouvet FE, Vande Berg BC, Melghem J, et al. MR imaging of the acetabular labrum: variations in 200 asymptomatic hips. AJR Am J Roentgenol. 1996;167:1025–8.

52. Cotten A, Boutry N, Demondion X, et al. Acetabular labrum: MRI in asymptomatic volunteers. J Comput Assist Tomogr. 1998;22:1–7.

53. Byrd JWT. Labral lesion: an elusive source of hip pain: case reports and review of the literature. Arthroscopy. 1996;12:603–12.

54. Notzli HP, Wyss TF, Stoecklin CH, et al. The contour of the femoral head-neck junction as a predictor for the risk of anterior impingement. J Bone Joint Surg. 2002;84-B:556–60.

55. Byrd JWT, Jones KS. Hip arthroscopy for labral pathology: prospective analysis with 10-year follow-up. Arthroscopy. 2009;25:365–8.

56. Cerezal L, Kassarjian A, Canga A, et al. Anatomy, biomechanics, imaging, and management of ligamentum teres injuries. Radiographics. 2010;30:1637–51.

57. Byrd JWT, Jones KS. Traumatic rupture of the ligamentum teres as a source of hip pain. Arthroscopy. 2004;20:385–91.

58. Gray AJR, Villar RN. The ligamentum teres of the hip: an arthroscopic classification of its pathology. Arthroscopy. 1997;13:575–8.

59. Beltran J, Knight CT, Zueler WA, et al. Core decompression for avascular necrosis of the femoral head: correlation between long-term results and preoperative MR staging. Radiology. 1990;175:533–6.

60. Shimizu K, Moriya H, Akita T, et al. Prediction of collapse with magnetic resonance imaging of avascular necrosis of the femoral head. J Bone Joint Surg. 1994;76A:215–23.

61. Iida S, Harada Y, Shimizu K, et al. Correlation between bone marrow edema and collapse of the femoral head in steroid induced osteonecrosis. AJR Am J Roentgenol. 2000;174:735–43.

62. Evans PD, Wilson C, Lyons K. Comparison of MRI with bone scanning for suspected hip fracture in elderly patients. J Bone Joint Surg Br. 1994;76:158–9.

63. Schultz E, Miller TT, Boruchov SD, et al. Incomplete intertrochanteric fractures: Imaging features and clinical management. Radiology. 1999;211:237–40.

64. Chung CB, Robertson JE, Cho GJ, et al. Gluteus medius tendon tears and avulsive injuries in elderly women: imaging findings in six patients. AJR Am J Roentgenol. 1999;173:351–3.

65. Kingzett-Taylor A, Tirman PFJ, Feller J, et al. Tendinosis and tears of gluteus medius and minimus muscles as a cause of hip pain: MR imaging findings. AJR Am J Roentgenol. 1999;173:1123–6.

66. Cabarrus MC, Ambekar A, Lu Y, et al. MRI and CT of insufficiency fractures of the pelvis and proximal femur. AJR Am J Roentgenol. 2008;191:995–1001.

67. Slocum KA, Gorman JD, Puckett ML, et al. Resolution of abnormal MR signal intensity in patients with stress fractures of the femoral neck. AJR Am J Roentgenol. 1997;168:1295–9.

68. Lee SK, Suh KJ, Kim YW, et al. Septic arthritis versus transient synovitis at MR imaging: preliminary assessment with signal intensity alterations of bone marrow. Radiology. 1999;211:459–65.

69. Schaberg JE, Harper MC, Allen WC. The snapping hip syndrome. Am J Sports Med. 1984;12:361–5.

70. Jacobson T, Allen WC. Surgical correction of the snapping iliopsoas tendon. Am J Sports Med. 1990;18:470–4.

71. Byrd JWT. Snapping hip. Oper Tech Sports Med. 2005;13:46–54.

My Approach to Athletic Pubalgia

4

Michael Brunt and Raymond Barile

Groin injuries are a common problem in sports and can be a diagnostic and management challenge for treating athletic trainers, therapists, and physicians for a number of reasons. The symptoms may be diffuse, the onset is often insidious, the regional anatomy in the groin is complex, and multiple causes may coexist. As a result, they can be difficult to diagnose and treat accurately. In addition, these injuries may result in a significant loss of playing time, and it can be difficult to predict the time frame for return to play.

Groin injuries occur most commonly in sports that have sudden, repetitive twisting, turning, and kicking motions at high speed. Therefore, sports such as soccer, ice hockey [1], and football are particularly prone to these types of injuries. Epidemiologic studies have shown that groin injuries occur in up to 5–23% of soccer players and, in one study, accounted for 8% of all injuries over one season [2]. Most are soft tissue injuries with the adductor muscle group being the most common site injured. Unlike other athletic injuries, they do not typically result from direct physical contact. As stated by Smodlaka [3] 30 years ago, groin injuries may be "brought on by a single injury or gradually by multiple micro traumas caused by overuse."

Anatomic Considerations

Evaluation of the athlete with groin pain requires a thorough understanding of the anatomy around the groin and pelvis, which is among the most complex biomechanically in the entire musculoskeletal system. The pelvis acts as a fulcrum around which the powerful abdominal and thigh muscles attach. It includes all of the soft tissue attachments around the pubis and pubic rami, exclusive of the hip joint. The relevant abdominal musculature includes the rectus abdominis, which attaches to the superior pubic rami and whose aponeurosis is in continuity with that of the adductor longus attachment. The obliques attach laterally to the rectus and inferiorly form the inguinal canal through which the spermatic cord and ilioinguinal and genital nerves course. The adductor muscle group actually comprises six different muscles (adductor longus, adductor brevis, adductor magnus, gracilis, pectineus, and obturator externus). Of these, the adductor longus is the most frequently injured and may undergo complete avulsion from the pubis (Fig. 4.1). The anatomy of the rectus abdominis-adductor aponeurosis is best visualized on a sagittal MRI view which is shown in Fig. 4.2.

Differential Diagnosis

The differential diagnosis of athletic groin pain is broad and includes injuries to the bony pelvis, muscular strains, hip injuries, sports hernia/athletic pubalgia, classic inguinal hernia, and nonathletic causes of groin pain. A detailed discussion of the various entities that cause athletic groin pain is beyond the scope of this chapter and can be found in several recent reviews on this subject [4–6]. However, these include pelvic stress fracture, osteitis pubis, rectus abdominis and oblique strains, hip flexor strains, and adductor muscle strains. Associated hip injuries must also be excluded including labral tears, femoral acetabular impingement, and hip osteoarthritis. Inguinal hernia is usually easily excluded on

M. Brunt, M.D. (✉)
Section of Minimally Invasive Surgery, Barnes-Jewish Hospital,
Washington University School of Medicine,
660 S. Euclid Avenue, Campus Box 8109,
St. Louis, MO, 63103, USA
e-mail: bruntm@wustl.edu

R. Barile, M.S., ATC
Head Athletic Trainer
St. Louis Blues Hockey Club, Scottrade Center,
1401 Clark Ave., St. Louis, MO, 63103, USA
e-mail: rbarile@stlblues.com

J.W.T. Byrd (ed.), *Operative Hip Arthroscopy*,
DOI 10.1007/978-1-4419-7925-4_4, © Springer Science+Business Media New York 2013

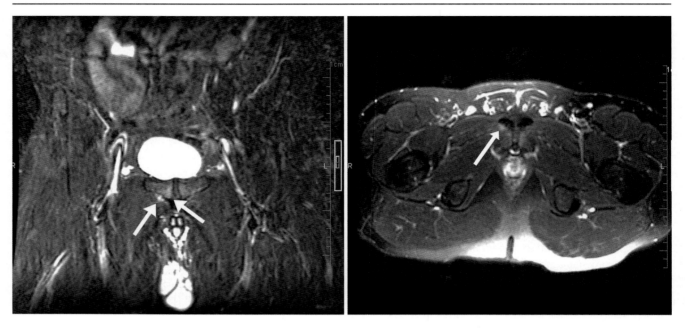

Fig. 4.1 Coronal and axial MRI sequences of right adductor longus tear (*arrows*) near the insertion onto the pubis. Marrow edema in the adjacent pubis is also present

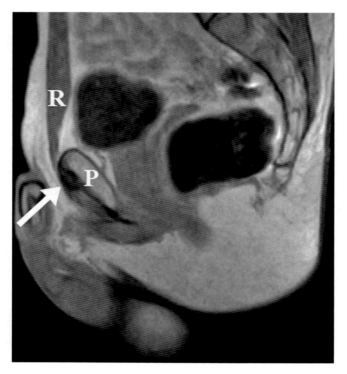

Fig. 4.2 Sagittal T1-weighted MRI of normal rectus-adductor aponeurosis complex and attachment at the pubis. *R* rectus abdominis, *P* pubis; *arrow* points to normal rectus-adductor aponeurosis

physical exam. Nonathletic causes should be suspected if there are any associated gastrointestinal, genitourinary, or gynecologic symptoms particularly in females.

Adductor strains represent one of the most common injuries in sports. In one series, 62% of sports groin injuries involved the adductor longus [7]. Adductor injuries may range from mild strains to complete disruption of the tendon unit from the inferior pubis. Acute adductor injuries are generally managed conservatively. The time frame to recovery can be quite variable from days to 5–6 weeks or more. In one study in NFL players, conservative management was associated with a shorter time to return to play than open repair [8]. Chronic adductor injuries can be quite problematic in some athletes and recalcitrant to conventional conservative management. These injuries commonly occur in conjunction with athletic pubalgia or sports hernia. Meyers has advocated a surgical approach to this problem and performs a partial adductor compartment release in selected athletes.

A number of risk factors have been identified that may predispose an athlete to groin injury. In one study of NHL players, a decrease in adductor to abductor strength ratio was significantly associated with an increase risk of injury [9]. Players with adductor strength less than 80% of abductor strength were 17 times more likely to sustain an adductor strain. In addition, an adductor strengthening program reduced the incidence of these injuries from 3.2/1,000 player game exposures to 0.71/1,000 player game exposures. Emery and colleagues [10] prospectively studied risk factors for groin injury over one NHL training camp and regular season. Those factors that were significantly associated with groin injury included less than 18 sport-specific training sessions off-season (RR 3.4), a history of a previous groin or abdominal strain (RR 2.9), and veteran player status (veteran > rookie RR 5.7).

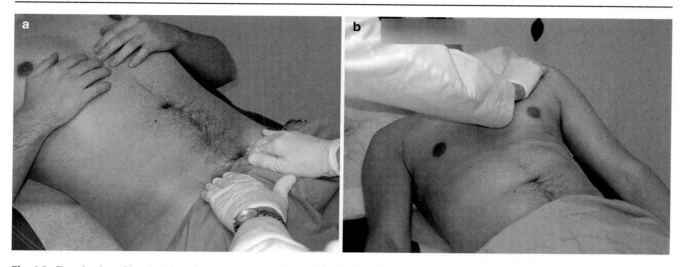

Fig. 4.3 Examination of inguinal floor for sports hernia pubalgia. (**a**) The floor is examined supine and during a sit-up for areas of weakness and tenderness. (**b**) Testing of oblique muscles. The athlete is asked to rotate their shoulders toward the opposite hip against resistance

Chronic groin pain in the athlete can be a special diagnostic and therapeutic challenge. A careful history should be obtained to determine the nature of the injury. Factors that should be specified include the duration of the pain, the precise location, and whether it is unilateral, bilateral, midline, or diffuse, whether the pain occurred as a result of specific precipitating event or had a more gradual, insidious onset, and whether it involves the inner thigh/adductor region and/ or hip. Activities which worsen the pain should be identified including running, sprinting, cutting movements, sudden starts or stops, shooting (as in ice hockey), kicking (e.g., soccer), and sneezing and coughing. The degree of limitation should be specified, and it should be determined whether the pain occurs at rest or improves with rest. For athletes in whom a diagnosis of sports hernia pubalgia is being considered, it is important that they be evaluated by a sports orthopedist prior to referral to a hernia surgeon to first exclude the hip and other orthopedic sources of pain and to ensure that an appropriate trial of conservative management and physical therapy has been undertaken.

For the classic sports hernia or athletic pubalgia presentation, symptoms typically consist of chronic inguinal and lower abdominal pain along the lateral distal rectus/medial inguinal floor area. The pain tends to occur during the extremes of exertion such as with sudden starts, turns, or cutting movements, propulsive skating movements, and kicking and may be aggravated by sneezing or coughing. The pain limits these sudden accelerating movements and, thereby, adversely impacts the athlete's ability to successfully compete. Associated adductor symptoms are commonly present, and the onset is typically insidious without a specific precipitating event. Athletes often note that their groins felt sore following a game or the day after a game and then progressively worsened or failed to resolve.

Exam findings are often minimal or subtle. An inguinal hernia bulge should be excluded. In the classic sports hernia, there is tenderness at the medial inguinal canal/ distal lower rectus abdominis near the pubis. There may be a dilated external ring and often is a palpable gap over the inguinal floor. There may be pain with resisted trunk rotation or resisted sit-ups (Fig. 4.3). Examination of the lower extremities for strength and pain with resisted movements should be carried out for the hip flexors, adductors, abductors, and other muscle groups as clinically indicated. The hip should be examined as part of the evaluation as well. The most common exam findings preoperatively in the athletes we have diagnosed with sports hernia pubalgia have been a weak inguinal floor (>90%), tenderness over the medial inguinal floor/lower lateral rectus (80%), pain with a resisted sit-up (64%) or trunk rotation (73%), and pain with resisted adduction (57%) [11].

Diagnostic imaging is indicated in athletes who fail to respond to initial conservative management or in whom there is suspicion of a high-grade injury acutely. Plain AP (anterior-posterior) pelvis x-rays may be useful for screening hip and bony pelvis abnormalities. The most useful imaging test in this author's experience for athletes with chronic groin pain is a pelvic MRI. This should include T1-weighted and fat-suppressed imaging sequences and should be carried out in coronal, axial, and sagittal planes; axial/oblique sequences may be useful for better delineating origin of the adductor tendon insertion sites. Findings associated with a sports-hernia-type pubalgia include focal marrow edema within the parasymphyseal pubis, a secondary cleft sign (Fig. 4.4), tear in the rectus abdominis insertion, adductor tears, or a tear in the rectus-adductor complex where it inserts on the pubis. In part, the MRI is done to exclude other pathology, and imaging findings in some athletes are minimal despite a supporting history and physical

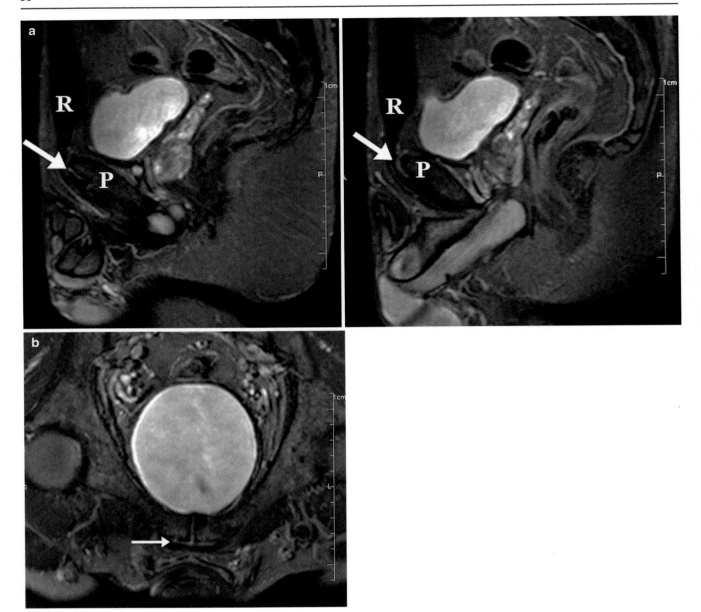

Fig. 4.4 MRI of pelvis in an athlete with athletic pubalgia. Shown are (**a**) sagittal images and (**b**) oblique axial image. The *arrow* points to the fluid cleft (*white line*). *R* rectus, *P* pubis

exam criteria for the diagnosis. Dynamic ultrasound has been used by some investigators [12] and may allow identification of a bulge in the posterior inguinal floor. This technique is highly operator dependent and is not often utilized in North America.

Local injection therapy may also be considered both for diagnostic and therapeutic reasons. For patients with midline pubic symphysis pain in whom imaging supports the diagnosis of osteitis pubis, fluoroscopic injection of local anesthetic plus corticosteroid into the symphysis joint space

may be indicated if conservative treatment measures fail [13]. The author has also used local injections under various other circumstances that may include (1) athletes with well-circumscribed symptoms and exam findings that are not typical for sports hernia pubalgia to help differentiate the etiology of the pain and for possible therapeutic benefit; (2) recalcitrant chronic adductor tendinopathy that does not occur in conjunction with sports hernia involving the lower abdominal inguinal floor, especially when it occurs in season; and (3) focal pain symptoms that occasionally arise postoperatively. Typically, a mixture of 0.5% bupivacaine (9 ml) and triamcinolone (1 ml) is used. No data are available on the use of other agents such as platelet-rich plasma for the athlete with chronic groin pain.

Pathophysiologic Mechanisms

The pathophysiology of sports hernia is subject to debate and may involve multiple mechanisms of injury, which are not exclusive of each other and may coexist in the athlete. Meyers has suggested that an imbalance in forces across the "pubic joint" may result in increased stress across the pubis and tearing or weakening of the rectus at or near its insertion on the pubis [14, 15]. Tears may also occur at the common rectus-adductor aponeurosis at the pubis and from increased pressure within or tension on the adductor compartment. Meyers has described 17 various combinations of these muscle and tendon injuries that may be a source of athletic pubalgia [16]. A second common finding is a weakened or deficient posterior inguinal floor and external oblique aponeurosis which occurs for similar reasons and may lead to increased tension across the rectus insertion and pubis. In addition, in some athletes, entrapment of the ilioinguinal or iliohypogastric nerves through tears in the external oblique [17, 18] or pressure on the genital nerve by a bulging posterior inguinal floor may occur [19]. This finding has led some groups to adapt a liberal approach toward nerve resection as a part of the repair.

Surgical Indications

The indications for surgical treatment of sports-hernia-type pubalgia are (1) symptoms that limit athlete performance; (2) failure of a period of conservative management, usually a minimum of 6–8 weeks but often longer; and (3) exclusion of other diagnoses or pathology such as underlying hip pathology. The question often arises as to whether these symptoms would eventually resolve with more extended periods of rest and conservative treatment. This issue was addressed in a study by Ekstrand et al. [20] and colleagues in soccer players with chronic groin pain. They prospectively randomized 66 soccer players with chronic athletic groin pain who had failed initial nonoperative treatment to surgery or further conservative management that consisted of various physical therapy regimens. All athletes had chronic groin pain that was 3 months or more in duration. Only the surgically treated group showed substantial and statistically significant improvement over the course of this study.

Surgical Approaches

Three broad categories of surgical repairs for sports hernia pubalgia have been described. These are (1) open primary pelvic floor repair, (2) open anterior tension-free mesh repair, and (3) laparoscopic posterior mesh repair. The two principal methods advocated for primary pelvic floor repair are the primary pelvic flood repair as performed by Meyers [16, 21] and the "minimal" repair technique described by Muschawek [12]. The Meyers technique is described as a primary pelvic floor in which the inferolateral border of the rectus abdominis fascia is suture plicated to the pubis and inguinal ligament. This repair is somewhat analogous to a Bassini hernia repair but differs in the way the sutures are oriented. A partial adductor release is also performed in some athletes. In the minimal repair technique described by Muschawek [12, 19], the posterior inguinal floor is stabilized using a nearly tension-free suture method. The genital nerve is also resected in selected cases. These procedures are described in detail elsewhere in this book.

Tension-free mesh repairs began to replace primary suture repair of inguinal hernia in the surgical practice in the early 1990s. This shift occurred for two reasons principally – first, primary suture repairs had a higher rate of hernia recurrence, and secondly, the tension-free mesh approach allowed an earlier return to unrestricted activity. As a result, the author's approach has been to utilize the open anterior tension-free mesh repair preferentially for patients with sports-hernia-type pubalgia. This approach is similar to the technique described by Lichtenstein [22] and may, in some cases, be accompanied by an ilioinguinal neurectomy. Theoretically, the potential advantages of this approach are an earlier return to activity because of the tension-free nature of the repair and potentially better durability of the repair, although for athletes this has not been proven. The principal other tension-free mesh approach is that described by the Montreal group. In their approach, a polytetrafluoroethylene (PTFE) patch is placed just below the external oblique aponeurosis to reinforce that layer. Separate tears in the external oblique are repaired primarily. In addition, ilioinguinal and/or iliohypogastric neurectomies are frequently performed in their athletes.

The third category of repair is the laparoscopic posterior mesh repair. This repair is technically identical to the laparoscopic inguinal repair for inguinal hernia and can be done totally extraperitoneal (TEP) or as a transabdominal preperitoneal procedure. The entire inguinal floor, particularly the area of the medial floor and distal rectus insertion, is covered in a tension-free mesh fashion. For adults with a conventional inguinal hernia, this approach has the advantages of less early postoperative pain and

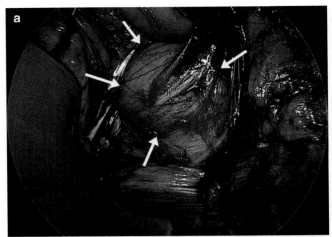

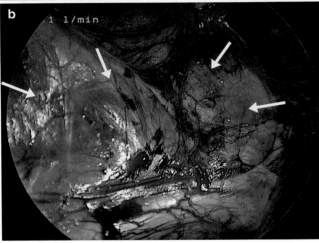

Fig. 4.5 Defect with thinning and bulging (*arrows*) in the posterior inguinal floor associated with sports hernia pubalgia as seen from (**a**) the open anterior view and (**b**) the posterior laparoscopic view. On the posterior laparoscopic view (**b**), the superior ramus of the pubis is the white bony structure at the inferior margin of the image with the weakened posterior inguinal floor and distal rectus indicated by the *arrows*

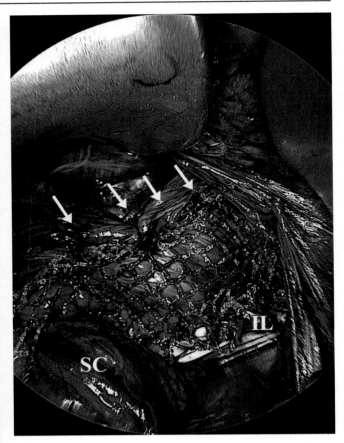

Fig. 4.6 Tension-free mesh repair of inguinal floor with lightweight polypropylene mesh. The *arrows* point to the medial suture line along the healthy transversalis fascia and rectus sheath. *SC* spermatic cord, *IL* inguinal ligament

potentially a more rapid recovery. However, anecdotally, it appears that there may be more recurrences related to this approach [15], and it is unclear as to whether this adequately addresses the pathophysiology of the underlying injury as comprehensively as do the open repair techniques.

Author's Approach

The preferred approach of this author is to use an open tension-free mesh repair using lightweight polypropylene mesh (Video 4.1: http://goo.gl/XCUnl). This procedure is typically done under local anesthesia with intravenous sedation as an outpatient procedure. The principal goal of the operation is to repair the defect in the posterior inguinal

floor as shown in Fig. 4.5. Therefore, the floor is reconstructed by suturing the mesh medially to the transversalis aponeurosis and laterally to the inguinal ligament. Proximally, the mesh is split into two limbs which are sutured above the internal ring to the inguinal ligament in order to maintain the proper conformity of the mesh to the posterior inguinal floor. The mesh is also anchored to the lateral rectus to help stabilize the rectus attachment to the pubis (Fig. 4.6). If there is any suggestion of ilioinguinal nerve entrapment (e.g., exiting a slit in the external oblique away from the external ring at an acute angle), an ilioinguinal neurectomy is then performed (Fig. 4.7). Likewise, the nerve is also resected if it appears it would be tethered by the mesh in order to preclude it from becoming a source of postoperative pain. Finally, the defect in the external oblique aponeurosis (Fig. 4.8) is closed primarily with absorbable suture. Over the last 15 months, the author has added a partial adductor compartment release to the inguinal floor repair in selected athletes. This release consists of incision of the anterior epimysial fibers of the adductor longus 2–3 cm from their insertion into the pubis via a separate incision over the proximal adductor tendon. A total of 5–7 cuts into the epimysium are made, and the adductor muscle intact and attachment to the pubis are left intact.

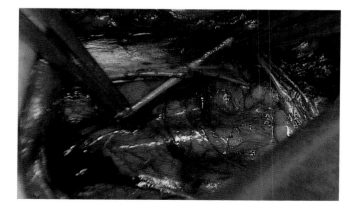

Fig. 4.7 Ilioinguinal nerve undergoing an acute angle turn as it exits a separate slit in the external oblique aponeurosis separate from the external ring in an athlete undergoing sports hernia repair. The external oblique has already been opened through the external ring to expose the spermatic cord

For athletes with sports hernia pubalgia in whom a previous open inguinal repair has been done, whether for inguinal hernia or past sports hernia repair, but who now has recurrent symptoms, the author prefers to use a laparoscopic approach in order to avoid the scar tissue in the groin from the previous dissection (Fig. 4.9). In this setting, the downside to a laparoscopic approach is minimal, and the risks of reoperating in a scarred inguinal canal, especially if prior mesh has been placed, may be considerable with risks of injury to cutaneous nerves, the vas deferens, and testicular blood supply.

Surgical Outcomes

The results of the various tension-free mesh approaches to repair of sports hernia pubalgia are listed in Table 4.1. Brown and colleagues [23] retrospectively reviewed outcomes of 107 repairs in 98 professional hockey players. All had PTFE mesh repairs and ilioinguinal nerve resection. Three of these

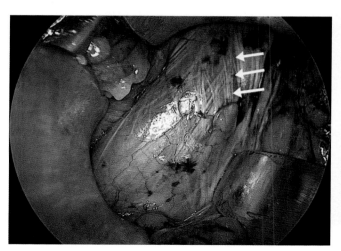

Fig. 4.8 Defect in the external oblique aponeurosis that is commonly seen at operation in sports hernia pubalgia. Stranding of some of the external oblique fibers can be seen (*arrows*)

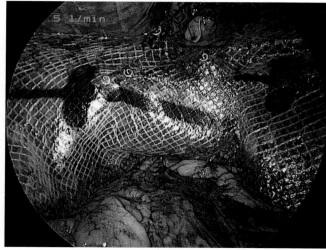

Fig. 4.9 Laparoscopic repair using total extraperitoneal approach. The lightweight polypropylene mesh covers the entire inguinal floor including posterior rectus sheath and its insertion on the pubis and is anchored in place with small titanium tacks

Table 4.1 Results of tension-free mesh approaches to sports hernia pubalgia

	Center	N	Duration of follow-up	Interval for return to play	Return to sport (%)
Open mesh repairs					
Joesting [25]	Minnesota	45	12 months	–	90
Brown [23]	Montreal	98	–	–	97
Brunt [24]	St. Louis	132	13.6 months	7 weeks	91
Laparoscopic repairs					
Paajanen [26]	Helsinki	41	50 months	1 month	95
Van Veen [27]	Rotterdam	55	24 weeks	3 months	91
Ziprin [18]	London	17	–	42 days	94
Evans [28]	UK	287	3 months–4 years	4 weeks	90

athletes had undergone prior laparoscopic repairs. Return of play was achieved in 97 of 98 athletes, and there were three recurrences (3%) that required re-repair. The interval for return to play was not specified.

In the Washington University Medical Center experience, repairs have been performed in 132 athletes [24].

Football, hockey, and soccer accounted for over 70% of the primary sports played by the athletes in this series, and the level of play was professional or collegiate in two-thirds, high school in 7%, and recreational in c. 30%. Over 90% were male, and the mean duration of symptoms prior to repair was 9.7 months. The majority of repairs were carried out in the off-season for the primary sport. In 87% of cases, repairs were unilateral and in 13% bilateral; however, subsequent repair of the contralateral side was undertaken in six athletes (4.5%) at a mean interval of 14.1 months after the initial procedure. In over 90% of cases, the repairs were performed under local anesthesia with sedation. At a mean interval of 13.6 months after surgical repair, 91% of athletes were able to successfully return to athletic competition at or near pre-injury level. In only one case was abdominal re-repair due to recurrent lower abdominal symptoms undertaken by the author. However, five other athletes underwent subsequent adductor procedures elsewhere for ongoing or recurrent adductor symptoms that limited athletic performance. The failure of some athletes because of chronic ongoing adductor symptoms only has led us to incorporate a partial adductor release similar to that described by Meyers into our management algorithm for selected athletes as described above.

The reported results of laparoscopic mesh series indicate similar outcomes of ≥90% successful return to play. Evans and associates reported that 90% of 278 athletes were able to return to play at an interval of approximately 4 weeks after surgery. One small, prospective, randomized trial has compared outcomes of laparoscopic and open approaches in rugby players. In this series, the open repairs consisted of a mix of primary sutured (non-mesh) and tension-free mesh repairs. The rate of return to training at 4 weeks was somewhat higher in the laparoscopic group; one failure due to recurrent pain was noted in each group. Occult hernias were observed at laparoscopic repair in 36% of 55 athletes in one study. The finding of occult hernias in this report likely reflects the perception of the posterior inguinal floor deficiency as viewed under the effects of laparoscopic insufflation rather than a true inguinal hernia.

Postoperative Rehabilitation and Physical Therapy

A postoperative rehabilitation program after repair of sports hernia pubalgia is important in guiding therapists and athletic trainers and in assisting the athlete toward a successful return to sports activities. Due to the lack of any established detailed protocols, our group developed a postoperative rehabilitation program several years ago which we have recently revised and updated that is focused on core abdominal strengthening, stabilization, and flexibility as well as lower body and hip strength, flexibility, and balance. The program is outlined in detail in Table 4.2 and Fig. 4.10, the essential features of which are a graduated return to full activity with an emphasis initially on building core and lower extremity strength and flexibility followed by sport-specific activities. Scar mobilization and deep tissue massage of the surrounding hip and leg musculature is also utilized. In addition, rehabilitation of adductor-related symptoms and pathology is essential and may extend the recovery phase in cases in which there is a significant adductor component to their injury. Sport-specific activities (e.g., running light football drills, catching/throwing, dribbling a soccer ball, skating) should commence at 3 weeks or as soon as the athlete can comfortably perform these activities.

The postoperative rehabilitation program is structured as a progressive series of stages with a timetable that is conservative and should be individualized; ultimately, athletes should be allowed to progress in the program according to their pain and comfort level rather than rigidly adhering to a time-based format. Muschawek [12] has advocated an accelerated timetable for return to play in patients undergoing a minimal repair technique, allowing for a return to play as early as 3–4 weeks postoperatively. Our experience has demonstrated that return to play is feasible within 5–8 weeks, but other variables may impact this timetable, including whether the repair is in-season versus off-season and whether there are other associated injuries, such as to the adductor group or others pelvic structures. The tension-free technique of the repair should, however, allow for a more aggressive progression to sport activity without increasing the risk of re-injury.

To examine the usefulness of the rehabilitation exercises, we surveyed a group of treating athletic trainers and physical therapists [11]. On the whole, they felt the rehabilitation exercises used by our group were highly useful and not overly sports specific. Most also felt the timetable for return to play was appropriate, although a majority of the patients they treated were in the off-season for their specific sport.

Summary

Groin injuries are a common problem in high-performance athletes. Injuries that fail to resolve with standard conservative management measures are best approached in a multidisciplinary team approach that includes the sports orthopedist, athletic trainer, and general surgeon who is knowledgeable about athletic groin injuries and sports hernia pubalgia. Surgical treatment should be reserved for highly selected athletes who have failed conservative treatment measures. A variety of surgical approaches are available to consider; in properly selected

Table 4.2 Abdominal Repair Rehab Program

Abdominal Repair Rehab Program				
L. Michael Brunt, M.D., St. Louis Blues Team Physician				
Ray Barile, M.S., A.T.C., St. Louis Blues Head Athletic Trainer				
Phase 1: Week 1				
Sets	Reps	Resistance	Freq	Fig. 4.10a
1	5–60 min	3–5 MPH	4× a week	
Note:	Walking, starting with short distances, progressing up to 45–60-min walks once per day			
	Use patient walking as an indicator to begin light stretching			
	When patient is able to walk 30 min continuous, begin light hamstring, quad, calf, and low back stretching as tolerated			
	Simple wound care, monitor for infection			
Phase 2: Week 2				
Sets	Reps	Resistance	Freq	Fig. 4.10b
1	8	As tolerated	6× a week	
Note:	Active hip range of motion exercises (leg swings in four planes)			
	Walking on inclined treadmill with emphasis placed on full extension on walking gait			
	Backward walking to 20 min			
	Begin bike workouts at week 2, start with slow continuous programs of 15, 20, 30, 40, and 60 min, and then progress to interval sprint work			
	Wall sits with Swiss ball			
	Light hip flexor stretch off plinth with a bent leg			
	Light hamstring, calf, and low back strengthening			
	Abdominal drawing-in maneuver			
Phase 3: Week 3				
Sets	Reps	Resistance	Freq	Fig. 4.10c
1	8	As tolerated	6× a week	
Note:	Continue exercises from Phase 2			
	Begin scar mobilization of surgical site Active release technique (A.R.T.) or deep tissue massage of surrounding hip and leg musculature			
	Pool walking as per wound healing. Begin monitored sport-specific skill development activities: ball dribbling and striking, stick handling, ball hitting progression, rowing progression, skating edgework			
Phase 4: Week 4				
Sets	Reps	Resistance	Freq	Fig. 4.10d
1	8	As tolerated	6 × week	
Note:	Continue exercises from Phase 3			
	Advance hip flexor stretching with progression into resistance strengthening			
	Quadruped stabilization exercises			
	Supportive PREs (progressive resistive exercises) – wall sits with ball, ball bridging			
	Standing stabilization with sport cords			
	Increase PREs for lower extremity body weight squats, step-ups, split squats, Thera-Band walks, single-leg slide board			
	Begin increasing sport-specific activities			
	Initiate more intense skating drills, running sprints, reintroduce football pads and individual contact drills			
	Advance throwing program to pre-practice levels			
	End-stage ball bridging			
	End-stage quadruped exercises			
	Initiate lower abdominal strengthening			
Phase 5: Week 5 and 6				
Sets	Reps	Resistance	Freq	Fig. 4.10e
1	8	As tolerated	7× a week	
Note:	Continue exercises from Phase 4			
	Transition return to weight room and strength and conditioning program			
	Positive findings presurgery now negative			
	Full practice, scrimmage, with team			
	End-stage exercises with an emphasis placed on maintaining proper muscle length and abdominal strength through adherence of a core stabilization program			
	Medical clearance, return to play authorization by surgeon and team physician			

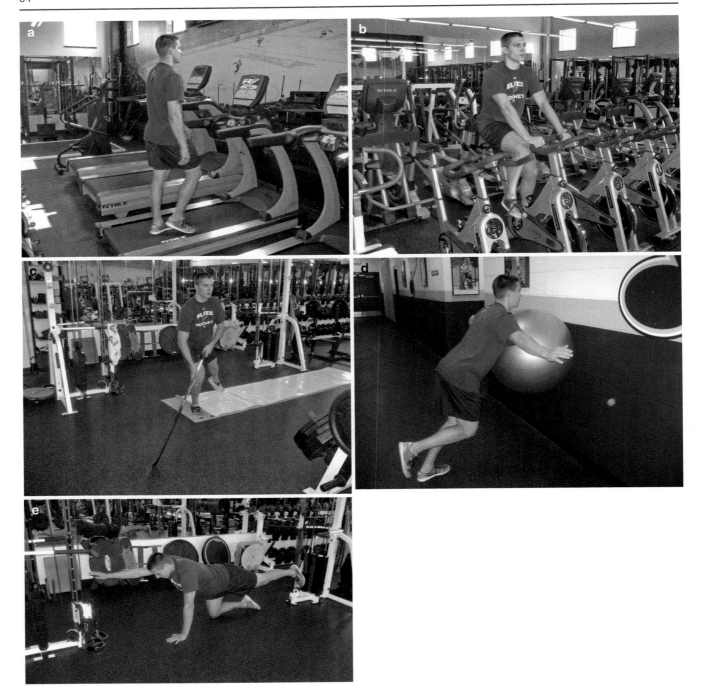

Fig 4.10 Rehabilitation program for abdominal core strengthening. Shown are (**a**) treadmill walking, (**b**) stationary bike, (**c**) slide board progression with stable core, (**d**) single-leg ball squat, and (**e**) core stabilization (quadruped exercise progression)

athletes, a tension-free mesh repair results in early rehabilitation and a consistent outcome. The use of a structured postoperative rehabilitation program can be helpful in guiding treating athletic trainers and therapists in the postoperative period.

References

1. Pettersson R, Lorenzton R. Ice hockey injuries: a 4 year prospective study of a Swedish elite ice hockey team. Br J Sports Med. 1993;27:251–4.

2. Ekstrand J, Hilding J. The incidence and differential diagnosis of acute groin injuries in male soccer players. Scand J Med Sci Sports. 1999;9:98–103.
3. Smodlaka VN. Groin pain in soccer players. Phys Sports Med. 1980;8:57–61.
4. Anderson K, Strickland AM, Warren R. Hip and groin injuries in athletes. Am J Sports Med. 2001;29:521–33.
5. Caudill P, Nyland J, Smith C, Yerasimides J, Lach J. Sports hernias: a systematic literature review. Br J Sports Med. 2008;42:954–64.
6. Nam A, Brody F. Management and therapy for sports hernia. J Am Coll Surg. 2008;206:154–64.
7. Renstrom P, Peterson L. Groin injuries in athletes. Br J Sports Med. 1980;14:30–6.
8. Schlegel TF, Bushnell Bd, Godfrey J, Boublik M. Success of non-operative management of adductor longus tendon ruptures in National Football League athletes. Am J Sports Med. 2009;37:1394–9.
9. Tyler TF, Nicholas SJ, Campbell RJ, McHugh MP. The association of hip strength and flexibility with the incidence of adductor muscle strains in professional ice hockey players. Am J Sports Med. 2001;29:124–8.
10. Emery CA, Meeuwisse WH. Risk factors for groin injuries in hockey. Med Sci Sports Exerc. 2001;33:1423–33.
11. Brunt LM, Quasebarth MA, Bradshaw J, Barile R. Outcomes of a standardized approach to surgical repair and postoperative rehabilitation of athletic hernia. In: AOSSM annual meeting 2007, Calgary; 2007.
12. Muschawek U, Berger L. Minimal repair technique of sportsmen's groin: an innovative open-suture repair to treat chronic groin pain. Hernia. 2010;14:27–33.
13. O'Connell MJ, Powell T, McCaffrey NM, O'Connell D, Eustace SJ. Symphyseal cleft injection in the diagnosis and treatment of osteitis pubis in athletes. AJR Am J Roentgenol. 2002;179:955–9.
14. Meyers WC, Greenleaf R, Saad A. Anatomic basis for evaluation of abdominal and groin pain in athletes. Oper Tech Sports Med. 2005;13:55–61.
15. Meyers WC, Yoo E, Devon ON, et al. Understanding "sports hernia" (athletic pubalgia): the anatomic and pathophysiologic basis for abdominal and groin pain in athletes. Oper Tech Sports Med. 2007;15:165–77.
16. Meyers WC, McKechnie A, Philippon MJ, Horner MA, Zoga AC, Devon ON. Experience with "sports hernia" spanning two decades. Ann Surg. 2008;248:656–65.
17. Irshad K, Feldman L, Lavoie C, Lacroix V, Mulder D, Brown R. Operative management of "hockey groin syndrome": 12 years experience in National Hockey League players. Surgery. 2001;130:759–66.
18. Ziprin P, Williams P, Foster ME. External oblique aponeurosis nerve entrapment as a cause of groin pain in the athlete. Br J Surg. 1999;86:566–8.
19. Muschawek U, Berger LM. Sportsmen's groin – diagnostic approach and treatment with the minimal repair technique. Sports Health. 2010;2:216–21.
20. Ekstrand J, Ringbog S. Surgery versus conservative treatment in soccer players with chronic groin pain: a prospective, randomized study in soccer players. Eur J Sports Traumatol Rel Res. 2001;23:141–5.
21. Meyers W, Foley D, Garrett W, Lohnes J, Mandelbaum B. Management of severe lower abdominal or inguinal pain in high-performance athletes. Am J Sports Med. 2000;28:2–8.
22. Amid PK, Lichtenstein IL. Technique facilitating improved recovery following hernia repair. Contemp Surg. 1996;49:62–6.
23. Brown R, Mascia A, Kinnear DG, Lacroix VJ, Feldman L, Mulder DS. An 18 year review of sports groin injuries in the elite hockey player: clinical presentation, new diagnostic imaging, treatment, and results. Clin J Sports Med. 2008;2008:221–6.
24. Brunt LM. Management of sports hernia and athletic pubalgia. In: Kingsnorth AN, LeBlanc KA, editors. Management of abdominal wall hernias. New York: Springer; 2011.
25. Joesting DR. Diagnosis and treatment of sportsman's hernia. Curr Sports Med Rep. 2002;1:121–4.
26. Paajanen H, Syvähuoko I, Airo I. Totally extraperitoneal endoscopic (TEP) treatment of sportsman's hernia. Surg Laparosc Endosc Percutan Tech. 2004;14:215–8.
27. van Veen RN, de Baat P, Heijboer MP, et al. Successful endoscopic treatment of chronic groin pain in athletes. Surg Endosc. 2007;21:189–93.
28. Evans DS. Laparoscopic transabdominal pre-peritoneal (TAPP) repair of groin hernia: one surgeons' experience of a developing technique. Ann R Coll Surg Engl. 2002;84:393–8.

Current Understanding of Core Muscle Injuries (Athletic Pubalgia, "Sports Hernia")

5

William C. Meyers, Adam Zoga, Tina Joseph, and Marcia Horner

The term *athletic pubalgia (AP)* is accurate but difficult to articulate, so we recommend the term *core muscle injuries*. The purpose of this chapter is to provide some nuts-and-bolts clarity concerning current understanding of career-threatening soft tissue injuries of the pelvis. Recent well-publicized injuries to a number of prominent athletes have raised the level of attention to this subject. The poor term "sports hernia" may mislead physicians and surgeons into incorrect management plans.

The best way to think about musculoskeletal injuries of the anterior pelvis is to consider injuries that occur either inside or outside of the "ball-in-socket" hip joint [1]. These injuries have true biomechanical bases. Most of these are hyperextension/hyperabduction injuries. One must eliminate from one's thinking process what the terms sports hernia and "sportsman's hernia" mistakenly imply with respect to the pathophysiology – occult hernia as the incipient injury. The latter term has been around for at least half a century and led to many unsuccessful surgeries.

W.C. Meyers, M.D. (✉)
Departments of Surgery, Duke University Health System,
Drexel University College of Medicine, and Thomas Jefferson
University, Vincera Core Physicians, 4623 S. Broad St Quarters M-1,
Philadelphia, PA 19112, USA

Duke University Health System, Durham, NC, USA

Core Performance Physicians,
4623 S. Broad St Quarters M1, Philadelphia, PA, USA
e-mail: wmeyers@vinceracorephysicians.com

A. Zoga, M.D.
Department of Radiology, Thomas Jefferson University,
132 South 10th St., 1083A, Philadelphia, PA, USA
e-mail: adam.zoga@jefferson.edu

T. Joseph, M.D.
Department of Surgery, Drexel University, College of Medicine/
Hahnemann Hospital, 245 North Road Street,
New College Suite 7150, Philadelphia, PA 19102, USA
e-mail: tj.tinajoseph@gmail.com

M. Horner, BA
Vincera Core Physicians, 4623 S. Broad St, Quarters M1,
Philadelphia, PA USA
e-mail: mhorner@vinceracorephysicians.com

Let us expand a bit more on the deceptive use of the word hernia. It conveys two huge false assumptions about athletic pubalgia injuries: (1) that the cause of this set of injuries has something to do with occult hernias and (2) that these injuries can be lumped into one explanation and treated the same way. In one series, we saw 121 different sets of pathology that accounted for the various injuries [2]. We currently reoperate on three to four patients per week after unsuccessful conventional hernia repairs, with or without mesh, for treatment of career-threatening, pubic-area pain, and this number is increasing.

So, if these are not hernias, what are these injuries? What might go on outside the ball-in-socket hip joint? Certainly, there is a great deal of obvious biomechanical activity there. The activity occurs relatively symmetrically around the pubic bone. That is why we introduced the term "pubic bone joint" or "pubic joint." This joint needs to be distinguished from the pubic symphyseal joint. One needs to think in terms of the entire right and left pubic symphyses acting together as the center of a great deal of motor activity in the normal situation. Many soft tissue structures distribute forces symmetrically around this bony pivot point. Disruption of the apparatus causes changes in both primary and opposing forces.

Some More General Thoughts

The anatomy of the pelvis is obviously complex, and if one keeps in mind the above concept (the two joints), understanding the anatomy becomes much simpler. The anterior pelvis, where most of these injuries reside, is intimately associated with the anatomy of the "core" [3]. We shall go more deeply into this anatomy. A variety of structures can be (and are) injured, and precise diagnoses usually lead to successful results. In our population of patients, we see a 10–15% frequency of "combination" injuries, i.e., debilitating injuries involving simultaneously both the hip and the pubic joints [4].

J.W.T. Byrd (ed.), *Operative Hip Arthroscopy*,
DOI 10.1007/978-1-4419-7925-4_5, © Springer Science+Business Media New York 2013

Accurate diagnosis of the athlete with pelvic pain remains challenging, particularly considering the possible visceral diagnoses. Recent progress has shed light on this topic, and care of these patients has greatly improved. Several years ago, the senior author published a review of his experience over the previous two decades [2]. During this period of time, we saw dramatic improvements in recognition of the injuries and identification of the various injury types, diagnosis, and treatments.

An easy way to think about the various diagnoses that must be considered in disabling pelvic pain in the athlete is to think in terms of three separate "buckets" of diagnoses. The buckets are (1) core muscle injury (CMI, athletic pubalgia), (2) hip disorders (H), and (3) the "other" diagnoses (O). The other diagnoses refer to the gastrointestinal, genitourinary, gynecologic or other systems, noninjury musculoskeletal diagnoses, or malignancy. Nearly all the diagnoses of the various clinical entities can be made on the basis of detailed histories and physical examinations and supported by the new magnetic resonance imaging (MRI) techniques [5–10].

With proper diagnosis, most of the injuries and other problems can be treated successfully. The threats out there in surgical practice related to managed care and pressure for surgical volumes may contribute to the misdiagnosis of occult hernia and treatment with conventional hernia repair. As has been taught for decades in surgical training programs for decades, the success rate of hernia repairs for pelvic pain in patients without easily demonstrable hernias remains suboptimal. Despite the conclusions (based on poor follow-up) of some papers in the literature, this is not the best care. Understanding the anatomy and likely mechanical bases for these injuries is central for successful diagnosis and treatment.

Anatomy

The Core

One way to think about the core and the muscles involved in these injuries is to divide the anatomy into (a) the "back" (paraspinous muscles), (b) the "side" (transversus, multifidi, and oblique muscles), (c) the "deep" (gluteus, rotator, flexor-extensor muscles), and (d) the "front (pubic joint attachments and support structures) muscles" [11]. For example, it is generally accepted that the transversus abdominis is the first muscle activated prior to the upper limb motion of pitching and that this set of muscles acts in coordination with the back. Therefore, it would seem that these muscles and the spine might be worth special attention and strengthening in the prevention of injury in baseball.

One might also think of all these muscles as a box, with the abdominal muscles and the specific adductors and flexors that attach to or cross the pubis as the front; the paraspinals and gluteals posteriorly as the back; the diaphragm on top; and the pelvic floor and para-hip musculature on the bottom, with the oblique musculature and iliac wings as the sides. Within this box are 29 muscles which work together to stabilize the spine and pelvis during the movements involved in most athletic activities.

The Bony Anatomy – Now superimpose the above concept of "the core" onto the pertinent anatomy. The bony pelvis essentially has two main functions: (1) to transfer weight to and from the appendicular and the axial skeleton and (2) to disperse compression forces resulting from its support of body weight [12]. To fulfill both functions, the bony pelvis depends on the attachments of powerful muscles. Four bones comprise the pelvis: two innominate "hip" bones, the sacrum, and the coccyx. The two innominate bones are joined anteriorly at the pubic symphysis and posteriorly at the sacrum. Together, the bony pelvis with its junctions sometimes is called the "pelvic girdle."

Besides the junctions of the major bones, the pelvis also contains many "micro-joints" that allow it to articulate and shift positions minimally in many ways with muscular contractions. The joints of the pelvis include the lumbosacral joints, the sacrococcygeal joint, the sacroiliac joints, and the pubic symphyseal joint. Most of the injuries that are the focus of this chapter involve the anterior half of the pelvis. The obturator canal has its own set of unusual syndromes, but these are all somewhat rare in the athlete. The attachments of the rectus abdominis and three central adductors onto a fibrocartilaginous plate that envelops the pubic symphysis are important elements of the anterior injuries. Slightly deep to this, the anterior edge of the inferior pubic ramus has spiny projections that can rub anteriorly against the proximal tendons in the adductor compartments, causing considerable pain and tearing. The iliopsoas tendon, which attaches to the lesser trochanter, is also a relatively commonly involved structure in both genders.

A number of conventional ligaments help stabilize these complex micro-joints and the grander pubic joint. Any of these ligaments can be the source of compensatory pain or inflammation complicating diagnoses of primary problems. For example, attachments such as the iliofemoral ligament, the iliotibial tract, the pubofemoral ligament, and the iliopsoas tendon act somewhat like "strap" muscles that stabilize the anterior pelvis that is the focus of many athletic pubalgia problems.

The Pubic Anatomy – A key part of the anterior pelvic anatomy that forms the fulcrum for many of the movements is the pubic symphysis. The two sides of the pubic symphysis join via a fibrocartilaginous disc. The traditional ligaments that join the symphyseal joint are the superior pubic ligament, the inferior pubic ligament, and the arcuate ligament, spanning the anteroinferior aspect of the pubic symphysis from pubic tubercle to pubic tubercle. This medium-sized joint is strengthened by the decussating fibers of the rectus abdominis and external oblique fibers, and ligamentous injury often accompanies lesions involving the rectus abdominis and adductor tendons. But remember, the symphyseal joint is only a tiny part of the overall dynamics. In contrast, the muscles that attach to the pubic symphysis play a huge role in the stabilization of the entire complex which is at the center of most pelvic activity. The interaction of these muscles and their attachments anterior to the pubic symphysis is much more important than the intersymphyseal disc.

In the median plane, the rectus abdominis muscles directly oppose the adductor attachments. In fact, these muscles interdigitate as they attach onto the fibrocartilaginous plate investing the symphyses. There is not usually much in the way of traditional tendon attachments here, contrary to the depiction in most anatomic textbooks. The rectus abdominis creates superoposterior tension, while the adductors create inferoanterior tension. When one considers the entire pelvis, contraction of these muscles creates an anterior tilt [1]. Action of the latter two muscle groups together creates tremendous force, an action that has been grossly underappreciated in the literature (Fig. 5.1a, b). The orientation of sutures in the repairs of injuries in these locations takes into account these normal anatomic orientations.

The Muscles

The muscles that originate and/or insert onto the bony pelvis play important roles in pelvic stability. They stabilize the pubic joint and at the same time functionally anchor the pelvis so that more distal parts of the body can move. The rectus abdominis, on each side, flexes the trunk as it compresses abdominal viscera and forms the anchor for considerable abduction and adduction, as well as internal and external hip rotation. The rectus abdominis originates at the pubic aponeurotic/cartilaginous plate and pubic crest and inserts on the xiphoid process and costal cartilages. The fibers of the rectus abdominis fan out and bind superiorly with the intercostal muscles, forming extensive complex insertions onto the ribs and costochondral cartilages. Laterally, the rectus abdominis attaches to the obliques via pure fibrous connections, enveloping complexes of nerves and tiny vascular structures.

The thigh muscles also play an important role in stability and primary or compensatory core injury. The posterior compartment [12] is comprised primarily of the hamstring muscles: the long and short heads of the biceps femoris, the semitendinosus, and the semimembranosus. Additional structures include a portion of the adductor magnus, several nerves from the sciatic trunk, and the profunda femoris artery. Fibers of muscles from the posterior compartment

bind with the medial compartment in the perineum and at the anterior ischial tuberosity.

The medial or adductor compartment is the most important in the thigh with respect to stability of the anterior pelvis and pubic joint. Three adductors – the pectineus, the adductor longus, and the adductor brevis – play a primary role in core stability. The next most important "adductor" seems to be the obturator externus. The adductor magnus inserts more laterally, and the gracilis is so small and posterior that these muscles are rarely involved significantly despite a considerable literature on "adductor magnus" and "gracilis" syndromes [13]. The gracilis arises from the pubic arch and inserts on the proximal tibia. The most important adductors with regard to core injury originate from the pubic symphysis and less important ones from the rami. They all insert onto the linea aspera of the femur. Interestingly, the anterior obturator nerve innervates all the adductors except the magnus, consistent with the cooperative function of these muscles regarding this joint.

The anterior compartment of the thigh does not involve the pubic symphysis directly but does provide a supportive function for the pubic joint. This compartment comprises the following muscles: sartorius, iliacus, psoas, vastus lateralis, vastus medialis, vastus intermedius, and rectus femoris. The sartorius arises from the anterior superior iliac spine and inserts onto the proximal medial tibia to form part of the pes anserinus. The relatively lateral location of the sartorius may account for an apparently more important role in stabilization of the female pelvis. The lateral femoral cutaneous nerve exits the bony pelvis near the origin of the sartorius and must be remembered in releases, repairs, or other surgery in this region. The rectus femoris has two heads, the more important of which attaches at the anterior inferior iliac spine. Distally, the rectus femoris fibers blend with the vastus intermedius. The iliacus and psoas interdigitate and insert onto the lesser trochanter of the femur after becoming intimate with the anterior capsule of the hip joint.

Most of the muscles of the medial compartment, and some in the anterior compartment, have directly opposing actions to portions of the abdominal and more lateral musculature. When the medial compartment muscles contract, the thigh moves towards the midline. When the rectus abdominis weakens, the adductor longus, pectineus, and/or brevis contract in relatively unopposed fashions, which can lead to painful compartment syndromes [2]. Other muscles such as the obturator internus, quadratus femoris, and biceps femoris may occasionally play primary or secondary roles in injury, involving the pelvic ilium, ischium, ischial tuberosity, or crest of the femur. Some of the back muscles can play primary roles in injury such as the quadratus lumborum, which we often see strained or torn after backpedaling maneuvers as in dancers and baseball outfielders [11].

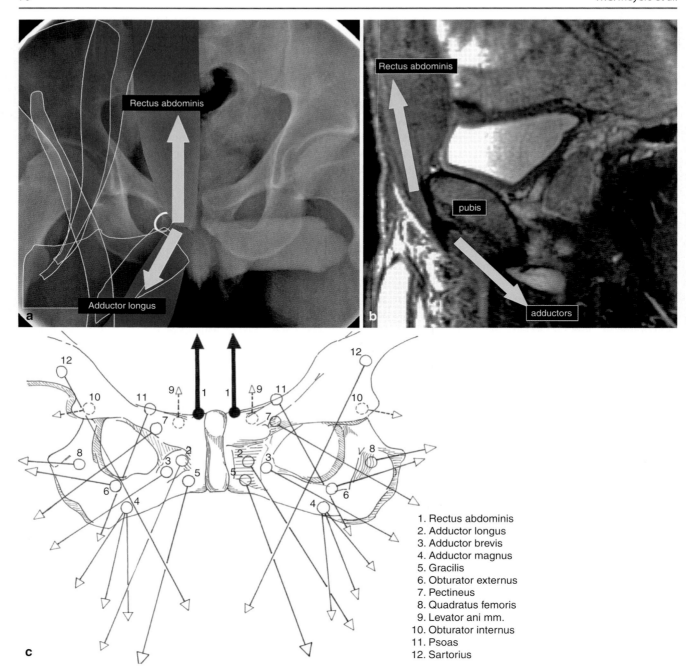

1. Rectus abdominis
2. Adductor longus
3. Adductor brevis
4. Adductor magnus
5. Gracilis
6. Obturator externus
7. Pectineus
8. Quadratus femoris
9. Levator ani mm.
10. Obturator internus
11. Psoas
12. Sartorius

Fig. 5.1 (**a**) This diagram superimposed on an AP pelvic radiograph depicts the major core muscle attachments at the anterior pelvis. The rectus abdominis flexes the trunk with a cranial-caudal biomechanical vector, while the adductor longus opposes the rectus abdominis tangentially. Note the close proximity between the attachments of these two structures anterior to the pubis and the superficial inguinal ring (0). (**b**) A diagram superimposed on a sagittal or lateral MR image shows the site at which the rectus abdominis origin blends with the adductor longus origin and the anterior pubic ligaments and capsule, a frequent site of musculoskeletal injury in core muscle injury. (**c**) Bony skeleton and forces of the pubic joint. The pubic symphysis is at the center of the forces created by these muscles. Signs and symptoms distribute around this axis

Pathophysiology

In athletes, tremendous torque occurs at the level of the pelvis. The anterior pelvis takes the brunt of most of the forces, and as mentioned, the pubic bone functionally serves as a fulcrum around which many of the forces are connected. Contraction of both large and small muscles here can create tremendous force. When one of these muscles weakens, it results in an inequality of forces on the pelvis, which can lead to pain, or athletic pubalgia. One can think of this part of the anterior pubis as the "pubic joint," and the more central attachments, e.g., the rectus abdominis and the three main adductors, as very important in terms of stability. The more lateral attachments including both muscles and other soft tissues that cross the joint such as the rectus femoris, iliopsoas, and iliotibial band also play supportive or "strap"-like roles. One analogy might be to the knee: with injury to the central attachments (e.g., anterior cruciate) being most important and more often requiring surgery, while injury to the more lateral attachments (e.g., collateral ligaments) is most often treated conservatively without fear of chronic joint instability (Fig. 5.1c).

Differences in the male and female pelvis probably explain why males more often develop the athletic pubalgia syndromes than women [1, 4]. These differences may include the thicker, heavier male pelvis causing greater shifts in force, the narrower male subpubic angle leading to a different distribution of force, the narrower pubic symphysis disc in males leading to decreased flexibility of the pelvis, and the narrower, probably less stable pelvis of the male in general. Further, the fibrocartilaginous pubic aponeurosis is more confluent and robust in the central portion in females without passage of the spermatic cord structures. Females are more likely to develop sartorius, psoas, and hip injuries, probably also reflecting the relatively wider pelvis and greater dependence on these "strap" muscles for stability.

The way to analyze each injury is to identify which muscles or groups of muscles have been weakened and which are overcompensating. As with ligamentous instability in the knee, the initial injury may be to one particular ligament, but the instability can result in pain and damage to the menisci and cartilage because of the inability of other structures about the knee to compensate for the instability. In the hip and pelvis, the more central attachments (e.g., rectus abdominis, attaching adductors) are more important to overall stability than the lateral attachments (e.g., rectus femoris, psoas, sartorius). The torque that causes most injuries results from hyperextension of the abdomen and hyperabduction of the thighs.

The most common mechanism of injury is a tear or a series of micro-tears of the pubic attachments as they insert onto the cartilaginous plate of the pubis. One way to think about the pathology associated with the more common injuries is to imagine pulling on two ends of a rope pulled taut over a stone. The pathology most evident on direct observation is fraying of the superficial aspects of the rope. The sides that get most torn depend on the direction of forces associated with the torque. Although we see the pathology on the superficial aspect of the rope (i.e., muscular sheath), this may be deceiving with respect to the depth of the pathology since the outside aspect of the rope is all that we can see. We must assume that the inside of the rope is also injured. The most severe portion of the injury is usually anterior and medial

because of the hyperextension/hyperabduction mechanisms involved. We classify the resultant pathology as follows: grade 1, single or multiple small identifiable tears; grade 2, partial avulsion/detachments(s); or grade 3, complete avulsion/detachments(s) (Fig. 5.2a–c).

The tears may also occur suddenly in any athletic activity with huge force shifts. The most dramatic of these shifts may occur in bull-riding owing to the position of the rider and unpredictable nature of the bull, leading to extreme, rapid extension and rotation at the waist simultaneously with forced thigh abduction. Some huge force shifts may be predictable and can cause a predominance of certain types of injury according to sport or even the position that the athlete plays.

An example is baseball. Perhaps the most studied mechanics of all sports are for the pitcher and batter. Both have "transition periods" after they finish their follow-throughs when they are susceptible to certain very specific injuries. We call these the transition phases of pitching and batting [11].

Diagnosis

With experience, diagnoses of the various clinical entities can be made primarily on history and physical examination [4] and supported by the new magnetic resonance imaging (MRI) techniques [5–10]. More recently, the authors have published sensitivities and specificities of MRI for athletic pubalgia lesions as well as a dedicated athletic pubalgia MRI protocol and a series of reproducible MR imaging patterns specific to this patient group. Histories are conducted with careful attention to the three "buckets" of diagnoses mentioned above: CMI (core muscle injury), H (hip problems), and O (other diagnoses). Because CMI results primarily from muscular disruption, the pain of AP is primarily exertional and often predictable with initiation of forceful activities such as sprinting and changes of direction. The pain can also affect normal activities such as coughing, sneezing, or rolling over in bed at night time. The pain can also vary from side to side, depending on patterns of compensation, and involve multiple sites of soft tissue attachments such as the rectus abdominis and specific adductor muscles. The inflammatory response associated with the osteitis pubis that sometimes accompanied athletic pubalgia can cause tenderness and pain particularly after cessation of activities [4].

In contrast, patients with H usually describe pain with or after minimal activity such as prolonged standing, walking or jogging, or with certain postures such as prolonged sitting, going up and down stairs, or internally/externally rotating the extremity while in a supine position, with more sporadic and less predictable episodes of pain.

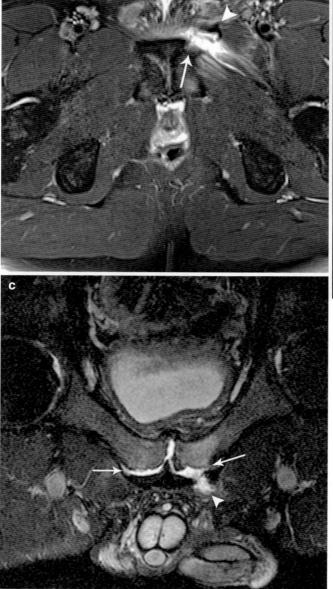

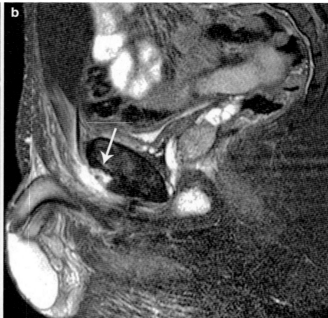

Fig. 5.2 (**a**) An axial T2-weighted fat-suppressed MR image at the level of the pubic symphysis shows a large defect in the fibrocartilaginous aponeurosis anterior to the pubic tubercle in an American football player with an acute left-sided groin injury (*arrow*). The defect predominately pertains to a rectus abdominis origin tear, but the adductor longus is avulsed and displaced anteroinferiorly. (**b**) A sagittal T2-weighted fat-suppressed MR image at the same level, just to the left of midline in the same patient, shows the detachment of the entire aponeurosis from the periosteum at the anteroinferior pubis (*arrow*), with extension into the adductor longus. (**c**) A coronal oblique T2-weighted fat-suppressed MR image at the anterior pubic symphysis shows an elongated detachment of the fibrocartilaginous aponeurotic plate spanning midline and near complete detachment of both rectus abdominis origins (*arrows*). The injury in this professional sprinter propagates into the adductor longus origin on the *left* (*arrowhead*), but not on the *right*

Pains from O causes often have historical clues such as genitourinary, gastrointestinal, or gynecological symptoms or past problems, or continuous or sporadic pain totally unrelated to physical activity. However, an important caution is to remember that some O patients also have benign musculoskeletal injuries at the same time, which can make accurate diagnosis of the more serious pathologies particularly perilous.

Physical examinations should be conducted with careful attention to the same three categories of diagnoses. For AP, we developed resistance tests for each of the muscles attaching to

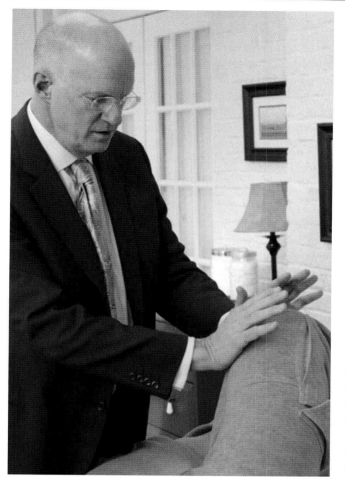

Fig. 5.3 The pectineus maneuver

plus numerous other rotational or hyperflexion or hyperextension tests that could isolate anterior, posterior, or lateral impingements or other pathology. Localized tenderness, of course, is sometimes helpful for specific diagnoses, although the tenderness associated with various types of bony or soft tissue inflammation also can be confusing. Extreme pain with light touch may be a clue to the existence or coexistence of CRPS (chronic regional pain syndrome)/RSD (reflex sympathetic dystrophy) [14, 15]. Comprehensive physical examinations, sometimes with internal pelvic or rectal examinations, are important, of course, to detect the nonmusculoskeletal diagnoses.

Specialized pelvic MRI and MRI hip arthrography have become increasingly accurate in demonstrating pathology that correlates with the history and physical examinations. The initially reported MRI sensitivity and specificity of 68% and 100%, respectively, for rectus abdominis injury and 86% and 89% for adductor injury [9, 10] are even better with a dedicated athletic pubalgia MRI protocol and a musculoskeletal radiologist. The technique uses a phased array send-receive surface coil, as well as new angles of plane selection optimized for visualization of the most frequently involved structures. This objective way of demonstrating injuries has provided convincing evidence of the multiplicity of soft tissue injuries as well as the overlap with ball-in-socket hip injuries. Similarly, MR arthrography has become increasingly sensitive in the diagnosis of intrinsic hip pathology and increasingly accurate with employment of dedicated intra-articular contrast and anesthetic protocols.

Some Other Clinical Considerations

We recently published a number of clinical observations made over the past two and a half decades [2]. For example, the number of sports, women, and nonathletes recognized with the injuries has all increased. Certain sports have a predominance of more severe injuries (e.g., football, bull-riding) compared to other sports (e.g., soccer). We have also recognized multiple clear patterns of injury according to sport or even specific positions within a sport. For example, baseball pitchers and hockey goalies have a predisposition for a certain type of adductor injury (Fig. 5.4), and certain types of dancers get very specific injuries deep in the pelvis. The main point is to remember that there are many specific diagnoses and treatments in the consideration of disabling abdominal and pelvic pain in the athlete. One cannot simply lump these injuries into one specific disorder. Just like knee pain, there are many potential causes. And musculoskeletal core anatomy at the pelvis is much more complex than that of the knee, so there are many more potential diagnoses. The diagnoses can be tricky and treatments do not always involve surgery [16].

or crossing the pubic symphysis or joint. These tests involve resistance against the primary action of each muscle. Interpretation of each test involves three considerations: (1) Does the test cause pain? (2) does the resultant pain correlate to the muscle being tested? and (3) does the resultant pain re-create the pain causing the athlete's disability.

For example, Fig. 5.3 depicts an example of a resistance test for soft tissue injury of athletic pubalgia. In this case, the maneuver is for a pectineus injury. The patient is supine with his knee flexed and is adducting against resistance. If (1) pain is evoked, (2) the evoked pain is at the pectineus insertion site, and (3) the pectineus insertion site is a site of complaint, then the patient most likely has a pectineus injury. One must also consider that severe osteitis of the pubic symphysis can sometimes masquerade as a pectineus injury and that osteitis may also coexist with a pectineus injury.

For H, the examination involves primarily range of motion tests without interference from contraction of muscles. These include the standard FABER and FADIR tests,

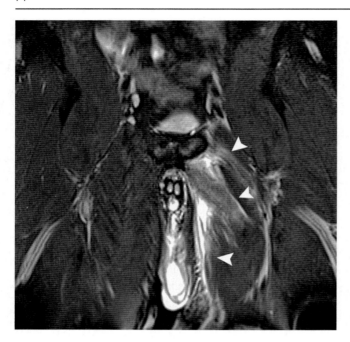

Fig. 5.4 A coronal STIR (short TE inversion recovery) MR image of the anterior pelvis in a professional hockey goalie with acute or chronic groin pain shows feathery soft tissue edema throughout the left thigh adductor compartment (*arrowheads*) involving multiple adductor muscles and centered distal to their origins at their myotendinous junctions

Treatment

For simplicity, we shall focus here on the types of surgery that may be employed in these injuries. We shall not go into detail with respect to the nonoperative methods of treatment or specific rehabilitation protocols that we feel have the greatest benefits. That would be too exhaustive considering the number of different problems that we encounter and should be explored in its own dedicated text.

Recently, we identified 26 different procedures and 121 different combinations of procedures that we had performed on a certain group of patients [2]. In fact, those numbers have increased. We list a number of those procedures in Table 5.1.

The surgical procedures include various types of reattachments and/or releases of soft tissues that normally attach or cross the pubic symphyses. They may also include portions of the same set of muscles relatively remote from the attachments. The precise procedures depend on the specific injuries and are based on an understanding of the anatomy described above. Basically, the injuries are presumed to cause instability of the pubic joint, and the procedures are designed to either tighten and/or broaden the attachments of various structures that normally attach to the pubic symphysis and/or loosen the attachments or other supporting structures via selective epimysiotomy and scar division.

For the repairs, we use for the most part simple suturing techniques. The techniques should not be thought as modifications of traditional hernia repairs. The specific technique depends on the specific muscles, other soft tissues, and portions of the muscles involved. There is little rationale for the use of mesh. Mesh use evolves from the misnomer sports hernia and does not address the injury directly. When the techniques of laparoscopic hernia repairs were developing in the late 1980s and there was uncertainty about the causes of athletic pubalgia, we performed a number of laparoscopic mesh repairs on athletes and were not happy with the results. Any degree of success then or now related to mesh hernia repairs probably can be attributed to intense scar induction and secondary stabilization of the joint. Patient selection, of course, also enters into this assessment. Adductor and other components of the injury cannot logically be addressed via a hernia technique. We see many patients with temporary, partial, or no relief from these procedures. We have also interviewed some patients who returned to levels of successful play, and all complained to some degree about "stiffness" or discomfort. As mentioned, we continue to see many patients who had unsuccessful hernia repairs with or without mesh. Fortunately, the success rate when we reoperate is high.

Likewise, the techniques of releases depend on the specific muscles, other soft tissues, and portions of the muscles involved. These are almost all compartmental releases comparable to the treatment of calf compartment syndrome in runners except in smaller, more focal compartments. Experience enters tremendously into the judgment with respect to what to loosen and what not to loosen. Rarely is any muscle actually divided in any of the release techniques.

Sometimes, we actually perform repairs and releases on the same muscles or groups of muscles. For example, as described above, we classify the pathologies on the basis of degree of avulsion. Grade 3 injuries can occur to any of the three principal adductors either in isolation or in combination, and repairs often involve mobilization and compartmental release as well as direct suturing of the avulsed muscle into intact components. One grade 3 injury type involves all three principal adductors with avulsion of the portion of the cartilaginous plate connecting the three. Anatomically, this means there has to be a simultaneous grade 3 injury of the rectus abdominis muscle. In this case, one may be able to suture the two cartilaginous pieces directly together and back onto the remaining pubic plate (see Fig. 5.5). Of course, one has a much better chance of doing such a repair soon after an acute injury. The latter repairs have been highly successful, and all the competitive athletes who had these repairs returned to preinjury levels of play (by their own subjective assessments) 6 weeks to 3 months after repair.

Table 5.1 Athletic pubalgia syndromes and possible procedures

Syndrome	Defect	Possible indicated procedure

Unilateral RA/unilateral AD
   Adductor longus (AL)
   Adductor pectineus (AP)
   Adductor brevis (AB)
	Tear and compartment syndrome (CS)	Repair and release

Pure AD syndromes	Normally CS	Release and/or repair
Bilateral RA/bilateral AD	Aponeurotic plate disruption; tear and CS	Repair and release
Unilateral/bilateral RA	Tear(s)	Repair
Osteitis pubis variant	Usually tears, CS, bone edema	Repair, release, steroid injection
Unilateral/bilateral	Combination tear(s) and CS	Repair(s) and Release(s)
Iliopsoas variant	Impingement and bursitis	Release
Baseball pitcher hockey goalie	AD tear and muscle belly	CS Release
Quadratus lumborum variant	Tear	Repair
Spigelian and high RA	Tear	Repair
Rectus femoris variant	Impingement	Release
Female variant	Medial disruption; lateral thigh compensation	Repair and release(s)
Round ligament syndrome	Inflammation with tear	Repair and excision
Dancer's variant	Obturator internus/externus	Release(s)
Rower's rib syndrome	Subluxation	Excision and mesh
Avulsions	Usually acute adductor injury	Repair and/or release(s)
AD/RA calcification syndromes	Chronic avulsions	Excision, release
Midline RA variant	Tears and muscle separation	Repair
Anterior ischial tuberosity variant	Posterior perineal inflammation, gracilis, hamstrings	Release
Complete symphyseal disruption	Muscle avulsions and symphyseal joint disruption	Direct muscle repairs, relocation of joint and arcuate ligament repair
AD contractures	Often associated with hip pathology	Release and hip repair
More uncommon variants	E.g. gracilis, quadratus, iliotibial band	Variable

Any of the soft tissues attached or crossing the pubic symphysis can be involved alone or in combination with other injuries. One can count the actual number of syndromes in various ways. For example, we see all the combinations of rectus abdominis injury and specific adductor injury, and both rectus abdominis and adductor injuries can be unilateral or bilateral. Note that a patient can have more than one variant

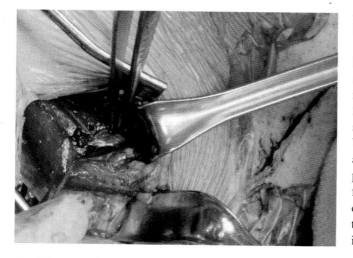

Fig. 5.5 A completed repair of simultaneous grade 3 avulsions of the rectus abdominis and the entire adductor apparatus with their fibrocartilaginous plate fragments. A similar repair has already been completed on the *left side* (Note the closed incision on the *left part* of the patient's body, i.e., *right side* of the photograph.) For orientation purposes, consider that an umbilical tape retracts the right spermatic cord laterally, and the lower retractor reveals the adductor area. The sutures represent where the two fibrocartilaginous plate fragments are joined together with the intact pubic symphyseal plate

Rehabilitation

Rehabilitation and performance protocols have evolved that are relatively specific for the various injuries and sports. The rehab protocols call for return to play somewhere between 3 days and 3 months postoperatively depending on the specific injury, sport, position, or choice of management. When three teams that strictly adhered to the protocols were analyzed, 18 of the 22 players were able to achieve return to play within the ascribed period. Eight of the 18 achieved full-play status ahead of the recommended time [2]. New concepts of core stability training have evolved that relate to the new pathophysiological understandings. We shall not go into these different protocols in this chapter.

Results and Return to Play

Over the past two and a half decades, we have seen tremendous progress in not only identification of the different types of injuries and the treatments but also in the specific and overall success rates. One must be careful, of course, in assessing success rates in this group of patients owing to a number of factors. The factors include type and severity of injury, classification of the injuries according to specific anatomy involved, short- (return-to-play data) versus long-term success rates, defining the intervals of follow-up, competitive versus noncompetitive status, workmen's compensation claims, concomitant hip injuries, contract negotiations, methods of assessment, and carefully defining the injury(ies) that one is talking about (e.g., just abdominal injuries versus including the other problems of AP).

In an early report, we found a 95.4% 2-year success rate in returning athlete patients to what they felt subjectively were their previous levels of performance [16, 17]. As we have continued to follow patients closely, the (long-term) success rates remain about the same despite a much wider range of indications and patients, plus lumping the "competitive" and "noncompetitive" athletes and "nonathletes" together in the same analysis groups. Most of the "nonsuccess" patients reported that they were "considerably better" but "not all the way better." The bulk of the latter patients had either concomitant hip problems that had not yet been addressed or pending workmen's compensation claims. Overall in the entire group of slightly over 11,000 surgeries, we have seen 33 clear recurrences. This represents 25 years and it should be considered that almost 30% of the overall group is either lost to follow-up or retired from sports. All the recurrences were between 1 and 11 years after the original surgeries with the majority occurring after 4 years. The most common reason for reoperation was development of contralateral problems after unilateral surgery.

A pending report on severe adductor, rectus abdominis, and other avulsion injuries with careful follow-up, interestingly, shows an overall 98% 2-year success rate, i.e., higher than the overall population. This group, by nature, represents the most severe of all the injuries. The surgery included many adductor repairs. Some of the patients also required concomitant hip surgery. All the patients with AP surgery alone returned to full play at previous levels of performance by 3 months after surgery. Thirty-two percent were back at 3 weeks, and over half were back at 6 weeks despite the severity of the injuries.

Of course, with the pressures on individual athletes and teams to return to play as early as possible after injury, the timing of return to play has garnered more attention. In certain play-off and other situations, we have returned patients to full play within 3–5 days after certain limited surgeries aimed at limited repair and division of nerve branches involved in the pain (after nonoperative measures such as simple injection blocks did not help). In a close assessment of 20 patients with selected injuries who chose 14- or 21-day protocols, 18 of the 20 patients were able to play at full strength by their own assessments within that time frame.

Reoperation

Three years ago, we reported on a seemingly alarming increase in a number of patients who had failed traditional hernia operations done at other institutions for athletic pubalgia. Over a 3-month period in 2007, we identified 47 such patients who underwent subsequent repair according to techniques. Fortunately, 40 of those 47 were able to return to full play within 3 months of subsequent surgery. During longer-term follow-up, 46 of the 47 have returned to full play, two of which required concomitant hip surgery. As mentioned, we are seeing an increasing number of similar patients requiring redo surgery at a pace of almost four patients per week. These patients include both open, mesh, or laparoscopic hernia repairs as well as the so-called "minimal" operations designed to return the players to full play as early as possible. MRI again plays an important role here in identifying the region and nature of the initial surgery as well as the salient lesion that might be a source of recurrent or new pain [10].

Conclusions

We have come a long way from the vague occult hernia concept in diagnosing and treating effectively the soft tissue and bony injuries of the pelvis. Appreciation of the complex anatomy is key, and then the various pathophysiologies and diagnostic and imaging techniques become almost intuitive. Successful outcomes result from precise diagnosis and therapy tailored to the individual patient and pathology.

References

1. Meyers WC, Yoo E, Devon ON, Jain N, Horner MA, Lauencin C, et al. Understanding "sports hernia" (athletic pubalgia): the anatomic and pathophysiologic basis for abdominal and groin pain in athletes. Oper Tech Sports Med. 2007;15:165–77.
2. Meyers WC, McKechnie A, Philippon MJ, Horner MA, Zoga AC, Devon ON. Experience with "sports hernia" spanning two decades. Ann Surg. 2008;248(4):656–65.
3. Escamilla R. Core trunk and stabilization in sports medicine in baseball. Sports Medicine of Baseball, eds Altcheck, DW, Andrews J, Dines J et al. Lippincott, Williams and Wilkins, Philadelphia, 2012.
4. Meyers WC, Kahan D, Joseph T, Butrymowicz A, Poor AE, Schoch S, Zoga AC. A current analysis of women athletes with pelvic pain. Med Sci Sports Exerc. 2011;43(8):1387–93.
5. Kavanagh EC, Koulouris G, Ford S, et al. MR imaging of groin pain in the athlete. Semin Musculoskelet Radiol. 2006;10:197–207.
6. Kavanagh EC, Zoga AC, Omar I, Koulouris G, Gopez A, Bergin D, Morrison WB, Meyers WC. MR imaging of the rectus abdominis/adductor aponeurosis: findings in the 'sports hernia'. Proceedings of the American Roentgen Ray Society. AJR Am J Roentgenol. 2007;188:A13–6.
7. Putschar WG. The structure of the human symphysis pubis with special consideration of parturition and its sequelae. Am J Phys Anthropol. 1976;45(3 pt 2):589–94.

8. Zajick DC, Zoga AC, Omar IM, Meyers WC. Spectrum of MRI findings in clinical athletic pubalgia. Semin Musculoskelet Radiol. 2008;12:3–12.

9. Zoga AC, Kavanaugh EC, Omar IM, et al. Athletic pubalgia and the "sports hernia": MR imaging findings. Radiology. 2008;247(3): 797–807.

10. Zoga AC, Morrison WB, Roth CG, Horner M, Meyers WC. MR findings in athletic pubalgia: normal postoperative appearance and reinjury patterns after pelvic repairs and releases for 'sports hernia'. In: Proceedings of the radiologic society of North America, Chicago; 2009.

11. Meyers WC, Thompson M, Coleman S, Zoga AC. Thoraco-abdominal and pelvic injuries (including athletic pubalgia, a.k.a. "sports hernia"). Sports Medicine of Baseball, eds Altcheck, DW, Andrews J, Dines J et al. Lippincott, Williams and Wilkins, Philadelphia, 2012.

12. Meyers WC, Greenleaf R, Saad A. Anatomic basis for evaluation of abdominal and groin pain in athletes. Oper Tech Sports Med. 2005;13(1):55–61, Elsevier.

13. Mora SA, Mandelbaum BR, Meyers WC. Abdomen and pelvis athletic injuries. Clinical Sports Medicine. Elsevier; Philadelphia, 2006.

14. Schwartzman RJ, Alexander GM, Grothusen J. Pathophysiology of complex regional pain syndrome. Expert Rev Neurother. 2006;6(5):669–81.

15. Schwartzman RJ, Erwin KL, Alexander GM. The natural history of complex regional pain syndrome. Clin J Pain. 2009;25(4): 273–80.

16. Meyers WC, Foley DP, Garrett WE, Lohnes JH, Mandlebaum BR, PAIN Study Group. Management of severe lower abdominal or inguinal pain in high-performance athletes. Am J Sports Med. 2000;28(1):2–8.

17. Taylor DC, Meyers WC, Moylan JA, et al. Abdominal musculature abnormalities as a cause of groin pain in athletes. Inguinal hernias and pubalgia. Am J Sports Med. 1991;19(3):239–42.

Sportsmen's Groin: Groin Pain: Always a Case for the Orthopedic Surgeon?

Ulrike Muschaweck and Luise Berger

Introduction

There are various pathologic changes which can result in groin pain, like hip injuries, muscular strain/avulsion trauma, sportsmen's groin, and a good many others. The sportsmen's groin (synonyms: "sportsman's hernia," "athletic hernia," "sports hernia," "(athletic) pubalgia," "incipient hernia," or "cryptic hernia") is one of the most frequent sports injuries and represents a severe clinical problem, especially in athletes. It presents with acute or chronic inguinal pain exacerbated with physical activity. The pain can be so intense that athletes are impaired, severely constrained, or even completely prevented from training and practicing sport.

Pathophysiology

Currently, there is little consensus regarding the pathophysiology. There have been many attempts to explain the cause of groin pain, like imbalance between the comparatively stronger hip adductor muscles and the comparatively weaker lower abdominal muscles [1, 2]. Weakness, poor endurance, reduced extensibility, or poor coordination of the muscular synergists necessary for effective dynamic hip motion control may precipitate functional instability, overuse, and injury at comparatively weaker noncontractile structures [1].

Among other theories, the entrapment of the genital branch of the genitofemoral nerve, the ilioinguinal, lateral femoral cutaneous, or obturator nerves may be responsible for the pain

U. Muschaweck, M.D., Ph.D. (✉)
Surgical Chief, Hernia Center Munich,
Hernienzentrum Dr. Muschaweck, Arabellastrasse 17,
Munich, Bavaria 81925, Germany
e-mail: um@hernien.de

L. Berger, M.D.
Department of Plastic Surgery and Hand Surgery,
Klinikum rechts der Isar, Ismaninger Str. 22,
Munich 81675, Bavaria, Germany
e-mail: lui.berger@web.de

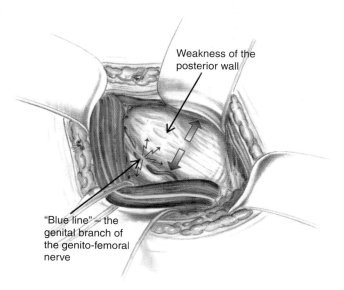

Fig. 6.1 Sportsmen's groin: A right-sided surgical view illustrates a localized bulge in the posterior inguinal wall with compression of the genital branch of the genitofemoral nerve

[3–5]. Principally, we agree with this assumption that the genital branch of the genitofemoral nerve is compressed by a localized bulge due to a circumscribed weakness in the posterior wall of the inguinal canal during the Valsalva maneuver (Fig. 6.1).

Additionally, as a consequence of the widened groin canal, the rectus muscle is retracted medially and cranially. This retraction causes an increased tension at the pubic bone. This pathomechanism is responsible for the pain at the symphysis pubis, also known as (athletic) pubalgia.

Diagnosis

Diagnosis should be made by an experienced examiner because it may be difficult to distinguish the symptoms between different problems. Through obtaining a careful history, physical examination, and dynamic ultrasonography, a correct diagnosis can be obtained.

Labels in Fig. 6.1: Weakness of the posterior wall; "Blue line" – the genital branch of the genito-femoral nerve

J.W.T. Byrd (ed.), *Operative Hip Arthroscopy*,
DOI 10.1007/978-1-4419-7925-4_6, © Springer Science+Business Media New York 2013

Medical History

Sportsmen's groin presents with acute or chronic groin pain exacerbated with physical activity. The patient usually reports pain (dull, diffuse, sharp, and burning) in the groin, often with radiation down the inner thigh, the scrotum, the testicle, and the pubic bone. In the early stages, the pain typically does not occur during competition but gives rise to aching after. Pain is aggravated by kicking, sudden changes in movement, coughing, and other "Valsalva"-type maneuvers [6, 7].

Physical Examination

The examination is carried out with the patient in upright position. When the inguinal canal is palpated, the patient usually confirms that the pain is getting worse. A sportsmen's groin is diagnosed when no inguinal hernia can be found, but there is a localized bulge in the posterior wall of the inguinal canal during the Valsalva maneuver (Fig. 6.1).

Dynamic Ultrasonography

Every patient should be explored with a dynamic ultrasound scan in supine position using a high-frequency transducer (5–13 MHz). Care should be taken not to compress the inguinal canal with excessive transducer pressure. The motion of the inguinal canal and its walls is observed during the Valsalva maneuver, and the size of the defect can be measured (about 2 cm on average). Sportsmen's groin is diagnosed if a convex anterior bulge of the posterior inguinal wall is observed during stress. Magnetic resonance imaging is reported to have good diagnostic potential [7, 8], but the examination is done with the patient in recumbent position. In our opinion, this explains the high rate of false-negative results with MRI and supports dynamic ultrasound scan as diagnostically conclusive, if it is done by an experienced examiner.

Treatment of Sportsmen's Groin: The Minimal Repair Technique

The literature suggests that sportsmen's groin rarely improves without surgery [2, 6, 9–12]. To avoid the development of chronic groin pain, surgical repair should be considered when conservative treatment over a period of 6–8 weeks has failed and when careful examination has excluded other potential pain sources [13–16].

In 2003, we introduced an innovative open-suture repair, called "Minimal Repair" technique [17]. This technique was

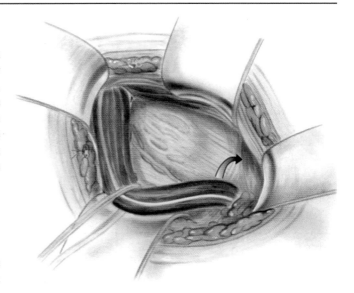

Fig. 6.2 Cranial and medial displacement of the rectus abdominis muscle (*arrow*) with increasing tension at the pubic bone

developed especially to exactly fit the needs of professional athletes with the intention to minimize the risks and traumatization of the patient.

The aim of the Minimal Repair technique is to eradicate groin pain by decompression of the genital branch of the genitofemoral nerve. The posterior wall is stabilized by a nearly tension-free suture without enlarging the defect of the posterior wall of the inguinal canal by the dissection. No prosthetic meshes are used to sustain full elasticity and the slide-bearing function (i.e., mobility and movability of the three layers of the abdominal wall) of abdominal muscles after surgery.

The Minimal Repair technique is performed under local anesthesia. The approach is carried out through a small inguinal incision, dissection of subcutaneous tissue, and splitting of the external oblique aponeurosis. The repair starts with testing the strength of the posterior inguinal wall by digital palpation. Typically, a circumscribed weakness is found in the posterior wall with the surrounding tissue firm and intact. The fascia transversalis is split, beginning in the area of the defect towards the deep internal ring. The length of the incision encloses only the area of fascial weakness; the surrounding tissue is kept intact (Fig. 6.2). The genital branch of the genitofemoral nerve should be assessed and, if necessary because of nerve damage, partly removed. Then, a continuous suture is placed from medial towards the deep inguinal ring creating a free fascia lip out of the iliopubic tract. There, the suture reverses towards the pubic bone. The free lip is included in the suture and brought to the inguinal ligament. The rectus abdominis muscle is lateralized with suture II to counteract the increased tension at the pubic bone caused by the retraction of the rectus muscle in the superior and medial direction. The pampiniform plexus is protected against mechanical irritation by creating a muscular collar at the deep ring with the lateral section of the internal oblique muscle (Fig. 6.3).

Conventional nonsteroidal anti-inflammatory drugs (NSAIDs) are used for postoperative pain relief. All patients are discharged on the day of operation. Patients are allowed to lift up to 20 kg (44 lb) immediately after surgery, to resume running/cycling on the second postoperative day (POD), to begin specific training on POD 3–4, and to fully train on POD 5. This is possible because the nearly tension-free suture does not cause pain.

In 2009, a prospective cohort study was carried out to evaluate the clinical outcome after operation under the Minimal Repair technique [17]. The primary endpoints were time to resume low-level training, full training/competing, and to complete pain relief. All patients felt that the operation had improved their symptoms considerably. All 86 of 86 athletes (100%) and 41 out of 42 nonathletes (97.6%)

reported, 4 weeks after operations in "Minimal Repair" technique, that they would have decided to undergo the operation in "Minimal Repair" technique again (Table 6.1). Of all patients, 78.9% reported that they were completely free of pain (median 14 days, IQR 6–28 days). Pain scores indicated a marked improvement in their level of pain ($p < 0.0001$). The pain score decreased from 6 (IQR 3.75–7) to 1 (IQR 0–2) 4 weeks after operation in "Minimal Repair" technique [17].

Comparing the groups of "athletes" and "nonathletes," there was a significant difference ($p < 0.05$) in "time to resumption of sport" and "return to peak performance." Athletes resumed their training earlier (median 7, IQR 4–14) than nonathletes (median 8.5, IQR 6.25–14) ($p = 0.002$). Furthermore, 83.7% of athletes already returned to peak performance within 4 weeks after operations in "Minimal Repair" technique, whereas 59.5% of nonathletes did so at this point of time ($p = 0.004$). The other parameters did not show significant differences [17] (Fig. 6.4).

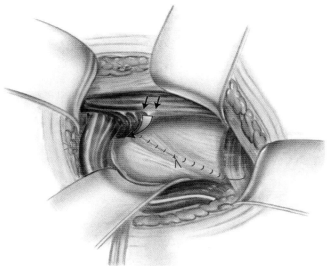

Fig. 6.3 The lateral section of the internal oblique muscle (*black arrows*) creates a muscular collar (*open arrow*) to protect the pampiniform plexus and nerves from mechanical irritation

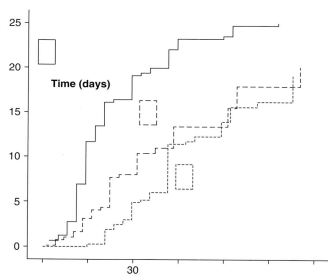

Fig. 6.4 Resumption of sport, pain release, and full exercise capacity in athletes

Table 6.1 Outcome 4 weeks after operation under the Minimal Repair technique

4 weeks after Minimal Repair	Athletes	Nonathletes	*p*-value
Resumption of sport within 28 days (%)	85/86 (98.8%)	39/42 (92.8%)	0.330
Time to resumption of sport (days)	7 (4–14)	8.5 (6.25–14.0)	0.002
Full return to sport within 28 days (%)	72/86 (83.7%)	25/42 (59.5%)	0.004
Time to full return to sport (days)	14 (10–28)	21 (14–28)	0.056
Complete relief of pain within 28 days (%)	68/86 (79.1%)	33/42 (78.6%)	1.00
Time to complete pain relief (days)	13 (7–28)	14 (5.25–28.0)	0.860
Perfect satisfaction of Minimal Repair	86/86 (100%)	41/42 (97.6%)	0.328
Pain scale (0–10) 4 weeks after Minimal Repair	0.5 (0–2)	1 (0–2.75)	0.064

Advantages of the Minimal Repair Technique

With Minimal Repair technique, the preparation and doubling of the fascia transversalis encloses only the area of fascial weakness and does not affect surrounding sound tissue like standard suture repairs (e.g., Shouldice repair) [17]. Commonly used surgical procedures include open repairs (e.g., Shouldice, Lichtenstein repairs) as well as laparoscopic repairs (e.g., transabdominal preperitoneal [TAPP] procedure, total extraperitoneal [TEP] procedure).

In comparison with the latter methods, the Minimal Repair technique has the following advantages: (1) no insertion of prosthetic mesh, (2) general anesthesia is not required, (3) less traumatization, (4) lower risk of severe complications, and (5) equal to or even faster convalescence.

Especially in athletes who require full elasticity and movement in their abdominal muscles, meshes should be avoided since inserted meshes result in localized stiffening of the abdominal muscles and, therefore, restricted movement. Since Minimal Repair technique does not make use of meshes, patients are not prone to mesh-related complications, such as infections with chronic groin sepsis and fistula formation which sometimes requires the removal of mesh [18], mesh migration and penetration into the bladder or bowel [19, 20], and foreign body reaction with decrease of arterial perfusion and testicular temperature [21] with consecutive secondary azoospermia [22]. Of note, 35% of open and 100% of laparoscopic procedures use mesh [13]. Concerning the recurrence of pain, we have had so far not one case within our uncontrolled clinical review. Overviewing over 2,000 Minimal Repairs in athletes since 2003, we have notice of only three patients in which pain could not be alleviated permanently.

The laparoscopic approach always requires general anesthesia. This is not the case with open procedures, including the Minimal Repair technique, so patients are not exposed to the side effects of general anesthesia. Existing data from large consecutive patient series and randomized studies have shown local anesthesia to be advantageous [23].

Open repairs were shown to be less traumatic than laparoscopic approaches [24]. Schwab et al. determined the systemic inflammatory response after endoscopic vs. Shouldice groin repair by monitoring cytokine activities (CRP, PGF1a, neopterin, IL-6). The immune trauma was significantly higher in the group with laparoscopic hernia repair than in the group who received a Shouldice repair. Therefore, the repair of groin hernias using a laparoscopic technique should not be regarded as a minimally invasive procedure that is less traumatic than conventional approaches [24]. Since the Minimal Repair technique does not split the whole posterior inguinal wall, as is the case with a Shouldice repair, it can be considered as even less invasive in respect to tissue damage.

Severe visceral and vascular complications were more often reported with laparoscopic techniques [25] as compared with open-repair techniques. A common problem after laparoscopic repair is postoperative urinary retention (22.2% after laparoscopic inguinal hernia procedures) [26]. The number of surgeons using laparoscopic procedures has been increasing in the last few years [10, 27–31]. With the Minimal Repair technique, neither minor nor major complications were observed during follow-up.

After laparoscopic repair, recovery generally took 6–8 weeks before full return to competition was permitted [6, 13, 31–33]. The recovery times in other studies varied from 2 to 3 weeks [27, 34], 4 weeks [35], 3–6 weeks [36], and up to 12 weeks [28, 31]. In a meta-analysis, Caudill et al. found postsurgical recovery times (based on sports activity) of 17.7 weeks for patients who underwent open approaches and 6.1 weeks for laparoscopic repairs [13]. Compared with these data, the convalescence after operation under the Minimal Repair technique is faster than after the customary procedures.

References

1. Biedert RM, Warnke K, Meyer S. Symphysis syndrome in athletes: surgical treatment for chronic lower abdominal, groin, and adductor pain in athletes. Clin J Sport Med. 2003;13:278–84.
2. Farber AJ, Wilckens JH. Sports hernia: diagnosis and therapeutic approach. J Am Acad Orthop Surg. 2007;15:507–14.
3. Akita K, Niga S, Yamato Y, Muneta T, Sato T. Anatomic basis of chronic groin pain with special reference to sports hernia. Surg Radiol Anat. 1999;21:1–5.
4. Bradshaw C, McCrory P, Bell S, Brukner P. Obturator nerve entrapment. A cause of groin pain in athletes. Am J Sports Med. 1997;25:402–8.
5. Rab M, Ebmer And J, Dellon AL. Anatomic variability of the ilioinguinal and genitofemoral nerve: implications for the treatment of groin pain. Plast Reconstr Surg. 2001;108:1618–23.
6. Hackney RG. The sports hernia: a cause of chronic groin pain. Br J Sports Med. 1993;27:58–62.
7. Swan Jr KG, Wolcott M. The athletic hernia: a systematic review. Clin Orthop Relat Res. 2007;455:78–87.
8. Meyers WC, McKechnie A, Philippon MJ, Horner MA, Zoga AC, Devon ON. Experience with "sports hernia" spanning two decades. Ann Surg. 2008;248:656–65.
9. Ekstrand J, Ringborg S. Surgery versus conservative treatment in soccer players with chronic groin pain: a prospective randomised study in soccer players. Eur J Sports Traumatol Rel Res (Testo stampato) (ISSN 1592–3894). 2001;23:141–5.
10. Ingoldby CJ. Laparoscopic and conventional repair of groin disruption in sportsmen. Br J Surg. 1997;84:213–5.
11. Moeller JL. Sportsman's hernia. Curr Sports Med Rep. 2007;6:111–4.
12. Polglase AL, Frydman GM, Farmer KC. Inguinal surgery for debilitating chronic groin pain in athletes. Med J Aust. 1991;155: 674–7.
13. Caudill P, Nyland J, Smith C, Yerasimides J, Lach J. Sports hernias: a systematic literature review. Br J Sports Med. 2008;42:954–64.
14. Ekberg O, Persson NH, Abrahamsson PA, Westlin NE, Lilja B. Longstanding groin pain in athletes. A multidisciplinary approach. Sports Med. 1988;6:56–61.

15. Joesting DR. Diagnosis and treatment of sportsman's hernia. Curr Sports Med Rep. 2002;1:121–4.

16. Van Der Donckt K, Steenbrugge F, Van Den Abbeele K, Verdonk R, Verhelst M. Bassini's hernial repair and adductor longus tenotomy in the treatment of chronic groin pain in athletes. Acta Orthop Belg. 2003;69:35–41.

17. Muschaweck U, Berger L. Minimal repair technique of sportsmen's groin: an innovative open-suture repair to treat chronic inguinal pain. Hernia. 2010;14(1):27–33.

18. Avtan L, Avci C, Bulut T, Fourtanier G. Mesh infections after laparoscopic inguinal hernia repair. Surg Laparosc Endosc. 1997;7:192–5.

19. Bodenbach M, Bschleipfer T, Stoschek M, Beckert R, Sparwasser C. Intravesical migration of a polypropylene mesh implant 3 years after laparoscopic transperitoneal hernioplasty. Urologe A. 2002;41:366–8.

20. Lange B, Langer C, Markus PM, Becker H. Mesh penetration of the sigmoid colon following a transabdominal preperitoneal hernia repair. Surg Endosc. 2003;17:157.

21. Peiper C, Junge K, Klinge U, Strehlau E, Ottinger A, Schumpelick V. Is there a risk of infertility after inguinal mesh repair? Experimental studies in the pig and the rabbit. Hernia. 2006;10:7–12.

22. Shin D, Lipshultz LI, Goldstein M, Barme GA, Fuchs EF, Nagler HM, McCallum SW, Niederberger CS, Schoor RA, Brugh 3rd VM, Honig SC. Herniorrhaphy with polypropylene mesh causing inguinal vasal obstruction: a preventable cause of obstructive azoospermia. Ann Surg. 2005;241:553–8.

23. Kehlet H, Aasvang E. Groin hernia repair: anesthesia. World J Surg. 2005;29:1058–61.

24. Schwab R, Eissele S, Bruckner UB, Gebhard F, Becker HP. Systemic inflammatory response after endoscopic (TEP) vs Shouldice groin hernia repair. Hernia. 2004;8:226–32.

25. Grant AM. Laparoscopic versus open groin hernia repair: meta-analysis of randomised trials based on individual patient data. Hernia. 2002;6:2–10.

26. Koch CA, Grinberg GG, Farley DR. Incidence and risk factors for urinary retention after endoscopic hernia repair. Am J Surg. 2006;191:381–5.

27. Genitsaris M, Goulimaris I, Sikas N. Laparoscopic repair of groin pain in athletes. Am J Sports Med. 2004;32:1238–42.

28. Kluin J, den Hoed PT, van Linschoten R, IJzerman JC, van Steensel CJ. Endoscopic evaluation and treatment of groin pain in the athlete. Am J Sports Med. 2004;32:944–9.

29. Paajanen H, Heikkinen J, Hermunen H, Airo I. Successful treatment of osteitis pubis by using totally extraperitoneal endoscopic technique. Int J Sports Med. 2005;26:303–6.

30. Susmallian S, Ezri T, Elis M, Warters R, Charuzi I, Muggia-Sullam M. Laparoscopic repair of "sportsman's hernia" in soccer players as treatment of chronic inguinal pain. Med Sci Monit. 2004;10:CR52–4.

31. van Veen RN, de Baat P, Heijboer MP, Kazemier G, Punt BJ, Dwarkasing RS, Bonjer HJ, van Eijck CH. Successful endoscopic treatment of chronic groin pain in athletes. Surg Endosc. 2007;21:189–93.

32. Ahumada LA, Ashruf S, Espinosa-de-los-Monteros A, Long JN, de la Torre JI, Garth WP, Vasconez LO. Athletic pubalgia: definition and surgical treatment. Ann Plast Surg. 2005;55:393–6.

33. Kumar A, Doran J, Batt ME, Nguyen-Van-Tam JS, Beckingham IJ. Results of inguinal canal repair in athletes with sports hernia. J R Coll Surg Edinb. 2002;47:561–5.

34. Azurin DJ, Go LS, Schuricht A, McShane J, Bartolozzi A. Endoscopic preperitoneal herniorrhaphy in professional athletes with groin pain. J Laparoendosc Adv Surg Tech A. 1997;7:7–12.

35. Paajanen H, Syvahuoko I, Airo I. Totally extraperitoneal endoscopic (TEP) treatment of sportsman's hernia. Surg Laparosc Endosc Percutan Tech. 2004;14:215–8.

36. Edelman DS, Selesnick H. "Sports" hernia: treatment with biologic mesh (Surgisis): a preliminary study. Surg Endosc. 2006;20:971–3.

Gross Anatomy

7

Oscar Fariñas Barberá and Ivan Sáenz Navarro

The hip has been the final challenge for arthroscopic treatment of the major joints in the body. Arthroscopy of the hip joint was initially performed by researchers in the 1930s [1, 2]. Nevertheless, it has evolved less than arthroscopy in other joints, compared with the shoulder or the knee. The reasons of this slower development are the technical requirements and instrumentation devices needed to access to the hip joint, as well as the anatomy of this specific joint. Many authors have also recognized that the depth of the hip joint acts as a limiting factor [3, 4].

Anatomical knowledge of the joint characteristics and surrounding structures (anatomical constraints, capsular reinforcements, peritrochanteric space, etc.) is basic for the surgical team to achieve good results avoiding iatrogenic lesions.

The hip can be divided arthroscopically into three compartments [5–8] that comprise different anatomical structures (Table 7.1). The first compartment was the first described in hip arthroscopy to diagnose and treat the different pathologies that affect the hip joint, and today this space is commonly known as the central compartment. The central compartment comprises the acetabular fossa, the lunate cartilage, the ligamentum teres, and the articular area of the femoral head. The peripheral compartment includes the femoral neck, the outer acetabular rim, synovial membrane, and the capsule including its capsular reinforcements (i.e., orbicularis zone). The acetabular labrum acts as a separator between central and peripheral compartment. The last compartment corresponds to the peritrochanteric compartment that lies between the iliotibial band and the proximal femur [9] and gives us the possibility to reach the deep gluteal

region. The access to this space provides the possibility to perform gluteus medius tendon repairs [8], trochanteric bursectomies [7], and the treatment of external snapping hip syndrome [10].

In order to describe adequately the different anatomical structures that compose the hip anatomy, we will organize them into compartments in comparison with arthroscopy (Table 7.1).

Central Compartment

Femoral Head

The femoral head has a rounded and smooth shape, representing approximately the two-thirds of a sphere. It is oriented upward, inward, and slightly forward.

At the level of the articular surface, it is located in a small and rough depression that corresponds to the fovea capitis (see Fig. 7.1). The fovea is slightly ovoid with an oblique, superior-to-posterior orientation [11]. The positioning of the fovea capitis is thought to be related with the disposition of the fibers of the ligamentum teres when they are tensed [12, 13].

The articular cartilage thickness decreases from the center to the periphery of the femoral head (see Fig. 7.2). This cartilage is more developed in the superior aspect than the inferior one, and it has its highest thickness just above the ligamentum teres attachment (2.5–3 mm) [14].

Some vessels penetrate into the femoral head through many small holes that are located at the bottom of the fovea capitis. These vessels come from an anterior branch of the obturator artery, but they are not patent in one-third of adults, so their contribution to the femoral head vascularization is variable [12, 13, 15].

The vascular supply of the femoral head is mainly provided by the medial femoral circumflex artery (MFCA) and its branches. The most important branch of the MFCA is the deep one that passes just deep to the external rotator

O. Fariñas Barberá, M.D. (✉)
Transplant Services Foundation, Musculoskeletal Tissue Unit,
Dr. Antoni Pujadas, 42, Sant Boi de Llobregat, Barcelona 08031, Spain
e-mail: obarbera@clinic.ub.es

I. Sáenz Navarro, M.D.
Department of Human Anatomy and Embriology, Facultat de Medicina,
C/Casanova 143, Barcelona, Spain
e-mail: ivansaenzn@hotmail.com

Table 7.1 Anatomical structures included in each arthroscopic hip compartment

Central compartment	Peripheral compartment	Peritrochanteric compartment
Lunate cartilage	Femoral neck	Proximal femur (including greater trochanter)
Acetabular fossa	Capsule (including ligament reinforcements)	Gluteus medius tendon
Ligamentum teres (of the head of the femur)	Synovial membrane (including synovial folds and plicae)	Iliotibial band
Acetabular labrum (inner acetabular labrum, central compartment; outer acetabular labrum, peripheral compartm ent)		Hip bursae
Femoral head		Sciatic nerve
		Inferior gluteal nerve

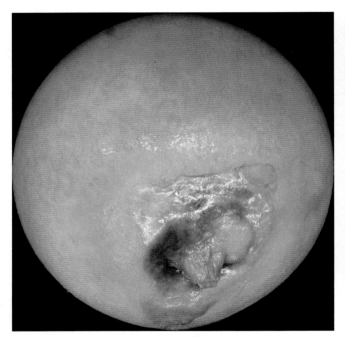

Fig. 7.1 Superior view of a right femoral head showing the position of the fovea capitis with the ligamentum teres attachment. Observe its typical ovoid morphology

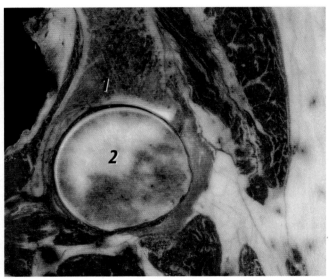

Fig. 7.2 Frontal cross section of a right hip joint. Observe the decrease of the femoral head articular cartilage from center to periphery. (*1*) Acetabulum. (*2*) Femoral head

muscles (piriformis, quadratus femoris, superior and inferior gemellus, internus obturator, and externus obturator muscles). The role of the lateral femoral circumflex artery is less important [16].

The MFCA has its origin from the deep femoral artery (83%) or the femoral artery (27%) [17]. The MFCA has usually five branches: ascending, descending, acetabular, superficial, and deep. The deep branch of the MFCA (see Fig. 7.3) is the most responsible for femoral head and neck vascularization [18]. It has its origin medially from the femoral artery between the pectineus and iliopsoas tendons, along the inferior border of externus obturator muscle. Afterward, the deep branch gives rise to the ascendant branch that passes in the space between quadratus femoris and inferior gemellus muscles (see Fig. 7.4). Then it passes

anterior to gemelli tendons and internus obturator muscle. Posteriorly, it penetrates the capsule at the level of superior gemellus m. and gives origin to 2–4 retinacular vessels (intracapsulary).

The role of the lateral femoral circumflex artery (LFCA) is less important [16], as well as its risk of injury, because most of the surgical approaches to the hip joint are performed in the posterior region (see Fig. 7.5).

Acetabulum

The acetabulum is a concave surface located in the lateral aspect of the hemipelvis as a result of the fusion of the three bones that form this bone: ilium, ischium, and pubis [19].

The morphology of the acetabulum has been described as a horseshoe-like articular surface, incompletely surrounding a quadrangular non-articular surface referred to as the acetabular

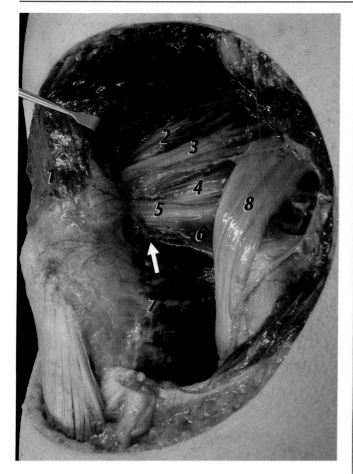

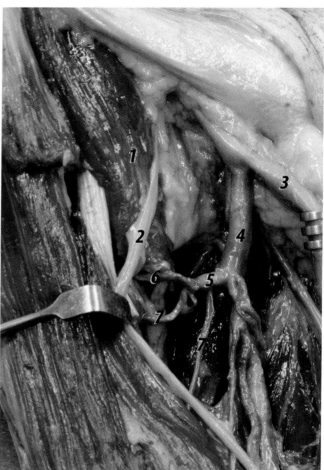

Fig. 7.3 Posterior view of left deep gluteus region showing pelvitrochanteric muscles and the course of the deep branch of the medial femoral circumflex artery (*white arrow*). (*1*) Gluteus medius m. (partially resected). (*2*) Gluteus minimus m. (*3*) Piriformis m. (*4*) Superior gemellus m. (*5*) Internus obturator m. (*6*) Inferior gemellus m. (*7*) Quadratus femoris m. (*8*) Sciatic nerve

Fig. 7.5 View of the right femoral triangle (Scarpa area). The sartorius and rectus femoris muscles have been partially removed. Observe the path of the lateral femoral circumflex artery. (*1*) Iliopsoas m. (*2*) Femoral nerve. (*3*) Femoral artery. (*4*) Deep femoral artery. (*5*) Lateral femoral circumflex artery. (*6*) Transverse branch. (*7*) Muscular branch

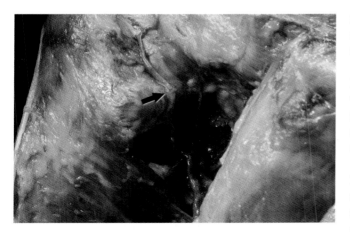

Fig. 7.4 Posterior view of the pelvitrochanteric muscles on a left hip. The quadratus femoris muscle has been partially removed to show the ascendant branch of the medial femoral circumflex artery. Observe the relationship between the artery and the medial aspect of the lesser trochanter of the femur (*black arrow*)

fossa [20]. The acetabulum is oriented forward forming an angle of 40° with the sagittal plane and downward forming an angle of 60° with the horizontal plane [21].

At the inferior border of the acetabular fossa, the acetabular rim decreases its size forming the acetabular notch that will be covered by the transverse acetabular ligament. The rest of the acetabulum corresponds to the lunate surface or cartilage. Covering the acetabular fossa, a small synovium can be identified (see Fig. 7.6).

The area of the lunate cartilage varies between 14.5 and 30.5 cm^2 [22]. In the study of Govsa et al. [22], they classified the different acetabular fossa morphologies according to the shape differences of the lunate cartilage. Four different types were described:

- Type I: The acetabular fossa had a cloverleaf-like form. This form was present in 60.62% of the cases.
- Type II: The acetabular fossa had a more semicircular shape. This form was observed in 28.76% of the cases.

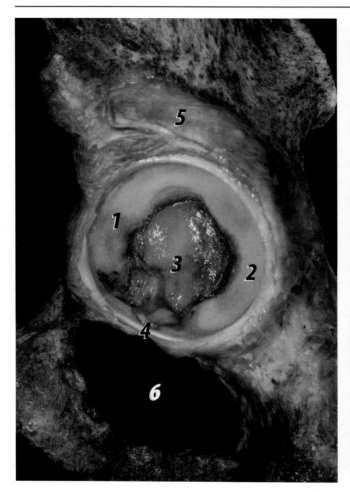 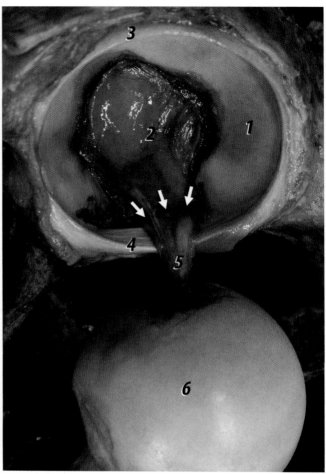

Fig. 7.6 Lateral view of a left hemipelvis focused on the acetabulum. Observe the synovial tissue that covers the acetabular fossa. (*1*) Anterior lunate cartilage, (*2*) Posterior lunate cartilage. (*3*) Acetabular fossa. (*4*) Transverse acetabular ligament. (*5*) Reflected tendon of the rectus femoris muscle. (*6*) Obturator foramen

Fig. 7.7 Lateral view of a left hip joint showing the ligamentum teres. Observe the origin of ligamentum teres from the inferior border of the transverse acetabular ligament and the superior border of the acetabular notch (*white arrows*). The hip joint has been dislocated. (*1*) Lunate cartilage. (*2*) Acetabular fossa. (*3*) Acetabular labrum. (*4*) Transverse acetabular ligament. (*5*) Ligamentum teres. (*6*) Femoral head

- Type III: The acetabular fossa had a smooth compact spongy bony surface that covered the floor. It was present in 1.77% of the cases.
- Type IV: It was determined an isolated defect above the superior lobe. The area of the superior lobe appeared as a spongy surface in 8.85% of the cases.

Unusual facets on the acetabulum have been described [22, 23]. A smooth facet placed in the non-articular part of the acetabulum, inferior to the anterior end of the lunate surface, was observed in 15.2–44.8% of the specimens with a higher incidence in males (67.7%). The shape of these facets was variable: oval (32.2–56.3%), piriform (22.9–45.1%), and elongated (20.8–22.5%).

Ligamentum Teres

Recently, the ligamentum teres lesions have increased its importance because of its role in hip pain and stability.

The ligament teres, also called the ligament of the head of the femur, has its main origin from the transverse acetabular ligament and along the inferior margin of the acetabulum (acetabular notch) (see Fig. 7.7). It is attached to the periosteum by two fascicles, which are located along the anterior and posterior border of the acetabular notch [12, 13, 24].

The attachment site of ligamentum teres is in the fovea capitis of the femur with an overall length, although it exists a great variability, of 30–35 mm [12, 13, 25]. The shape of ligamentum teres is pyramidal and somewhat flattened on its origin but gently transitions into a round or ovoid shape and attaches as an ovoid ligament [11].

In 2007, Demange et al. [26] published that the ligamentum teres is composed by three bundles: anterior, posterior, and medial. The strongest bundle is the posterior one, while the medial bundle is the thinnest.

The ligament of the head of the femur acts as a strong intrinsic stabilizer of the hip joint. Different theories have been developed about the role of this ligament. Rao and Bardakos [12, 13] stated that ligamentum teres plays a mechanical role in hip stabilization because their fibers are more taut when the hip is in flexion, abduction, and external rotation. Leunig et al. [27] postulated that the ligament may play a proprioception role preventing excessive movement. Finally, Gray and Villar [28] proposed that ligamentum teres helps to distribute the synovial fluid by the way of the "windshield wiper" effect.

Acetabular Labrum

The acetabular labrum is a fibrocartilaginous structure attached to the periphery of the osseous acetabular rim. It has been classically described with a prismatic and triangular shape, but different studies demonstrated some variations on it. Lecouvet et al. [29], using coronal MR images, mentioned that labral shapes were found to be triangular (66%), round (11%), flat (9%), or absent (4%), depending on the individuals and sites. Won et al. [30] performed a cadaveric study and concluded that the labrum shape was triangular in 93.1% of the cases (54 acetabula).

At the anterior-inferior portion of the acetabular labrum is located the transverse acetabular ligament as a consequence of the acetabular notch presence (point of fusion between ischium and pubis) (see Fig. 7.8).

The main functions of the acetabular labrum are to increase the joint depth enhancing the articular stability and congruity [31] as well as to provide a seal for protection of the articular cartilage of the hip [32].

The vascularization of the acetabular labrum has been well studied due to its implication in the prognosis and evolution of the labral tears. The blood supply comes mainly from the superior and inferior gluteal arteries although there is a small contribution from the medial and lateral circumflex arteries and the intrapelvic vasculature. All of these arteries form a periacetabular vascular ring from where different radial branches arise, pass over the capsular aspect of the acetabular labrum, and terminate near the free edge of the labrum [33, 34]. Kalhor et al. [33] studied the vascular supply of 35 acetabular labrums and concluded that the highest concentration of vessels was found in the posterior half of the labrum, the posterosuperior quadrant appeared to have a slightly higher density of vessels than the posteroinferior quadrant, and the anteroinferior quadrant had a higher density of radial branches than anterosuperior one. The main responsible of the blood supply of the superior and posterosuperior quadrant is the superior gluteal artery, while the posterior and posteroinferior parts are mainly vascularized by the inferior gluteal artery. According to these data, the labrum blood supply remains intact when the labral tear affects the articular aspect (most of the cases), but it is interrupted when a labral detachment occurs.

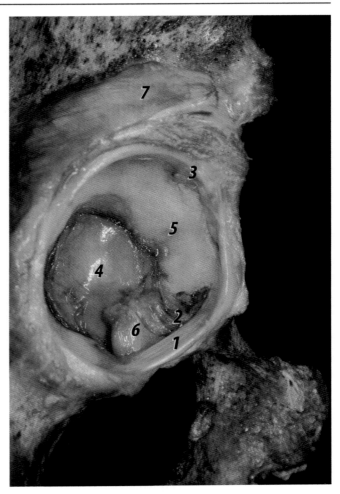

Fig. 7.8 Posterolateral view of a right acetabulum. Note the origin and attachment of the transverse acetabular ligament. (*1*) Transverse acetabular ligament. (*2*) Acetabular notch. (*3*) Acetabular labrum. (*4*) Acetabular fossa. (*5*) Anterior lunate cartilage. (*6*) Ligamentum teres (resected). (*7*) Reflected tendon of the rectus femoris muscle

Peripheral Compartment

Femoral Neck

The femoral neck is the distal continuation of the femoral head. The transition area between both structures is quite irregular because it is composed of two curve lines that are joined at the anterosuperior part of the femoral head as well as at its posterior aspect.

The femoral neck adopts a flatten cylinder morphology showing two different aspects:
- Anterior aspect that is almost flat
- Posterior aspect that is convex in a longitudinal direction and concave in a transverse direction

Proximally the femoral neck is wider in order to maintain the femoral head, and it presents many vascular holes.

Distally the femoral neck continues with two reliefs: the greater trochanter and lesser trochanter.

The femoral neck forms an angle of 130° with the diaphyseal axis of the femur, and it is 10–30° anteversed.

Capsule

The hip capsule is a thick and fibrous cover that is attached around the acetabulum proximally (acetabular rim, lateral aspect of the acetabular labrum, and transverse ligament of the acetabulum) and the femoral neck distally. Special attention is required to the distal insertion of the capsule [14] because of the multiple surgical involvements:

- Anteriorly the capsule is strongly attached to the anterior intertrochanteric line (spiral line of the femur).
- Posteriorly the capsule is attached to the femoral neck. This attachment represents an asymmetry between the anterior and posterior capsule not only regarding the insertion points but also the higher laxity of the posterior one.
- Superiorly the capsule is attached in an oblique line that joins the anterior and posterior capsular attachment.
- Inferiorly the capsule is attached from the anterior intertrochanteric line to the posterior capsule, passing over the lesser trochanter.

Two different fibers compose the joint capsule: longitudinal and circular. The longitudinal fibers, located superficially, take a superior-inferior direction to cross with the circular fibers and being mingled with the capsular reinforcement ligaments. Meanwhile, the circular fibers are located deeply and take perpendicular direction to the axis of the femoral head. These circular fibers are well visualized at the posterior and inferior aspect of the joint.

The capsular reinforcement ligaments are the iliofemoral, ischiofemoral, and the femoral arcuate ligament [35, 36].

The iliofemoral ligament (also named Y-ligament of Bigelow) originates from the anterior-inferior iliac spine (below the direct head of the rectus femoris muscle) and the acetabular rim (see Fig. 7.9), and it is divided into two fascicles (superior and inferior) as it crosses the joint. The superior fascicle attaches proximally along the anterior intertrochanteric line (just below the gluteus minimus tendon). The inferior fascicle is thinner and inserts distally to the superior fascicle at the level of the anterior intertrochanteric line. The iliofemoral ligament restricts the hip extension allowing the erect posture to be maintained. This ligament is the most resistant of the reinforcement ligaments.

The ischiofemoral ligament arises from the ischiatic rim of the acetabulum, follows the spiral direction of the iliofemoral ligament, and attaches to the posterior aspect of the femoral neck (see Fig. 7.10). Due to its posterior position, the main function is to restrict the internal rotation, but also the adduction when the hip is flexed.

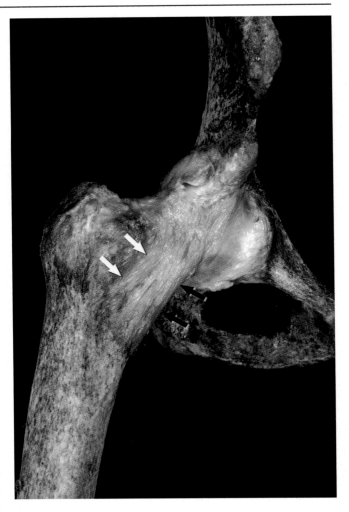

Fig. 7.9 Anterior view of the right hip capsule. Observe the presence of the iliofemoral ligament with its two components: superior (*white arrows*) and inferior fascicle (*black arrows*)

The femoral arcuate ligament originates at the greater trochanter, passes deep to the ischiofemoral ligament, around the posterior aspect of the femoral neck, and attaches to the lesser trochanter (see Fig. 7.10). This ligament acts tensioning the capsule in extreme flexion and extension of the hip. Previously this ligament was described as orbicularis zone because of the direction of its fibers.

Synovial

The synovial membrane of the hip joint arises from the free border of the acetabular labrum, and it attaches close to the border of the articular cartilage of the femoral head.

Along its surface, the synovial membrane presents some specific modifications of its morphology that are called synovial folds. The incidence of the labral plicae increases with age [37] and has been related to synovial disease [6].

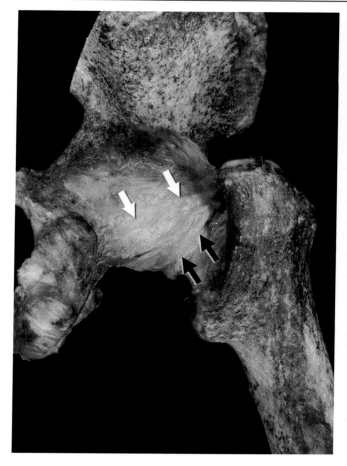

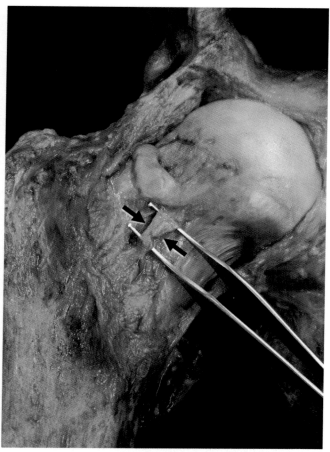

Fig. 7.10 Posterior view of the right hip joint. Observe the presence of the ischiofemoral ligament (*white arrows*) and femoral arcuate ligament (*black arrows*) that passes below the first one

Fig. 7.11 Anterior view of the right hip joint with arthritis. An anterior capsulotomy has been performed. Observe the placement of the anterior synovial fold (*black arrows*)

Three synovial folds have been described: anterior, medial, and lateral [38].

The anterior synovial fold is placed in the anterior aspect of the femoral neck being adherent to it. It is identified as single fibers covering the neck (see Fig. 7.11).

The medial synovial fold is located at the medial aspect of the neck being not adherent to it. It passes proximal from the medial border of the femoral head distally to the lesser trochanter (see Fig. 7.12). It is the more prominent synovial fold in the hip joint.

Finally, the lateral synovial fold runs from the greater trochanter upward to the lateral margin of the head, just along the lateral aspect of the femoral neck.

Peritrochanteric Space

The peritrochanteric space was initially described as area between the iliotibial band and the proximal femur [9], but actually we can expand this concept to those areas we can reach using the peritrochanteric portals, like the deep gluteal region [8] or the iliopsoas tendon.

Proximal Femur

Peritrochanteric portals were first described to diagnose and treat the pathologies that were grouped into the "greater trochanteric pain syndrome." A better knowledge of the great trochanter anatomy will help the surgeons to identify arthroscopically the different structures and treat their pathologies.

The typical morphology of the greater trochanter is produced by the architecture of the abductor mechanism [39, 40].

Pfirrmann et al. [41] described the presence of four different facets in the greater trochanter (see Fig. 7.13):

- The anterior facet can be identified on the anterolateral surface of the trochanter and corresponds to the attachment of the gluteus minimus tendon. Is oval in shape and shares a medial border with the intertrochanteric line. The anterior border is formed by the intertrochanteric line just posterior to the capsular insertion of the hip.
- The superoposterior facet is located in the top of the greater trochanter and has an oblique transverse orientation. It gives attachment to the gluteus medius tendon.

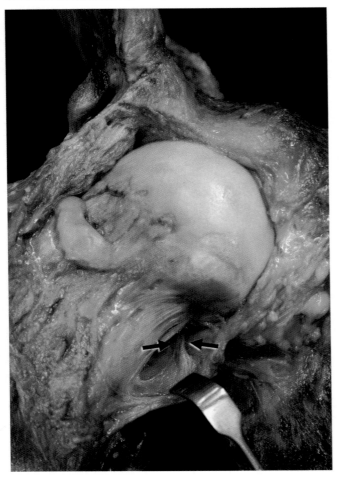

Fig. 7.12 Anterior view of the right hip joint with arthritis. An anterior capsulotomy has been performed. Observe the placement of the medial synovial fold (*black arrows*)

- The lateral facet has an inverted triangular shape. It is in contact with the superoposterior facet through its posterior-superior border. In the same way that superoposterior facet it is completely covered by the gluteus medius tendon.
- The posterior facet is placed in the posterior aspect of the greater trochanter. It is in close contact with the lateral and superoposterior facets through its superior border. This facet does not receive any tendon attachment, but it is covered by the trochanteric bursa.

Hip Bursae Complex

Three different peritrochanteric bursae have been described: trochanteric bursa, subgluteus medius bursa, and subgluteus minimus bursa [39, 42, 43]. The description of the "bursae complex" was performed by Pfirrmann et al. [41]:

- The trochanteric bursa is the largest hip bursa. It is located beneath the gluteus maximus muscle and iliotibial tract. Its function is to cover the posterior facet of the greater trochanter, the gluteus medius tendon, and the proximal part of the vastus lateralis origin.
- The subgluteus medius bursa is placed deep to the lateral part of the gluteus medius tendon.
- The subgluteus minimus bursa lays beneath the gluteus minimus tendon, in a medial and superior position. It covers partially the anterior area of the hip capsule.

Deep Gluteal Region

The deep gluteal region includes the gluteus medius muscle, gluteus minimus muscle, piriformis muscle, superior and

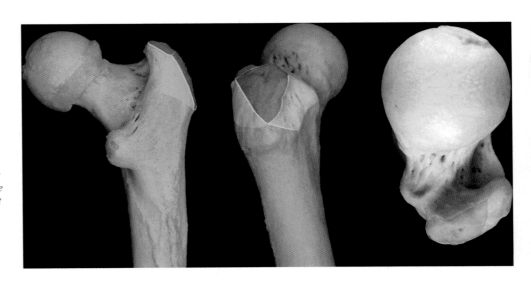

Fig. 7.13 Placement representation of the greater trochanter facets. Posterior view (*left image*), lateral view (*middle image*), and superior view (*right image*) of the proximal femur. (*Blue*) Superoposterior facet. (*Green*) Posterior facet. (*Red*) Lateral facet. (*Yellow*) Anterior facet

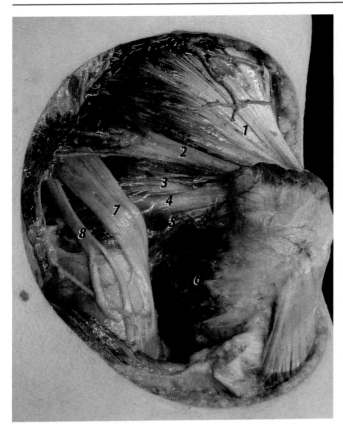

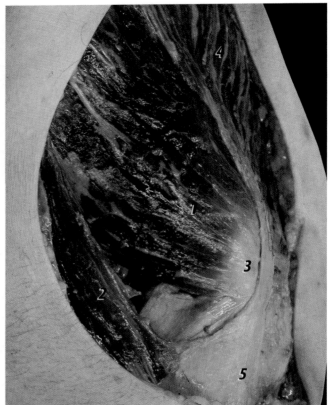

Fig. 7.14 Posterior view of right deep gluteus region. The gluteus medius muscle has been removed to show the gluteus minimus muscle. (*1*) Gluteus minimus m. (*2*) Piriformis m. (*3*) Superior gemellus m. (*4*) Internus obturator m. (*5*) Inferior gemellus m. (*6*) Quadratus femoris m. (*7*) Sciatic nerve. (*8*) Posterior femoral cutaneous nerve

Fig. 7.15 Posterior view of the right gluteus region. The gluteus maximus has been partially resected to show the gluteus medius main attachment into the superoposterior facet of the greater trochanter. (*1*) Gluteus medius m. (*2*) Gluteus maximus m. (*3*) Greater trochanter. (*4*) Tensor fascia latae m. (*5*) Iliotibial band

inferior gemelli muscles, obturator internus muscle, obturator externus muscle, and quadratus femoris muscle (see Fig. 7.14) that are also named as "pelvitrochanteric muscles." All of these muscles are covered by the gluteus maximus muscle.

The gluteus medius muscle has three different groups of fibers [14] that act over the hip joint in a different way: anterior fibers produce an abduction and internal rotation of the hip, posterior fibers produce also abduction but external rotation of the hip, and finally the middle fibers only produce abduction. The gluteus medius attachment can also be divided into three parts [41]:

• The main tendon arose from the central posterior portion of the muscle, and it is attached to the superoposterior facet of the greater trochanter (see Fig. 7.15). The thickness of this main tendon is not homogeneous, so the medial part is thicker than the lateral one.
• The lateral part of the tendon takes its origin from the undersurface of the gluteus medius muscle, and it is usu-

ally thin. It is attached into the lateral facet of the greater trochanter and continues anteriorly covering the insertion of the gluteus minimus tendon.
• The anterior part of the tendon is surrounded and attached by the gluteus minimus muscle.

The gluteus minimus muscle, which is covered by the gluteus medius muscle, attaches to the greater trochanter through two different components [41] (see Fig. 7.16). The main tendon is attached mainly in the anterior (lateral and inferior aspect) facet of the greater trochanter. The fibers that compose this main tendon are the anterior muscle fibers. The secondary part of the gluteus minimus is attached through a muscular insertion into the anterior and superior aspect of the hip capsule.

Some intrapelvis neurovascular structures arise into the deep gluteal region from the intrapelvic area. They can be divided depending on its relationship with the piriformis muscle.

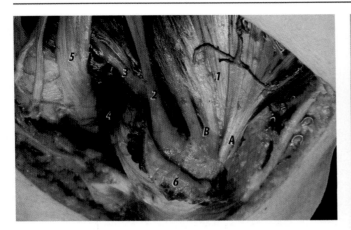

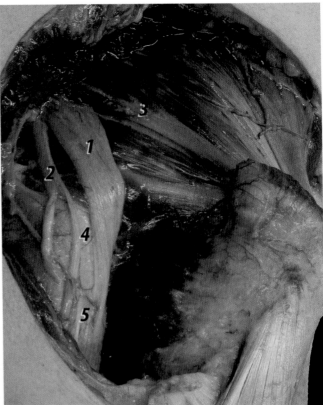

Fig. 7.16 Cranial view of the gluteus minimus attachment. Differentiate the two components: (*A*) main tendon attached to the anterior facet of the greater trochanter and (*B*) secondary attachment to the hip capsule. (*1*) Gluteus minimus m. (*2*) Piriformis m. (*3*) Internus obturator m. with both gemelli. (*4*) Quadratus femoris m. (*5*) Sciatic nerve. (*6*) Gluteus medius m. (resected)

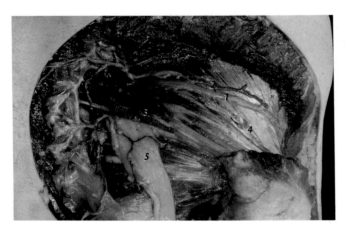

Fig. 7.17 Posterior view of the right deep gluteal region (gluteus medius m. has been resected). Path of the superior gluteal nerve and artery after pass superior to the piriformis muscle. (*1*) Superior gluteal nerve. (*2*) Superior gluteal artery. (*3*) Piriformis m. (*4*) Gluteus minimus m. (*5*) Sciatic nerve

Fig. 7.18 Posterior view of the right deep gluteal region (gluteus medius m. has been resected). Observe the location of sciatic nerve and its close relationship with the ischiatic tuberosity and the proximal origin of hamstrings. (*1*) Sciatic nerve. (*2*) Posterior femoral cutaneous nerve. (*3*) Piriform muscle. (*4*) Ischiatic tuberosity. (*5*) Proximal origin hamstrings

The superior gluteal nerve passes superior to the piriformis muscle. It courses with the superior gluteal artery between the gluteus medius and minimus muscles (see Fig. 7.17). At a variable distance from the greater sciatic notch, it divides into a superior and an inferior branch [44]. The superior branch accompanies the upper branch of the deep division of the superior gluteal artery and innervated the gluteus minimus muscle, gluteus medius muscle, and tensor fascia latae muscle. The inferior branch runs with the lower branch of the division of the superior gluteal artery across the gluteus minimus muscle and also innervates the gluteus medius muscle as well as the tensor fascia latae muscle.

The sciatic nerve exits the pelvis through the greater sciatic notch just inferior to the piriformis muscle and being covered by the gluteus maximus muscle. It passes between the ischial tuberosity and the greater trochanter lying close to the posterior capsule of the hip [45]. Miller et al. [46] performed a cadaveric study and concluded that the sciatic nerve is located at a mean distance of 1.2 ± 0.2 cm from the most lateral aspect of the ischial tuberosity, and it has an intimate relation with proximal origin of the hamstrings like the inferior gluteal nerve and artery (see Fig. 7.18).

The inferior gluteal nerve leaves the pelvis through the greater sciatic notch, just inferior to the piriformis muscle and medial regarding the sciatic nerve. After its pass inferior to the piriform muscle, it divides into different branches which pass posteriorly into the deep surface of the gluteus maximus muscle (the number of branches can vary from 3 to 7) [47]. Apaydin et al. [47] measured the mean distance between the closest branch to the greater trochanter and the greater trochanter, and the result was 0.8 cm (0–2.2 cm). Ling and Kumar [48] reported that the inferior gluteal nerve entered into the deep surface of the gluteus maximus muscles approximately at 5 cm from the tip of the greater trochanter of the femur, over the inferior one-third of the belly of the gluteus maximus muscle.

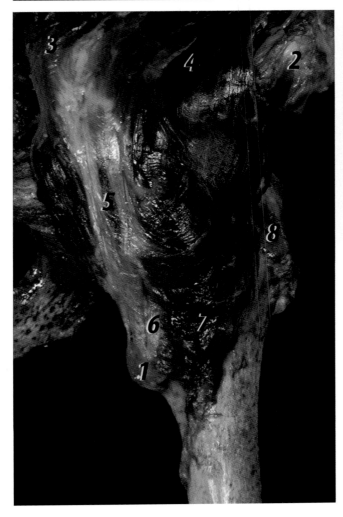

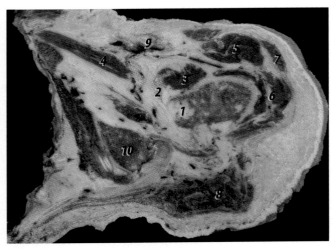

Fig. 7.20 Transverse cross section of a right hip joint at level of the lesser trochanter showing the attachment of the iliopsoas tendon on it. (*1*) Lesser trochanter. (*2*) Iliopsoas tendon. (*3*) Iliopsoas muscle. (*4*) Pectineus muscle. (*5*) Rectus femoris muscle. (*6*) Vastus lateralis muscle. (*7*) Tensor fasciae latae muscle. (*8*) Gluteus maximus muscle. (*9*) Femoral artery and nerve. (*10*) Ischiatic tuberosity

Fig. 7.19 Anterior view of a left iliopsoas muscle. Other muscles have been removed. Observe the attachment of the iliopsoas tendon into the lesser trochanter as well as its three components described by Tatu et al. [52]. (*1*) Lesser trochanter. (*2*) Anterior-inferior iliac spine. (*3*) Psoas major muscle. (*4*) Iliacus muscle. (*5*) Main tendon or psoas major tendon (split into two bundles). (*6*) Accessory tendon or iliac tendon. (*7*) Proper muscular fibers of the iliacus muscle. (*8*) Greater trochanter

Iliopsoas Tendon

The iliopsoas tendon is involved in the internal snapping hip syndrome caused by its slipping either over the femoral head, iliofemoral ligament, or iliopectineal ridge, or sometimes can be produced by anatomical variations like a bifid iliopsoas tendon [49, 50]. An endoscopic release of the iliopsoas tendon can be done at the level of the hip capsule or at its attachment in the lesser trochanter [51].

The iliopsoas tendon is formed by the confluence of the muscle bellies of the psoas major and iliacus muscles, being attached to the lesser trochanter. This tendon can be divided into three components: main tendon or psoas major tendon, accessory tendon or iliac tendon, and the proper fibers of the iliacus muscle [52] (Fig. 7.19):

- The psoas major tendon (main tendon) originates above the inguinal ligament. It is proximally oriented in a frontal plane, but it presents a rotation which transforms its anterior surface into a medial surface and its posterior surface into a lateral surface. After this rotation, the tendon spreads out and attaches into the lesser trochanter (Fig. 7.20). Sometimes, it can be partially split into two bundles (Fig. 7.19).
- The iliac tendon (accessory tendon) is located laterally to the psoas major tendon. While the most medial fibers of the iliacus muscle are joined with the main tendon, the most lateral fibers form an accessory tendon than it is attached to the lesser trochanter.
- The muscular fibers from the iliacus muscle, wich are not taking part in the accessory tendon, ended up on the anterior surface of the lesser trochanter and in the infratrochanteric area.
- Two important anatomical relationships of the iliopsoas tendon have to be considered for arthroscopic procedures in this area:
- The posterior surface of the iliopsoas muscle and tendon is in close contact with the anterior capsule of the hip. This close relationship allows to perform an iliopsoas tenotomy from the peripheral compartment of the hip (Fig. 7.21).
- Some branches from the femoral nerve are directly over the anterior surface of the iliopsoas muscle (Fig. 7.22). These branches are at risk when a release of the iliopsoas tendon is performed, although in a more distal position they are protected by the presence of the iliopsoas bursae and the vastus intermedius [51].

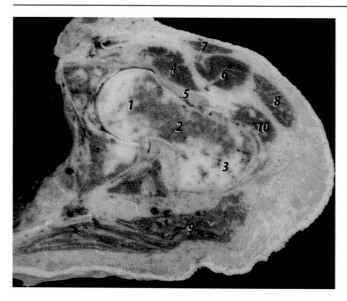

Fig. 7.21 Transverse cross section of a right hip at level of femoral neck showing the close relationship between the iliopsoas muscle and the anterior capsule of the hip. (*1*) Femoral head. (*2*) Femoral neck. (*3*) Greater trochanter. (*4*) Iliopsoas muscle. (*5*) Anterior capsule of the hip. (*6*) Rectus femoris muscle. (*7*) Sartorius muscle. (*8*) Tensor fasciae latae muscle. (*9*) Gluteus maximus muscle. (*10*) Gluteus medius muscle

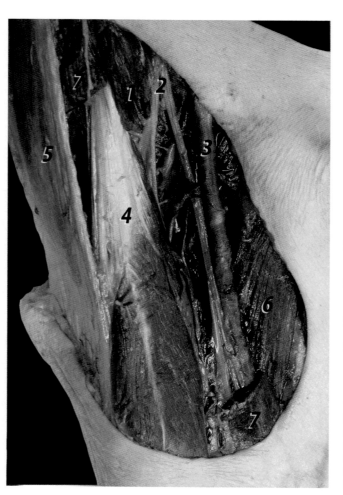

References

1. Birscher E. Die arthroendoskopie. Zbl Chir. 1921;48:1460–1.
2. Burman MS. Arthroscopy or the direct visualization of joints: an experimental cadaver study. J Bone Joint Surg. 1931;13:669–95.
3. Kim S-J, Choi N-H, Kim H-J. Operative hip arthroscopy. Clin Orthop. 1998;353:156–65.
4. Dvorak M, Duncan CP, Day B. Arthroscopic anatomy of the hip. Arthroscopy. 1990;6:264–73.
5. Dorfmann H, Boyer T. Hip arthroscopy utilizing the supine position. Arthroscopy. 1996;12:264–7.
6. Dorfmann H, Boyer T. Arthroscopy of the hip: 12 years of experience. Arthroscopy. 1999;15:67–72.
7. Wiese M, Rubenthaler F. Early results of endoscopic trochanter bursectomy. Int Orthop. 2004;28:218–21.
8. Voos JE, Rudzki JR, Shindle MK, et al. Arthroscopic anatomy and surgical techniques for peritrochanteric space disorders in the hip. Arthroscopy. 2007;23:1246.e1–e5.
9. Robertson WJ, Kelly BT. The safe zone for hip arthroscopy: a cadaveric assessment of central, peripheral, and lateral compartment portal placement. Arthroscopy. 2008;24:1019–26.
10. Ilizaliturri Jr VM, Martinez-Escalante FA, Chaidez PA, et al. Endoscopic iliotibial band release for external snapping hip syndrome. Arthroscopy. 2006;22:505–10.
11. Cerezal L, Kassarjian A, Canga A, et al. Anatomy, biomechanics, imaging, and management of ligamentum teres injuries. Radiographics. 2010;30:1637–51.
12. Rao J, Zhou YX, Villar RN. Injury to the ligamentum teres: mechanism, findings, and results of treatment. Clin Sports Med. 2001;20:791–9.
13. Bardakos NV, Villar RN. The ligamentum teres of the adult hip. J Bone Joint Surg Br. 2009;91:8–15.
14. Testut L, Latarjet A. Anatomía humana. 4th ed. Barcelona: Salvat editores SA; 1990. p. 660–76.
15. Chandler SB, Kreuscher PH. A study of the blood supply of the ligamentum teres and its relation to the circulation of the head of the femur. J Bone Joint Surg. 1932;14:834–46.
16. Lavigne M, Kalhor M, Beck M, et al. Distribution of vascular foramina around the femoral head and neck junction: relevance for conservative intracapsular procedures of the hip. Orthop Clin North Am. 2005;36:171–6.
17. Gautier E, Ganz K, Krugel N, et al. Anatomy of the medial femoral circumflex artery and its surgical implications. J Bone Joint Surg Br. 2000;82:679–83.
18. Carliouz H, Pous JG, Rey JC. Les epiphysiolyses femorales superrieures. Rev Chir Orthop Reparatice Appar Mot. 1968;54:388–481.
19. Kapandji AI. Fisiología articular. Miembro inferior. 5th ed. Buenos Aires: Editorial Médica Panamericana; 1998. p. 14–72.
20. Feugier P, Fessy MH, Bejui J, et al. Acetabular anatomy and the relationship with pelvic vascular structures. Surg Radiol Anat. 1997;19:85–90.
21. Fernández-Fairén M. Biomecánica de la cadera. In: Viladot A, editor. Lecciones básicas de biomecánica del aparato locomotor. 1st ed. Barcelona: Springer; 2001. p. 185–96.
22. Govsa F, Ozer MA, Ozgur Z. Morphologic features of the acetabulum. Arch Orthop Trauma Surg. 2005;125:453–61.
23. Gupta V, Choudhry R, Tuli A, et al. Unusual facets on the acetabulum in dry adult human coxal bones: a morphological and radiological study. Surg Radiol Anat. 2001;23:263–7.

Fig. 7.22 Anterior view of a femoral triangle. Observe the relationship between the branches of the femoral nerve and the iliopsoas muscle. The sartorius muscle has been partially removed. (*1*) Iliopsoas muscle. (*2*) Femoral nerve. (*3*) Femoral artery. (*4*) Rectus femoris muscle. (*5*) Tensor fasciae latae muscle. (*6*) Pectineus muscle. (*7*) Sartorius muscle

24. Sampatchalit S, Barbosa D, Gentili A, et al. Degenerative changes in the ligamentum teres of the hip: cadaveric study with magnetic resonance arthrography, anatomical inspection, and histologic examination. J Comput Assist Tomogr. 2009;33:927–33.

25. Chen HH, Li AF, Li KC, et al. Adaptations of ligamentum teres in ischemic necrosis of human femoral head. Clin Orthop Relat Res. 1996;328:268–75.

26. Demange MK, Kakuda CM, Pereira CA, et al. Influence of the femoral head ligament on hip mechanical function. Acta Orthop Bras. 2007;15:187–90.

27. Leunig M, Beck M, Stauffer E, et al. Free nerve endings in the ligamentum capitis femoris. Acta Orthop Scand. 2000;71:452–4.

28. Gray AJ, Villar RN. The ligamentum teres of the hip: an arthroscopic classification of its pathology. Arthroscopy. 1997;13:575–8.

29. Lecouvet F, Vande Berg BC, Malghem J, et al. MR imaging of the acetabular labrum: variations in 200 asymptomatic hips. AJR. 1996;167:1025–8.

30. Won Y-Y, Chung I-H, Chung N-S, et al. Morphological study on the acetabular labrum. Yonsei Med J. 2003;44:855–62.

31. Ferguson SJ, Bryant JT, Ganz R, et al. The influence of the acetabular labrum on hip joint cartilage consolidation: a poroelastic finite element model. J Biomech. 2000;33:953–60.

32. Ferguson SJ, Bryant JT, Ganz R, et al. The acetabular labrum seal: a poroelastic finite element model. Clin Biomech. 2000;15:463–8.

33. Kalhor M, Beck M, Huff TW, et al. Capsular and pericapsular contributions to acetabular and femoral head perfusion. J Bone Joint Surg Am. 2009;91:409–18.

34. Beck M, Leunig M, Ellis T, et al. The acetabular blood supply: implications for periacetabular osteotomies. Surg Radiol Anat. 2003;25:361–7.

35. Martin HD, Savage A, Braly BA, et al. The function of the hip capsular ligaments: a quantitative report. Arthroscopy. 2008;24:188–95.

36. Hewitt JD, Glisson RR, Guilak F, et al. The mechanical properties of the human hip capsule ligaments. J Arthroplasty. 2002;17:82–9.

37. Fu Z, Peng M, Peng Q. Anatomical study of the synovial plicae of the hip joint. Clin Anat. 1997;10:235–8.

38. Dienst M, Gödde S, Seil R, et al. Hip arthroscopy without traction: in vivo anatomy of the peripheral hip joint cavity. Arthroscopy. 2001;17:924–31.

39. Beck M, Sledge JB, Gautier E, et al. The anatomy and function of the gluteus minimus muscle. J Bone Joint Surg Br. 2000;82:358–63.

40. Gottschalk F, Kourosh S, Leveau B. The functional anatomy of tensor fasciae latae and gluteus medius and minimus. J Anat. 1989;166:179–89.

41. Pfirrmann CWA, Chung CB, Theumann NH, et al. Greater trochanter of the hip. Attachment of the abductor mechanism and a complex of three bursae – MR imaging and MR bursography in cadavers and MR imaging in asymptomatic volunteers. Radiology. 2001;221:469–77.

42. Bywaters EGL. The bursae of the body. Ann Rheum Dis. 1965;24:215–8.

43. Duparc F, Thomine JM, Dujardin F, et al. Anatomic basis of the transgluteal approach to the hip-joint by anterior hemimyotomy of the gluteus medius. Surg Radiol Anat. 1997;19:61–7.

44. Lavigne P, de Loriot Rouvray TH. The superior gluteal nerve. Anatomical study of its extrapelvic portion and surgical resolution by trans-gluteal approach. Rev Chir Orthop Reparatrice Appar Mot. 1994;80:188–95.

45. Martin HD, Shears SA, Johnson JC, et al. The endoscopic treatment of sciatic nerve entrapment/deep gluteal syndrome. Arthroscopy. 2011;27:172–81.

46. Miller SL, Gill J, Webb GR. The proximal origin of the hamstrings and surrounding anatomy encountered during repair. A cadaveric study. J Bone Joint Surg Am. 2007;89:44–8.

47. Apaydin N, Bozkurt M, Loukas M, et al. The course of the inferior gluteal nerve and surgical landmarks for its localization during posterior approaches to hip. Surg Radiol Anat. 2009;31:415–8.

48. Ling ZX, Kumar VP. The course of the inferior gluteal nerve in the posterior approach to the hip. J Bone Joint Surg Br. 2006;88:1580–3.

49. Shu B, Safran MR. Bifid iliopsoas tendon causing refractory internal snapping hip. Clin Orthop Relat Res. 2011;469:289–93.

50. Deslandes M, Guillin R, Cardinal E, et al. The snapping iliopsoas tendon: new mechanisms using dynamic sonography. AJR Am J Roentgenol. 2008;190:576–81.

51. Ilizaliturri VM, Villalobos FE, Chaidez PA, et al. Internal snapping hip syndrome: treatment by endoscopic release of the iliopsoas tendon. Arthroscopy. 2005;11:1375–80.

52. Tatu L, Parratte B, Vuillier F, et al. Descriptive anatomy of the femoral portion of the iliopsoas muscle. Anatomical basis of anterior snapping of the hip. Surg Radiol Anat. 2001;23:371–4.

Portal Anatomy

8

Oscar Fariñas Barberá and Ivan Sáenz Navarro

The improvement of the arthroscopic equipment and the technical development have allowed surgeons to carry out diagnoses and arthroscopic treatments that were performed using open procedures since that moment.

The constant description of new techniques requires a precise knowledge of the hip anatomy and common portal placement. In spite of that, the major part of complications described in the literature [1–5] is related to the distraction of the joint and patient positioning (transient neuropraxia of the pudendal, sciatic, and perineal nerves, abdominal pain, perineal hematoma, etc.); some of them are directly connected with portal establishment (extravasation of fluids, iatrogenic labral and chondral damage, dysesthesias of the lateral femoral cutaneous nerve, etc.). The reported complication rates associated with hip arthroscopy range from 0.5% to 6.4% [1–5]. Byrd in a combined review of 1,491 cases reported only one permanent nerve injury [6]. The most common iatrogenic injuries related to portal placement are the labrum, which is susceptible to perforation, and the chondral surface, which can be scratched by the instrumentation [7].

In addition to the anatomical characteristics of the hip joint (anatomical constraints, capsular reinforcements, peritrochanteric space, etc.), two specific details have been taken into account:

- The depth of the hip joint acts as a limiting factor to access the articular space [8, 9], and for this reason, a special instrumentation is needed. Monllau et al. [10] performed a tomographic study of the most common

approaches to the hip joint analyzing the needed depth to reach the joint or surrounding structures. They conclude that the average distance for the anterolateral portal to the joint was 11.26 cm, 9.8 cm for the anterior portal, and 12.41 cm for the posterolateral (paratrochanteric) portal. This depth distance multiplies the risk of iatrogenic damage due to the increased number of anatomical structures that are crossed during portal establishment.

- In comparison to most of the joints where arthroscopic procedures are performed (wrist, shoulder, knee) in the hip arthroscopy, there are significant neurovascular structures at risk in both anterior and posterior aspects (femoral nerve, lateral femoral cutaneous nerve, lateral femoral circumflex artery, superior gluteal nerve, etc.) (Table 8.1).

The portal placement and structures at risk of the most common portals used to access the different hip arthroscopic compartments (central, peripheral, and peritrochanteric) are described.

Central Compartment

The most common portals used to access the central compartment are the anterolateral portal, anterior portal, and posterolateral portal (see Fig. 8.1). Other accessory portals have been described in the literature: mid-anterior portal [11] and distal accessory lateral portal [12].

Anterolateral Portal

This portal, also named anterior paratrochanteric portal, is located most centrally in the "safe zone" for arthroscopy [13] and usually is the first portal to be established under image intensifier control (Table 8.2).

The anterolateral portal is placed directly over the superior margin of the greater trochanter at its anterior border

O. Fariñas Barberá, M.D. (✉)
Transplant Services Foundation, Musculoskeletal Tissue Unit,
Dr. Antoni Pujadas, 42, Sant Boi de Llobregat,
Barcelona 08031, Spain
e-mail: obarbera@clinic.ub.es

I. Sáenz Navarro, M.D.
Department of Human Anatomy and Embriology,
Facultat de Medicina,
C/Casanova 143, Barcelona, Spain
e-mail: ivansaenzn@hotmail.com

J.W.T. Byrd (ed.), *Operative Hip Arthroscopy*,
DOI 10.1007/978-1-4419-7925-4_8, © Springer Science+Business Media New York 2013

Table 8.1 Structures at risk during placement of hip portals

Portal	Structures at risk
Anterolateral portal	Superior gluteal nerve
	Acetabular labrum
	Articular cartilage
Posterolateral portal	Sciatic nerve
	Deep branch of the medial femoral circumflex artery
	Acetabular labrum
	Articular cartilage
Anterior portal	Lateral femoral cutaneous nerve
	Femoral nerve
	Ascending branch of the lateral femoral circumflex artery
Mid-anterior portal	Lateral femoral cutaneous nerve
	Ascending branch of the lateral femoral circumflex artery
	Femoral nerve
Mid-anterolateral portal	Lateral femoral cutaneous nerve
	Femoral nerve
	Ascending branch of the lateral femoral circumflex artery
Distal lateral accessory portal	Lateral femoral cutaneous nerve
	Ascending branch of the lateral femoral circumflex artery
Accessory anterolateral portal	Transverse branch of the lateral femoral circumflex artery
Superolateral portal	Superior gluteal nerve
Distal anterolateral accessory portal	Transverse branch of the lateral femoral circumflex artery
Auxiliary posterolateral portal	Superior gluteal nerve

Table 8.2 Anterolateral portal summary

Placement	1 cm anterior and 1 cm superior to the tip of the greater trochanter
Pathway	Medial or through the tensor fascia lata muscle. It penetrates the gluteus medius muscle
Structures at risk	Superior gluteal nerve and artery (average distance of 4.4–6.4 cm) [11, 13]
	Acetabular labrum and articular cartilage (can be avoided accessing from the peripheral compartment) [22, 23]
Comments	Commonly accepted as the first portal to be established
	A more superior portal has been described [14]

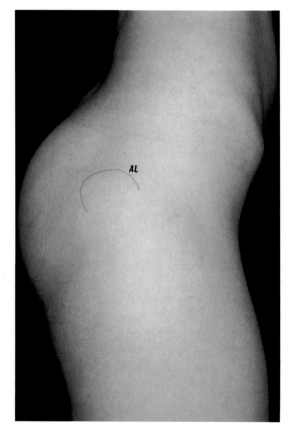

Fig. 8.2 Lateral view of a right hip showing the topographic placement of the anterolateral portal over the superior margin of the greater trochanter at its anterior border. (1) Greater trochanter (delimited by a *black line*), *AL* anterolateral portal

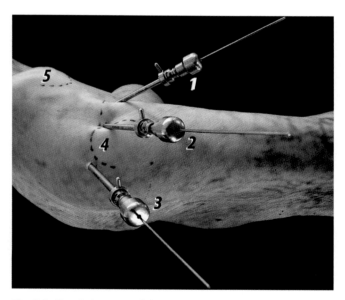

Fig. 8.1 Portal placement of the most common hip arthroscopy portals on a right hip. The anterolateral portal is placed 1 cm superior and 1 cm anterior to the tip of the greater trochanter. The posterolateral portal is placed 1 cm superior and 1 cm posterior to the tip of the greater trochanter. The anterior portal is placed at the intersection of a vertical line descending from the anterior-superior iliac spine and a horizontal line from the tip of the greater trochanter. (*1*) Anterior portal, (*2*) anterolateral portal, (*3*) posterolateral portal, (*4*) greater trochanter, (*5*) anterior-superior iliac spine

[14] although other authors place it 1 cm superior and 1 cm anterior to the tip of the greater trochanter [15] (see Fig. 8.2). From this point, it passes just medial or through the tensor fascia lata muscle, and afterward, it penetrates the gluteus medius muscle to reach the lateral aspect of the capsule at its anterior margin [13]. We must assure a neutral rotation of the hip in order to place the cannula directly to the femoral head due to its anteversed position [14].

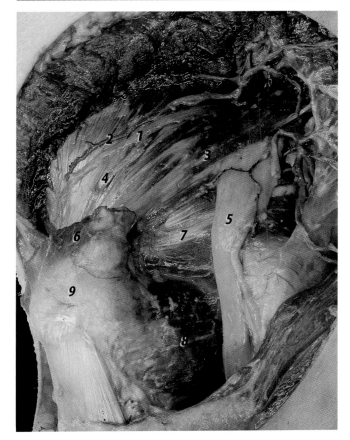

Fig. 8.3 Posterior view of a left hip showing the superior gluteal nerve and artery path (the gluteus maximus and medius muscles have been resected). (*1*) Superior gluteal nerve, (*2*) superior gluteal artery, (*3*) piriformis m., (*4*) gluteus minimus m., (*5*) sciatic nerve, (*6*) gluteus medius m., (*7*) obturator internus m., (*8*) quadratus femoris m., (*9*) greater trochanter

The structures at risk during anterolateral portal placement are the acetabular labrum and articular cartilage, as well as the superior gluteal nerve. In spite of the risk of lesion of these structures, this portal is the safest with respect to neurovascular bundles medially and posteriorly [13].

The superior gluteal nerve exits the pelvis through the greater sciatic foramen (sciatic notch), just superior to the piriformis muscle (sometimes the superior gluteal nerve can perforate the piriformis muscle [16], with the superior gluteal vascular pedicle). It runs horizontal, from posterior to anterior, between the gluteus medius and minimus muscles, to terminate into the tensor fascia lata (supplying all of them) (see Fig. 8.3). The superior gluteal nerve is divided into several branches that usually are two (superior and inferior), although some authors described three branches [17, 18]. The inferior branch is thicker than superior one, and it supplies the tensor fascia lata muscle.

The average distance of the superior gluteal nerve to the anterolateral portal varies from 4.4 to 6.4 cm (range 3.2–8.1 cm) depending on the authors [11, 13]. The tip of the

Table 8.3 Posterolateral portal summary

Placement	1 cm superior and 1 cm posterior to the tip of the greater trochanter
Pathway	It penetrates the gluteus maximus, medius, and minimus muscles
	It is placed superior and anterior to the piriformis muscle
Structures at risk	Sciatic nerve (average distance of 21.8–30 mm) [11, 13, 27]
	Deep branch of the medial circumflex artery [12]
	Acetabular labrum and articular cartilage (can be avoided accessing from the peripheral compartment or placing the portal as far as possible from the acetabular margin)
Comments	Used as the first portal to be established by some authors [26]
	Avoid the external rotation and flexion of the hip [13, 27, 33]

greater trochanter can act as a landmark to determine the position of the superior gluteal nerve. Different authors have measured the distance between both structures obtaining average distances of 51.25, 45, and 30 mm (range 10–65 mm) [19–21]. For this reason, the "safe zone" should be considered 2–3 cm from the tip of the greater trochanter [22].

The acetabular labrum and articular cartilage of the femoral head are also structures at risk of injury during portal placement to the central compartment of the hip. Despite the description of current techniques to avoid the lesion of these structures [7], sometimes it is unavoidable. One alternative, with significantly fewer potential risks, is to establish the anterolateral portal to the peripheral compartment being directed to the transition of the anterior femoral head and femoral neck [23, 24]. At this point, the femoral head is free of cartilage, the acetabular labrum is located proximally at 2–3 cm, and the capsule is separated from the neck [25].

A more superior portal has been described [26], but it presents a higher risk of lesion of the superior gluteal nerve, and it can have some access limitations due to the presence of the lateral acetabular rim.

Dorfmann et al. [27] also described a variation of anterolateral portal that was placed midway on a line connecting the anterior-superior iliac spine and the anterior-superior corner of the greater trochanter.

Posterolateral Portal

This portal, also named posterior paratrochanteric portal, is the first to be established by some authors [28] (Table 8.3).

The posterolateral portal is placed similar to the anterolateral portal except at the posterior margin of the greater trochanter [14] although other authors move it 1 cm superior and 1 cm posterior to the tip of the greater trochanter [15]

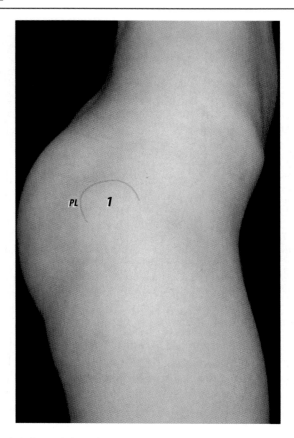

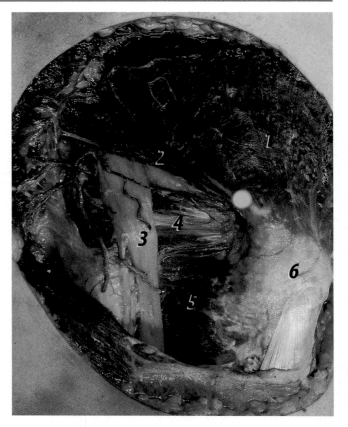

Fig. 8.4 Lateral view of a right hip showing the topographic placement of the posterolateral portal over the superior margin of the greater trochanter at its posterior border. (*1*) Greater trochanter (delimited by a *black line*), *PL* posterolateral portal

Fig. 8.5 Right gluteal region showing the posterolateral portal placement (*blue dot*). The gluteus maximus muscle has been resected. (*1*) Gluteus medius m., (*2*) piriformis m., (*3*) sciatic nerve, (*4*) obturator internus m., (*5*) quadratus femoris m., (*6*) greater trochanter

(see Fig. 8.4). From this point, it penetrates the gluteus maximus, medius, and minimus muscles to reach the lateral capsule at its posterior margin [13] (see Fig. 8.5). The piriformis muscle is placed inferior and posterior to the portal pathway (see Fig. 8.6). The orientation of the cannula is 5° cephalad and 5° anterior in a neutral position of the hip.

The structures at risk during posterolateral portal placement are the acetabular labrum and articular cartilage, as well as the sciatic nerve and the deep branch of the medial circumflex artery.

The distance of the sciatic nerve to the posterolateral portal have been studied by different authors reporting an average measurement of 21.8 mm (range 11–38 mm) [11], 29 mm (range 20–43 mm) [13], and 30 mm [29] (see Fig. 8.5).

The deep branch of the medial circumflex artery is the most responsible for femoral head and neck vascularization [30] (see Chap. 5 for description). Sussmann et al. [31] reported that the deep branch of the medial circumflex artery lies at a mean distance of 10.1 mm from the posterolateral portal when it passes close to the piriformis tendon, and emphasized the role of the posterior bony border of the greater trochanter as a safe landmark at the moment of portal

placement in order to avoid the lesion of this artery. Special attention to the terminal branches of this artery (lateral retinacular vessels) that perforate the joint capsule and run along the posterior and lateral aspects of the femoral neck (see Fig. 8.7) is given. These lateral retinacular vessels can be injured during posterolateral portal establishment at level of the head-neck junction [32, 33].

In the same way that establishing anterolateral portal, the acetabular labrum and articular cartilage of the femoral head are at risk of injury during posterolateral portal placement. One solution could be to establish the posterolateral portal from the peripheral compartment or to ensure the portal is as far distal to the acetabular margin as possible without damaging the femoral head [28].

This portal appears to be safe but some considerations must be taken into account about patient positioning:

- Some authors suggested that, in order to relax the capsule and to make easy the distraction of the joint, a slight flexion of the hip can be performed [34]. This maneuver will also place the sciatic nerve in a more tensioned position, being closer to the posterior aspect of the hip joint and increasing its risk of injury [13].

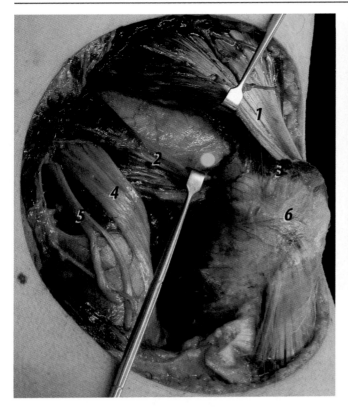

Fig. 8.6 Posterior view of a right deep gluteal region. The gluteus minimus and piriformis muscles have been retracted. Observe the placement of the posterolateral portal at level of the posterior hip capsule (*blue dot*) and its relationship with the piriformis muscle. (*1*) Gluteus minimus m., (*2*) piriformis m., (*3*) gluteus medius m. (resected), (*4*) sciatic nerve, (*5*) posterior femoral cutaneous nerve, (*6*) greater trochanter

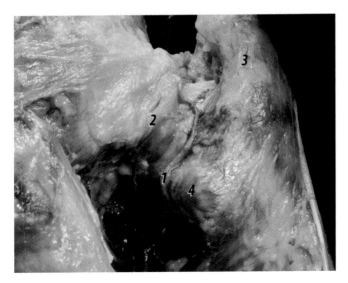

Fig. 8.7 Posterior view of a right hip joint (most of the muscles have been resected). Observe the path of the deep branch of the medial circumflex artery and its close relationship with the posterior and lateral capsule where the artery arises to the lateral retinacular vessels. (*1*) Deep branch of the medial circumflex artery, (*2*) posterior capsule, (*3*) greater trochanter, (*4*) lesser trochanter

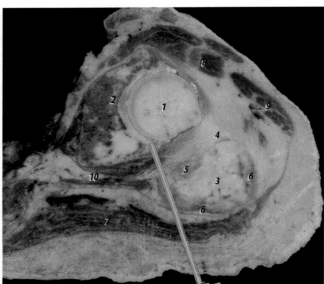

Fig. 8.8 Transverse cross section of a right hip joint. Observe the approximate relationship between the posterolateral portal and the sciatic nerve. If the hip is placed in external rotation, the posterior border of the greater trochanter goes closer to the sciatic nerve. (*1*) Femoral head, (*2*) acetabulum, (*3*) greater trochanter, (*4*) gluteus minimus tendon, (*5*) piriformis tendon, (*6*) gluteus medius tendon, (*7*) gluteus maximus m., (*8*) rectus femoris m., (*9*) tensor fascia lata m., (*10*) sciatic nerve

- External rotation must be avoided before the posterolateral portal establishment because it will move the greater trochanter more posteriorly. This position will place the sciatic nerve at a significant risk of lesion [13, 27, 28] (see Fig. 8.8).

Anterior Portal

The anterior portal is typically placed at the intersection of a vertical line descending from the anterior-superior iliac spine and a horizontal line from the tip of the greater trochanter to the previously mentioned line [35] (see Fig. 8.9) (Table 8.4). This position lies an average distance of 6.3 cm distal to the anterior-superior iliac spine [13]. The cannula must be directed approximately 45° cephalad and 30° toward the midline [14]. Some slight variations of the anterior portal placement have been described by different authors (see Fig. 8.9): 1 cm lateral and 1 cm distal from the intersection of a sagittal line drawn down the middle of the anterior thigh and a transverse line drawn from the tip of the greater trochanter to the superior aspect of the pubic bone [29], 1 cm lateral to the anterior-superior iliac spine and in line with the anterolateral portal [11], or 4–6 cm distal to the anterior-superior iliac spine [25].

The portal placement needs the aid of direct visualization from the anterolateral portal due to the possibility of presence

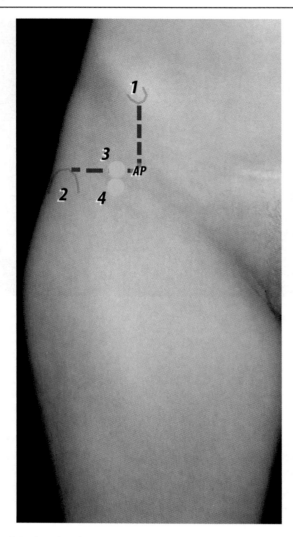

Table 8.4 Anterior portal summary

Placement	Intersection of a vertical line descending from the anterior-superior iliac spine and a horizontal line from the tip of the greater trochanter to the previously mentioned line [34]
	Placed under direct arthroscopic visualization
Pathway	It passes through the interval between the gluteus minimus and rectus femoris muscles before reaching the anterior capsule
	It can penetrates the sartorius or tensor fascia lata depending on a more medial or lateral establishment
Structures at risk	Lateral femoral cutaneous nerve (average distance of 3 mm [13], 15.4 mm [11])
	Femoral nerve (average distance of 32 mm [13])
	Ascending branch of the lateral circumflex artery (average distance 31–37 mm [11, 13])
Comments	Best way to avoid the lesion of the lateral femoral cutaneous nerve is to apply a blunt dissection during portal establishment
	Minor blood supply of the lateral femoral circumflex artery to the head and neck of the femur

Fig. 8.9 Anterior view of right hip showing the common placement of the anterior portal. The cannula must be oriented 35° cephalad and 35° posterior. Two portal establishment variants are marked (*blue dots*). (*1*) Anterior-superior iliac spine, (*2*) greater trochanter, (*3*) variant by Robertson et al. [11], (*4*) variant by Bond et al. [29]

of anatomical variations. Ilizaliturri et al. [35] described a guide to assist the anterior portal establishment using the common anatomical landmarks and a reference point inside the hip joint (anterior capsule of the joint where the entrance of the anterior portal is preferred).

From its point of entrance, the anterior portal passed through the interval between the gluteus minimus and rectus femoris muscles before entering the joint through the anterior capsule (see Figs. 8.10 and 8.11). Depending on variations of its placement, more medial or lateral, it also penetrates the tensor fascia lata muscle (laterally) [11] or the sartorius and rectus femoris muscles (medially) [13].

The structures at risk during anterior portal placement are the lateral femoral cutaneous nerve, femoral nerve, and the ascending branch of the lateral circumflex artery. Glick et al.

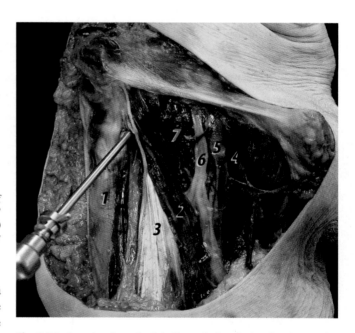

Fig. 8.10 Anterior view of a right femoral triangle showing the anterior portal placement. Observe the portal is located just lateral to the rectus femoris muscle and between the sartorius and tensor fascia lata muscles. (*1*) Tensor fascia lata m., (*2*) sartorius m., (*3*) rectus femoris m., (*4*) femoral vein, (*5*) femoral artery, (*6*) femoral nerve, (*7*) iliopsoas m.

[36] recommend to palpate and mark the femoral artery prior to positioning and draping the patient in order to avoid its injury.

The lateral femoral cutaneous nerve exits the pelvis, under the inguinal ligament, through an opening medial to the anterior-superior iliac spine at an average distance of 6–73 mm from it [37]. Once in the thigh, it turns laterally and downward

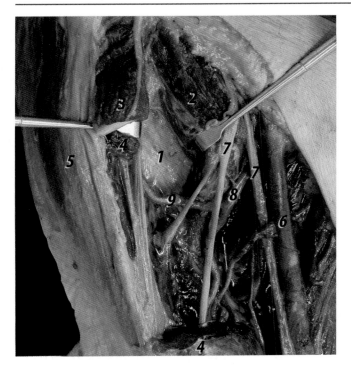

Fig. 8.11 Anterior view of a right hip showing the anterior capsule. The sartorius and rectus femoris muscles have been resected. (*1*) Anterior capsule, (*2*) iliopsoas m., (*3*) sartorius m., (*4*) rectus femoris m., (*5*) tensor fascia lata m., (*6*) femoral artery, (*7*) femoral nerve branches, (*8*) lateral circumflex artery, (*9*) ascendant branch of the lateral circumflex artery

to be divided mainly into anterior and posterior nerves over the sartorius muscle approximately at 5 cm inferior to the anterior-superior iliac spine. These branches crossed the lateral border of the sartorius ranged from 2.2 to 11.3 cm inferior to the anterior-superior iliac spine [37]. The function of the posterior branches is to innervate the skin from the level of the greater trochanter to the middle of the thigh, whereas the anterior branches divided into lateral and medial segments to descend subcutaneously reaching the knee (see Fig. 8.12).

In opposite to the consistent course of the lateral femoral cutaneous nerve, its branching pattern varies extremely. The number of branches varies from 0 to 5, being the most frequent numbers of 2–3 branches [11, 13, 37]. This great variability represents an increased risk of injury of this nerve (mainly its medial branches) during the anterior portal establishment.

Byrd et al. [13] reported the anterior portal pierces the sartorius muscle close to the lateral femoral cutaneous nerve branching site and passes approximately 3 mm medial to its most medial branch [2, 10, 13, 15]. Robertson et al. [11] reported an average distance 15.4 mm (range 1–28 mm) of the anterior portal to the lateral femoral cutaneous nerve.

Different alternatives have been proposed to decrease the risk of lesion of the lateral femoral cutaneous nerve. Robertson et al. [11] routinely place the anterior portal 1 cm

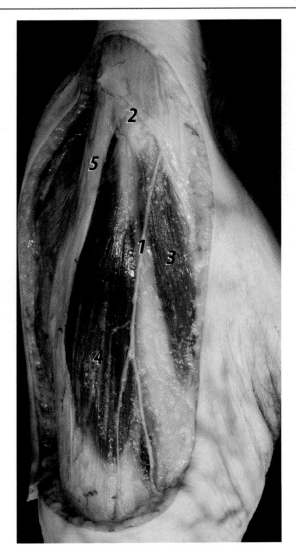

Fig. 8.12 Anterior view of a right hip showing the course of the lateral femoral cutaneous nerve. Take special attention into its relationship with the anterior-superior iliac spine and the point it crosses the lateral border of the sartorius muscle. (*1*) Lateral femoral cutaneous nerve, (*2*) anterior-superior iliac spine, (*3*) sartorius m., (*4*) rectus femoris m., (*5*) tensor fascia lata m.

lateral to its traditional placement, and for this reason, the mean distance to the lateral femoral cutaneous nerve branches increased to 15 mm. Byrd et al. [13] stated this lateral displacement of the anterior portal does not avoid the lateral femoral cutaneous nerve because of the variability on the number of branches and the broad area covered by them. The best way to minimize the risk of lesion is to apply a proper technique like blunt dissection of the subcutaneous tissue with a hemostat.

The femoral nerve after its pass under the inguinal ligament is located into the femoral triangle, lateral to the femoral artery (separated by a portion of iliopsoas muscle). At this point, it splits into an anterior and posterior division.

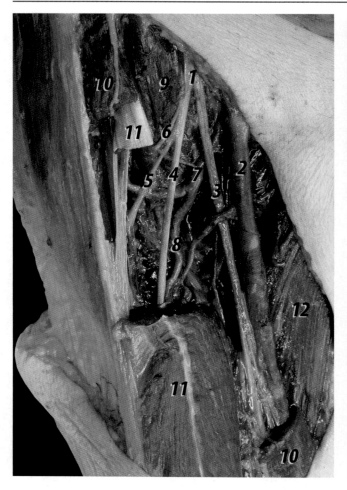

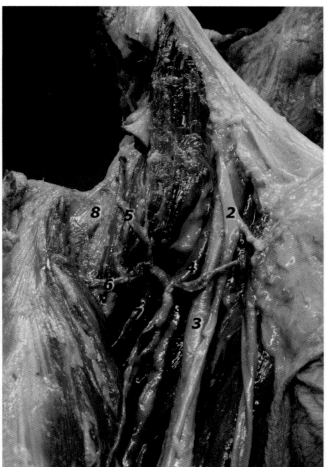

Fig. 8.13 Anterior view of a right femoral triangle showing the different branches of the femoral nerve and its relationships with the surrounding structures. The rectus femoris and sartorius muscles have been partially resected. (*1*) Femoral nerve, (*2*) femoral artery, (*3*) saphenous nerve and muscular branch to the vastus medialis m., (*4*) muscular branch to the vastus lateralis m., (*5*) muscular branch to the rectus femoris m., (*6*) muscular branch to the sartorius m., (*7*) lateral femoral circumflex artery, (*8*) descending branch of the lateral femoral circumflex artery, (*9*) iliopsoas m., (*10*) sartorius m., (*11*) rectus femoris m., (*12*) pectineus m.

Fig. 8.14 Anterior view of the femoral neck showing the distribution of the different branches of the lateral femoral circumflex artery (LFCA) (*right hip*). (*1*) Iliopsoas m., (*2*) femoral nerve (resected), (*3*) femoral artery, (*4*) deep femoral artery, (*5*) ascending branch of the LFCA, (*6*) transverse branch of the LFCA, (*7*) descending branch of the LFCA, (*8*) anterior capsule

The anterior division gives off different cutaneous branches (medial, intermediate, and lateral cutaneous nerves) as well as muscular branches to pectineus and sartorius muscles.

The posterior division of the femoral nerve mainly gives origin to the muscular branches to the four components of the quadriceps femoris muscle and the saphenous nerve that accompanies the femoral artery along the thigh and terminates into the foot. The muscular branch to the rectus femoris muscle enters the upper part of the deep surface of the muscle, supplying a filament to the hip joint. The muscular branch to the vastus lateralis muscle is located next to the descending branch of the lateral circumflex artery along the thigh. The muscular branch to the vastus medialis muscle runs with the saphenous nerve and femoral artery until the middle of the thigh where it enters the muscle (see Fig. 8.13).

Byrd et al. [13] measured the distance from the anterior portal to the lateral border of the femoral nerve. The peculiarity of this measurement was that performed at three levels (sartorius muscle, rectus femoris muscle, and capsule) because the distance varied depending on the level of depth. The minimum distance of these three measurements averaged 32 mm (range 27–50 mm) being slightly closer at the capsular level (average distance of 37 mm). Robertson et al. [11] performed the same measurement obtaining similar results at the capsular level but higher distances at sartorius and rectus femoris muscle levels due to the 1-cm lateral displacement of the anterior portal point of entry.

The lateral femoral circumflex artery arises from the lateral side of the deep femoral artery most of the cases. From this point, it goes to a lateral position just behind the sartorius and rectus femoris muscles and between the divisions of the femoral nerve. At this level, it gives origin to the ascending, transverse, and descending branches (see Fig. 8.14).

Table 8.5 Other portals to the central compartment

Mid-anterior portal	
Placement	Distal vertex of an equilateral triangle formed with the anterior and anterolateral portal
Pathway	It penetrates the tensor fascia lata and passes between the gluteus minimus and rectus femoris muscles
Structures at risk	Lateral femoral cutaneous nerve (average distance 25.2 mm [11])
	Terminal branches of the ascending branch of the lateral femoral circumflex artery (average distance 10.1 mm [11])
	Femoral nerve at capsular level (average distance 39.9 mm [11])
Comments	A proximal mid-anterior can be placed proximally
Mid-anterolateral portal	
Placement	Halfway between the anterior and anterolateral portals, about 2 cm distal to a line connecting both portals
Pathway	It penetrates the tensor fascia lata and gluteus medius muscles
Structures at risk	Same that anterior and anterolateral portals
Distal lateral accessory portal	
Placement	1 cm anterior and 4 cm distal to the anterolateral portal
Pathway	It penetrates the tensor fascia lata muscle and the capsule at the orbicularis zone
Structures at risk	Lateral femoral cutaneous nerve and the ascending branch of the lateral femoral circumflex artery

Commonly the ascending and transverse branches have a common conduit and subsequently divide with the ascending branch supplying the vastus lateralis, tensor fascia lata, and minor gluteal muscles. Finally, the lateral circumflex artery surrounds the vastus lateralis muscle and anastomoses with the deep branch of the medial femoral circumflex artery.

The ascending branch of the lateral circumflex artery is located at a mean distance of 89 mm (range 75–115 mm) distal to the anterior-superior iliac spine on the line drawn from this bone landmark to the lateral border of the patella [38–40].

The anterior portal lies proximal to the artery at a mean distance of 31–37 mm (range 10–60 mm) depending on authors [11, 13]. Sometimes a small terminal branch can be identified that extends proximally toward the anterior portal placement. The variability on the presence and course of this terminal branch of ascending branch of the lateral femoral circumflex artery produces divergences in the measurements obtained by Byrd et al. [13] where the distance to the anterior portal was 2–4 mm and Robertson et al. [11] where the distance was 2–33 mm, although the authors coincide in the closest distance.

In addition to the relatively safe position of the ascending branch of the lateral femoral circumflex artery, we have to take into account that the role of this artery in the femoral head and neck vascularization is less important than the medial femoral circumflex artery [41].

Other Portals to the Central Compartment

The mid-anterior portal is placed drawing an equilateral triangle with the anterior and anterolateral portal (one portal on each vertex of the triangle), being the new portal placed distally to the previous ones (Table 8.5). The insertion angle approximate is 35° cephalad and 25° posterior [11]. If the same process is repeated proximally, the new placement corresponds to the proximal mid-anterior portal (see Fig. 8.15). The mid-anterior portal penetrates the tensor fascia lata muscle and passes through the interval between the gluteus minimus and rectus femoris muscles. The major structures at risk during portal placement are the lateral femoral cutaneous nerve at a mean distance of 25.2 mm (range 9–38 mm) and the ascending branch of the lateral femoral circumflex artery at a mean distance of 19.2 mm (range 5–42 mm) although its terminal branches are closer (average distance 10.1 mm). The femoral nerve is far from the portal (closest average distance 39.9 mm corresponds to the capsular level) [11].

The mid-anterolateral portal is halfway between the anterior and anterolateral portals, about 2 cm distal to a line connecting both portals [29]. From this point, it penetrates the tensor fasciae latae and gluteus medius muscles. The structures at risk of this portal are the same than for the anterior portal. It is typically used in labral repairs and femoral neck debridement.

Philippon et al. [12] described an additional distal lateral accessory portal placed approximately 1 cm anterior and 4 cm distal to the anterolateral portal. It penetrates the tensor fascia lata muscle and the capsule through the orbicularis zone. This portal is established under direct visualization from the anterior portal to visualize the anterior femoral head and neck. The main structures at risk are the lateral femoral cutaneous nerve and the ascending branch of the lateral femoral circumflex artery.

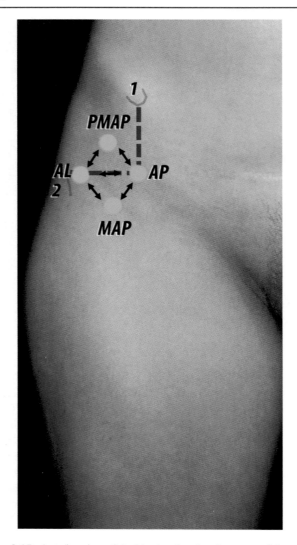

Fig. 8.15 Anterior view of the hip showing the placement of the mid-anterior and proximal mid-anterior portals. Observe the relationship with the anterolateral and anterior portals as well as the equidistant distance between all of them. *AP* anterior portal, *AL* anterolateral portal, *MAP* mid-anterior portal, *PMAP* proximal mid-anterior portal, (*1*) anterior-superior iliac spine, (*2*) greater trochanter

Peripheral Compartment

In addition to the specific portals described to access the peripheral compartment (ancillary anterolateral portal, superolateral portal) [28, 42] (Table 8.6), some portals usually used to access to the central compartment can be used just redirecting its orientation to the femoral neck or the transition between it and the femoral head (anterolateral portal, posterolateral portal, mid-anterior portal) [11, 25, 28, 29, 42, 43] (Table 8.7) (Fig. 8.16).

Two portals are routinely used to access the peripheral compartment: the anterolateral portal and an ancillary anterolateral portal [42].

Table 8.6 Specific portals to the peripheral compartment

Accessory anterolateral portal	
Placement	3–5 cm distal to the anterolateral portal along the anterior border of the greater trochanter
Pathway	It penetrates the tensor fascia lata and passes between the gluteus minimus and rectus femoris muscles
Structures at risk	Transverse branch of the lateral femoral circumflex artery
Superolateral portal	
Placement	Superior apex of an equilateral triangle formed by the standard anterolateral and posterolateral portals
Pathway	It perforates the iliotibial band and the gluteus medius muscle
Structures at risk	Superior gluteal nerve

Table 8.7 Differences of orientation of the standard portals to the central and peripheral compartments [11, 14]

Portal	Central compartment	Peripheral compartment
Anterolateral portal	15° cephalad	15° caudad
	15° posterior	5° posterior
Posterolateral portal	5° cephalad	25° caudad
	5° anterior	15° anterior
Mid-anterior portal	35° cephalad	15° cephalad
	25° posterior	20° posterior

The location of anterolateral portal placement to the peripheral compartment is found by palpating a soft spot one third the distance of a line drawn from the anterior-superior iliac spine to the tip of the greater trochanter [25]. It is oriented perpendicular to the femoral neck axis to the junction between the femoral head and neck on its anterior aspect just below the zona orbicularis (15° caudad and 5° posterior). In this area, the femoral head is free of cartilage, the capsule is separated from the neck, and the anterior acetabular labrum is located 2–3 mm proximally [25].

The ancillary or accessory anterolateral portal is placed approximately 3–5 cm distal to the anterolateral portal along the anterior border of the greater trochanter [29]. It is usually established by direct visualization from the anterolateral portal and under image intensifier guidance [42]. It penetrates the tensor fascia lata and passes through the interval between the gluteus minimus and rectus femoris muscles. The only one neurovascular structure at risk is the transverse branch of the lateral femoral circumflex artery.

The superolateral portal is located at the superior apex of an equilateral triangle formed by the standard anterolateral and posterolateral portals [28]. This portal is directed to the superior aspect of the head-neck transition. It perforates the iliotibial band and the gluteus medius muscle. The superior gluteal nerve is at risk during this portal placement due to its

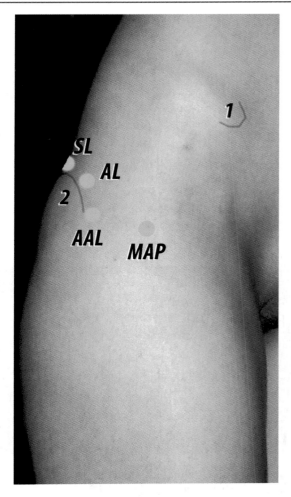

Fig. 8.16 Oblique anterior view of a right hip showing the topographic location of the most common used portals to the peripheral compartment (excepting the posterolateral portal). *AL* anterolateral portal, *MAP* mid-anterior portal, *SL* superolateral portal, *AAL* accessory anterolateral portal, (*1*) anterior-superior iliac spine, (*2*) greater trochanter

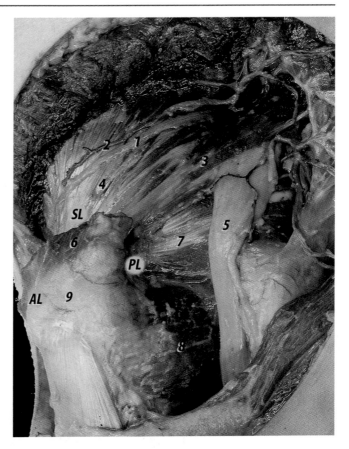

Fig. 8.17 Posterior view of a left deep gluteal region showing the approximate location of the superolateral portal, forming an equilateral triangle with the anterolateral and posterolateral portals. Observe the close relationship with the superior gluteal nerve and artery. *SL* superolateral portal, *AL* anterolateral portal, *PL* posterolateral portal, (*1*) superior gluteal nerve, (*2*) superior gluteal artery, (*3*) piriformis m., (*4*) gluteus minimus m., (*5*) sciatic nerve, (*6*) gluteus medius m., (*7*) obturator internus m., (*8*) quadratus femoris m., (*9*) greater trochanter

average distance of 30–51 mm to the tip of the greater trochanter [19–21] (see Fig. 8.17). The function of this portal is mainly for viewing purposes.

The posterolateral portal to the peripheral compartment is redirected to the posterior aspect of the femoral neck or the posterior junction of the femoral head and neck. The cannula is oriented 25° caudad and 15° anterior. It penetrates the same structures than the posterolateral portal to the central compartment (gluteus maximus, medius, and minimum muscles). This portal is placed at an average distance of 34 mm to the sciatic nerve. This higher distance in comparison to the posterolateral portal to the central compartment is attributed to the more anterior course of the portal pathway [11]. The deep branch of the medial femoral circumflex artery is also at risk although the posterior border of the greater trochanter acts as a bony protector.

The mid-anterior portal to the peripheral compartment is reoriented, forming an insertion angle of approximately 15° cephalad and 20° posterior. In the same way as the mid-anterior portal to the central compartment, it penetrates the tensor fascia lata muscle being placed through the interval between gluteus minimus and rectus femoris muscles. The closest neurovascular structures at risk during portal establishment are the terminal branches of the lateral femoral circumflex artery at an average distance of 14.7 mm (range 1–30 mm) [11].

Peritrochanteric Space

Different portals have been described to access the peritrochanteric space. Basically, we can divide these portals into two groups: (1) standard portals redirected to the peritrochanteric space (anterolateral, anterior, and posterolateral

Table 8.8 Specific portals to the peritrochanteric space

Proximal anterolateral accessory portal	
Placement	Directly posterior to the proximal mid-anterior portal
Pathway	It perforates the junction of the gluteus maximus and tensor fascia lata to form the iliotibial band
Peritrochanteric space portal	
Placement	At the level of the mid-anterior portal in a more posterior location just anterior to the anterior border of the greater trochanter
Pathway	It passes through the interval between the tensor fascia lata muscle and the iliotibial band
Distal anterolateral accessory portal	
Placement	Distally to the peritrochanteric space portal at the same distance that exists between the proximal anterolateral accessory and peritrochanteric space portals
Pathway	It passes just anterior to the iliotibial band
Structures at risk	Transverse branch of the lateral femoral circumflex artery

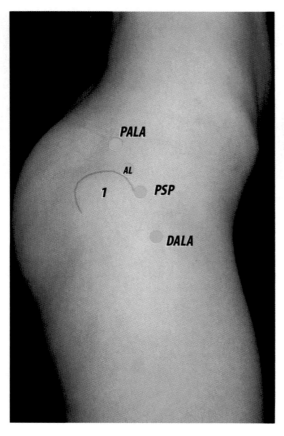

Fig. 8.18 Lateral view of the hip showing the placement of the most common used peritrochanteric portals. *AL* anterolateral portal, *PALA* proximal anterolateral accessory portal, *PSP* peritrochanteric space portal, *DALA* distal anterolateral accessory portal, (*1*) greater trochanter (*outlined*)

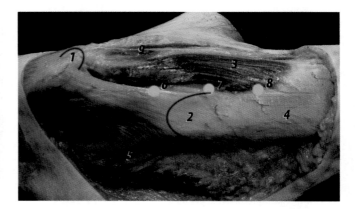

Fig. 8.19 Lateral view of the hip showing the placement of the common peritrochanteric portals (*blue dots*). The anterior-superior iliac spine and greater trochanter have been outlined. (*1*) Anterior-superior iliac spine, (*2*) greater trochanter, (*3*) tensor fascia lata m., (*4*) iliotibial band, (*5*) gluteus maximus m., (*6*) proximal anterolateral accessory portal, (*7*) peritrochanteric space portal, (*8*) distal anterolateral accessory portal, (*9*) lateral femoral cutaneous nerve

The proximal anterolateral accessory portal is placed directly posterior to the proximal mid-anterior portal. It perforates the junction of the gluteus maximus and tensor fascia lata to form the iliotibial band, entering into the peritrochanteric space.

The peritrochanteric space portal is established at the level of the mid-anterior portal in a more posterior location just anterior to the anterior border of the greater trochanter. It passes through the interval between the tensor fascia lata muscle and the iliotibial band.

The distal anterolateral accessory portal is placed distally to the peritrochanteric space portal at the same distance that exists between the first two portals (proximal anterolateral accessory and peritrochanteric space portals). It penetrates into the peritrochanteric space just anterior to the iliotibial band. This portal is the only one which has a structure at risk, the transverse branch of lateral femoral circumflex artery (see Fig. 8.14). This artery courses in close proximity to the distal anterolateral accessory portal before going deep into

portals) and (2) portals described to access the peritrochanteric space (proximal anterolateral accessory portal, distal anterolateral accessory portal, peritrochanteric space portal, auxiliary posterolateral portal) (Table 8.8).

The three portals commonly used to access the peritrochanteric space according to Robertson et al. [11] are the proximal anterolateral accessory, distal anterolateral accessory, and peritrochanteric space portals (see Figs. 8.18 and 8.19).

the vastus lateralis muscle. Robertson et al. [11] located this artery at a mean distance of 23.4 mm (range 17–40 mm) medially to the portal.

Some authors access the peritrochanteric space through standard portals described to be used into the central compartment, that are redirected to the greater trochanter and surrounding areas [44, 45].

The anterior portal described to access into the peritrochanteric space [45] is placed 1 cm lateral to the anterior-superior iliac spine within the interval between the tensor fascia lata and sartorius muscles. The cannula is oriented toward the peritrochanteric space with the leg in full extension, 0° of abduction, and 10–15° of internal rotation.

Other described portals to the peritrochanteric space are:

- Distal posterior portal [45]: It is placed midway between the tip of the greater trochanter and the vastus tubercle along the posterior one third of the greater trochanter midline.
- Proximal to the tip of the greater trochanter in line with the distal posterior portal [45].
- Auxiliary posterolateral portal [44]: It is placed 3 cm posterior and 3 cm superior to the greater trochanter. It allows a better visualization of the sciatic nerve up to the sciatic notch. There a significant risk of injury of the superior gluteal nerve if the gluteus medius muscle is perforated with the cannula by error.

References

1. McCarthy JC, Lee JA. Hip arthroscopy: indications, outcomes, and complications. Instr Course Lect. 2006;55:301–8.
2. Byrd JWT. Surgical techniques: hip arthroscopy. J Am Acad Orthop Surg. 2006;14:433–44.
3. Sampson TG. Complications of hip arthroscopy. Clin Sports Med. 2001;20:831–6.
4. Clarke MT, Arora A, Villar RN. Hip arthroscopy: complications in 1054 cases. Clin Orthop Relat Res. 2003;406:84–8.
5. Rodeo SA, Forster RA, Welland AJ. Current concepts review. Neurological complications due to arthroscopy. J Bone Joint Surg. 1993;75-A:917–26.
6. Byrd JT. Complications associated with hip arthroscopy. In: Byrd JT, editor. Operative hip arthroscopy. 2nd ed. New York: Thieme; 1998. p. 171–6.
7. Byrd JWT. Avoiding the labrum in hip arthroscopy. Arthroscopy. 2000;16:770–3.
8. Kim S-J, Choi N-H, Kim H-J. Operative hip arthroscopy. Clin Orthop. 1998;353:156–65.
9. Dvorak M, Duncan CP, Day B. Arthroscopic anatomy of the hip. Arthroscopy. 1990;6:264–73.
10. Monllau JC, Solano A, Leon A, et al. Tomographic study of the arthroscopic approaches to the hip joint. Arthroscopy. 2003;19:368–72.
11. Robertson WJ, Kelly BT. The safe zone for hip arthroscopy: a cadaveric assessment of central, peripheral, and lateral compartment portal placement. Arthroscopy. 2008;24:1019–26.
12. Philippon MJ, Schenker ML. Arthroscopy for the treatment of femoroacetabular impingement in the athlete. Clin Sports Med. 2006;25:299–308.
13. Byrd JWT, Pappas JN, Pedley MJ. Hip arthroscopy: an anatomic study of portal placement and relationship to the extra-articular structures. Arthroscopy. 1995;11:418–23.
14. Byrd JT. Portal anatomy. In: Byrd JT, editor. Operative hip arthroscopy. 2nd ed. New York: Thieme; 1998. p. 110–6.
15. Philippon MJ, Stubbs AJ, Schenker ML, et al. Arthroscopic management of femoroacetabular impingement: osteoplasty technique and literature review. Am J Sports Med. 2007;35:1571–80.
16. Akita K, Sakamoto H, Sato T. Arrangement and innervation of the glutei medius and minimus and the piriformis: a morphological analysis. Anat Rec. 1994;238:125–30.
17. Diop M, Parratte B, Tatu L, et al. Anatomical bases of superior gluteal nerve entrapment syndrome in the piriformis foramen. Surg Radiol Anat. 2002;24:155–9.
18. Thomine JM, Duparc F, Dujardin F, et al. Abord transglutéal de hanche par hémimyotomie antérieure du gluteus medius. Rev Chir Orthop. 1999;85:520–5.
19. Duparc F, Thomine JM, Dujardin F, et al. Anatomic basis of the transgluteal approach to the hip joint by anterior hemimyotomy of the gluteus medius. Surg Radiol Anat. 1997;19:61–7.
20. Bos JC, Stoeckart R, Klooswijk AIJ, et al. The surgical anatomy of the superior gluteal nerve and anatomical radiologic bases of the direct lateral approach to the hip. Surg Radiol Anat. 1994;16:253–8.
21. Pascarel X, Dumont D, Nemme B, et al. Arthroplastie totale de la hanche par voie de Hardinge. Résultat Clinique de 63 cas. Rev Chir Orthop. 1989;75:98–103.
22. Miguel Perez M, Llusa M, Ortiz JC, et al. Superior gluteal nerve: safe area in hip surgery. Surg Radiol Anat. 2004;26:225–9.
23. Dienst M, Goedde S, Seil R, et al. Hip arthroscopy without traction: in vivo anatomy of the peripheral hip joint cavity. Arthroscopy. 2001;17:924–31.
24. Dienst M, Goedde S, Seil R, et al. Diagnostic arthroscopy of the hip joint. Orthop Traumatol. 2002;10:1–14.
25. Dienst M, Seil R, Kohn DM. Safe arthroscopic access to the central compartment of the hip. Arthroscopy. 2005;12:1510–4.
26. Ide T, Akamatsu N, Nakajima L. Arthroscopic surgery of the hip joint. Arthroscopy. 1991;7:204–11.
27. Dorfmann H, Boyer T, Henry P, et al. A simple approach to hip arthroscopy. Arthroscopy. 1988;4:141–2.
28. Simpson J, Sadri H, Villar R. Hip arthroscopy technique and complications. Orthop Traumatol Surg Res. 2010;96(8 Suppl):S68–76. Epub 2010 Oct 30.
29. Bond JL, Knutson ZA, Ebert A, et al. The 23-point arthroscopic examination of the hip: basic setup, portal placement, and surgical technique. Arthroscopy. 2009;25:416–29.
30. Carliouz H, Pous JG, Rey JC. Les epiphysiolyses femorales superrieures. Rev Chir Orthop Reparatice Appar Mot. 1968;54:388–481.
31. Sussmann PS, Zumstein M, Hahn F, et al. The risk of vascular injury to the femoral head when using the posterolateral arthroscopy portal: cadaveric investigation. Arthroscopy. 2007;23:1112–5.
32. Gautier E, Ganz K, Krugel N, et al. Anatomy of the medial femoral circumflex artery and its surgical implications. J Bone Joint Surg. 2000;82-B:679–83.
33. Lavigne M, Kalhor M, Beck M, et al. Distribution of vascular foramina around the femoral head and neck junction: relevance for conservative intracapsular procedures of the hip. Orthop Clin N Am. 2005;36:171–6.
34. Frich L, Lauritzen J, Juhl M. Arthroscopy in diagnosis and treatment of hip disorders. Orthopaedics. 1989;12:389–91.
35. Ilizaliturri VM, Valero FS, Chaidez PA, et al. An aiming guide for anterior portal placement in hip arthroscopy. Arthroscopy. 2003;19(9):E125–7.
36. Glick JM, Sampson TG, Gordon RB, et al. Hip arthroscopy by the lateral approach. Arthroscopy. 1987;3:4–12.
37. Grothaus MC, Holt M, Mekhail AO, et al. Lateral femoral cutaneous nerve. An anatomic study. Clin Orthop Relat Res. 2005;437:164–8.
38. Gurunluoglu R. The ascending branch of the lateral circumflex femoral vessels: review of the anatomy and its utilization as

recipient vessel for free-flap reconstruction of the hip region. J Reconstr Microsurg. 2010;26:359–66.

39. Saadeh FA, Haikal FA, Abdel-Hamid FA. Blood supply of the tensor fasciae latae muscle. Clin Anat. 1998;11:236–8.

40. Little III JW, Lyons JR. The gluteus medius-tensor fasciae latae flap. Plast Reconstr Surg. 1983;71:366–71.

41. Rouviere H, Delmas A, editors. Anatomia humana descriptiva, topográfica y funcional. Barcelona: Elsevier-Masson; 2005.

42. Byrd JWT. Hip arthroscopy: evolving frontiers. Oper Tech Orthop. 2004;14:58–67.

43. Byrd JWT. Hip arthroscopy, the supine approach: technique and anatomy of the intraarticular and peripheral compartments. Tech Orthop. 2005;20:17–31.

44. Martin HD, Shears SA, Johnson JC, et al. The endoscopic treatment of sciatic nerve entrapment/deep gluteal region. Arthroscopy. 2011;27:172–81.

45. Voos JE, Rudzki JR, Shindle MK, et al. Arthroscopic anatomy and surgical techniques for peritrochanteric space disorders in the hip. Arthroscopy. 2007;23:1246.e1–5.

Arthroscopic Anatomy of the Hip

Carlos A. Guanche

Introduction

As hip arthroscopy becomes more common, it is vital that accurate knowledge of the anatomy of the hip and how to establish the common portals is combined with correct patient selection, sound preoperative planning, and consistent arthroscopic technique in order to maximize clinical outcomes. Even though arthroscopy of the hip was first performed as early as 1931 [1], its clinical application has developed rather slowly [2, 3].

From an arthroscopic point of view, Dorfmann and Boyer [4] divided the hip into two compartments separated by the acetabular labrum (central and peripheral). The central compartment includes the acetabular fossa, ligamentum teres, lunate cartilage, and articular surface of the femoral head in the weight-bearing area. The peripheral compartment includes the non-weight-bearing cartilage of the femoral head, the femoral neck with its synovial folds, and the joint capsule. To access and visualize the central compartment, traction must be applied to the joint, whereas the peripheral compartment is examined without traction [5, 6]. As it is common for hip joint pathologies to affect both compartments, the surgeon should be accustomed to performing the technique both with and without traction.

General Considerations

It is important to recognize a series of surface landmarks that must be located once the patient is correctly positioned and with the hip in traction. The iliac crest, the anterior superior iliac spine, and the symphysis pubis are easily palpable even in most patients. The prominence of the greater trochanter is another important reference point.

C.A. Guanche, M.D.
Southern California Orthopedic Institute,
6815 Noble Avenue, Van Nuys, Los Angeles, CA 91405, USA
e-mail: cguanche@scoi.com

The working area is defined by a series of lines that must be marked on the skin [7] (Fig. 9.1). A transverse line is drawn from the superior border of the trochanter to the superior border of the pubic bone. The majority of the accessory portals will be made distal to this transverse line, as this will provide correct orientation for access to both compartments of the joint. A sagittal line starting at the anterior superior iliac spine (ASIS) is drawn distally down the anterior aspect of the thigh. This sagittal line is the limit of the safe area for the creation of anterior portals; the femoral neurovascular bundle (deep femoral nerve and the femoral artery and vein) and the main branch of the femoral cutaneous nerves are situated medial to this line. As orthopedic surgeons become more comfortable with hip arthroscopy, the indications are increasing. Knowledge of the anatomy will allow safe access and adequate visualization as most structures are at a safe distance from the portals [8].

Intracapsular Anatomy of the Hip and Arthroscopic Examination

The interior of the joint capsule of the hip is occupied not only by the acetabulum and the head and neck of the femur but also by several anatomic structures that need to be recognized: the acetabular labrum, ligamentum teres, and synovial folds. These structures are a fundamental part of pathological conditions, and it is therefore necessary to be able to recognize their normal appearance and differentiate them from abnormal states.

The Acetabular Labrum

The acetabular labrum is found on the rim of the bony acetabulum. The labrum is a fibrocartilage with a triangular cross section; it increases the depth and coverage of the acetabulum, thus favoring stability of the hip joint by forming slightly more than a hemisphere. The labrum has three surfaces: The base or

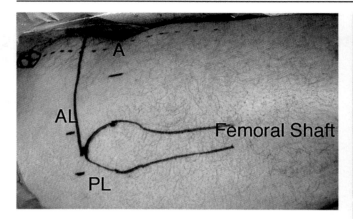

Fig. 9.1 Surface anatomy of the hip. A transverse line drawn from the superior border of the trochanter to the superior border of the pubic bone defines the working area. The majority of the accessory portals will be made distal to this transverse line. A sagittal line starting at the anterior-superior iliac spine drawn distally down the anterior aspect of the thigh defines the safe area for the creating the anterior portals (*A* anterior portal, *AL* anterolateral portal, *PL* posterolateral portal)

adherent surface is the part that attaches onto the rim of the acetabulum; the internal or articular surface is continuous with the articular surface of the acetabulum, such that it is occasionally difficult to distinguish on simple arthroscopic vision; and finally, the external surface attaches to the joint capsule, leaving a free border that can be observed during arthroscopic examination. The size of the labrum varies; it is thicker superiorly and posteriorly than it is inferiorly and anteriorly [9, 10]. Classic anatomic studies observed variations of between 6 and 10 mm in the height of the labrum. Superiorly, there is a slight separation between the attachment of the capsule and the acetabular rim, creating a space between the labrum and the capsule known as the paralabral sulcus, labrum-capsular sulcus, or perilabral recess [10, 11]. It is important to get used to the normal arthroscopic appearance of the paralabral sulcus (Fig. 9.2).

On the inner lip of the acetabulum lies the chondrolabral junction, which is the most common site for labral pathology. However, it must be remembered that a partial separation of the labrum may be observed at the superior part of the acetabulum as an anatomic variant [12]. This separation is called the sublabral sulcus and should not be confused with a labral lesion. In vivo observation by hip arthroscopy shows the most common site for labral injury to be the anterior and anterosuperior regions [12–14]. Lesions of the posterior labrum are less common and are due to an axial impact with the hip flexed [12]. However, the distinction between the sublabral sulcus and a labral lesion is not always clear; a labral lesion should be considered when there are compatible symptoms or when there is an associated image of labral hemorrhage in acute disorders or granulation tissue indicating attempted healing in chronic disorders [12].

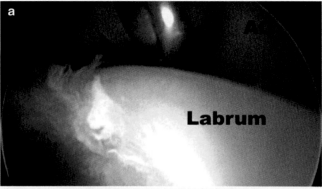

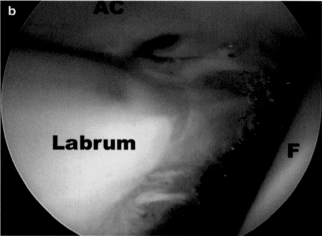

Fig. 9.2 The paralabral sulcus. There are several variants including a relative sulcus of about 1 cm, as seen in (**a**). In others, there is an obliterated sulcus, as seen in (**b**)

The Ligamentum Teres

The ligamentum teres or ligamentum capitis femoris [15] is an intra-articular ligament that attaches the head of the femur to the acetabulum. It arises in the inferior part of the acetabular fossa and runs inferiorly and anteriorly across the joint space to insert into the fovea capitis of the head of the femur.

The ligamentum teres is trapezoid; its base, which is thickened into two bands, inserts onto the border of the acetabular notch and onto the transverse ligament of the acetabulum. As it runs toward the femoral head, it becomes progressively round or oval in shape before inserting into the fovea capitis at a site slightly posterior and inferior to the true center of the head.

In cross section, the ligamentum teres is pyramidal, with a fascicular appearance formed by anterior and posterior bundles; it follows a spiral course from its acetabular attachment to its femoral insertion.

Dynamic hip examination shows that the ligament becomes taut during external rotation of the hip and relaxed with internal rotation (Fig. 9.3). A recent arthroscopic study

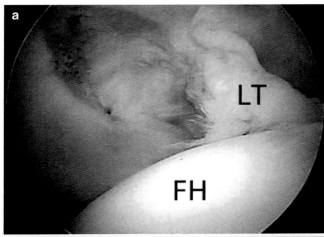

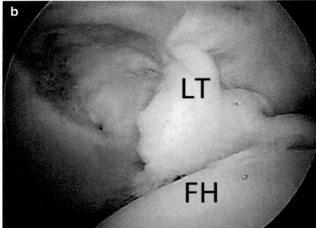

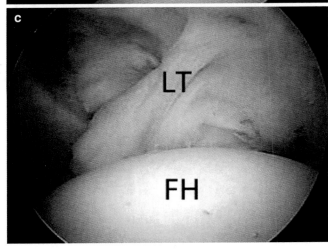

Fig. 9.3 Arthroscopic views of the ligamentum teres through accessory distal anterior portal during (**a**) internal rotation, (**b**) neutral rotation, and (**c**) external rotation (the view is of a left hip, viewed from the anterior portal) (*LT* ligamentum teres, *FH* femoral head)

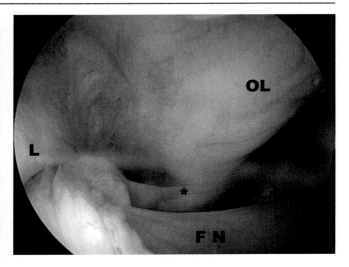

Fig. 9.4 Medial synovial fold (*) is the medial extent typically used for femoral neck resection (*OL* orbicular ligament, *FN* femoral neck, *L* labrum)

function similar to that of the anterior cruciate ligament in the knee [17].

The Synovial Folds

As the neck of the femur is intracapsular, a synovial membrane covers it. This tissue forms a series of folds that descend along the femoral neck, from the border of the cartilage of the femoral head to the insertion of the joint capsule on the femur. These folds are variable in number and size, and it is important to distinguish them from possible adhesions. Synovial folds, which may be large, are usually observed medially and laterally; an anterior fold is less common.

The medial synovial fold is an important reference for initial orientation and usually indicates the medial limit for performing osteochondroplasty in cases of femoroacetabular impingement, while the lateral fold marks the lateral limit for this resection (Fig. 9.4). The lateral fold indicates the site of entry of the perforating arterioles, which are important for vascularity of the femoral head [18] (Fig. 9.5).

The medial synovial fold can be affected by an impingement disorder called pectineofoveal impingement [19]. Clinically, these patients refer mechanical pain in the hip with movements of flexion and rotation; this can force them to reduce or stop sporting activities. Complementary studies are usually normal, and the diagnosis must be made by arthroscopy, which reveals trapping of this synovial fold with the medial soft tissues (zona orbicularis and psoas muscle tendon). In consequence, the synovial fold becomes hypertrophic, rubbing against the femoral neck during the sporting activity. Treatment consists of excision of the thickened synovial fold.

of high-level athletes revealed hypertrophic changes of the ligamentum teres, suggesting a relationship with chronic instability of the hip [16]. The ligamentum teres may have a

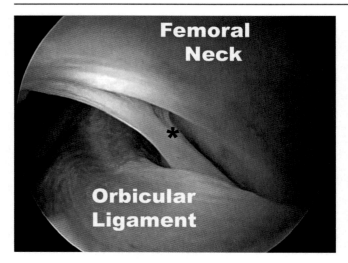

Fig. 9.5 Lateral synovial fold (*) is the lateral (or posterior) extent of femoral neck resections. The fold includes the critical vessels (medial femoral circumflex) that contribute to vascularity of the femoral head

Systematic Arthroscopic Exam of the Hip

A systematic arthroscopic examination (*Vid. 9.1*: http://goo.gl/Rjh1Q of the central and peripheral compartments of the hip increases the accuracy and reproducibility of each hip arthroscopy. With this approach, and employing a three portal technique (anterolateral, posterolateral, and anterior), there are several points that are essential to examine and document (Table 9.1) [20]. The use of a standardized, approach ensures that all components of the hip are carefully inspected and makes it possible to document the procedure correctly, making retrospective analysis possible. Moreover, a methodical technique allows us to compare arthroscopic findings with clinical presentations, further enhancing our diagnostic capabilities.

The anterolateral (AL) portal is always the first portal to be established. The procedure is performed under traction in order to examine the central compartment. This is followed by arthroscopy without traction for evaluation of the peripheral compartment. One technique that is important to keep in mind is that of extending the capsular entry point with the use of either an arthroscopic blade or an electrocautery ablator (Fig. 9.6). Regardless of the method chosen, a capsulotomy is the key to allowing free access to all of the critical areas that may need to be addressed in any given procedure.

Examination of the Central Compartment

The central compartment must be explored starting from the central region of the joint, by way of the AL portal. The structures visualized are, in order, the acetabular fossa, the

Table 9.1 The 23 points of hip arthroscopy

Central compartment—anterolateral portal
1. Cotyloid fossa, pulvinar, ligamentum teres
2. Posterior medial acetabulum and labrum
3. Anterior triangle—anterior capsule, anterior labrum, femoral head
4. Anterior labrum, paralabral sulcus
5. Lateral labrum, capsular sulcus
6. Posterior capsule, zona orbicularis
7. Femoral head

Central compartment—anterior portal
8. Ligamentum teres
9. Posterior transverse ligament, posteromedial labrum
10. Anterior transverse ligament, anterior labrum loose bodies, labral tears
11. Superior articular cartilage
12. Lateral labrum
13. Posterolateral capsule

Central compartment—posterolateral portal
14. Inferior gutter
15. Weight-bearing dome of the acetabulum
16. Anterolateral labrum
17. Femoral head

Peripheral compartment—anterolateral portal
18. Medial femoral neck, orbicular ligament, medial synovial fold
19. Medial gutter
20. Anterior labrum
21. Lateral labrum
22. Lateral femoral neck, orbicular ligament
23. Anterior femoral neck, anterior synovial fold

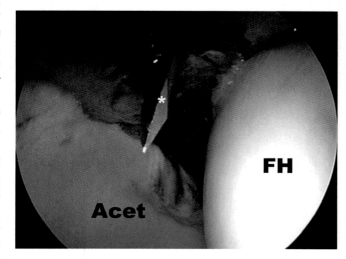

Fig. 9.6 Arthroscopic view of the controlled capsulotomy (this view is of a right hip, viewed from the AL portal and working via the anterior portal) (*FH* femoral head, *Acet* acetabular wall)

posteromedial acetabular cartilage and labrum, the anterior triangle, the anterior labrum and paralabral sulcus, the posterolateral labrum, the posterior capsule, and the femoral head.

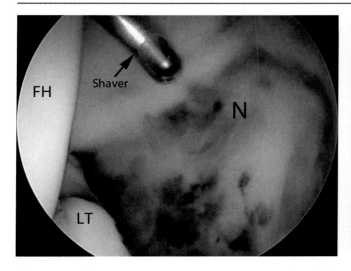

Fig. 9.7 Point 1 in the 23-point examination (left hip) is the area of the ligamentum teres insertion in the notch (*LT* ligamentum teres, *FH* femoral head, *N* notch)

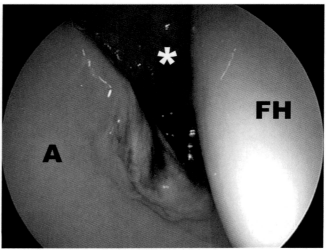

Fig. 9.8 Anterior triangle (point 3) in a right hip. This *asterisk* demarcates the point of entry in the anterior capsule (*FH* femoral head, *A* acetabulum)

Beginning with the 70° arthroscope introduced through the anterolateral portal into the central compartment, the first landmark includes the components of the medial wall of the acetabulum, including the acetabular or cotyloid fossa, pulvinar, and ligamentum teres (Fig. 9.7). It is important to use this view for general orientation; in addition, synovitis of the acetabular fossa and tears of the ligamentum teres are commonly seen from this position [21].

By rotating the scope, one can visualize the posteromedial acetabular cartilage and labrum. With adequate distraction, the posterior capsular reflection can also be seen. The lens is then rotated anteriorly, and the scope is raised and retracted to visualize the anterior triangle, which is composed of the anterior capsule, anterior labrum, and femoral head (Fig. 9.8).

The anterior triangle is a very helpful landmark and will give direct visualization when establishing the anterior portal. Once the anterior portal is established, the camera is withdrawn further and the anterior labrum and paralabral sulcus come into view. It is important to learn the normal anatomy of the labrum in order to be able to detect pathological changes. The triangular anterior labrum usually fuses with the acetabular cartilage inferiorly and the paralabral sulcus superiorly. This is a common area to find labral tears and degeneration.

There are some anatomic variants that are important to note. The most common is a superior extension of the notch which has been termed the "keyhole complex" and appears to be somewhat cystic in nature, when probed (Fig. 9.9). This complex appears, most commonly, in younger patients.

Another variant is an extension in several directions of the notch. These extensions appear to be remnants of the triradiate epiphysis (ilioischial and iliopubic grooves) and also

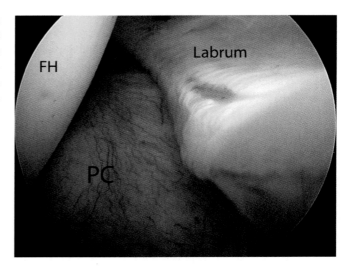

Fig. 9.9 The posterior capsule and posterior acetabulum (point 14). This is the most important area to visualize for loose bodies and possible ligamentum teres disruptions (*Acet* acetabulum, *FH* femoral head, *Post* posterior capsule)

appear in younger patients, with occasional observation in somewhat older patients (Fig. 9.10) [22].

After further withdrawal of the arthroscope, the lens can be rotated inferiorly to view the lateral labrum and its attachment to the capsular sulcus. Pushing the camera inferiorly and rotating the lens superiorly will show the posterior capsule from its acetabular attachment to the concentric fibers of the zona orbicularis at the junction of the femoral head and neck. Retracting the scope so that the cartilage of the femoral head can be examined from its inferior to superior margins documents the final landmark of the AL portal. The leg can be gently rotated internally and externally during this

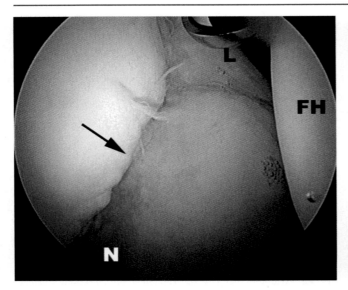

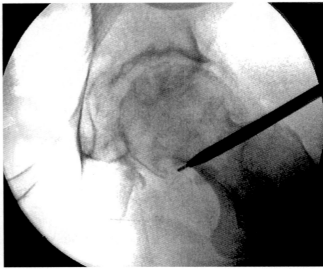

Fig. 9.10 Iliopubic groove (*arrow*) in a right hip observed from the anterolateral portal (*FH* femoral head, *L* labrum, *N* notch)

Fig. 9.11 Entry into the peripheral compartment from the AL skin entry and redirecting toward the medial physeal scar remnant

inspection in order to provide as wide a view as possible. Once these structures are documented, the scope is moved to the anterior (A) portal.

This portal gives the best view of the ligamentum teres as it arises from the posteroinferior margin of the acetabulum and inserts onto the medial aspect of the femoral head [23]. Even minor tears can be diagnosed with gentle rotation of the lower extremity. With adequate distraction, the scope can be maneuvered posteriorly to view the posterior aspect of the transverse ligament where it inserts onto the posteromedial labrum. This is a site where articular loose bodies can lodge.

Pulling the scope back (anterior to the ligament) reveals the anterior aspect of the transverse ligament and its attachment to the anterior labrum. By rotating the lens laterally, the superior acetabular cartilage is seen. This part of the examination ends at the lateral labrum and point of entry for the AL portal. This view provides an excellent angle to aid in the diagnosis and debridement or repair of most labral tears. From this vantage point, the posterolateral (PL) portal can be safely established.

The PL portal gives a good view of the posterior capsule, the weight-bearing part of the acetabulum, the anterolateral labrum, and the femoral head. From the medial notch, the arthroscope is slowly withdrawn and moved inferiorly over the posterior labrum into the inferior gutter, which runs from the capsular attachment on the posterior and medial acetabulum to the thickened cylindrical sleeve of the orbicular ligament that surrounds the femoral neck (Fig. 9.9). The lens of the scope is then rotated cranially and advanced to see the weight-bearing dome of the acetabulum. Cartilage degeneration and cyst formation within the acetabulum are often best appreciated in this area. The camera is then moved

superiorly to view the anterolateral labrum from a different angle. Finally, rotating the lens, the posterior aspect of the femoral head can be examined. The camera should be drawn tangentially over the surface of the cartilage in an effort to observe as much of the femoral head as possible.

Examination of the Peripheral Compartment

After the appropriate treatment of any condition diagnosed in the central compartment, the limb is taken out of traction and the hip is positioned in approximately 45° of flexion. This relaxes the anterior capsuloligamentous complex and permits adequate inspection of the peripheral compartment to be performed. Using a method similar to the one described by Dienst et al., a spinal needle is directed from the AL portal toward the medial physeal scar of the femoral head (Fig. 9.11) [5].

Once inside the peripheral compartment, the visual field should be moved from medial to lateral over the femoral head and then from lateral to medial along the femoral neck. There are six landmarks commonly inspected within the peripheral compartment: the medial femoral neck, the medial femoral head, the anterior femoral head, the lateral femoral head, the lateral femoral neck, and the anterior femoral neck.

Upon entering the peripheral compartment from the AL portal, the initial view is typically of the medial neck. If the camera is oriented so that it is looking down upon the femoral neck, the first anatomic complex is a very consistent landmark, comprising the orbicular ligament, medial synovial fold, and femoral neck (Fig. 9.4).

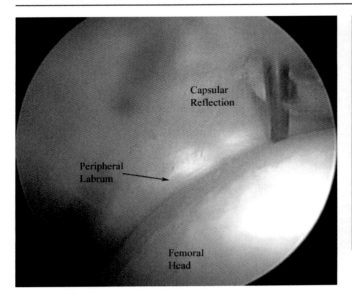

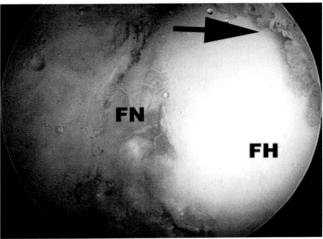

Fig. 9.13 View of the lateral femoral head and acetabular labrum (*arrow*) on a left hip, in a patient with cam impingement (*FH* femoral head, *FN* femoral neck)

Fig. 9.12 The peripheral labrum and anterior capsule as well as the sublabral recess can easily be seen from the AL in most patients. This view is from the AL portal in a right hip

Like the acetabular fossa and the ligamentum teres in the central compartment, the medial synovial fold and orbicular ligament serve as excellent landmarks. This is very important, as good orientation is the basis for correct arthroscopic diagnosis and treatment.

From the medial neck, the camera is directed superiorly and is slowly withdrawn as it is gently maneuvered under the orbicular ligament, sliding into the medial gutter. It is not uncommon to find hidden loose bodies in this area. After viewing the medial gutter, the scope can be rotated laterally, sliding along the entirety of the anterior femoroacetabular interface to visualize the anterior and lateral labrum and femoral head (Fig. 9.12).

The anterior capsule is usually too stiff to allow inspection past the lateral aspect of the labrum and femoral head. The posterolateral aspect of the peripheral compartment is therefore not included in the routine examination. Occasionally, the hip can be flexed and abducted to 45°, allowing the arthroscope to pass between the lateral synovial fold and the orbicular ligament into the posterolateral area. This area is small as the insertion of the posterior joint capsule is 2–3 cm proximal to that of the anterior capsule [24]. This posterior area is easier to access after adequate capsular release and femoral neck debridement.

From the lateral aspect of the femoral head, the camera is withdrawn distally to reach the lateral aspect of the femoral neck. From here, fibers of the orbicular ligament can be seen from the peripheral compartment side and correspond well to the previous view from the central compartment.

This is also the most common area for cam lesions commonly seen with femoroacetabular impingement [6, 25–29].

While viewing of the lateral femoral neck, the leg is flexed and internally rotated to document impingement of the femoral neck with the lateral acetabulum (Fig. 9.13).

From the lateral neck, the arthroscope is rotated medially to view the anterior neck. Unlike the medial and lateral synovial folds, the anterior synovial fold is tightly adherent to the anterior femoral neck and only rarely forms a distinct anatomic entity. The arthroscope is then pushed toward the medial neck where the orbicular ligament and medial synovial fold come into view again. This is the final portion of the systematic approach to the hip joint.

Summary

Currently, there is unprecedented enthusiasm for hip arthroscopy, as this modality is transforming the management of hip injuries. Careful preoperative planning, precise portal placement, a knowledge of the potential complications, and a methodical sequence of arthroscopic examination, progressing from one part of the joint cavity to another systematically in each case, are essential for effective hip arthroscopy.

A systematic arthroscopic examination of the central and peripheral compartments ensures that all components of the hip are carefully inspected and increases the accuracy and reproducibility of diagnostic hip arthroscopy. This standard also helps differentiate normal structures from their pathological counterparts. Furthermore, it allows us to correlate arthroscopic findings with clinical presentations, enhancing our diagnostic abilities and providing better clinical outcomes. As new indications and techniques are developed, this standardized approach to diagnostic hip arthroscopy provides a solid ground in the technique.

References

1. Burman M. Arthroscopy or the direct visualization of joints. J Bone Joint Surg. 1931;4:669–95.
2. Kelly BT, Riley III JW, Philippon MJ. Hip arthroscopy: current indications, treatment options, and management issues. Am J Sports Med. 2003;31:1020–37.
3. Byrd JWT. The role of hip arthroscopy in the athletic hip. Clin Sports Med. 2006;25:255–78.
4. Dorfmann H, Boyer T. Hip arthroscopy utilizing the supine position. Arthroscopy. 1996;12:264–7.
5. Dienst M, Gödde S, Seil R, Hammer D, Kohn D. Hip arthroscopy without traction. In vivo anatomy of the peripheral hip joint cavity. Arthroscopy. 2001;17:924–31.
6. Guanche CA, Bare AA. Arthroscopic treatment of femoroacetabular impingement. Arthroscopy. 2006;22:95–106.
7. Byrd JWT. Hip arthroscopy utilizing the supine position. Arthroscopy. 1994;10:275–80.
8. Byrd JW, Pappas JN, Pedley MJ. Hip arthroscopy: an anatomic study of portal placement and relationship to the extra-articular structures. Arthroscopy. 1995;11:418–23.
9. Petersilge CA, Haque MA, Petersilge WJ, Lewin JS, Lieberman JM, Buly R. Acetabular labral tears: evaluation with MR arthrography. Radiology. 1996;200:231–5.
10. Ghebontni L, Roger B, El-Khoury J, Brasseur JL, Grenier PA. MR arthrography of the hip: normal intra-articular structures and common disorders. Eur Radiol. 2000;10:83–8.
11. Petersilge CA. MR arthrography for evaluation of the acetabular labrum. Skeletal Radiol. 2001;30:423–30.
12. Byrd JWT. Labral lesions: an elusive source of hip pain case reports and literature review. Arthroscopy. 1996;12:603–12.
13. Fitzgerald Jr RH. Acetabular labrum tears: diagnosis and treatment. Clin Orthop. 1995;311:60–8.
14. McCarthy J, Noble P, Aluisio FV, Schuck M, Wright J, Lee J. Anatomy, pathologic features, and treatment of acetabular labral tears. Clin Orthop. 2003;406:38–47.
15. Brewster S. The development of the ligament of the head of the femur. Clin Anat. 1991;4:245–55.
16. Guanche CA, Sikka RS. Acetabular labral tears with underlying chondromalacia: a possible association with high-level running. Arthroscopy. 2005;21:580–5.
17. Wenger D, Miyanji F, Mahar A, et al. The mechanical properties of the ligamentum teres. A pilot study to assess its potential for improving stability in children's hip surgery. J Pediatr Orthop. 2007;4:408–10.
18. Beaulé P, Campbell P, Lu Z, et al. Vascularity of the arthritic femoral head and hip resurfacing. J Bone Joint Surg. 2006;88A:85–96.
19. Dorfmann H, Boyer T. Arthroscopy of the hip: 12 years experience. Arthroscopy. 1999;15:67–72.
20. Bond JL, Knutson ZA, Ebert A, et al. The 23-point arthroscopic examination of the hip: basic set-up, portal placement and surgical technique. Arthroscopy. 2009;25:416–29.
21. Byrd JWT. Avoiding the labrum in hip arthroscopy. Arthroscopy. 2000;16:770–3.
22. Paliobeis CP, Villar RN. Arthroscopic identification of iliopubic and ilioischial grooves in a single adult acetabulum. BMJ Case Rep. 2010. doi:10.1136/bcr.03.2010.2857.
23. Glick JM. Hip arthroscopy: the lateral approach. Clin Sports Med. 2001;20:733–47.
24. Byrd JWT. Gross anatomy. In: Byrd JWT, editor. Operative hip arthroscopy. 2nd ed. New York: Springer; 2005. p. 69–83.
25. Ganz R, Parvizi J, Beck M. Femoroacetabular impingement: a cause for osteoarthritis of the hip. Clin Orthop. 2003;417:112–20.
26. Ito K, Minka M, Leunig M. Femoroacetabular impingement and the cam-effect. J Bone Joint Surg Br. 2001;83B:171–6.
27. Lavigne M, Parvizi J, Beck M. Anterior femoroacetabular impingement. Part I: technique of joint preserving surgery. Clin Orthop. 2004;413:61–6.
28. Beck M, Leunig M, Parvizi J. Anterior femoroacetabular impingement. Part II: midterm results of surgical treatment. Clin Orthop. 2004;418:67–73.
29. Murphy S, Tannast M, Kim YJ. Debridement of the adult hip for femoroacetabular impingement: indications and preliminary clinical results. Clin Orthop. 2004;429:178–81.

Position and Distraction Options

10

Allston J. Stubbs and Austin V. Stone

Most complications in hip arthroscopy are due to too much or too little distraction.

—*James Glick, MD*

The patient must be properly positioned for the procedure to go well. Poor positioning will assure a difficult procedure.

—*J.W.T. Byrd, MD*

Introduction

While hip arthroscopy has advanced and become more utilized over the last two decades, the importance of proper patient positioning and hip joint distraction has not diminished. The constrained nature of the hip joint with a complex soft tissue envelope necessitates a predictable and reproducible method of access for even the most experienced hip surgeon and arthroscopist. As noted by Dr. Jim Glick early in the modern phase of hip arthroscopy, the adage still holds true that most procedural complications are associated with too much or too little distraction of the hip joint [1].

In the 1931, Dr. Burman was the first surgeon to comment in the literature that needle access between the head of the femur and the acetabulum was "manifestly impossible" [2]. Fortunately for the modern hip arthroscopist, hip joint access has evolved into a reproducible procedure that Dr. Burman would certainly appreciate today. Two primary patient positions – supine and lateral – have evolved over the last two decades to provide predictable access to most hip intra-articular and extra-articular anatomy. Despite the emergence of newer procedures and the improved recognition of pathology, the supine and lateral approaches have stood the test of time as safe, effective, and reproducible. Current hip arthroscopists have the luxury of deciding whether to perform in the supine or lateral position based on surgeon preference, patient factors, and the availability of operative equipment.

The purpose of this chapter is to review the principles and practice of both the supine and lateral positions for hip arthroscopy including anesthesia and operating room setup.

The risks and benefits as well as pearls and pitfalls will be reviewed for each. Further discussion will be made of distraction options that facilitate central compartment access in both positions. Portal access with either approach will be addressed in a future chapter. The goals of this chapter are to familiarize the reader with the historical and modern perspectives on hip arthroscopy positioning, the challenges of hip joint access with enumerated solutions, and the roles of hip joint distraction and "tractionless" hip arthroscopy.

Preoperative Planning: A Team Approach

Any discussion on the operative management of the hip arthroscopy patient should reassure the surgeon and promote a deliberate and team approach. Before a patient is ever introduced into the operative theater for a hip arthroscopy procedure, there should be a definitive understanding of the surgeon's expectations and the operative process from preinduction anesthesia to postoperative care. While hip arthroscopy is "an arthroscopic procedure," it is a new type of experience for most operating room staff. Keeping this fact in mind, the hip arthroscopist has already thought through the variety of procedural issues that may arise before ever starting the case. It is wise for the operative surgeon to hold "in-service-type" events with critical members of the team such as the anesthesiologist, circulating nurse, scrub assistant, industry representative, and preoperative and postoperative nursing. A well-rested and educated team will ensure the best possible outcome for the patient and the least amount of stress for the operating surgeon.

Anesthesia Planning

Fortunately, most hip arthroscopy procedures utilize anesthesia techniques common to hospitals and outpatient centers that perform orthopedic procedures. Several pieces of

A.J. Stubbs, M.D. (✉)
Department of Orthopaedic Surgery, Wake Forest University,
131 Miller Street, Winston-Salem, NC 27103, USA
e-mail: astubbs@wakehealth.edu

A.V. Stone, M.D.
Department of Orthopaedic Surgery, Wake Forest University,
Medical Center Boulevard, Winston-Salem, NC 27517, USA
e-mail: austin.stone@gmail.com

J.W.T. Byrd (ed.), *Operative Hip Arthroscopy*,
DOI 10.1007/978-1-4419-7925-4_10, © Springer Science+Business Media New York 2013

information about the hip arthroscopy procedure should be shared with the anesthesia team. The first and most important concern should be airway management – specifically how the patient will be positioned during the procedure, supine or lateral. Additionally, the position of the arms is important for IV access and blood pressure monitoring.

Second is the type of anesthesia requested. It is important to emphasize the importance of muscle relaxation and lack of patient movement during the procedure. The most predictable method to achieve relaxation is via general anesthesia with muscle paralytics. This approach works best in the patients with more advanced hip disease resulting in more difficult distraction, longer case times, and greater amounts of pathology to treat. Regional anesthesia techniques such as a lumbar plexus sciatic block can be employed for adjuvant relaxation and postoperative pain control. In centers where regional anesthesia is not available, spinal or epidural anesthesia may be sufficient as either a primary anesthesia plan or supplemental to general anesthesia.

Third is the importance of patient monitoring during the procedure. Specifically, maintaining euthermia may be difficult during long cases or centers without fluid warming capabilities. Also, blood pressure management may affect visualization during the procedure. We recommend maintaining the patient's mean arterial pressure (MAP) at approximately 65 mmHg or less. This MAP should be equal to or less than the arthroscopic pump pressure. Finally, educating the anesthesia team on signs of intra-abdominal or retroperitoneal fluid extravasation will help to reduce the morbidity of this complication.

Essential Operating Room Equipment

Several items are consistent in every hip arthroscopy case including access cannula systems, fluid management, radiofrequency (RF) devices, and fluoroscopy. Current cannula systems accommodate the standard large joint 4-mm arthroscope and may offer standard and long-length options depending on the thickness of the hip soft tissue envelopment. A standard axial MRI scan of the operative hip will allow the surgeon to accurately measure the depth of the joint from various points about the outer hip. These measurements can be compared to the operative cannula length of the system being used to ensure the greatest chance of success with cannula access. Hip arthroscopy cannula systems typically rely on an arthroscopic bridge that provides effective length to the cannula systems as well as fluid inflow and outflow ports. It is recommended that surgeons utilize a bridge that rotates separately from the arthroscope and camera head to avoid conflict between the fluid inflow/outflow and the fiber-optic light cord.

Fluid management is one of the most critical aspects of the case and should be monitored for both visualization and

patient safety. While gravity-fed systems may be sufficient, it is recommended that a third-generation fluid management system pump be utilized to ensure higher-flow/lower-pressure capability. More specifically, these newer pump designs are outflow dependent and as such limit the risk of continual fluid delivery to the thigh compartment, intra-abdominal compartment, or retroperitoneal space. As there are different pump systems available, no absolute values of fluid pressure or flow are recommended. However, the surgeon should utilize the settings that offer the most visibility and flexibility during the procedure while limiting the risk of fluid extravasation and RF overheating complications.

Third, RF devices have become a mainstay of arthroscopic procedures, and hip arthroscopy is no different. Fixed angle and flexible RF devices are available that allow the surgeon to achieve hemostasis, resect/ablate tissue, and assess tissue in a probe-like fashion. Successful use of the RF device relies on the surgeon to appreciate the amount of energy that each device emits. The way that a particular RF device behaves in the knee or shoulder joint will not necessarily predict the behavior within the hip joint. More specifically, the constrained nature of the hip joint makes RF access and control more challenging. A good rule of thumb is to limit RF use to the lowest energy setting possible and in the most conservative method possible. Ultimately, RF use around the hip joint has not been studied extensively and common sense is recommended.

Finally, fluoroscopic imaging is essential to ensuring that all efforts to obtain hip joint access are successful. A standard size fluoroscope is recommended to allow full circumferential access around the operative site. Mini-C-arm fluoroscopes common to small joint procedures are not recommended as they lack a diameter appropriate to access around most distraction systems. Generally speaking, the fluoroscope should be brought in from the side of the operative table opposite to the surgeon. Anticipated fluoroscope positions during the case should be assessed prior to initiating traction to ensure that anatomic views specific to the procedure are available. As with all procedures, for both the surgeon's, staff's, and patient's health, the amount of fluoroscopic exposure should be limited to only views and time needed to gain access, assess instrumentation position, and finalize procedural details.

Patient Positioning: Supine

Supine patient positioning for hip arthroscopy has been recommended as a less difficult position for OR staff and anesthesia team, more accessible for access to the anterior hip region, and more predictable surgeon positioning on fracture table. For certain surgeons and operating environments, it may be a faster setup than the lateral position [3].

Supine Positioning with Standard Table

The patient is placed supine on a standard fracture table or Jackson table with traction attachment (Fig. 10.1). The upper extremities may be wrapped together in a papoose fashion across the patient's chest or with the operative side arm draped individually across the chest. Circulation to the upper extremity or upper extremities is optimized by spacing over a small stack of blankets which allows the elbow(s) to be flexed less than 90°. As there is a chance of positional ischemia to the upper extremity placed across the chest, we recommend a pulse oximeter to a finger to ensure good perfusion during the case. The arm on the nonoperative side, if not positioned across the chest, can be placed on an arm board for improved anesthesia vascular access. The grounding pad for the RF device is attached to the patient's skin across the abdomen or nonoperative thigh.

The fracture table or distraction attachment should have the option to lateralize the perineal post toward the operative side. This lateral post placement should be secured before moving the patient to the operative table. The patient's pelvis is subsequently positioned against a well-padded perineal post. The padded post will abut against the medial thigh of the operative hip. This additional padding with a transverse force vector against the thigh minimizes the potential of pudendal nerve neurapraxia.

The patient's feet are padded and placed in the traction boots in neutral rotation with the hips flexed 15° and abducted to approximately 25° (Fig. 10.2a). Hip distraction with excessive flexion increases the tension on the sciatic nerve and may result in sciatic injury. The nonoperative limb is positioned with three things in mind: to provide adequate room for hip visualization with the C-arm fluoroscope, to stabilize the pelvis and torso with a mild counterforce, and to avoid any undue stress on the nonoperative limb and hip joint. The nonoperative limb is allowed to rotate to its natural rotation, and this rotation is secured for the remainder of the operation. A slight countertraction of 10–20 lb is applied to the nonoperative leg to stabilize the pelvis and torso. All bony prominences should be well padded with foam or towels, with specific attention placed on the contralateral ischial tuberosity and sacrum which may rest or be at risk for resting on exposed plastic or metal bed parts.

A surgical time-out is typically done before the application of traction to the operative lower extremity. All traction to the operative leg is done in a gentle and deliberate fashion.

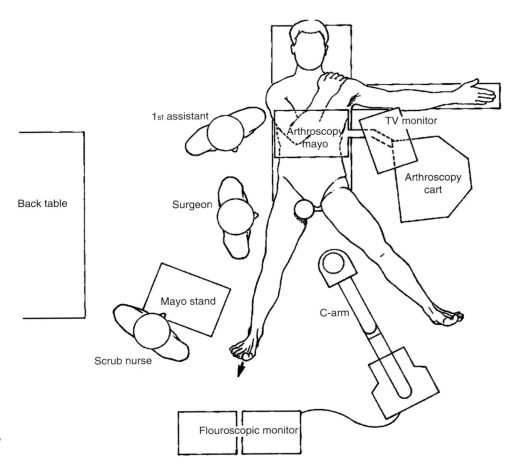

Fig. 10.1 Operating room setup supine schematic. (Courtesy of J.W. Thomas Byrd, MD, Nashville, TN)

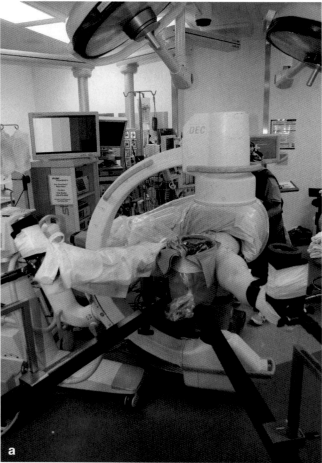

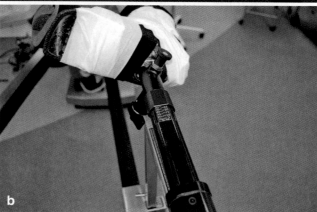

Fig. 10.2 (**a**) Operating room setup supine: Note padded perineal post, padded and reinforced feet, papoosed upper extremity, and relative position of critical equipment. (**b**) Tensiometer for table distraction: Note that this may be useful for operative and nonoperative leg in supine position

Adequate anesthesia including muscle paralysis is checked at this point. We recommend the application of traction before the operative hip is prepped and draped for the procedure. This application is done to ensure that the operative setup is secure and will provide the appropriate amount of distraction to access the hip joint.

To apply traction, the operative knee is brought into full extension with the foot in neutral rotation. The abduction/adduction movement of the operative hip is allowed to move freely. The operative lower extremity is then brought into neutral adduction against the padded perineal post. A fluoroscopic view of the operative hip is taken, and the operative surgeon looks for a radiographic lucency (vacuum) between the femoral head and acetabular roof known as the crescent sign [4]. If a crescent sign is visualized on the fluoroscopic view, then the operative leg is secured in this neutral rotation. If there is no crescent sign, then additional traction is gently applied through the traction boot until the crescent sign appears on the adducted fluoroscopic view. In an adequately relaxed patient, most hip joints will distract with approximately 25–50 lb of traction [5] – effectively the weight of a small child (Fig. 10.2b). Hyperlaxity patients may require less traction. Arthritic patients may require more traction. While not required, a tensiometer may be helpful in monitoring and assessing the amount of relative traction used to distract a hip joint.

Approximately 10–15 mm of fluoroscopic joint space is sufficient at initial distraction since the hip capsule and associated soft tissues will relax and accommodate the new tensile forces applied through the joint. Traction may be relaxed while the operative hip is prepped and draped and then reapplied. Alternatively, prior to the application of traction to the hip, the hip can be prepped and draped to allow venting of the capsule with a spinal needle to decrease the intrinsic negative pressure vacuum between the femoral head and acetabulum. This needle venting may decrease the amount of force necessary to initiate the fluoroscopic crescent sign seen with joint distraction. The surgeon, assistant, and scrub technician stand on the operative side of the patient with the fluoroscopy and arthroscopy monitors located opposite the surgeon.

Patient Positioning: Lateral

Lateral positioning of the patient offers an alternative to the supine position (Fig. 10.3). The position is familiar to most orthopedic surgeons because it is similar to the lateral decubitus positioning for total hip arthroplasty. One advantage of the lateral position is ease of access to the hip in obese patients because gravity pulls the panniculus away from the operative field [6–9]. The earliest proponents of the lateral position were Drs. Glick and Sampson who noted that the entry to the hip is simpler than the supine technique because the approach into the hip is in a straight line over the greater trochanter [6]. In cases where there are large anterior hip osteophytes, one may find the lateral position and entry to be necessary. Instrumentation placement and surgical assistant location across from the surgeon may also be facilitated by

Fig. 10.3 Operating room setup lateral schematic

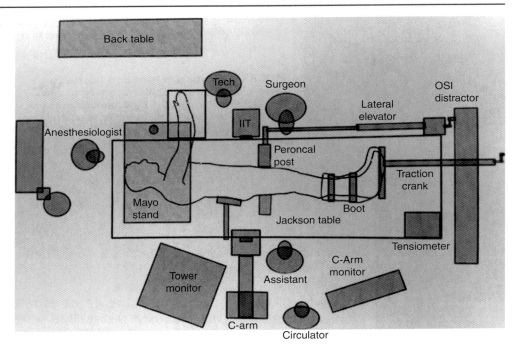

lateral positioning. The extra time spent in positioning the patient is a frequently cited concern; however, Sampson has noted that surgeries in the lateral position were completed more quickly despite the extra time spent in positioning the patient [1].

Lateral Positioning with Standard Table

In the lateral position, the patient is placed in the lateral decubitus position on a standard operating table with the involved hip upward (Fig. 10.4) [6, 9]. The upper extremities are placed out from the patient with an axillary roll placed under the dependent axilla. The upper torso is secured with a beanbag device or padded bolsters and straps. A heavily padded (at least 9-cm) perineal post is secured to the table such that it projects eccentrically skyward to ensure an adequate axial vector against the perineum and lateral vector against the operative medial thigh. The operative lower extremity is padded along the foot and ankle and placed in a traction boot and positioned such that the operative medial thigh rests against the perineal post. The contralateral limb remains well padded and resting dependently on the table without any additional preparation.

Like the supine approach, the anterior capsule is relaxed by placing the hip in sight flexion (15°), but as with the supine position, care must be exercised to avoid excessive tension on the sciatic nerve. Flexion beyond 20° is not beneficial and places the sciatic nerve at risk. In similar fashion to the supine position, traction should be tested under fluoroscopic visualization prior to sterile prep and draping to

ensure adequate distraction can be achieved. Gentle traction is applied through the operative limb until a crescent sign is noted on the fluoroscopic image intensifier [4]. A tensiometer may be used to monitor the relative traction across the extremity. Additionally, the hip capsule may be vented in a sterile fashion before the application of traction. The C-arm fluoroscope should remain nearby for use to visualize the hip until the portals are placed. During portal placement, the operative limb remains in neutral rotation to maximize the distance to the sciatic nerve from the posterior portal. The surgeon stands on the front side of the patient with an assistant across the operative field. A scrub technician is closer to the patient's feet and behind the surgeon.

Distraction Options

Ultimately, distraction of the hip is critical to the success of central compartment hip arthroscopy. Traction allows for portal placement and enables instrumentation to be efficiently and effectively maneuvered. Initial reports of distraction forces needed approached 200 lb; however, more recent investigation determined that proper anesthesia and release of the intra-articular vacuum in the hip joint significantly reduce the distraction force [10, 11]. The importance of decompressing the joint by puncturing the joint capsule and injecting normal saline was first estimated in nonanesthetized volunteers and then confirmed in a cadaveric study [10–12]. By releasing the intra-articular vacuum and properly anesthetizing the patient, effective distraction can be achieved at more reasonable forces under 50 lb [10].

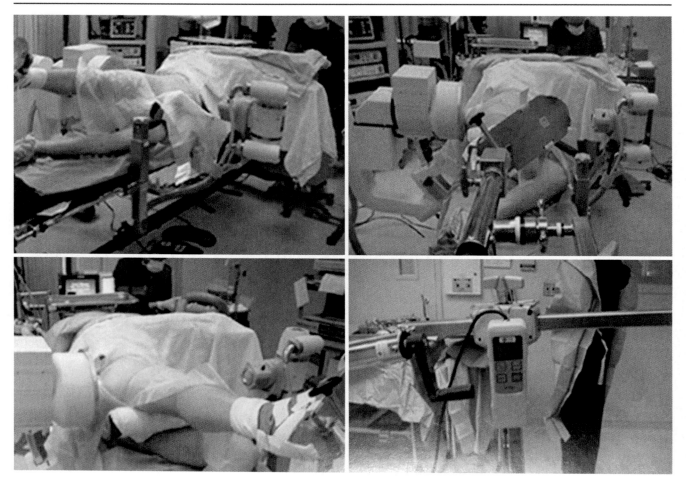

Fig. 10.4 Operating room setup lateral: Note padded perineal post, padded and reinforced feet, draped upper extremity, and relative position of critical equipment. Images courtesy of Thomas Sampson, MD, San Francisco, CA

Some devices are designed for use with standard operating tables, rather than the fracture table. The use of these devices maybe beneficial in centers where fracture tables are limited or unavailable and where patient characteristics and surgeon preference preclude their use. These distraction devices have not been comparatively reviewed, so surgeon preference, surgical center availability, and training are the primary determining factors.

In addition to standard hip fracture tables such as the Maquet table (Getinge Group AB, Solna, Sweden) and Amsco OrthoVision table (Steris, Inc, Mentor, OH, USA), commercially available "noninvasive" hip distractors are present for both the lateral and supine positions. The Smith and Nephew Hip Positioning System (Andover, MA, USA), the OSI hip distractor (Union City, CA, USA), the Spider Hip Position System (Tenet Medical, Calgary, Canada), and the Arthrex Hip Distractor System (Arthrex, Inc., Naples, FL, USA) can all be used for either the supine or lateral positions; the McCarthy Hip Distractor by Innomed (Savannah, GA, USA) is for the lateral position only. Additionally, two "inva-

sive" hip distraction systems are also available. The first, the DR Hip Distractor (DR Medical AG, Solothurn, Switzerland) can be used in both supine and lateral positions. The second, the Dahners Hip Distractor from Medical Products Resource (Burnsville, MN) is used for the lateral position only.

The Smith and Nephew Endoscopy Hip Positioning System attaches to a standard operating table for use with either the supine or lateral position. Its system is radiolucent and contains an enlarged perineal post to minimize the opportunity for nerve compression. The Arthrex Hip Distractor System attaches to a standard operating table and may be used with either position, too. Also, it may be autoclaved.

The DR Medical Hip Distractor operates as a sterile, external fixator device that does not require a perineal post. It is beneficial in cases with expected traction times over 2 h due to early surgeon experience and complex central compartment work. As an external fixation system, it requires pin placement into the pelvis and femur but avoids complications involving sciatic nerve stretch injury or skin complications along the foot and ankle [13].

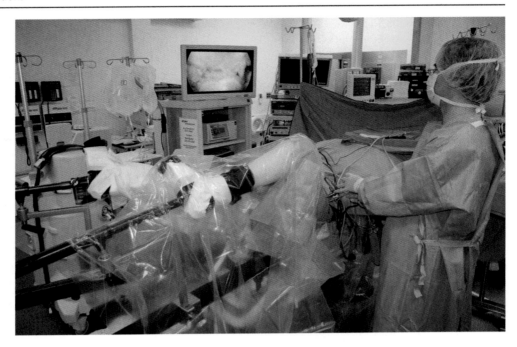

Fig. 10.5 Tractionless hip arthroscopy: Note position of operative extremity in approximately 40° of hip flexion

The Dahners Hip Distractor is unique in that it uses skeletal traction through a distal femoral K-wire and is also an independent sterile component in the operative field [14, 15]. This autoclavable distractor system allows the surgeon to manipulate the traction device intraoperatively and remain sterile. The use of this skeletal traction system also avoids complications with skin compression along the foot and ankle region.

Tractionless Hip Arthroscopy

Both supine and lateral positioning allows for tractionless hip arthroscopy; however, different distraction systems may facilitate or inhibit its use. In theory, hip arthroscopy without traction is like surgery without a tourniquet. In selective situations, it can be less stressful, lower risk, and more flexible. Hip arthroscopy without traction is primarily utilized to approach the peripheral compartment space to manage loose bodies, synovial disorders, labral disorders, and CAM morphology along the femoral head and neck junction. Further use of the hip arthroscope in an endoscopic fashion allows visualization of the lesser trochanteric space to perform iliopsoas release, the greater trochanteric space to manage the abductor compartment and greater trochanteric bursa, and the subgluteal space to manage nerve entrapment and piriformis conditions.

A hip arthroscopy within the capsule and hip endoscopy outside the capsule may begin out of traction from the peripheral compartment, or it may follow central compartment work in traction. To facilitate entry into the peripheral compartment space, one must flex the hip approximately 40° to relax the anterior capsule of the hip [16] (Fig. 10.5). This hip flexion is performed without any distraction across the hip joint. The peripheral compartment space may be entered directly from the central compartment after the release of traction or may be entered de novo with the assistance of fluoroscopy to identify the trajectory of the femoral neck. In the de novo approach, a Seldinger-type technique is used to guide the hip cannula to the intracapsular space. With a Seldinger-based approach, the surgeon via an accessory anterolateral portal and fluoroscopic guidance directs a spinal needle along the femoral neck through the capsule and into the peripheral compartment. A nitinol guidewire threaded through the spinal needle is subsequently used to guide dilator and cannula access into the peripheral compartment space. The most versatile hip positioning systems allow for full freedom of motion of the hip joint to completely evaluate the peripheral compartment space.

Further endoscopic approaches can be performed with the hip in neutral flexion. Approaches are facilitated to the lesser trochanter with the lower extremity in external rotation, the greater trochanter with the lower extremity in abduction, and the subgluteal space with the hip in more extension. Future chapters will detail specific access recommendations to these anatomic regions.

Complications

While there is a future chapter devoted to hip arthroscopy complications, there has been no significant difference in complication rates between hip arthroscopy attempted from the supine and lateral positions. Both positioning options are subject to the

Table 10.1 Patient position and distraction pearls

Develop and follow a positioning protocol for either supine or lateral position
Educate your operative team on the supine or lateral position
Obtain and maintain adequate anesthesia
Know your equipment and its limitations
Have essential instrumentation and equipment available before application of traction
Keep traction to approximately 1 h and less than 2 h continuous

Table 10.2 Avoiding and preventing position and distraction complications

Potential pitfalls	Avoiding pitfalls
Pudendal neurapraxia	Eccentrically located perineal post with >9-cm pad
	Limit traction time to 1–2 h
Genital injury	Check before, during, and after application of traction
	Eccentrically located perineal post with >9-cm pad
	Limit traction time to 1–2 h
Lower extremity skin injury	Well padded and secure traction boot
	Limit traction time to 1–2 h
Sciatic nerve injury	Do not flex the hip >20° in traction
	Limit traction time to 1–2 h
Articular surface damage	Achieve at least 12–15 mm of radiographic distraction
	Utilize atraumatic cannulae and fluoroscopy
	Appreciate feel of needle and cannula entry

same complications, including nerve palsy, genital injury, and skin compromise. The rate of these complications is below 5% and may be improving with more reliable distraction options and better surgeon awareness and education [17, 18].

Several pearls of wisdom have emerged over the last 20 years regarding the avoidance of complications with positioning and distraction. These suggestions are listed in Table 10.1. Most important of these observations are to maintain traction times around 1 h (absolute traction time of 2 h continuous), protect vulnerable areas, and use the least amount of force necessary to distract and maintain access the joint [19].

A report of 283 consecutive procedures reported by Byrd in the supine position noted just three complications (1%) [5]. One patient developed portal tract heterotopic ossification and a neurapraxia of a branch of the lateral femoral cutaneous nerve. A second patient experienced a partial transient neurapraxia of the lateral femoral cutaneous nerve that completely resolved. The author also reports that one patient felt that the surgery made her feel worse.

The majority of complications from hip arthroscopy are related to traction [5, 17, 18]; however, the vast majority of these complications are avoidable with careful consideration

of the amount of traction force and duration of traction [17, 19]. In Sampson's review of 530 cases at a single institution, the author reported 34 cases with complications (6.4%). Of the 27 transient complications, 20 were transient nerve injuries and were directly related to the prolonged traction times (>5 h) [17]. Only three of these cases were considered significant and none were related to traction. Reducing the amount of traction force and monitoring the time of traction and intermittent release during complicated cases will help avoid traction-related complications (Table 10.2).

Summary

Supine positioning and lateral positioning are two successful approaches to hip arthroscopy. Good outcomes and low complication rates are comparable for both methods. Each requires a dedicated surgical team approach involving anesthesia and nursing. The operative setup for hip arthroscopy comprises essential equipment and modern distraction systems. The hip arthroscopist should be familiar with available distraction options and operative resources to ensure reproducibility and the best patient outcome.

References

1. Sampson TG. The lateral approach. In: Byrd JWT, editor. Operative hip arthroscopy. 2nd ed. New York: Thieme; 2005. p. 129–44.
2. Burman MS. Arthroscopy or direct visualization of the joints: an experimental cadaver study. J Bone Joint Surg Am. 1931;13A:669–95.
3. Byrd JWT. The supine approach. In: Byrd JWT, editor. Operative hip arthroscopy. 2nd ed. New York: Thieme; 2005. p. 145–69.
4. Philippon MJ, Stubbs AJ, Schenker ML, Maxwell RB, Ganz R, Leunig M. Arthroscopic management of femoroacetabular impingement: osteoplasty technique and literature review. Am J Sports Med. 2007;35:1571–80.
5. Byrd JWT. Hip arthroscopy: the supine position. Clin Sports Med. 2001;20:703–31.
6. Glick JM. Hip arthroscopy: the lateral approach. Clin Sports Med. 2001;20:733–47.
7. Glick JM. Hip arthroscopy by the lateral approach. Instr Course Lect. 2006;55:317–23.
8. Glick JM. Hip arthroscopy using the lateral approach. Instr Course Lect. 1988;37:223–31.
9. Glick JM, Sampson TG, Gordon RB, Behr JT, Schmidt E. Hip arthroscopy by the lateral approach. Arthroscopy. 1987;3:4–12.
10. McCarthy JC. Hip arthroscopy: applications and technique. J Am Acad Orthop Surg. 1995;3:115–22.
11. Eriksson E, Arvidsson I, Arvidsson H. Diagnostic and operative arthroscopy of the hip. Orthopedics. 1986;9:169–76.
12. Dienst M, Gödde S, Seil R, Hammer D, Kohn D. Hip arthroscopy without traction: in vivo anatomy of the peripheral hip joint cavity. J Arthroscopy. 2001;17:924–31.
13. Simpson J, Sadri H, Villar R. Hip arthroscopy techniques and complications. Orthop Traumatol Surg Res. 2010;96(8 Suppl):S68–76.
14. Smart LR, Oetgen M, Noonan B, Medvecky M. Beginning hip arthroscopy: indications, positioning, portals, basic techniques, and complications. J Arthroscopy. 2007;23:1348–53.

15. Bushnell BD, Hoover SA, Olcott CW, Dahners LE. Use of an independent skeletal distractor in hip arthroscopy. J Arthroscopy. 2007;23:106.e1–4.

16. Dienst M. Hip arthroscopy without traction. In: Byrd JWT, editor. Operative hip arthroscopy. 2nd ed. New York: Thieme; 2005. p. 170–88.

17. Sampson TG. Complications of hip arthroscopy. Clin Sports Med. 2001;20:831–5.

18. Clarke MT, Arora A, Villar RN. Hip arthroscopy: complications in 1054 cases. Clin Orthop Relat Res. 2003;406:84–8.

19. Byrd JWT. Complications associated with hip arthroscopy. In: Byrd JWT, editor. Operative hip arthroscopy. 2nd ed. New York: Thieme; 2005. p. 229–35.

Routine Arthroscopy and Access: Central and Peripheral Compartments, Iliopsoas Bursa, Peritrochanteric, and Subgluteal Spaces

J.W. Thomas Byrd

Introduction

Hip arthroscopy first started with the central (intra-articular) compartment and evolved to include the peripheral compartment [1–3]. Iliopsoas bursoscopy was then developed to access the iliopsoas tendon [4]. Further endoscopic techniques have been formulated accessing the peritrochanteric space and then migrating into the subgluteal region, and early work has begun on endoscopic treatment of proximal hamstring lesions [5, 6]. This evolution is not yet complete.

Arthroscopy of the hip can be effectively performed with the patient in either the supine or lateral position. The selection is largely based on the surgeon's personal preference. Most surgeons have chosen to adopt the supine method. The qualities of this approach that we favor are as follows. Positioning of the patient is simple and can be accomplished in just a few minutes. The procedure can be performed on virtually any standard fracture table although special distractors are also available that are more readily available in an outpatient setting. Orientation of the joint is familiar to orthopedic surgeons accustomed to managing hip fractures, and the layout of the operating room is user-friendly for the surgeon, assistants, and operating room staff. There is reliable access for all standard portal placements, and it easily accommodates repositioning for arthroscopy of the peripheral compartment as well as iliopsoas bursoscopy and most other surrounding endoscopic techniques around the hip.

Dictums on Hip Arthroscopy

Regardless of the position or technique that is chosen for performing this procedure, there are several dictums that should be thoroughly understood. First, a successful outcome is

J.W.T. Byrd, M.D.
Nashville Sports Medicine Foundation,
2011 Church Street, Suite 100, Nashville, TN 37203, USA
e-mail: byrd@nsmfoundation.org

most clearly dependent on proper patient selection. A technically well-executed procedure will fail when performed for the wrong reason. This may include failure of the procedure to meet the patient's expectations. Second, the patient must be properly positioned in order for the case to go well. Poor positioning will assure a difficult procedure. Third, simply gaining access to the hip joint is not an outstanding technical accomplishment. The paramount issue is accessing the joint in as atraumatic a fashion as possible. Due to its constrained architecture and dense soft tissue envelope, the potential for inadvertent iatrogenic scope trauma is significant and, perhaps to some extent, unavoidable. Thus, every reasonable step should be taken to keep this concern to a minimum. Perform the procedure as carefully as possible and be certain that it is being performed for the right reason.

OR Setup

Anesthesia

The procedure is performed as an outpatient under general anesthesia. Epidural is an appropriate alternative but requires an adequate motor block to ensure muscle relaxation.

Patient Positioning

(See Video 11.1: http://goo.gl/E7JHa) A fracture table can be used, or a specially designed distractor can be adapted to a standard OR table (Fig. 11.1a, b). The patient is positioned supine. A heavily padded perineal post is used. The genitalia are carefully inspected to make sure that the area is not going to be harmed by the post during the application of traction. The post is positioned laterally against the medial thigh of the operative leg (Fig. 11.2). Lateralizing the perineal post adds a slight transverse component to the direction of the traction vector (Fig. 11.3). It also distances the post from the area of the pudendal nerve, lessening the risk of compression neurapraxia.

J.W.T. Byrd (ed.), *Operative Hip Arthroscopy*,
DOI 10.1007/978-1-4419-7925-4_11, © Springer Science+Business Media New York 2013

The operative hip is positioned in approximately 25° of abduction. Slight flexion (<10°) may relax the capsule and facilitate distraction, but excessive flexion should be avoided.

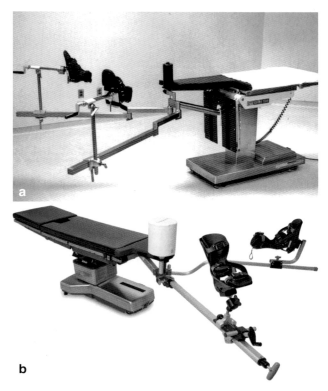

Fig. 11.1 (**a**) Most standard fracture tables can accommodate the needs of hip arthroscopy with a few modifications. (**b**) A specialized distractor provides versatility and is more practical for an outpatient ambulatory surgery setting. (All rights are retained by Dr. Byrd)

Increasing flexion places tension on the sciatic nerve and may increase the risk of traction neurapraxia and will also start to close off access to the anterior part of the hip. Neutral rotation of the extremity during portal placement is important for proper orientation, but freedom of rotation of the foot plate during the procedure facilitates visualization of the femoral head.

The contralateral extremity is abducted as necessary to accommodate positioning of the image intensifier between the legs. The image intensifier can be placed from the opposite side of the patient, but this eliminates the ability to obtain lateral or oblique views of the hip. Prior to distracting the operative hip, slight traction is applied to the nonoperative leg. This stabilizes the torso on the table and keeps the pelvis from shifting during distraction of the operative hip.

Traction is then applied to the operative extremity and distraction of the joint confirmed by fluoroscopic examination. Usually, about 50 lb of traction force is adequate. Sometimes more force is necessary for an especially tight hip but should be undertaken with caution. About 8–10 mm of joint space separation is needed for introduction of the instruments. Some hips can be easily distracted with only slight traction. Excessive joint space separation (greater than 1.5–2 cm) should be avoided. Traction neurapraxia can occur from excessive elongation as well as from excessive force.

If adequate distraction is not readily achieved, allowing a few minutes for the capsule to accommodate to the tensile forces often results in relaxation of the capsule and adequate distraction without excessive force. Also, a vacuum phenomenon will be apparent fluoroscopically. This is created by the negative intracapsular pressure caused by distraction. This seal will be released when the joint is distended with fluid at

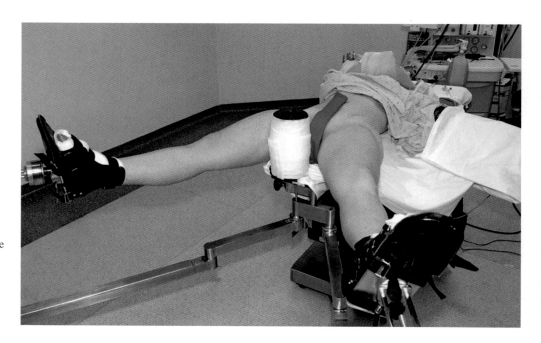

Fig. 11.2 The patient is positioned on the fracture table so that the perineal post is placed as far laterally as possible toward the operative hip resting against the medial thigh. (All rights are retained by Dr. Byrd)

Fig. 11.3 The optimal vector for distraction is oblique relative to the axis of the body and more closely coincides with the axis of the femoral neck than the femoral shaft. This oblique vector is partially created by abduction of the hip and partially accentuated by a small transverse component to the vector (Courtesy of J.W. Thomas Byrd, MD, Nashville, TN)

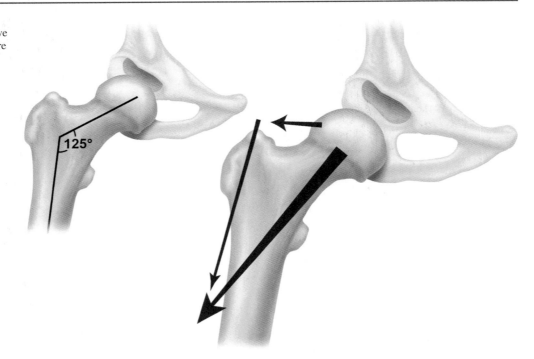

the time of surgery and may further facilitate distraction. However, the effect is variable and should not be depended on to overcome inadequate traction [7].

Once the ability to distract the hip joint has been confirmed, the traction is released. The hip is then prepped and draped and traction reapplied when ready to begin arthroscopy. The surgeon, assistant, and scrub nurse are positioned on the operative side of the patient. The monitor and arthroscopy equipment with a sterile Mayo stand containing the arthroscopes and power shaver are positioned on the contralateral side (Fig. 11.4).

Tips

If a hip has limited flexibility, it should not be forced to neutral rotation. This may unnecessarily tighten the capsule and create more challenges for distraction. Also, less abduction may be necessary in the presence of a varus femoral neck in order to adequately access the joint around the greater trochanter.

There are different descriptions on how best to position the leg and each may work well. Whichever is selected, it is important to position the patient the same way each time in order to become consistent in the technique of hip arthroscopy. Certain circumstances such as the patient's body type or joint configuration may require adjustments, but it is important to have a reproducible starting point from which these adjustments are made.

Normally, when applying traction to the hip, if a little joint space separation is achieved, this is an encouraging sign that sufficient separation will be accomplished once the vacuum seal has been released and the joint distended with fluid. When traction is applied and no joint separation occurs, this may be an indication of a tight hip which should be evident from the exam or may indicate that the labral seal is successfully functioning as a gasket. When applying traction, a noticeable pop may occur where the labral seal releases and the joint opens up. If not, when the joint is vented with the spinal needle, this will usually result in adequate distraction. If the joint space separation is limited despite application of traction and distension with fluid, this indicates a tight hip that may require special considerations for access. This is covered in Chap. 27.

Traction neurapraxias are usually deemed to be a consequence of traction force and time. In general, sufficient force is necessary to achieve adequate joint space separation for placing the instruments and avoiding iatrogenic injury. Most often, 2 h is described as an appropriate limit on the duration of traction [8]. This is equated to tourniquet time although there is no physiologic correlation between the two. If more prolonged periods of traction are necessary, the traction can be released, allowing the joint to rest, and then be reapplied.

Fig. 11.4 Schematic of the operating room layout showing the position of the surgeon, assistant, scrub nurse, arthroscopy cart, monitor and Mayo, scrub nurse's Mayo, C-arm, and back table (Courtesy of J.W. Thomas Byrd, MD, Nashville, TN)

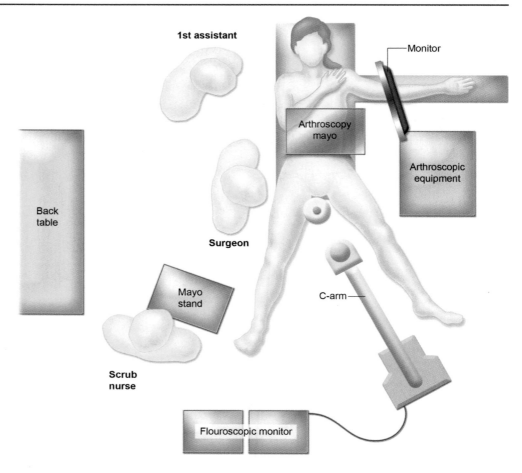

Equipment

Specialized distractors have been developed that can be applied to a standard operating room table (Fig. 11.1b). These are especially applicable in the outpatient setting where a fracture table would not normally be available. Otherwise, most standard fracture tables can accommodate the few specific needs of hip arthroscopy (Fig. 11.1a). A tensiometer is a helpful tool that can be incorporated into the foot plate. This is especially useful for monitoring the intraoperative ability to maintain adequate distraction. A large-sized perineal post with generous padding more safely distributes the pressure on the perineum and facilitates lateralization of the operative hip.

An image intensifier is used for all cases. This is important for assuring precise portal placement. Simply accessing the joint is often not difficult. More important is care and precision in portal placement to minimize the risk of iatrogenic damage.

Both the 30° and 70° arthroscopes are routinely used to optimize visualization. Interchanging the two scopes allows excellent visualization despite the limited maneuverability caused by the bony architecture of the joint and its dense soft tissue envelope. The 30° scope provides the best view of the central portion of the acetabulum and femoral head and the

superior portion of the acetabular fossa, while the 70° scope is best for visualizing the outer edges of the joint, the acetabular labrum, the capsule, and the inferior portion of the fossa.

A fluid pump provides significant advantages in the hip. A high flow system can provide optimal flow without having to use excessive pressure. This is important for visualization and safety. Adequate flow is essential for good visualization necessary in order to perform the procedure effectively and in an expedient manner. Flow cannot be as precisely modulated with a gravity system, creating difficulties both with visualization and extravasation. However, the surgeon must always be cognizant that the pump is functioning properly. Different pumps perform and behave differently, and it is important to be familiar with the traits of a given pump before using it during complex hip procedures.

Extra-length cannulas are specifically designed to accommodate the dense soft tissue envelope that surrounds the hip (Fig. 11.5). The extra length has been accomplished by shortening the accompanying bridge which allows these cannulas to be used with a standard arthroscope. For extremely large patients, there are also special extra long scopes (Fig. 11.6). Cannulated obturators allow passage of the cannula/obturator assembly over a nitinol guide wire prepositioned in the joint through 6-in., 17-gauge spinal needles (Fig. 11.7). The scrub

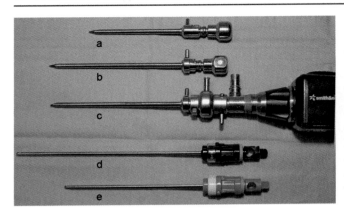

Fig. 11.5 A standard arthroscopic cannula (**a**) is compared to the extra-length cannula (**b**). A modified bridge (**c**) has been shortened to accommodate the extra-length cannula with a standard length arthroscope. Extra-length blades (**d**) are also available compared to the standard length blades (**e**). (All rights are retained by Dr. Byrd)

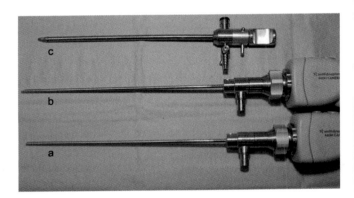

Fig. 11.6 Extra-length 30° (**a**) and 70° (**b**) scopes are available with an accompanying diagnostic cannula (**c**) to accommodate extremely dense soft tissues. (All rights are retained by Dr. Byrd)

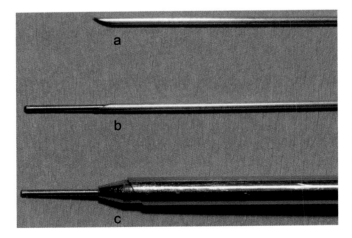

Fig. 11.7 The cannulated obturator system allows for greater ease in reliably establishing the portals once proper positioning has been achieved with the spinal needle. The 6" 17-gauge spinal needle (**a**, **b**) accommodates passage of a nitinol wire (**b**, **c**). Specially treated, the wire is resistant to kinking. The cannulated obturator allows for passage of the obturator/cannula assembly over the guide wire (**c**). (All rights are retained by Dr. Byrd)

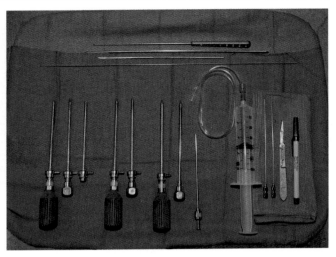

Fig. 11.8 The scrub nurse's Mayo stand contains basic instruments necessary for initiating the arthroscopic procedure including: a marking pen; #11 blade scalpel; 6" 17-gauge spinal needles; 60-cc syringe of saline with extension tubing; a nitinol guide wire; three 4.5-, two 5.0-, and one 5.5-mm cannulas with cannulated and solid obturators; a switching stick; a separate inflow adapter; and modified probe. (All rights are retained by Dr. Byrd)

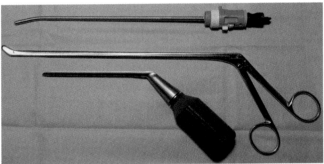

Fig. 11.9 A slotted cannula allows great versatility for curved shavers, large hand instruments, and numerous other needs around the hip. (All rights are retained by Dr. Byrd)

nurse's Mayo stand contains the instruments routinely needed for each case (Fig. 11.8). The 5.0-mm cannula is used for initial introduction of the arthroscope while the inflow is attached. The diameter allows adequate flow for the fluid management system attached through the bridge. Once all three portals have been established, the inflow can be switched to one of the other cannulas and the 5.0-mm cannula replaced with a 4.5-mm cannula. The use of three 4.5-mm cannulas allows complete interchangeability of the arthroscope, instruments, and inflow. The 5.5-mm cannula is available for larger shaver blades.

Extra-length blades are available. Curved designs can be useful for maneuvering within the spherical geometry of the joint. These can be passed through slotted cannulas (Fig. 11.9) which accommodate the curved shaver blades as well as other hand instruments.

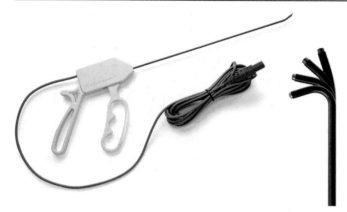

Fig. 11.10 A flexible radiofrequency device is an important adjunct to rigid instruments and shavers, which are restricted due to the constrained anatomy of the hip. (All rights are retained by Dr. Byrd)

Thermal devices demonstrate specific advantages in the hip. The small diameter and flexible designs allow access to recesses within the joint difficult to access with mechanical blades (Fig. 11.10). Also, because of the limits on maneuverability, it can be difficult for the shaver to excise damaged articular cartilage or labrum and create a stable edge. Thermal devices are often much more effective at creating a smooth transition zone, preserving more healthy tissue.

General Technique

The technique described here has proved to be effective and reproducible [9, 10]. Routine arthroscopy begins in the central compartment because it is the most common site of pathology that leads to painful symptoms precipitating the need for arthroscopy (Video 11.2: http://goo.gl/vps17). Usually, the procedure will include arthroscopy of the peripheral compartment and possibly other extra-articular areas. However, it is the findings of the central compartment that typically dictate the extent of the procedure that must be performed, for example, correction of FAI, as well as others.

Central Compartment

Portals

(See Video 11.3: http://goo.gl/kj83A) Three standard portals are utilized for arthroscopy of the intra-articular compartment: anterior, anterolateral, and posterolateral (Figs. 11.11 and 11.12) [11, 12]. The site of the anterior portal coincides with the intersection of a sagittal line drawn distally from the anterior superior iliac spine and a transverse line across the superior margin of the greater tro-

chanter. The direction of this portal courses approximately 45° cephalad and 30° toward the midline http://goo.gl/E7JHa). The anterolateral and posterolateral portals are positioned directly over the superior aspect of the trochanter at its anterior and posterior borders.

Another popular portal is the modified anterior position (Fig. 11.13) [13]. As the name implies, it is a modification of the standard description, with a more lateral and distal location. Variations of 1–2 cm on the anterior portal are common to achieve accurate triangulation into the joint. A more distal position may be chosen by some to give a better angle for placing anchors in the anterior rim of the acetabulum (Video 11.4: http://goo.gl/S58cw). However, this site may need to have a more extreme distal location in order to make sure that the anchors diverge from the articular surface of the acetabulum. A curved drill guide system can make this a little easier from the modified position. A more distal site has less utility for accessing other pathology of the central compartment. Also, there is a misperception that moving the portal more laterally avoids branches of the lateral femoral cutaneous nerve which is not the case [11].

Anterior Portal

The pathway of the anterior portal penetrates the muscle belly of the sartorius and the rectus femoris before entering the anterior capsule (Fig. 11.14). At the portal level, the lateral femoral cutaneous nerve has usually divided into three or more branches. Consequently, the portal usually passes within several millimeters of one of these branches. Because of the multiple branches, the nerve is not easily avoided by altering the portal position. Rather, it is protected by utilizing meticulous technique in portal placement. Specifically, the nerve is most vulnerable to a deeply placed skin incision which lacerates one of the branches. Therefore, the initial stab wound should be made carefully through the skin only. Passing from the skin to capsule, the anterior portal runs almost tangential to the axis of the femoral nerve and lies only slightly closer to it at the level of the capsule, with an average minimum distance of 3.2 cm. The relationship of the ascending branch of the lateral circumflex femoral artery is variable but averages 3.6 cm inferior to the anterior portal.

Anterolateral Portal

The anterolateral portal penetrates the gluteus medius prior to entering the lateral aspect of the capsule at its anterior margin (Fig. 11.15). The superior gluteal nerve lies an average of 4.4 cm superior to the portal.

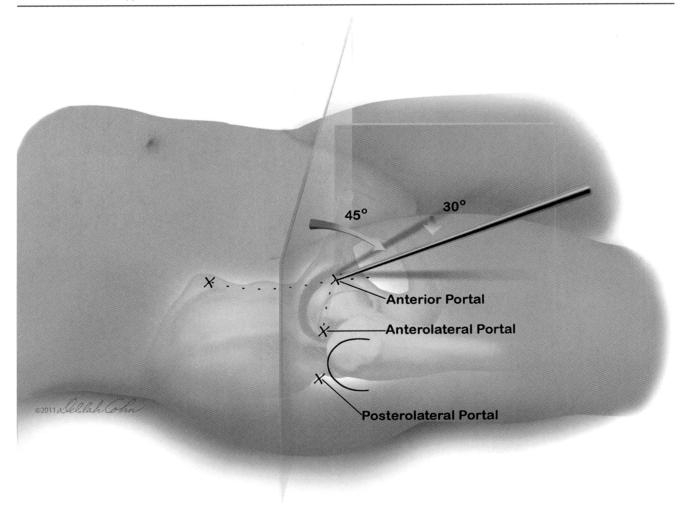

Fig. 11.11 The anterior portal roughly coincides with the intersection of a sagittal line drawn distally from the anterior superior iliac spine and a transverse line across the superior margin of the greater trochanter. Generally, it is directed approximately 45° cephalad and 30° toward the midline. Depending on the patient's anatomy, it may be chosen to place this slightly more lateral and distal in order to properly intersect the joint. The anterolateral and posterolateral portals are positioned at the anterior and posterior borders of the trochanteric tip, converging slightly as they enter the joint. (All rights are retained by Dr. Byrd)

Posterolateral Portal

The posterolateral portal penetrates both the gluteus medius and minimus prior to entering the lateral capsule at its posterior margin (Fig. 11.16). Its course is superior and anterior to the piriformis tendon. The portal lies closest to the sciatic nerve at the level of the capsule with the distance averaging 2.9 cm. An average distance of 4.4 cm separates the portal from the superior gluteal nerve.

Portal Placement

The anterolateral portal lies most centrally in the "safe zone" for arthroscopy and thus is the portal placed first [11, 12].

Subsequent portal placements are assisted by direct arthroscopic visualization. This initial portal is placed by fluoroscopic inspection in the AP plane. However, orientation in the lateral plane is equally important. With the leg in neutral rotation, femoral anteversion places the center of the joint just anterior to the center of the greater trochanter. Thus, the entry site for the anterolateral portal at the anterior margin of the greater trochanter corresponds with entry of the joint just anterior to its midportion. This correct entry site of the joint is achieved by keeping the instrumentation parallel to the floor during portal placement (Fig. 11.17).

When distracting the hip, a vacuum phenomenon will usually be present (Fig. 11.18a). Prepositioning for the anterolateral portal is performed with a 6" 17-gauge spinal needle under fluoroscopic control. Careful positioning of this needle

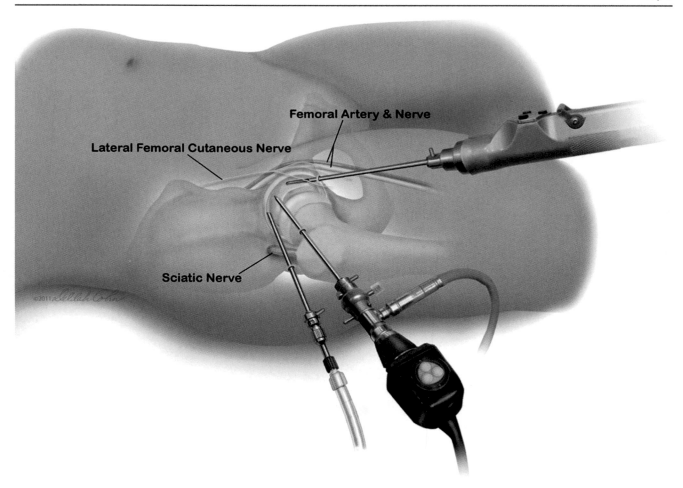

Fig. 11.12 The relationship of the major neurovascular structures to the three standard portals is demonstrated. The femoral artery and nerve lie well medial to the anterior portal. The sciatic nerve lies posterior to the posterolateral portal. Small branches of the lateral femoral cutaneous nerve lie close to the anterior portal. Injury to these is avoided by utilizing proper technique in portal placement. The anterolateral portal is established first since it lies most centrally in the safe zone for arthroscopy. (All rights are retained by Dr. Byrd)

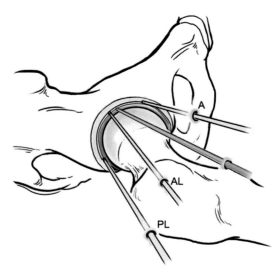

Fig. 11.13 The modified anterior portal (*green*) is described as being between the anterior (*A*) and anterolateral portals (*AL*) and slightly more distal. (All rights are retained by Dr. Byrd)

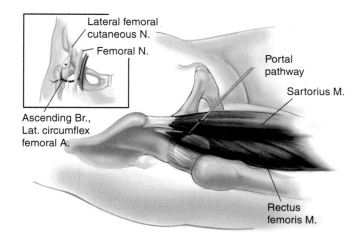

Fig. 11.14 Anterior portal pathway/relationship to lateral femoral cutaneous nerve, femoral nerve, and lateral circumflex femoral artery (Courtesy of Smith & Nephew, Inc., Andover, Massachusetts)

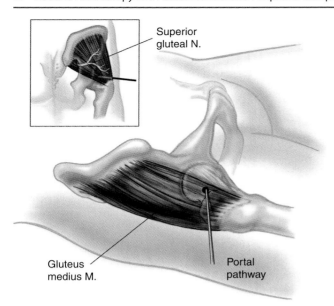

Fig. 11.15 Anterolateral portal pathway/relationship to superior gluteal nerve (Courtesy of Smith & Nephew, Inc., Andover, Massachusetts)

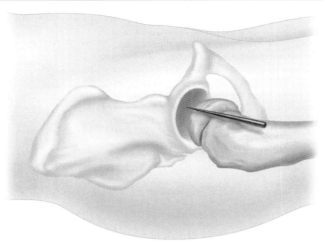

Fig. 11.17 With the patient supine, the hip is in neutral rotation with the kneecap pointing toward the ceiling. A needle placed at the anterior margin of the greater trochanter (anterolateral position) is maintained in the coronal plane by keeping it parallel to the floor as it enters the joint. Due to femoral neck anteversion, the entry site will be just anterior to the joint's center. If the entry site is too anterior, it becomes crowded with the anterior portal. If it is too posterior, it becomes difficult to properly visualize the entry site for the anterior portal (Courtesy of J.W. Thomas Byrd, MD, Nashville, TN)

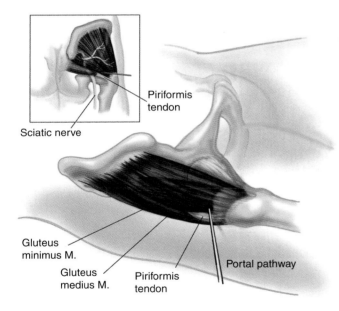

Fig. 11.16 Posterolateral portal pathway/relationship to the sciatic nerve and superior gluteal nerve (Courtesy of Smith & Nephew, Inc., Andover, Massachusetts)

is essential because, with the cannulated arthroscopy system, the cannula/obturator assembly will enter exactly where the needle has been placed. Release of the vacuum seal, by insertion of the needle, creates an air arthrogram affect, which may assist in silhouetting the outline of the lateral labrum (Fig. 11.18b) [14]. The tactile feel is important because greater resistance is felt if the labrum is inadvertently penetrated, more so than when just penetrating the capsule. Once

the needle has been placed, the joint is then distended with approximately 40 ccs of fluid and the intracapsular position confirmed by backflow of fluid. Distension of the joint enhances distraction (Fig. 11.18c). If it is felt that the needle may have pierced the labrum, once the joint has been distended, it is a simple process to back the needle out and reenter the capsule below the level of the labrum.

A stab wound is made through the skin at the needle. The guide wire is placed through the needle and the needle is removed. The cannulated obturator with the 5.0-mm arthroscopy cannula is passed over the wire into the joint (Fig. 11.18d).

While establishing the portal, the cannula/obturator assembly should pass close to the superior tip of the greater trochanter and then directly above the convex surface of the femoral head. It is important to keep the assembly off the femoral head to avoid inadvertent articular surface scuffing.

Once the arthroscope has been introduced, the anterior portal is placed next. Positioning is now facilitated by visualization from the arthroscope as well as fluoroscopy. The 70° scope works best for directly viewing where the instrumentation penetrates the capsule (Fig. 11.19). Prepositioning is again performed with the 17-gauge spinal needle, entering the joint directly underneath the free edge of the anterior labrum. As the cannula/obturator assembly is introduced, it is lifted up to stay off the articular surface of the femoral head while passing underneath the acetabular labrum.

If proper attention is given to the topographical anatomy in positioning the anterior portal, the femoral nerve lies well

Fig. 11.18 AP fluoroscopic view of a right hip.
(**a**) A vacuum effect is apparent due to the negative
intracapsular pressure created by distraction of the
joint (*arrows*). (**b**) A spinal needle is used in
prepositioning for the anterolateral portal. Venting the
joint with the needle releases the vacuum effect.
(**c**) Distension of the joint with fluid further facilitates
distraction. (**d**) The cannula/obturator assembly is
being passed over the nitinol wire that had been
placed through the spinal needle (Courtesy
of J.W. Thomas Byrd, MD, Nashville, TN)

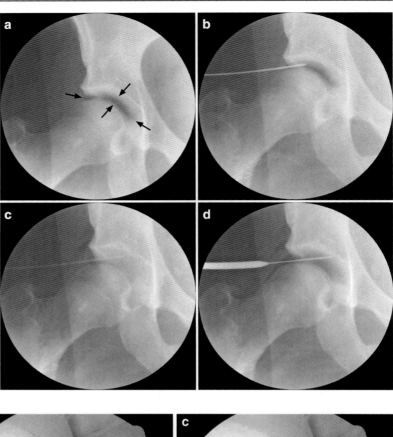

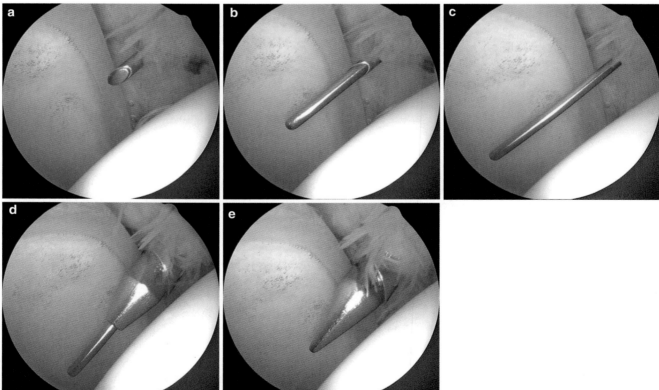

Fig. 11.19 Viewing anteriorly from the anterolateral portal, the anterior portal is positioned in the center of the triangle formed by the free
margin of the anterior labrum, femoral head, and edge of the arthroscope image. (**a**) Prepositioning is performed with a 17-gauge spinal
needle. (**b**) A nitinol guide wire is passed through the needle. (**c**) The
needle has been withdrawn, leaving the nitinol guide wire in place. (**d**)
The cannula/obturator assembly is delivered over the guide wire. (**e**)
Final positioning of the cannula for the anterior portal. (All rights are
retained by Dr. Byrd)

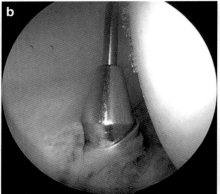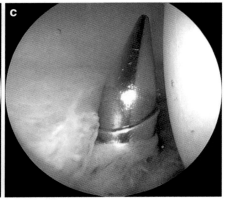

Fig. 11.20 Viewing posteriorly from the anterolateral portal, positioning is performed for the posterolateral portal in the similar triangle formed by the free margin of the posterior labrum, femoral head, and edge of the arthroscope image. (**a**) Prepositioning with the 17-gauge spinal needle. (**b**) The cannula/obturators assembly is delivered over the nitinol guide wire. (**c**) Final positioning for the posterolateral cannula. (All rights are retained by Dr. Byrd)

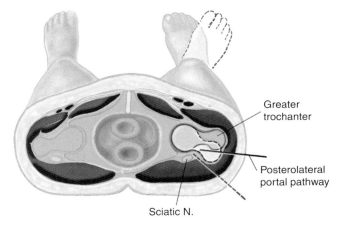

Greater trochanter

Posterolateral portal pathway

Sciatic N.

Fig. 11.21 Neutral rotation of the operative hip is essential for protection of the sciatic nerve during placement of the posterolateral portal (Courtesy of Smith & Nephew, Inc., Andover, Massachusetts)

medial to the approach [11, 12]. However, the lateral femoral cutaneous nerve lies quite close to this portal. It is best avoided by utilizing proper technique in portal placement. The nerve is most vulnerable to laceration by a skin incision placed too deeply.

Lastly, the posterolateral portal is introduced. The fluoroscopic guidelines are similar to the anterolateral portal. Rotating the lens of the arthroscope posteriorly brings the entry site underneath the posterior labrum into view (Fig. 11.20). Placement under arthroscopic control ensures that the instrumentation does not stray posteriorly, potentially placing the sciatic nerve at risk. The hip remains in neutral rotation during placement of the posterolateral portal. External rotation of the hip would move the greater trochanter more posteriorly, and, since this is the main topographical landmark, the sciatic nerve might be more at risk for injury (Fig. 11.21).

Tips

Placement of the first portal (anterolateral) for introduction of the arthroscope is critically dependent on needle placement that is guided only by fluoroscopy. It is important to avoid the labrum and assure that the portal is reasonably centered in the hip [14]. In the illustrative example (Fig. 11.22a), the spinal needle has been placed and the vacuum seal released, resulting in an air arthrogram effect silhouetting the lateral labrum. Once the joint is distended with fluid (Fig. 11.22b), the femoral head is noted to have migrated distally with distension, but the needle remains closer to the acetabulum. This can be an indication that the needle is held up because it has penetrated the labrum. Maintaining distension of the joint, the needle is backed out (Fig. 11.22c) and then repositioned further distally (Fig. 11.22d). Distension of the joint accomplishes two important feats. It may better separate the joint surfaces, and it also pushes the capsule away from the labrum, making it easier to place the needle through the capsule and not the labrum. In fact, for most cases, once the joint has been distended, we will reposition the needle at least once to avoid the labrum. We have found that, with this technique, there is a very low incidence of inadvertently perforating the labrum. As the needle is placed back through the capsule, the bevel is initially turned away from the labrum (Fig. 11.22d). The bevel is then spun to face the femoral head (Fig. 11.22e), so it is less likely to nick the articular surface of the femoral head as it is advanced. The nitinol guide wire is placed through the needle and is noted to pass to the medial side of the fossa (Fig. 11.22f). This indicates that the positioning is reasonably well centered in the joint. If the nitinol guide wire does not pass freely to the medial side of the joint that indicates that the position may be too anterior or posterior. In this circumstance, the surgeon should reposition the needle to accomplish better centering. Lastly, the cannula/obturator assembly is advanced over the guide wire (Fig. 11.22g). As it is advanced, it is good to periodically slide the guide wire back and forth to make sure that it does not kink. If the guide wire becomes kinked, it is a simple process to retrieve it by just removing the obturator from the cannula, bringing the guide wire with it. Advancing the assembly without recognizing that the guide wire is kinked will result in breaking the guide wire.

The standard description for the anterior portal is at the intersection of a sagittal line through the ASIS and a transverse line across the tip of the trochanter. However, actual placement of the anterior portal can be variable and is dictated by the angle of access necessary to intersect the joint, with a slightly cephalad angle passing underneath the anterior lip of the acetabulum. The sagittal line through the ASIS is simply a medial limit for the anterior portal. Placement lateral to this line is acceptable, but it should not be medial to this line because of risk to the femoral neurovascular structures. Commonly, the entry site will end up being somewhat more lateral and distal to achieve the optimal direction for entry to the joint.

If the initial entry site of the anterolateral portal is too posterior, it can make it difficult to visualize the entry site for the anterior portal. Conversely, if it is too anterior, it will crowd itself with the anterior portal. Also, if the labrum has been penetrated by the cannula, this can make it more difficult to clearly visualize the entry site for the subsequent portals. If it is better to view posteriorly than anteriorly, sometimes the posterolateral portal may be placed before the anterior portal.

Normally, the posterolateral portal is the easiest to place since it roughly parallels the anterolateral portal, converging slightly. In the supine position, adipose tissue falls posteriorly so, in obesity, this is the one portal that may exceed the length of normal hip arthroscopy instruments. It is also the least important of the three portals since the majority of hip pathology resides in the anterior half of the joint. However, it is important to use this portal for thorough inspection, and it is also important to be facile in its placement for the challenging cases where it may be more essential. The posterolateral portal complements the anterior portal for providing complete access to the medial side of the joint and the acetabular fossa.

Occasionally, hemorrhage in the joint may result in a bloody fluid field when the arthroscope is introduced. This cannot simply be flushed out. Unlike a knee or shoulder with more capacious compliant capsule that distends from the fluid and can then be flushed out of the cannula, the hip capsule is noncompliant and there is minimal flow without a separate site of egress. The fluid can be vented by positioning the needle for the anterior portal. With patience, the field of view can be cleared for placement of the other portals. As an alternative method, the fluid can be evacuated from the joint, providing a dry view of the entry site for the anterior portal (Fig. 11.23). Under all circumstances, we will distend the joint with fluid prior to placing the initial portal. This is an important step to protect the labrum. As we have noted, distension aids in separating the joint surfaces, but it also pushes the capsule away from the labrum, allowing a better opportunity for the needle to be placed through the capsule and avoid the labrum.

Diagnostic Arthroscopy

When preparing for hip arthroscopy, the surgeon formulates a tentative treatment plan based on the preliminary diagnosis. However, the definitive treatment strategy will be dictated by the findings observed at arthroscopy. With the current limitations of investigative techniques, the arthroscopic findings may differ significantly from those implied by the preoperative studies. Thus, a systematic and thorough initial inspection of the joint is imperative. Once all aspects of the intra-articular pathology have been identified, the surgeon can then embark on intervention with appropriate time management to address all aspects within the joint. The surgeon should avoid spending considerable time on one obvious aspect of the pathology to only then realize that there is other coexistent damage that needs to be addressed as well. Managing time within the joint is important, especially when traction is applied.

Using the three portal technique (anterior, anterolateral, and posterolateral), inspection begins from the anterolateral portal (Fig. 11.12) (Video 11.5: http://goo.gl/ZiUMW). This is the first portal established since it lies most centrally in the safe zone for arthroscopy. Inspection begins with the 70° scope as this provides the best view of the outer margins of the joint and is used for allowing direct arthroscopic visualization of where the other two portals are placed. The anterolateral portal provides the best view of the anterior portion of the joint (Fig. 11.24).

Next, the arthroscope is placed in the anterior portal. Viewing laterally, the relationship of the lateral two portals

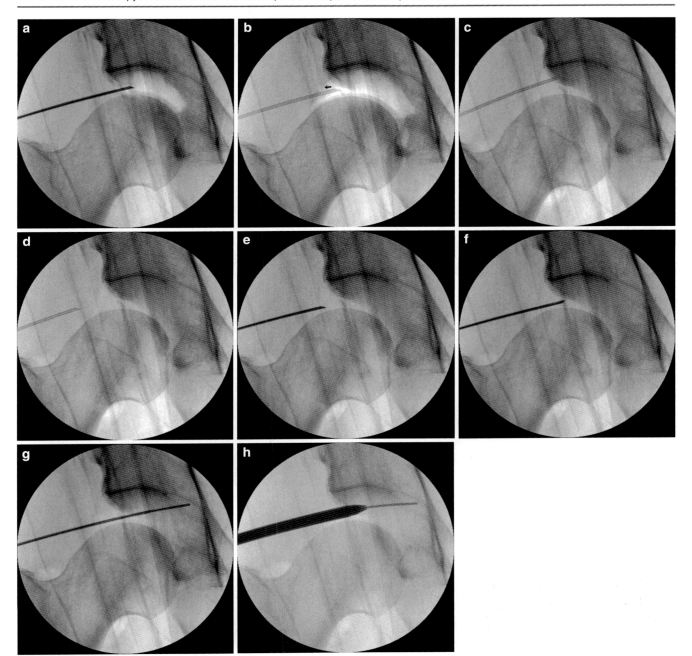

Fig. 11.22 Fluoroscopic image of a right hip. (**a**) The joint has been distracted and a spinal needle has been placed in the anterolateral position. (**b**) Removing the stylus releases the vacuum seal and creates an air arthrogram that silhouettes the lateral labrum (*arrow*). (**c**) The joint has been distended with fluid. The femoral head migrates distally but the needle remains in close approximation to the acetabulum, indicating that it may be held by having penetrated the labrum. (**d**) Maintaining distension, the needle has been backed out of the joint. (**e**) With the bevel turned away from the labrum, the needle is repositioned distally. (**f**) The bevel is then turned away from the femoral head as the needle is advanced, to avoid nicking the articular surface. (**g**) The nitinol guide wire passes freely through the needle to the medial side of the joint, indicating that it is centered in the hip. (**h**) The cannula/obturators assembly is advanced over the guide wire. (All rights are retained by Dr. Byrd)

underneath the lateral labrum is seen (Fig. 11.25). The surgeon should be especially cognizant to critique the entry site of the anterolateral portal since this is the one portal that is placed only under fluoroscopic guidance without benefit of arthroscopic visualization of where the portal enters the joint. Viewing medially from the anterior portal, the surgeon can see the most inferior limit of the anterior labrum (Fig. 11.26).

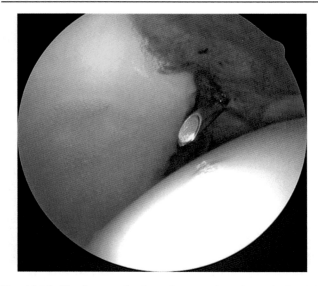

Fig. 11.23 Viewing anterior from the anterolateral portal of a right hip. The joint as been evacuated of fluid and a spinal needle is observed positioning for the anterior portal. (All rights are retained by Dr. Byrd)

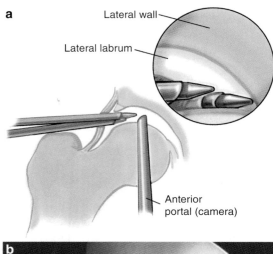

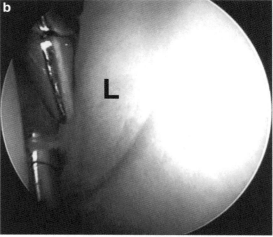

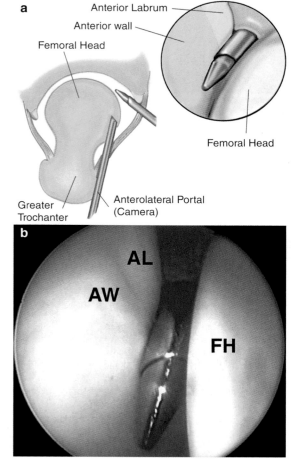

Fig. 11.24 (**a**) Arthroscopic view of a right hip from the anterolateral portal (Courtesy of Smith & Nephew, Inc., Andover, Massachusetts). (**b**) Demonstrated are the anterior acetabular wall (*AW*) and the anterior labrum (*AL*). The anterior cannula is seen entering underneath the labrum and the femoral head (*FH*) is on the right (Courtesy of J.W. Thomas Byrd, MD, Nashville, TN)

Fig. 11.25 (**a**) Arthroscopic view from the anterior portal (Courtesy of Smith & Nephew, Inc., Andover, Massachusetts). (**b**) Demonstrated are the lateral aspect of the labrum (*L*) and its relationship to the lateral two portals (Courtesy of J.W. Thomas Byrd, MD, Nashville, TN)

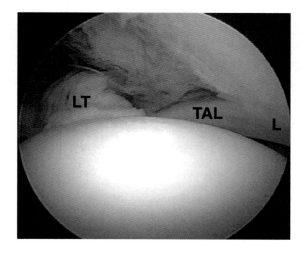

Fig. 11.26 Viewing inferomedially from the anterior portal demonstrates where the inferior aspect of the anterior labrum (*L*) becomes contiguous with the transverse acetabular ligament (*TAL*) below the ligamentum teres (*LT*) (Courtesy of J.W. Thomas Byrd, MD, Nashville, TN)

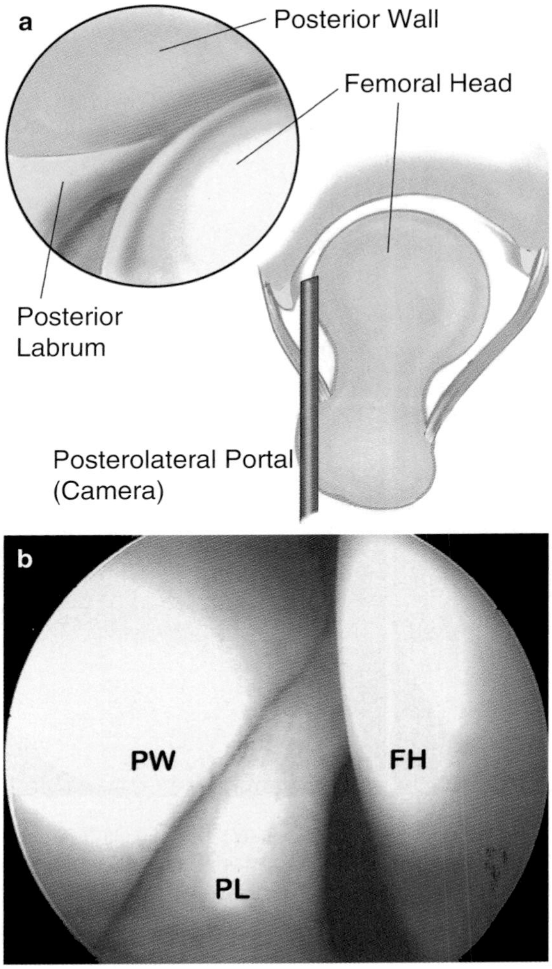

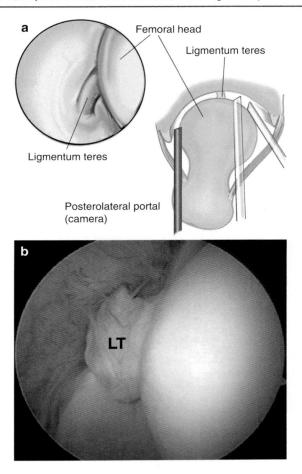

a Posterior Wall

Femoral Head

Posterior Labrum

Posterolateral Portal (Camera)

b

PW   FH

PL

a Femoral head

Ligamentum teres

Ligamentum teres

Posterolateral portal (camera)

b

LT

Fig. 11.28 (**a**) The acetabular fossa can be inspected from all three portals (Courtesy of Smith & Nephew, Inc., Andover, Massachusetts). (**b**) The ligamentum teres (*LT*), with its accompanying vessels, has a serpentine course from its acetabular to its femoral attachment (Courtesy of J.W. Thomas Byrd, MD, Nashville, TN)

Fig. 11.27 (**a**) Arthroscopic view from the posterolateral portal (Courtesy of Smith & Nephew, Inc., Andover, Massachusetts). (**b**) Demonstrated are the posterior acetabular wall (*PW*), posterior labrum (*PL*), and the femoral head (*FH*) (Courtesy of J.W. Thomas Byrd, MD, Nashville, TN)

The arthroscope is then placed in the posterolateral portal which provides the best view of the posterior regions of the joint, especially the posterior labrum (Fig. 11.27). The posterior labrum is the portion that is least often damaged and has the most consistent morphological appearance. Thus, viewing this area is often used as a reference in assessing variations of the anterior or lateral labrum and accompanying pathology.

Each of the three portals provides a different perspective on the acetabular fossa (Fig. 11.28). The 70° scope provides a direct view of the ligamentum teres which resides in the inferior portion of the fossa. The transverse acetabular ligament can also be partially viewed coursing underneath the ligamentum teres. After completing the inspection with the 70° scope, the 30° is then used, reversing the sequence of steps between the three portals. The 30°scope provides a better view of the central portion of the femoral head and acetabulum and the superior portion of the acetabular fossa.

Inspection and subsequent access to various recesses of the joint are facilitated by capsulotomies around the portals (Fig. 11.29). A single-piece construction arthroscopic knife is placed through the cannula and the cannula removed, so that transverse incisions several millimeters in each direction can be created. The cannula is then passed back over the knife into the joint. These are routinely performed around the anterolateral and anterior portals, improving maneuverability for the arthroscope in the anterolateral portal and medial access to the joint from the anterior portal. These small cuts should not create any troublesome problems with extravasation or instability of the joint.

Sometimes the iliopsoas tendon can be exposed from the central compartment (Video 11.6: http://goo.gl/RdQEp) [15]. This is accomplished by extending the capsulotomy medially from the anterior portal (Fig. 11.30a–c). This may require extensive medial dissection, and thus the iliopsoas is often best addressed from the peripheral compartment.

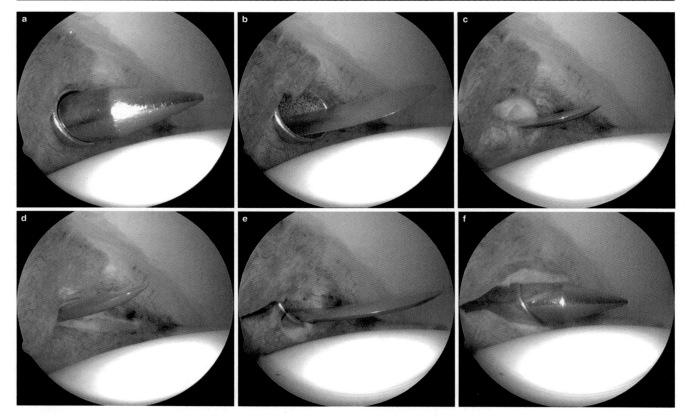

Fig. 11.29 Viewing from the anterior portal of this right hip, a capsulotomy is performed around the anterolateral portal. (**a**) The initial anterolateral portal has been placed. (**b**) An arthroscopic knife is introduced through the cannula. (**c**) The cannula has been removed to more freely maneuver the knife. (**d**) A transverse capsulotomy is performed going several millimeters in each direction. (**e**) The cannula is returned over the knife, which acts as a switching stick. (**f**) Freedom of movement of the cannula is substantially enhanced. (All rights are retained by Dr. Byrd)

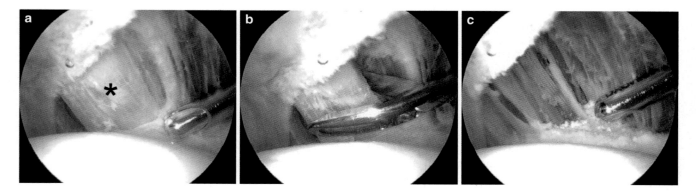

Fig. 11.30 (**a**) Viewing anteriorly from anterolateral portal of this right hip, the iliopsoas tendon has been exposed (*asterisk*). (**b**) The tendon is released with a cutting hand instrument. (**c**) The tendon has been released, revealing the muscular portion which is preserved. (All rights are retained by Dr. Byrd)

There are a few normal variants that are common enough to be worthy of mention for diagnostic arthroscopy of the joint.

The lateral and the anterior portions of the labrum are the most variable. Sometimes this portion of the labrum is thin, poorly developed, and hypoplastic and, at other times, may appear enlarged. In the presence of acetabular dysplasia, the lateral labrum is especially hypertrophic, having more of a stabilizing and weight-bearing role substituting for the absent lateral portion of the bony acetabulum. A labral cleft is sometimes present (Fig. 11.31) (Video 11.7: http://goo.gl/jRhAx) [16]. This is a normal finding and should not be misinterpreted as a traumatic detachment. The distinguishing

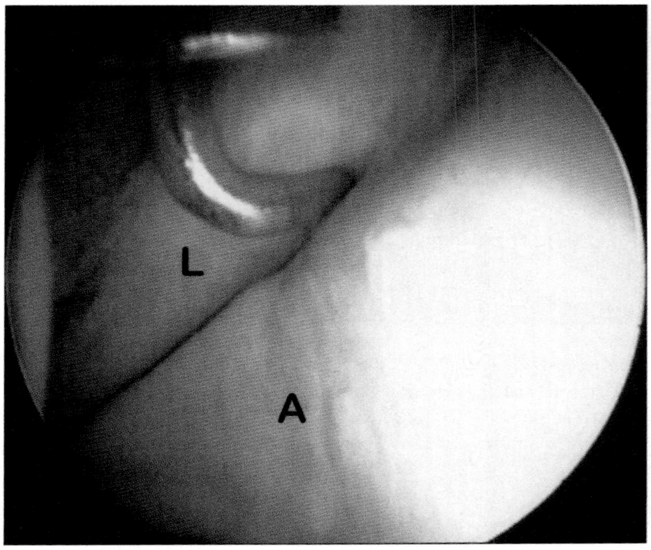

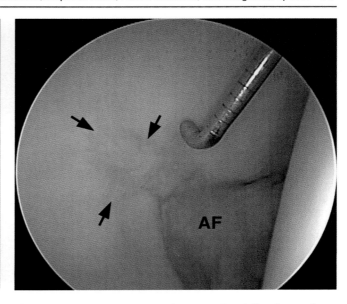

Fig. 11.33 The stellate crease is frequently found directly superior to the acetabular fossa (*AF*) characterized by a stellate pattern of chondromalacia (*arrows*). This appears to be a normally occurring process, even in young adults, without clear prognostic significance (Courtesy of J.W. Thomas Byrd, MD, Nashville, TN)

Fig. 11.31 The cleft identified by the probe sometimes separates the margin of the acetabular articular surface (*A*) from the labrum (*L*). This is a normal variant without evidence of trauma or attempted healing response (Courtesy of J.W. Thomas Byrd, MD, Nashville, TN)

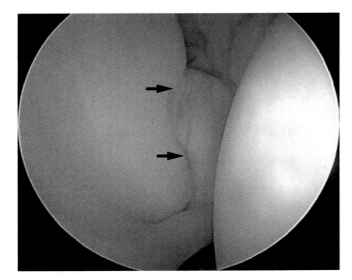

Fig. 11.32 The physeal scar (*arrows*) is an area devoid of articular surface that may extend posteriorly from the acetabular fossa (as shown here) or anteriorly demarcating the area of the old triradiate physis (Courtesy of J.W. Thomas Byrd, MD, Nashville, TN)

features are absence of damaged appearing tissue and absence of any attempted healing response that would be expected in the presence of trauma.

Remnants of the triradiate cartilage may be evident in adulthood as a physeal scar, void of overlying articular cartilage, extending in a linear fashion along the medial aspect of the acetabulum anterior and/or posterior to the fossa (Fig. 11.32) (Video 11.8: http://goo.gl/274Ce). This should not be misinterpreted as an old fracture line.

A commonly encountered observation in adults is a stellate-appearing articular lesion immediately above the acetabular fossa referred to as the stellate crease (Fig. 11.33) (Video 11.9: http://goo.gl/dvn3o) [17]. When seen, it is unlikely to be of clinical significance as a contributing cause of pain and is of uncertain long-term prognostic significance regarding susceptibility to future degenerative disease. Occasionally, this must be distinguished from traumatic articular lesions which can occur in this same area, especially from a lateral blow to the hip impacting the femoral head against the superomedial acetabulum.

A precursor to the stellate crease seen in teenagers and young adults is the supra-acetabular fossa (Video 11.10: http://goo.gl/JnTix) [18]. This is a bony recess that may be present in the supramedial acetabular surface. This is usually evident on plain films and, on MRI, will appear as a fluid filled defect (Fig. 11.34a, b). This defect should not be interpreted as an osteochondral lesion. This may persist late into the third decade of life but eventually fills with bone, covered by irregular fibrocartilage identified as the stellate crease in adulthood. Arthroscopically, the configuration of a smaller fossa above the proper acetabular fossa gives the appearance of an old-fashioned keyhole and has been described as the "keyhole complex." This is not described as a "lesion" since it is a normal developmental variation. Fibrous bands may extend down to the formal acetabular fossa (Fig. 11.34c), and debridement of these fibrotic bands may be necessary to fully visualize the underlying acetabular architecture. Presently, it is unclear whether these bands

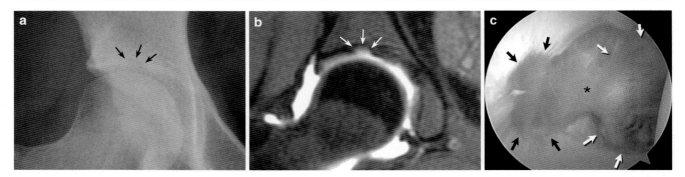

Fig. 11.34 The supra-acetabular fossa is a morphological variant. (**a**) AP radiograph of a right hip illustrates the typical appearance (*arrows*). (**b**) A coronal T1-weighted MRI image with gadolinium arthrography illustrates the typical defect (*arrows*) filled with contrast. (**c**) An arthroscopic view illustrates the supra-acetabular fossa (*black arrows*) with fibrotic bands (*asterisk*) extending down into the acetabular fossa proper (*white arrows*). The configuration gives the appearance of a "keyhole" (Courtesy of J.W. Thomas Byrd, MD, Nashville, TN)

may contribute to symptoms in some patients or if this is strictly an incidental finding.

> **Tips**
>
> After placing the portals in the hip, the first next step is to move the arthroscope to the anterior portal for evaluation of positioning of the original anterolateral portal. If the labrum is inadvertently perforated, this is the time that the cannula is repositioned before any further harm is done. If the anterolateral portal is too posterior or anterior, this is corrected by a capsulotomy extended in the direction necessary to rectify it.

Peripheral Compartment

At least two standard methods are available for accessing the periphery. The traditional method described first is normally used for less complex procedures that do not require extensive exposure and extensive capsulotomies [3]. Small capsulotomies around the portals of the central compartment improve maneuverability within the joint but do not accommodate moving the instruments directly from the central to the peripheral compartment.

More generous capsulotomies connecting the anterior and anterolateral portals are usually necessary for complex labral repairs and for correction of pincer and cam impingement [19]. With these capsulotomies, the instruments can simply be swept from the central to the peripheral area with less constraint. The morbidity of these capsulotomies is minimal but must be performed thoughtfully and correctly to avoid creating problems of instability [20].

When capsulotomies are not necessary, the traditional method provides an atraumatic technique for accessing the periphery.

Traditional Portal Placement for Peripheral Joint

(See Video 11.11: http://goo.gl/J2y1J) After completing arthroscopy of the interior of the hip, the instruments can be removed and traction released for access to the peripheral compartment [2, 3]. The hip is flexed approximately 45° which relaxes the anterior capsule (Fig. 11.35). From the anterolateral entry site, the spinal needle penetrates the capsule on the anterior neck of the femur under fluoroscopic control (Fig. 11.36a, b). Using the guide wire, the cannula obturator assembly is then placed (Fig. 11.36c). The 5-mm cannula is preferable with the inflow attached to the scope.

For instrumentation, an ancillary portal is placed 5 cm distal to the anterolateral portal. Once again, prepositioning is performed with the 17-gauge spinal needle, directly observing through the arthroscope where the needle enters the peripheral compartment (Fig. 11.36d). Many loose bodies reside in this area and can be retrieved. This also provides superior access to the synovial lining and capsule, which can be important for performing a thorough synovectomy.

This approach provides an excellent perspective of the peripheral compartment (Figs. 11.37 and 11.38), bringing into view structures that cannot be seen from inside the joint and also provides a different peripheral perspective on some of the intra-articular structures. The medial synovial fold is consistently visualized adjacent to the anteromedial neck of the femur.

If needed, the iliopsoas tendon can be readily exposed with this method (Video 11.12: http://goo.gl/zA1FO) [21, 22]. It can be found above the zona orbicularis at the level of the medial synovial fold. The capsule is usually thin and sometimes the iliopsoas tendon can be visualized through this thin capsule (Fig. 11.39a). A window through the capsule can be created for dividing the tendinous portion of the iliopsoas (Fig. 11.39b–d). For addressing cam impingement, this approach is too distal and anterior. Exposure would require more extreme dissection proximally and laterally.

Fig. 11.35 The operative area remains covered in sterile drapes, while the traction is released and the hip flexed 45°. *Inset*: Illustrates position of the hip without the overlying drape (Courtesy of Smith & Nephew, Inc., Andover, Massachusetts)

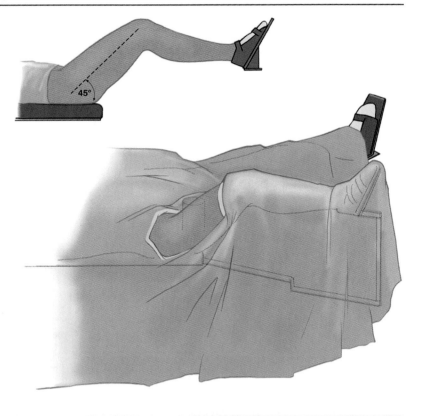

Fig. 11.36 AP fluoroscopic view of the flexed hip. (**a**) From the anterolateral entry site, the 17-gauge spinal needle has been repositioned on the anterior neck of the femur. The spinal needle can be felt perforating the capsule before contacting the bone. (**b**) The guide wire is placed through the spinal needle. It should pass freely to the medial capsule as illustrated. (**c**) The cannula obturator assembly is being placed over the guide wire. (**d**) The position of the 30° arthroscope is shown while a spinal needle is being placed for an ancillary portal (Courtesy of J.W. Thomas Byrd, MD, Nashville, TN)

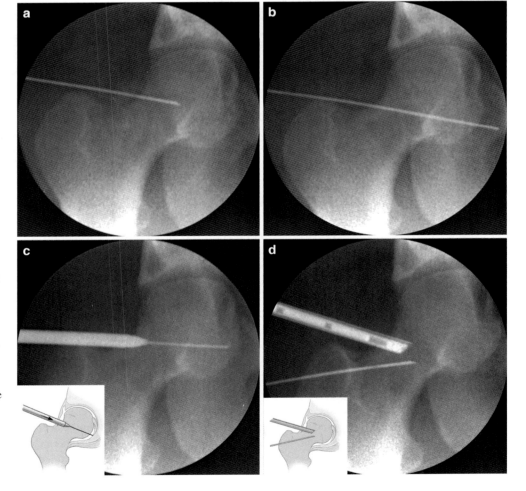

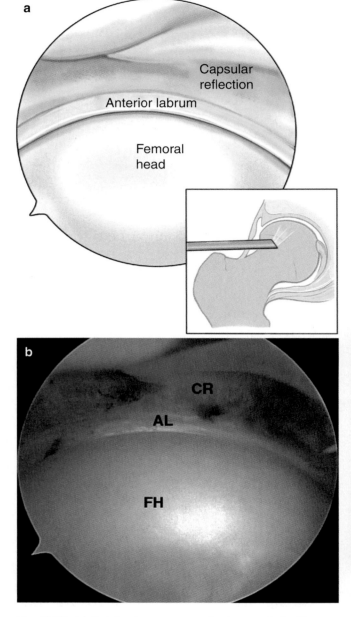

Fig. 11.37 (a) Peripheral compartment viewing superiorly (Courtesy of Smith & Nephew, Inc., Andover, Massachusetts). (b) Demonstrated is the anterior portion of the joint including the articular surface of the femoral head (*FH*), anterior labrum (*AL*), and the capsular reflection (*CR*) (Courtesy of J.W. Thomas Byrd, MD, Nashville, TN)

Peripheral Portal Access Via Capsulotomy

(See Video 11.13: http://goo.gl/RBuKf) A capsulotomy is performed by connecting the anterior and anterolateral portals (Fig. 11.40) [19, 23]. This can be as small as 1.5 cm but can be extended when more exposure is needed or as part of the treatment of a stiff hip. The posterolateral portal is removed. A 5-mm cannula is used for the arthroscope to accommodate placing the inflow on the scope cannula. The anterolateral and anterior portals are backed out peripheral to the labrum. The traction is released and the hip is flexed

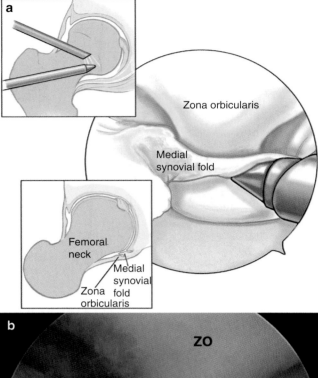

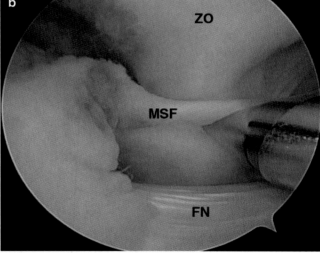

Fig. 11.38 (a) Peripheral compartment viewing medially (Courtesy of Smith & Nephew, Inc., Andover, Massachusetts). (b) Demonstrated are the femoral neck (*FN*), medial synovial fold (*MSF*), and the zona orbicularis (*ZO*) (Courtesy of J.W. Thomas Byrd, MD, Nashville, TN)

while maintaining the view between the two portals. Watching through the scope is important to keep within the working space as the peripheral compartment is brought into view. The amount of hip flexion is adjusted to the needs for exposure from the periphery. Most commonly, this technique is used to address a cam lesion. As the hip is flexed and the femoral head rotates into the acetabulum, the articular margin of the cam lesion is visualized. Usually, this is less than 35° of flexion. Greater flexion can cause the cam lesion to disappear within the acetabulum.

Once the peripheral space has been accessed, further exposure can be gained as needed. Other portals can be placed as necessary for operative procedures. We use a

Fig. 11.39 (**a**) Fibers of the iliopsoas tendon (*asterisk*) are visible through the thin medial capsule anterior to the femoral head (*FH*) and labrum (*L*). This is located directly above the zona orbicularis at the level of the medial synovial fold. (**b**) A small capsular window is created, exposing the iliopsoas tendon. (**c**) A cutting hand instrument is used to release the tendinous portion of the iliopsoas. (**d**) The tendon has been released, revealing the muscular portion of the iliopsoas, which is preserved (Courtesy of J.W. Thomas Byrd, MD, Nashville, TN)

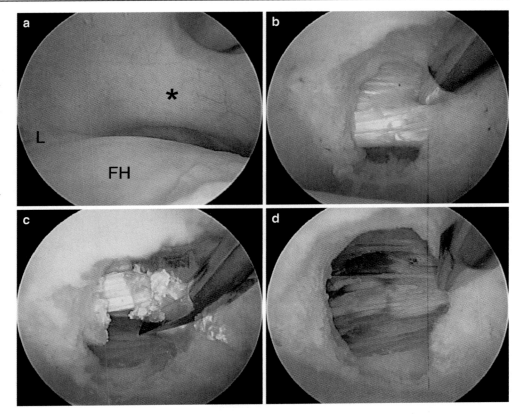

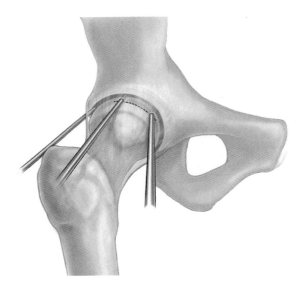

Fig. 11.40 The *dotted line* demarcates the capsulotomy performed by connecting the anterior and anterolateral portals. The extent of the capsulotomy is adjusted to the needs of the hip. In cases where instability is a concern, the capsulotomy is minimized. For stiff hips with severe impingement, an aggressive capsulectomy may be performed as part of the treatment to maximize motion. (All rights are retained by Dr. Byrd)

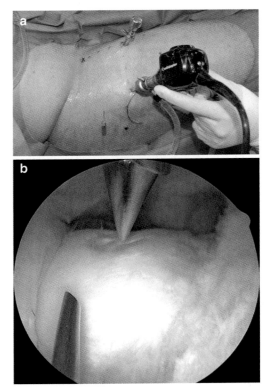

Fig. 11.41 (**a**) The posterolateral portal has been removed and the hip flexed with the arthroscope in the anterolateral portal. Prepositioning has been performed with a spinal needle for placement of a proximal anterolateral portal. (**b**) Viewing arthroscopically, the anterior cannula is in place and the spinal needle has been positioned. (All rights are retained by Dr. Byrd)

proximal (or cephalad) anterolateral portal for optimizing access to a cam lesion (Fig. 11.41). The anterior portal can be maintained or removed, depending on the procedure performed (Fig. 11.42). With the hip flexed, the proximal anterolateral portal is slightly more posterior, while the original

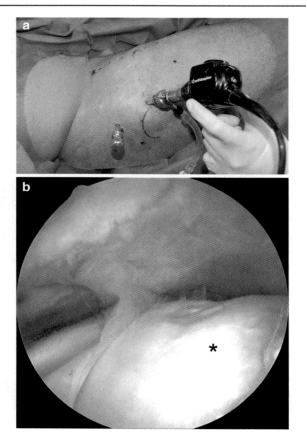

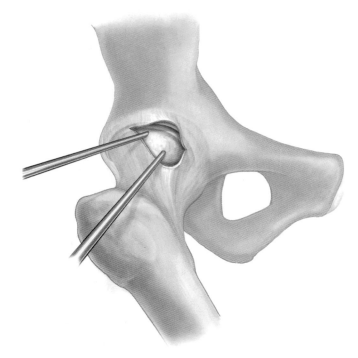

Fig. 11.43 Schematic illustrates the relationship of the proximal and distal anterolateral portals centered over a cam lesion, visualized through the capsulotomy. (All rights are retained by Dr. Byrd)

Fig. 11.42 (**a**) The anterior portal has been removed and substituted with a proximal anterolateral portal. (**b**) Viewing arthroscopically, the two portals are centered over a cam lesion (*asterisk*). (All rights are retained by Dr. Byrd)

anterolateral portal, which is now the more distal of the two, is more anterior.

This approach is ideal for placing the portals directly over the cam lesion, which is most commonly located over the anterolateral quadrant of the femoral head/neck junction (Fig. 11.43). Moving more medial, the medial synovial fold can come into view, and a separate capsular window can be made in the thin medial capsule to expose the iliopsoas tendon (Fig. 11.44). Sometimes with extensive capsulotomies, the tendon can simply be viewed through the capsulotomy (Fig. 11.45).

Iliopsoas Bursoscopy

(See Video 11.14: http://goo.gl/0Tlxn) Iliopsoas bursoscopy is performed without traction. The hip is flexed approximately 20° with maximal external rotation that moves the lesser trochanter more anterior and accessible to the portals. Two laterally based portals are needed for viewing and instrumentation within the bursa (Fig. 11.46a). These portals are distal to those used for the peripheral

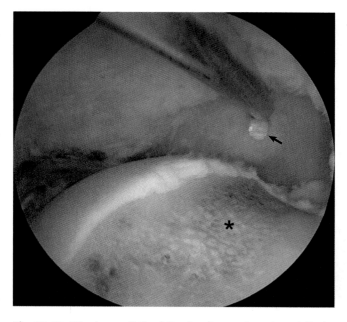

Fig. 11.44 Viewing medially, following femoroplasty (*asterisk*), the iliopsoas tendon has been exposed through a small medial capsular window (*arrow*). (All rights are retained by Dr. Byrd)

compartment and require fluoroscopy for precise positioning. They are also slightly more anterior to provide direct access over the area of the lesser trochanter. Angling from slightly above or below, the spinal needle is placed directly

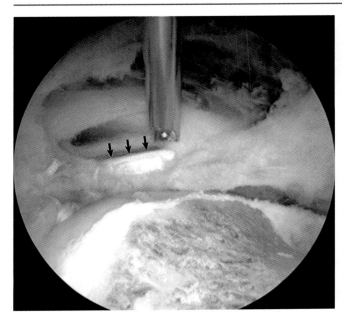

Fig. 11.45 In this example, following femoroplasty and labral refixation, the iliopsoas tendon (*arrows*) is visible through the medial extent of the capsulotomy. (All rights are retained by Dr. Byrd)

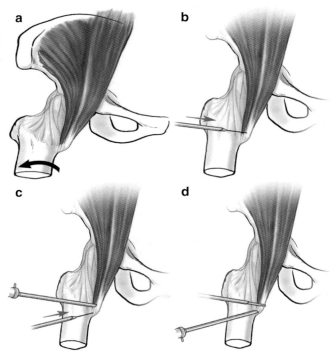

Fig. 11.46 Access to the iliopsoas bursa at the insertion of the tendon on the lesser trochanter is illustrated in this right hip. (**a**) The hip is flexed approximately 20° with full external rotation. (**b**) Angling down slightly, a laterally based portal is positioned on the lesser trochanter. (**c**) With the arthroscope in place, a second portal converges to the space over the lesser trochanter. (**d**) Switching between portals, bursal tissue and debris can be removed, clearing the space. (All rights are retained by Dr. Byrd)

on the lesser trochanter under fluoroscopy (Fig. 11.46b). With the arthroscope introduced, this allows room for a second portal to converge into the bursa (Fig. 11.46c). Adhesions or fibrinous debris within the bursa may need to be debrided in order to achieve clear visualization (Fig. 11.46d). Staying next to bone avoids straying into the anterior soft tissues.

Iliopsoas bursoscopy is most commonly performed for release of the iliopsoas tendon, but synovial disorders, including synovial chondromatosis and pigmented villonodular synovitis may exist and be treated within this area. Release of the iliopsoas tendon from the lesser trochanter was the first endoscopic method described (Fig. 11.47a–d) [4, 24]. This is a more complete tendon release than when performed in the periphery where a substantial muscular portion of the iliopsoas is preserved [21, 22]. The results are comparable, whether it is a fractional lengthening from the periphery or a complete release from its insertion. We have not encountered any permanent functional deficits among properly selected cases [25]. More concerning has been our observation of heterotopic ossification (HO), which is a recognized risk of any surgery on the iliopsoas tendon (Fig. 11.48) [25, 26]. In our experience, HO has not been encountered when releasing the tendon from the periphery, but this could be due to prophylaxis with nonsteroidal anti-inflammatory medication that we have employed since switching to the peripheral technique. We still use the technique from within the bursa for iliop-

soas impingement encountered secondary to total hip arthroplasty or resurfacing. It allows the surgeon to avoid the prosthesis and surgical scarring around the joint. For these cases, we use a single low-dose radiation treatment to reduce the risk of HO.

Trochanteric Bursoscopy (Peritrochanteric Space)

(See Video 11.15: http://goo.gl/T8BpK) Numerous disorders reside in the peritrochanteric space and can be addressed with endoscopic methods [5]. Positioning of the patient is the same as for arthroscopy of the central compartment, but no traction is needed. The hip is in extension and neutral rotation with slight abduction. Abduction relaxes the iliotibial band and opens the space within the peritrochanteric region. This is most easily accessed with anteriorly based portals directed posteriorly into the peritrochanteric space (Fig. 11.49).

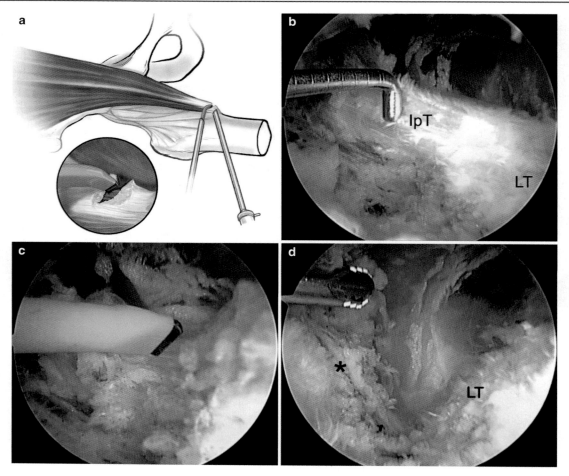

Fig. 11.47 (a) The two portals are useful for release of the tendinous portion of the iliopsoas. (b) Arthroscopic view of the iliopsoas tendon (*IpT*) being probed at its enthesis on the lesser trochanter (*LT*). (c) The enthesis is being released with a flexible RF device. (d) Division is complete with separation of the tendon (*asterisk*) from the lesser trochanter (*LT*). (All rights are retained by Dr. Byrd)

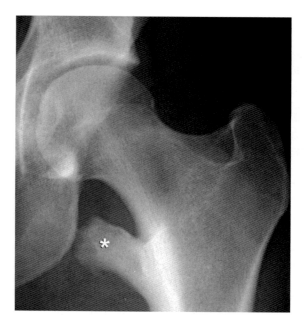

Fig. 11.48 Left hip AP radiograph of a 21-year-old intercollegiate basketball player reveals formation of heterotopic ossification (*asterisk*) at the lesser trochanter following previous endoscopic iliopsoas release from this location. (All rights are retained by Dr. Byrd)

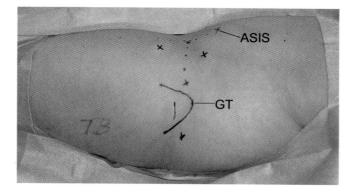

Fig. 11.49 Viewing this left hip, two portals (*red x's*) provide access to the peritrochanteric space from anterior. These are positioned proximal and distal to the vastus lateralis ridge which is marked on the surface by the *red line*. The greater trochanter (*GT*) and anterior superior iliac spine (*ASIS*) are marked, as well as the standard arthroscopy portals for the central compartment (*purple x's*) (Courtesy of J.W. Thomas Byrd, MD, Nashville, TN)

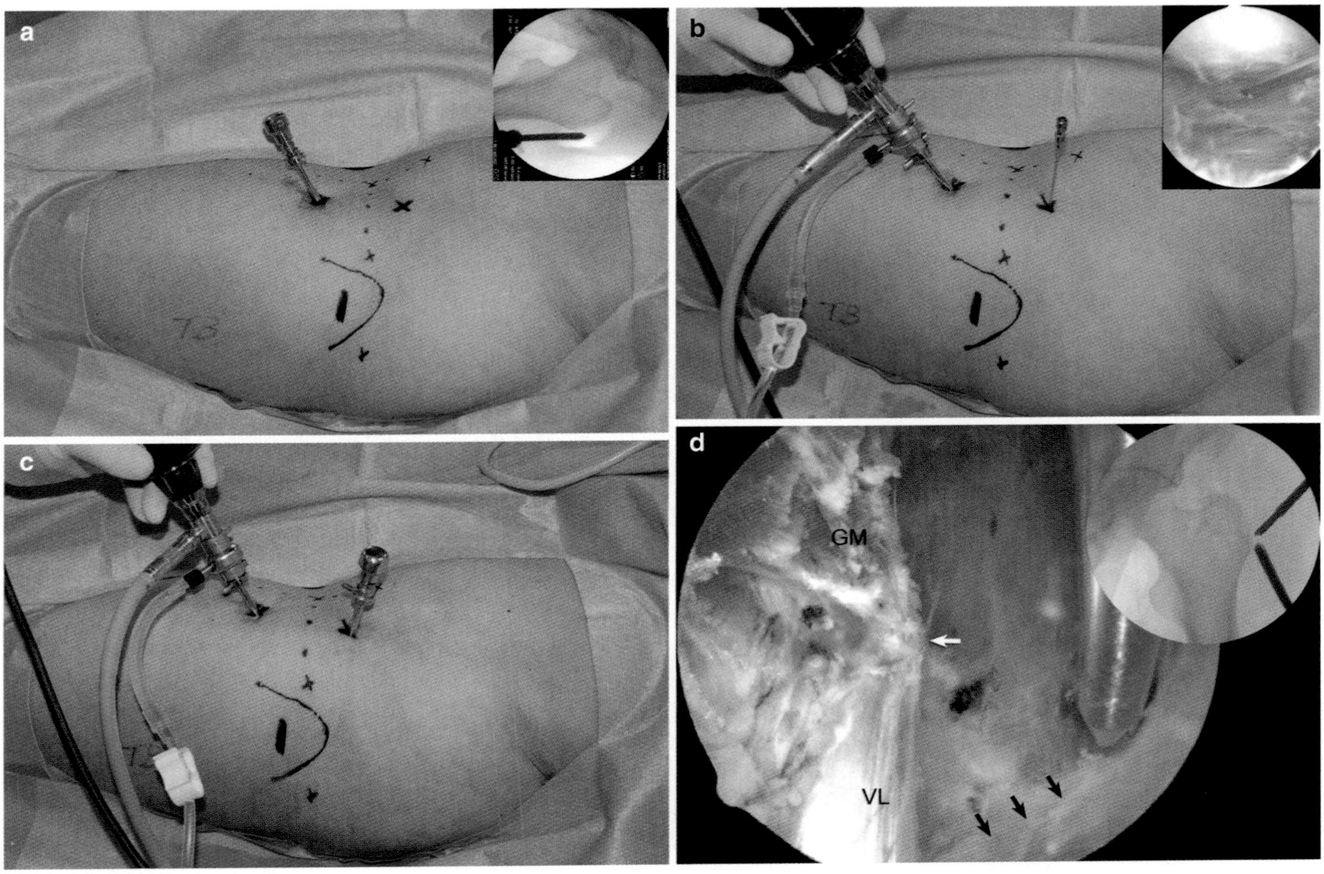

Fig. 11.50 (**a**) The distal portal is placed into the peritrochanteric space. The fluoroscopic image illustrates positioning of the portal underneath the iliotibial band at the vastus lateralis ridge, which is the lateral-most prominence of the greater trochanter. This location avoids penetrating the gluteus medius or vastus lateralis. (**b**) The second portal is then placed under direct arthroscopic visualization. Prepositioning is performed with a 17-gauge spinal needle. (**c**) A working portal has been established and arthroscopy is facilitated by switching the arthroscope and instruments between the two portals. (**d**) The convergence of the insertion of the gluteus medium (*GM*) and the origin of the vastus lateralis (*VL*) at the vastus ridge (*white arrow*) is in view. Posteriorly, the figures of the gluteus maximus (*black arrows*) course diagonally to its insertion on the posterior proximal femur (Courtesy of J.W. Thomas Byrd, MD, Nashville, TN)

The first portal is positioned at the anterior border of the tensor fascia lata (Fig. 11.50a). Under fluoroscopic control, it is directed posteriorly into the trochanteric bursa at the level of the vastus lateralis ridge. Placing the portal just lateral to this ridge aids in having the cannula pass underneath the iliotibial band but not perforate the muscular portion of the gluteus medius insertion or vastus lateralis origin that are just above and below the vastus ridge. Under direct arthroscopic visualization, a second portal is then placed vertically in line with the initial portal (Fig. 11.50b). It is best for these two portals to converge from above and below the vastus ridge to avoid crowding of the instrumentation (Fig. 11.50c). Debris is then removed and the peritrochanteric space is developed.

This suffices for simple trochanteric bursectomy. Other pathology may require laterally based portals that can then easily be positioned for addressing problems such as snapping of the iliotibial band (Fig. 11.51a–d) (Video 11.16: http://goo.gl/DBGNN) or abductor repair (Fig. 11.52a–f) (Video 11.17: http://goo.gl/zyd9G) [21, 27].

Subgluteal Space

The subgluteal space is a posterior extension of the peritrochanteric space, geographically separated by the insertion site of the gluteus maximus on the posterior aspect of the proximal femur. Access to the subgluteal region begins with development and inspection of the peritrochanteric region (Fig. 11.53a–d). Then, viewing from the peritrochanteric space, posterolaterally based portals can safely be positioned. These must be posterior enough to pass behind the posterior border of the greater trochanter. For this portion of the procedure, the hip is placed in full internal rotation, which brings the greater trochanter more anterior and eases access to the subgluteal region.

Traditionally recognized disorders such as piriformis syndrome, previously addressed with open procedures, can be treated endoscopically (Video 11.18: http://goo.gl/6PaqI) [28]. Endoscopy is also helping to define other disorders such as subgluteal syndrome [6].

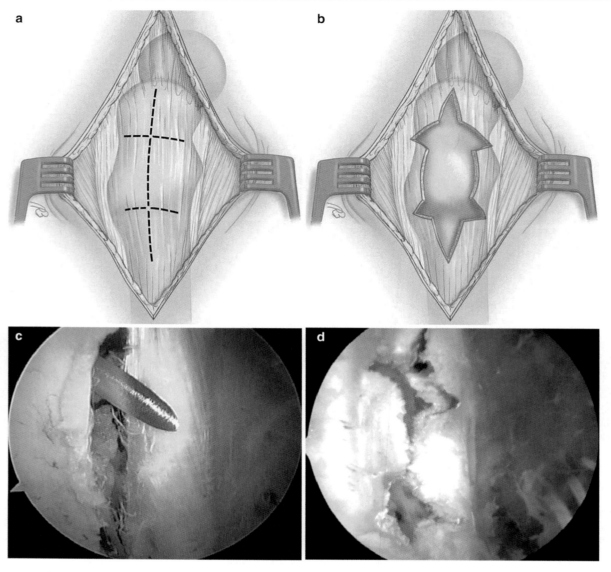

Fig. 11.51 (**a**) Illustration depicts the modified cruciate incision used to correct snapping of the iliotibial band. (**b**) The relaxing effect on the iliotibial band is illustrated. (**c**) Viewing the peritrochanteric space of a right hip from the anterior portal, the longitudinal limb of the modified cruciate incision is being created with an arthroscopic knife. (**d**) The modified cruciate incision has been completed with relaxation of the iliotibial band. (All rights are retained by Dr. Byrd)

Fig. 11.52 The left peritrochanteric space is being viewed. (**a**) The greater trochanter (*GT*) has been exposed by complete sleeve avulsion of the gluteus medius tendon (*arrows*). (**b**) The third of three double-loaded suture anchors is being placed. (**c**) All suture limbs have been passed in a mattress fashion. (**d**) The proximal row of mattress sutures has been secured, leaving single suture limbs for distal fixation. (**e**) A distal fixation device is being placed. (**f**) The proximal row of three anchors with double-limbed mattress sutures has been reinforced against three distal fixation devices. (All rights are retained by Dr. Byrd)

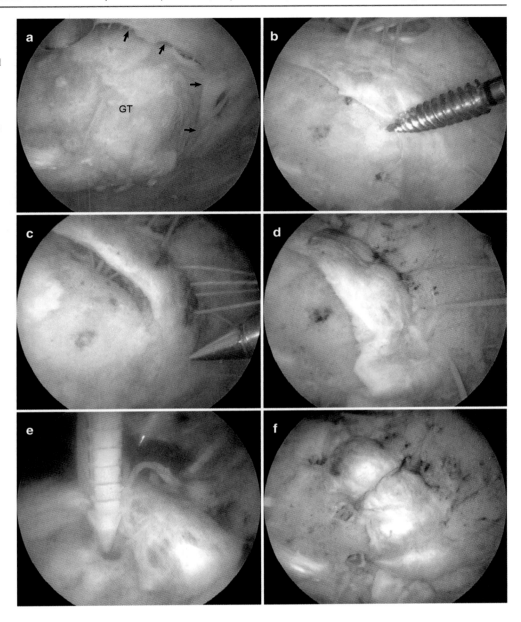

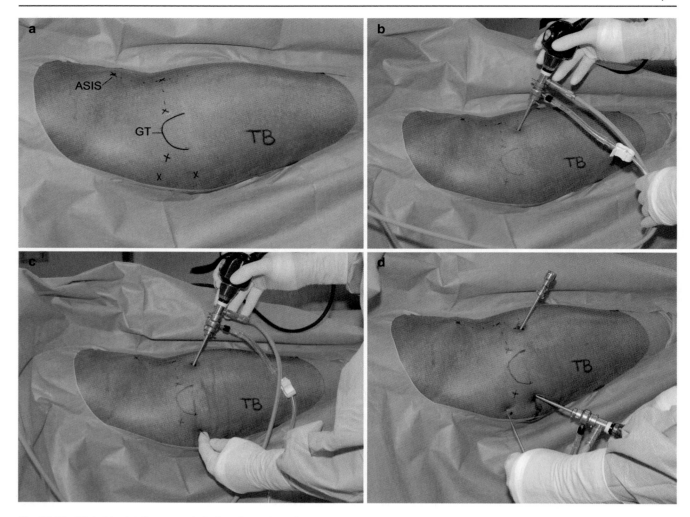

Fig. 11.53 Right hip. (**a**) Two posteriorly based portals (*red x's*) provide access to the subgluteal space. The greater trochanter (*GT*) and anterior superior iliac spine (*ASIS*) are marked, as well as the standard arthroscopy portals for the central compartment (*purple x's*). (**b**) The arthroscope is placed from anterior into the peritrochanteric space, allowing direct visualization for placement of the initial subgluteal portal. (**c**) Prepositioning is performed with a spinal needle for the initial subgluteal portal. (**d**) Now, with the arthroscope in the subgluteal space, positioning is performed for an additional subgluteal portal. (**e**) The peritrochanteric cannula has been removed, now with standard subgluteal portals for endoscopy. (**f**) Viewing posteriorly, the head is to the left and the foot to the right. The piriformis tendon (*PT*) is below the posterior margin of the gluteus medius (*G Med*) and gluteus minimus (*G Min*). A dense leash of fibrovascular bands (*FB*) inferior to the piriformis tethers the sciatic nerve (*SN*). The nerve is noted to lie on top of the rest of the short external rotators (*SE*). (**g**) In this case of piriformis syndrome, the piriformis tendon (*PT*) is divided with a hand basket. (**h**) The sciatic nerve (*SN*) has been decompressed from the remnant muscular stump of the piriformis (*Piri*) and the divided fibrovascular bands (*FB*). (All rights are retained by Dr. Byrd)

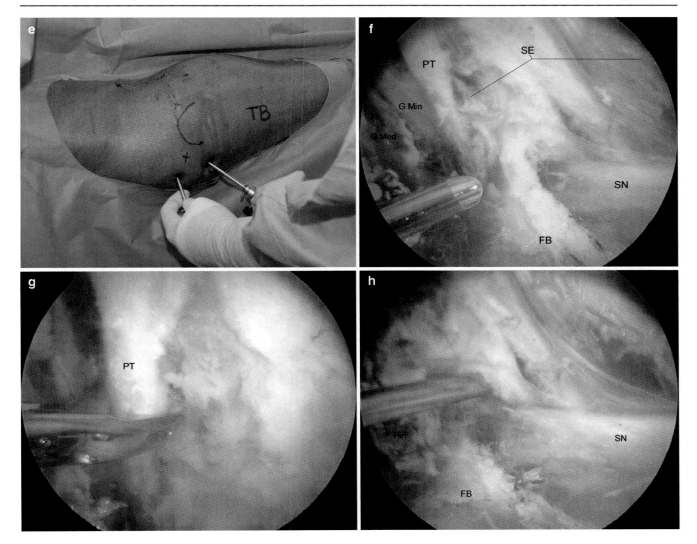

Fig. 11.53   (continued)

Conclusions

The popularity of the supine approach for hip arthroscopy is based on its proven efficacy and reproducibility. It allows optimal access for the central and peripheral compartments, accommodating joint position changes and intraoperative range of motion for dynamic assessment. It is also versatile for adapting to extra-articular procedures including iliopsoas bursoscopy and endoscopy of the peritrochanteric and subgluteal spaces.

References

1. Byrd JWT. Hip arthroscopy utilizing the supine position. Arthroscopy. 1994;10(3):275–80.
2. Dienst M, Godde S, Seil R, Hammer D, Kohn D. Hip arthroscopy without traction: in vivo anatomy of the peripheral hip joint cavity. Arthroscopy. 2001;17(9):924–31.
3. Byrd JWT. Hip arthroscopy, the supine approach: technique and anatomy of the intraarticular and peripheral compartments. Tech Orthop. 2005;20(1):17–31.
4. Byrd JWT. Snapping hip. Oper Tech Sports Med. 2005;13(1): 46–54.
5. Voos JE, Ranawat AS, Kelly BT. The peritrochanteric space of the hip. Instr Course Lect. 2009;58:193–201.
6. Martin HD, Shears SA, Johnson JC, et al. The endoscopic treatment of sciatic nerve entrapment/deep gluteal syndrome. Arthroscopy. 2011;27(2):172–81.
7. Byrd JWT, Chern KY. Traction vs distension for distraction of the hip joint during arthroscopy. Arthroscopy. 1997;13(3): 346–9.
8. Sampson TG. Complications of hip arthroscopy. Tech Orthop. 2005;20:63–6.
9. Byrd JWT. Hip arthroscopy. J Am Acad Orthop Surg. 2006;14: 433–44.
10. Byrd JWT, Jones KS. Hip arthroscopy in athletes. 10 year follow up. Am J Sports Med. 2009;37:2140–3. Originally published online August 14, 2009.
11. Byrd JWT, Pappas JN, Pedley MJ. Hip arthroscopy: an anatomic study of portal placement and relationship to the extra-articular structures. Arthroscopy. 1995;11(4):418–23.

12. Byrd JWT. Portal anatomy. In: Byrd JWT, editor. Operative hip arthroscopy. 2nd ed. New York: Springer; 2005. p. 110–6.

13. Kelly BT, Weiland DE, Schenker ML, Philippon MJ. Arthroscopic labral repair in the hip: surgical technique and review of the literature. Arthroscopy. 2005;21(12):1496–504.

14. Byrd JWT. Avoiding the labrum in hip arthroscopy. Arthroscopy. 2000;16(7):770–3.

15. Stubbs AJ. Intra-articular arthroscopic recession of the iliopsoas tendon: medial protection, 2011 Annual meeting multimedia education center, American Academy of Orthopaedic Surgeons, Chicago; 2011.

16. Byrd JWT. Labral lesions, an elusive source of hip pain: case reports and review of the literature. Arthroscopy. 1996;12(5):603–12.

17. Keene GS, Villar RN. Arthroscopic anatomy of the hip: an in vivo study. Arthroscopy. 1994;10(4):392–9.

18. Byrd JWT. Hip arthroscopy. Portal technique and arthroscopic anatomy. Orthopade. 2006;35(1):41–2. 44–50, 52–3.

19. Byrd JWT, Jones KS. Arthroscopic management of femoroacetabular impingement. Instr Course Lect. 2009;58: 231–9.

20. Ranawat AS, McClincy M, Sekiya JK. Anterior dislocation of the hip after arthroscopy in a patient with capsular laxity of the hip. A case report. J Bone Joint Surg Am. 2009;91(1):192–7.

21. Byrd JWT. Hip arthroscopy for non-structural hip problems. Ch 53. In: Berry DJ, Lieberman JR, editors. Surgery of the hip. Philadelphia: Elsevier (Saunders), 2013

22. Wettstein M, Jung J, Dienst M. Arthroscopic psoas tenotomy. Arthroscopy. 2006;22(8):907.e1–4.

23. Byrd JWT. Arthroscopic management of femoroacetabular impingement (FAI). Surg Tech Orthop Traumatol. 2011:67–80.

24. Byrd JWT. Evaluation and management of the snapping iliopsoas tendon. Instr Course Lect. 2006;55:347–55.

25. Byrd JWT, Polkowski GG, Jones KS. Endoscopic management of the snapping iliopsoas tendon (SS-33). Arthroscopy. 2009;25 Suppl 6:18.

26. Velasco AD, Allan DB, Wroblewski BM. Psoas tenotomy and heterotopic ossification after Charnley low-friction arthroplasty. Clin Orthop Relat Res. 1993;291:193–5.

27. Voos JE, Shindle Mk, Pruett A. Endoscopic repair of gluteus medius tendon tears of the hip. Am J Sports Med. 2009;37(4):743–7.

28. Byrd JWT. Piriformis syndrome. Oper Tech Sports Med. 2005;13(1): 71–9.

Loose Bodies: Tips and Pearls

12

Benjamin Domb and Itamar Botser

Introduction

Intra-articular loose bodies have been known as a source of articular pain for many years. During the nineteenth century, loose bodies were believed to form either as a result of traumatic breakage of the articular cartilage or from the synovial membrane [1]. However, removal of loose bodies at that time could have been fatal [1]. Today, there are many indications for hip arthroscopy, with loose bodies as one of the most common [2–4]. Moreover, hip arthroscopy is ideally set for the removal of loose bodies [2, 5].

In 1977, Milgram published a study on more than 300 different specimens in which one or more osteochondral bodies were found in surgery; he has classified loose bodies into three groups [6]. The first group included patients with post-traumatic osteochondral fractures, in which articular cartilage was found within the loose bodies, and in some cases, the concomitant chondral defect from which the loose body arose was found. The second class of loose body included those found in the presence of articular surface disintegration with degenerative joint disease and avascular necrosis (AVN); in these cases, articular surface damage was either noted in surgery or radiographically. The last group consisted of patients with myriads of free lose bodies, sometimes hundreds, and a grossly normal joint surface; these cases were presumed to be synovial chondromatosis. In addition to these classifications, Milgram also distinguished between loose bodies and attached osteochondral bodies. Nowadays, the nineteenth century theory is still valid; loose bodies can arise from tissue within the joint, the synovial membrane, or the articular surface. Once a loose body is lodged in the joint, a common sequence occurs: proliferation of bone and cartilage with subsequent resorption by osteoclasts on the surface [7].

While removal of symptomatic loose objects from the hip joint represents a clear indication for hip arthroscopy, not all loose bodies have to be removed. In some cases listed below, other measures should be taken.

Signs and Symptoms

Patients with loose bodies in the hip may complain of pain around the hip joint along with catching, locking, clicking, and grinding sensations.

Diagnosis

Diagnosis of loose bodies in the hip joint can be difficult; in many cases, concomitant injury may accompany loose bodies in the hip joint. The clinical history is most important for the diagnosis of intra-articular loose bodies. Legg-Calve-Perthes disease (LCPD) as a child may point toward an osteochondritis dissecans (OCD), while a fracture raises suspicion of an osteochondral fragment. Upon examination, the range of motion may be mechanically limited and clicking or catching may be noted.

The presence of a loose body on an imaging modality does not always indicate the source of the symptoms. Diagnostic intra-articular injection of anesthetic agent to the hip joint is often recommended before hip arthroscopy. Pain originating from intra-articular pathology will subside partially or fully following the injection.

Imaging

X-ray is usually the first imaging modality to be used; however, only loose bodies containing bone or calcium can be identified on X-ray [2]. We recommend a series of four views that includes an AP pelvis, Dunn view, cross table, and false profile of both hips. The combination of these X-rays gives a comprehensive view of the proximal femur and acetabulum. In many cases, a loose body can only be noticed on one view,

B. Domb, M.D. (✉) • I. Botser, M.D.
Hinsdale Orthopaedics Associates,
1010 executive ct. suite #250, Westmont, IL 60559, USA

Loyola Stritch School of Medicine,
Chicago, IL, USA
e-mail: dombsteam@gmail.com; itamar@botser.com

J.W.T. Byrd (ed.), *Operative Hip Arthroscopy*,
DOI 10.1007/978-1-4419-7925-4_12, © Springer Science+Business Media New York 2013

while remaining unseen on the others; loose bodies may be in the peripheral compartment or in the acetabular fossa.

Computed tomography (CT) can clearly image and pinpoint the location of loose body fragments in the hip joint; however, visualization of cartilaginous loose bodies may be limited. Magnetic resonance arthrography (MRA) can, however, visualize cartilaginous loose bodies. While MRA has a high specificity, its sensitivity for the detection of loose bodies has been shown to be less than 50% [8]. Nonetheless, MRA is reasonable before hip arthroscopy, as it allows more accurate diagnosis of concomitant injuries such as labral tears. A diagnostic intra-articular injection can be performed with the injection of anesthetic.

Although ultrasound is an excellent tool to assess foreign bodies in soft tissue and extra-articular space, it has limited functionality in the diagnosis of loose bodies inside the hip joint.

Posttraumatic Loose Bodies

Acetabular fractures and femoral head fractures are an etiology for loose fragments in the hip joint. Those posttraumatic fragments are a common cause of loose bodies in the hip joint [5]. The classic management is removal of the fragments. However, the removal of a large fragment might produce a noncongruent weight-bearing articular surface. Matsuda has recently published a case report of arthroscopic reduction and internal fixation of a large osteochondral fragment of the femoral head [9]. Evans et al. [10] have published a case report of a 32-year-old man with a symptomatic traumatic osteochondral defect of the femoral head. One year after the injury, with the failure of conservative treatment, he underwent subsequent arthroscopy using a fresh-stored osteochondral allograft plug via a trochanteric osteotomy. One year after the surgery, the patient is reported to be asymptomatic.

Posttraumatic Acetabular Rim Fracture: Case Presentation

A 22-year-old male student complaining of right hip pain for 4 years following a football injury where two other players' helmets collided into his right hip. He was diagnosed with a fracture of the acetabulum at that time and was treated conservatively. After having continued pain in the lateral side of the hip, incomplete healing of an acetabular rim fracture was seen on an AP pelvis X-ray (Fig. 12.1). The fragment was surgically resected due to the fact that the center-edge angle without the broken lateral rim measured 24°. At hip arthroscopy, a large chondral lesion was found which warranted a performed microfracture. Next, a small loose body was removed, and the acetabular rim fracture was excised which was followed by femoral osteoplasty. Following surgery, the patient continued to have pain; a residual cam lesion was noted, and a revision arthroscopic osteoplasty was done 1 year later.

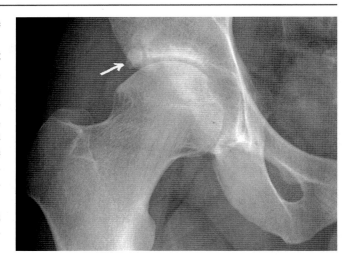

Fig. 12.1 Preoperative view of the right hip view showing unfused fracture of the acetabular rim (*arrow*)

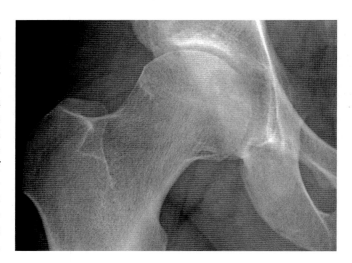

Fig. 12.2 Postoperative view of the right hip after removal of the unfused fragment

Even so, the pain did not resolve. At the last follow-up, two and a half years after the first surgery, the patient was still in pain. An updated X-ray showed borderline dysplasia with a center-edge angle of 20° and early arthritis (Fig. 12.2), which was felt to be the cause of his continued pain. This case highlights the potential for poor outcomes with a large acetabular rim fracture. In this setting, if the rim fracture is not reparable, peri-acetabular osteotomy may be considered.

Femoral Head Fracture After Anterior Hip Dislocation: Case Presentation [11]

A 22-year-old male involved in a snowboarding accident sustained an anterior hip dislocation with fracture of the femoral head. The hip was relocated 4 h post-injury, and the patient was referred for evaluation 1 week later. The presence

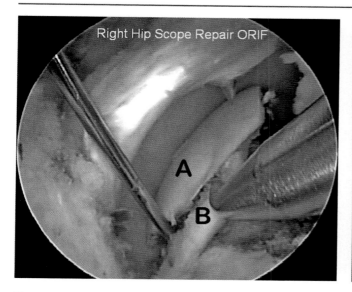

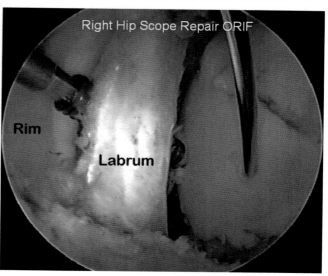

Fig. 12.3 Arthroscopic view of "clamshell" fracture being pried open with microfracture awl prior to arthroscopic osteosynthesis. The two cartilage surfaces of the folded-over fracture are represented by *A* and *B* (Courtesy of Dean Matsuda, MD, with permission from *Orthopedics Today*)

Fig. 12.4 Arthroscopic view of first headless screw being inserted after angle of approach has been improved with arthroscopic rim trimming. Note the cannulated screw being inserted between trimmed acetabular rim and detached labrum (Courtesy of Dean Matsuda, MD, with permission from *Orthopedics Today*)

of a large osteochondral fracture in a critical weight-bearing region favored arthroscopic osteosynthesis over resection; however, concurrent FAI morphology affected the arthroscopic management. During hip arthroscopy, the osteochondral fragment was found folded over itself in a "clamshell" configuration. The "clamshell" was pried open using a microfracture awl (Fig. 12.3). The fragment was reduced and fixated using two headless screws, but only after rim reduction and labral detachment permitted an improved angle of approach for screw fixation (Fig. 12.4). Arthroscopic labral refixation and femoral osteoplasty followed. One year postoperatively radiographs showed healing of the fracture (Fig. 12.5), and the patient was highly satisfied, able to return to snowboarding and tennis.

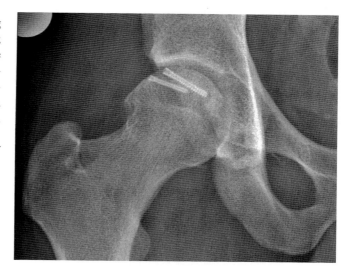

Fig. 12.5 One year postoperatively, the fracture is seen healed (Courtesy of Dean Matsuda, MD)

Synovial Chondromatosis

Synovial chondromatosis (Figs. 12.6 and 12.7) is one of the most common causes of loose bodies in the hip joint. Milgram [6] has identified three stages of the disease: (1) active intrasynovial disease with no loose bodies, (2) transitional phase, with intrasynovial nodules and free loose bodies, and (3) multiple loose bodies with no active intrasynovial disease. The disease is subtle in nature; by the time it becomes symptomatic and diagnosis is made, the synovial process is usually resolved and the source of the symptoms is the resulting loose bodies. X-ray will not show the loose bodies in most cases; however, MRI may show small loose bodies within the synovial fluid (Fig. 12.6). Boyer and Dorfmann [12] reported the results of 111 cases of primary synovial

chondromatosis in the hip that were treated arthroscopically. In their cohort with a follow-up of 1–16 years, more than half of the patients required at least one additional surgery.

Degenerative Joint Disease and Avascular Necrosis

Loose bodies are known to be related to degenerative joint disease (DJD) and to proliferate as the disease progresses. There are three mechanisms of loose body formation in the presence

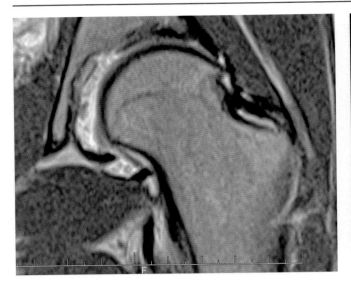

Fig. 12.6 Coronal cut of the left hip, via a proton density magnetic resonance with gadolinium showing loose bodies within the synovial fluid at the same patient with synovial chondromatosis

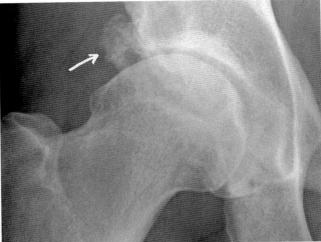

Fig. 12.8 Preoperative view of the right hip of a patient with hypertrophic osteoarthritis; large osteophyte is seen latterly (*arrow*)

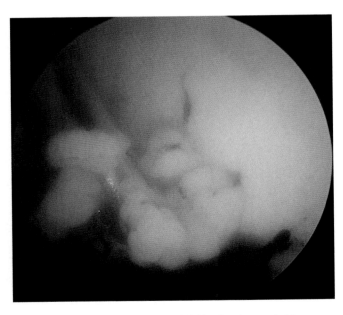

Fig. 12.7 Arthroscopic view of the left hip showing myriad loose bodies in a patient with synovial chondromatosis

Degenerative Joint Disease: Case Presentation

A 42-year-old man came to our clinic with complaint of right hip pain for 4 months; the pain was insidious in onset. He was an avid soccer player, and the pain was hindering his ability to play. He also complained of pain while walking long distances. On physical exam, he walked without a limp and had extreme pain and range of motion (ROM) limitation in flexion (up to 100°) and internal rotation (up to 5°). A positive anterior impingement test was noted. The X-rays (Fig. 12.8) showed joint space of 2.8 mm minimum on the lateral side, a large cam lesion, and large broken irregular osteophytes. During hip arthroscopy surgery, the broken osteophytes were removed (Fig. 12.9), the FAI morphology was addressed with acetabuloplasty and osteoplasty, and a labral tear was repaired. At 3 and 6 months postoperatively, the patient reported relief of the pain and was able to walk 5–10 miles every day at work. Fifteen months after the hip arthroscopy, the patient reported excruciating pain and soreness while walking and climbing stairs. On X-rays, increased osteoarthritic changes were noted; therefore, THR was advised. This case illustrates that arthroscopy for loose bodies in the setting of DJD may provide short-term relief; however, in the long-term, the DJD is expected to progress.

of DJD: (1) fragmentation of the joint surface, (2) fractured osteophytes, and (3) osteochondral nodule proliferation in the periarticular soft tissue [6]. Removal of loose bodies and osteophytes may address the mechanical symptoms; this will not, however, stop the progression of the disease. It has been shown in the past that joint space narrowing and high Tonnis grade are predictors of poor prognosis with hip arthroscopy. According to the authors' experience on 231 patients, hips which were graded as Tonnis 2 or 3 had satisfying results 3 months postoperatively, but worse results at following visits [13].

Osteochondritis Dissecans as a Sequela of Perthes Disease

Osteochondritis dissecans (OCD) in the hip is one of the four known sequelae of LCPD, which include coxa magna, coxa brevis, and coxa irregularis [14]. In most cases, the OCD will not appear solely, and treatment of one or more of the other

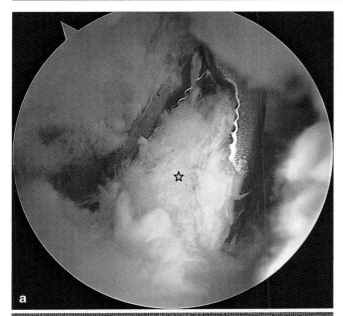

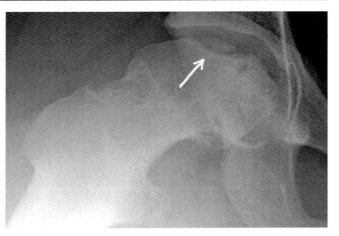

Fig. 12.10 Preoperative Dunn view of the right hip of a 24-year-old patient showing a large osteochondritis dissecans (OCD) lesion as a sequela of Legg-Calve-Perthes disease as a child (*arrow*)

OCD After LCPD: Case Presentation

Twenty-five-year-old female athletic trainer, presented with hip pain with a history of LCPD that was diagnosed at the age of 9. On examination, a marked ROM limitation was noted. The X-rays showed a deformation of the femoral head combined with large OCD (Fig. 12.10); the joint space, however, was intact. Via open surgical dislocation, the OCD was refixated using absorbable pins and osteoplasty of the head was done (Fig. 12.11 and Video 12.1: http://goo.gl/XyR7q). Three months after surgery, the patient was satisfied with an increased range of motion, reduced pain, and a very slight Trendelenburg gait; the X-ray showed healing of the OCD (Fig. 12.12).

Os Acetabuli

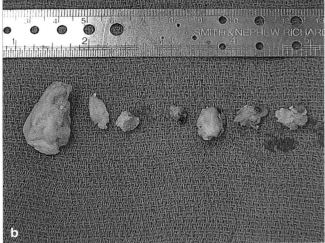

Fig. 12.9 (**a**) Arthroscopic removal of broken osteophyte (*star*) using a standard arthroscopic tool. View through the anterolateral portal, instrument through mid-anterior portal. (**b**) Seven osteophytes which were removed arthroscopically from the same patient

pathologies is warranted. In the case that the OCD is not in a weight-bearing area, arthroscopic removal of the lesion, debridement, and osteoplasty suffice. However, in the case the OCD is in a weight-bearing area, removal of the lesion will create a deformed femoral head; in that case, it is advised to either fix the OCD back to its place (see case presentation) or to use an osteochondral graft to fill the defect [14, 15]. The decision whether to use an open dislocation or an arthroscopic technique is dependent on the lesion size and concomitant pathology. For example, in the case of coxa brevis in which the neck is shortened and the greater trochanter has overgrown, open surgery may be indicated since greater trochanter advancement is beneficial [14].

Os acetabuli is an ossicle located at the acetabular rim. It was describe by Ponseti in 1978 as a secondary ossification center of the acetabulum and a normal stage in its development [16]. In some patients, the os acetabuli remains unfused even at adulthood, resulting in an os acetabuli. Some authors consider this to be a fatigue fracture due to stress overload [17]. It should be noted that radiographic appearance similar to an os acetabuli may stem from multiple other causes, as listed in Table 12.1.

On a retrospective study, Martinez et al. [17] have found large osseous fragments at the anterolateral acetabular rim in 18 hips (15 patients) out of 495 patients treated for FAI. All hips presented with a "cam"-type impingement, and 16 had additional anterior overcoverage of the acetabulum as reflected by a retroverted acetabulum.

Os acetabuli can be a source of hip pain and should be removed during surgery if suspected to be part of the

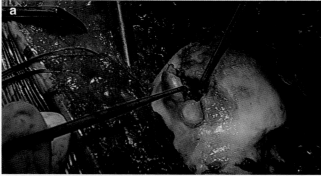

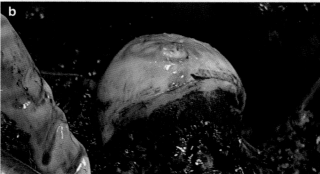

Fig. 12.11 (**a**) Microfracture of the OCD lesion via open surgical dislocation, the deformation of the femoral head is clearly seen. (**b**) Same patient after fixation of the OCD using absorbable pins and femoral neck osteoplasty

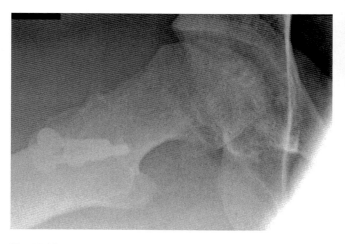

Fig. 12.12 Postoperative Dunn view of the right hip 3 months after the fixation of the OCD and femoral neck osteoplasty

Table 12.1 Pathologies with radiographic appearance of os acetabuli

1. Unfused secondary ossification center
2. Fatigue fracture due to stress overload (FAI morphology)
3. Acute acetabular rim fracture (Trauma)
4. Ossification of the labrum
5. Calcium deposit in the labrum
6. Fractured rim osteophyte
7. Adhesed loose body to the acetabular rim

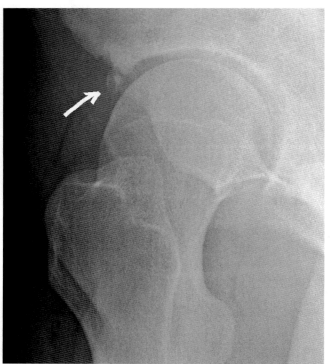

Fig. 12.13 False profile view of a left hip with anterior os acetabuli (*arrow*)

sion of the os, to determine whether removal of the os will leave acetabular undercoverage.

Os Acetabuli: Case Presentation

Nineteen-year-old male, presented with right hip pain that began gradually a couple of years earlier. On examination, a positive anterior impingement test was noted along with mild ROM limitations. On the false profile X-ray view of the right hip joint (Fig. 12.13), an os acetabuli was seen in the anterior aspect of the joint. Using an arthroscopic approach, the os acetabuli was removed (Video 12.2: http://goo.gl/HvD2w), a labral tear was repaired, and the bony FAI morphology of the

pathology. However, care should be taken in removing unfused secondary ossification centers, as removal of a large os may result in iatrogenic dysplasia. In order to prevent this, the lateral and anterior center-edge (CE) angles should be measured preoperatively with and without inclu-

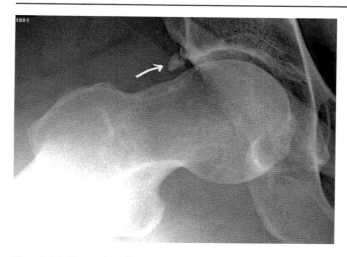

Fig. 12.14 Dunn view of a right hip, 1 year post-hip arthroscopy, demonstrating a calcific deposit in the acetabular labrum (*arrow*)

proximal femur was addressed with osteoplasty. Three months after the surgery, the patient was satisfied, with improved ROM.

Calcium Deposit Inside a Labral Tear

In some cases with labral tears, a calcium deposit inside the labrum can be seen on plain X-ray. Seldes et al. [18] in a milestone study regarding the acetabular labrum anatomy, found formation of peripheral osteophytes inside the labral tear between the articular margin and the detached labrum. The calcium deposit seen under X-ray is characterized by irregular borders and a popcorn appearance. The calcification can either be very small and hardly seen or large as in the next case presentation and video.

Calcium Deposit: Case Presentation

60-year-old female, referred for evaluation 1 year after hip arthroscopy with labral debridement and pain that did not resolve postoperatively. On physical exam, a limited range of motion was noted along with posterior hip pain at flexion and a modified Harris hip score (mHHS) of 67.2 points. On preoperative X-ray (Fig. 12.14), a calcium deposit is seen lateral to the joint. Additionally, lateral joint space narrowing and bone sclerosis was noted. Due to the arthritic stage of the joint, hip replacement was offered as an option. However, the patient selected hip arthroscopy in order to delay arthroplasty. During revision arthroscopy, a large calcium deposit was found in the labrum and removed using a probe (Video 12.3: http://goo.gl/rqcXU). Later, the labrum

was debrided, and acetabuloplasty and osteoplasty were done. After the surgery, the patient experienced relief of pain and symptoms, with postoperative mHHS of 95.7 points.

Foreign Bodies

Foreign bodies in the hip joint can be iatrogenic, e.g., breakage of a surgical tool, or penetration from the outside, such as bullets. There have been several reports about removal of bullets from the hip joint using arthroscopic devices [19–21]. There are several indications for bullet removal: (1) intra-articular lodging of the bullet, in order to prevent additional chondral damage; (2) neurovascular proximity; and (3) lead bullets, in order to prevent chronic lead poisoning.

The Authors' Experience

Over the last 728 hip arthroscopies performed by the senior author (B.G.D.), 87 cases (12%) involved removal of free bodies. The mean age of the patients with free bodies was 42 (range, 16–60), higher than the remaining population ($p=0.03$). Furthermore, the percent of male patients was higher ($p=0.002$), the Tonnis arthritic grade was higher ($p<0.0001$), and the labral tear size was larger ($p<0.0001$) for patients with loose bodies (Table 12.2).

As for the clinical status before the surgery, we found a difference in the preoperative pain, as reflected by the visual analog scale (VAS), which was higher in the presence of free bodies ($p=0.01$). A marginally significant lower score was found according to the non-arthritic hip score (NAHS); however, no difference was found according to the modified Harris score (mHHS). One year after the surgery, there was no significant difference in the improvement of the VAS, NASH, or mHHS results between patients with or without free bodies.

Tips and Pearls for Arthroscopic Free Body Removal

The first step in removal of free bodies from the joint is the diagnosis of their presence. In most cases, the diagnosis is made by preoperative imaging, i.e., an os acetabulum or a fracture. In other cases, smaller free bodies will be visible at the time of introduction to the joint, as in many cases of synovial chondromatosis. However, in some cases, the free bodies may not be immediately obvious upon insertion of the

Table 12.2 Authors' experience comparing procedures involving loose body removal to all other hip arthroscopies

		Loose body removal		
		+	−	*p* value
Number of patients (total 728)		87	641	
Mean age (years)		41.84	38.38	0.0351
Gender (*n*)	Male	52 (59.77%)	246 (38.38%)	0.0001
	Female	35 (40.23%)	395 (61.62%)	
Tonnis grade	0	31 (41.33%)	338 (67.74%)	<0.0001
	1	34 (45.33%)	116 (23.25%)	
	2	9 (12.00%)	45 (9.02%)	
	3	1 (1.33%)	0 (0%)	
Labral tear size (hours)		3.63	2.9	<0.0001
Preoperative VAS		6.70	6.1	0.0144
Mean 1 year VAS change		−3.21	−2.73	0.4344
Preoperative mHHS		60.41	60.04	0.8601
Mean 1 year mHHS change		+22.04	+21.00	0.8225
Preoperative NAHS		52.27	56.78	0.0675
Mean 1 year NAHS change		+19.03	+20.89	0.6678

arthroscope; common hiding places are the acetabular fossa, the inferior recess, and the distal to the zona orbicularis.

Accessing the loose body may be a hurdle in the hip joint. A majority of loose bodies, particularly those near the rim such as os acetabuli, can be accessed through the anterolateral and mid-anterior portals. However, some loose bodies such as those in synovial chondromatosis can float or adhere in the acetabular fossa. To access the fossa, additional direct anterior portal and posterolateral portal can be useful.

In general, three device types are used for free body removal: motorized shavers, hollow bore cannulas, and arthroscopic graspers. The size of the free body determines which device is used. Small free bodies or debris in the joint can be removed using a shaver. With the shaver suction on, small free bodies are easily sucked out of the joint. Medium-size free bodies can be extracted using a cannula; the hydrostatic pressure inside the joint creates "vacuum cleaner" effect at the end of the cannula, which allows the loose bodies to flow out of the joint. This is highly applicable in synovial chondromatosis. Large free bodies can usually be removed intact with a grasper. Extremely large loose bodies can be broken inside the joint into smaller fragments, which may then be individually removed with the grasper.

A major obstacle in retrieving loose bodies from the hip joint stems from the depth of the hip within its soft tissue envelope. In order to avoid dislodging the loose bodies in the soft tissues during retrieval, it is often useful to enlarge the portal tract at the capsule, fascia, and skin. Enlarging the portal tract can be accomplished using a long tonsil or hemostat clamp, by inserting the clamp, and then spreading as you pull back.

In summary, loose bodies may appear in many forms. A repertoire of multiple approaches, devices, and techniques will facilitate easy removal of most loose bodies with minimal surgical time or morbidity to the patient.

References

1. Marsh H. On the origin and structure of certain loose bodies in the knee-joint. Br Med J. 1888;1(1424):787–8.
2. Kelly BT, Williams RJ, Philippon MJ. Hip arthroscopy: current indications, treatment options, and management issues. Am J Sports Med. 2003;31(6):1020–37.
3. McCarthy JC, Lee JA. Arthroscopic intervention in early hip disease. Clin Orthop Relat Res. 2004;429:157–62.
4. Byrd JWT, Jones KS. Prospective analysis of hip arthroscopy with 10-year followup. Clin Orthop Relat Res. 2009;468(3):741–6.
5. Byrd JW. Hip arthroscopy for posttraumatic loose fragments in the young active adult: three case reports. Clin J Sport Med. 1996;6(2):129–33; discussion 133–124–129–133; discussion 133–124.
6. Milgram JW. The classification of loose bodies in human joints. Clin Orthop Relat Res. 1977;124:282–91.
7. Milgram JW. The development of loose bodies in human joints. Clin Orthop Relat Res. 1977;124:292–303.
8. Neckers AC, Polster JM, Winalski CS, Krebs VE, Sundaram M. Comparison of MR arthrography with arthroscopy of the hip for the assessment of intra-articular loose bodies. Skeletal Radiol. 2007;36(10):963–7.
9. Matsuda DK. A rare fracture, an even rarer treatment: the arthroscopic reduction and internal fixation of an isolated femoral head fracture. Arthroscopy. 2009;25(4):408–12.
10. Evans KN, Providence BC. Case report: fresh-stored osteochondral allograft for treatment of osteochondritis dissecans the femoral head. Clin Orthop Relat Res. 2009;468(2):613–8.
11. Matsuda DK. Hip arthroscopy for trauma: innovative techniques for a new frontier. Orthopedics Today. 2010;6:6–9.
12. Boyer T, Dorfmann H. Arthroscopy in primary synovial chondromatosis of the hip: description and outcome of treatment. J Bone Joint Surg Br. 2008;90(3):314–8.
13. Domb BG, Smith TW, Botser IB. In: The learning curve in hip arthroscopy: a Prospective Analysis of Importance of Surgeon

Experience. American Academy of Orthopaedic Surgeons, New-Orleans; 2010.

14. Anderson LA, Erickson JA, Severson EP, Peters CL. Sequelae of Perthes disease: treatment with surgical hip dislocation and relative femoral neck lengthening. J Pediatr Orthop. 2010;30(8):758–66.

15. Siebenrock KA, Powell JN, Ganz R. Osteochondritis dissecans of the femoral head. Hip Int. 2010;20(4):489–96.

16. Ponseti IV. Growth and development of the acetabulum in the normal child. Anatomical, histological, and roentgenographic studies. J Bone Joint Surg Am. 1978;60(5):575–85.

17. Martinez AE, Li SM, Ganz R, Beck M. Os acetabuli in femoro-acetabular impingement: stress fracture or unfused second- ary ossification centre of the acetabular rim? Hip Int. 2006;16(4):281–6.

18. Seldes RM, Tan V, Hunt J, Katz M, Winiarsky R, Fitzgerald RH. Anatomy, histologic features, and vascularity of the adult acetabular labrum. Clin Orthop Relat Res. 2001;382:232–40.

19. Singleton SB, Joshi A, Schwartz MA, Collinge CA. Arthroscopic bullet removal from the acetabulum. Arthroscopy. 2005;21(3):360–4.

20. Sozen YV, Polat G, Kadioglu B, Dikici F, Ozkan K, Unay K. Arthroscopic bullet extraction from the hip in the lateral decubitus position. Hip Int. 2010;20(2):265–8.

21. Gupta RK, Aggarwal V. Late arthroscopic retrieval of a bullet from hip joint. Indian J Orthop. 2009;43(4):416–9.

Labral Management: An Overview

J.W. Thomas Byrd

Introduction

Labral tears have long been an indication for hip arthroscopy and still represent the most common lesion encountered [1, 2]. Even back in the 1990s, we knew it was not normal for a labrum to tear and one should always look for some underlying predisposition [3]. However, at that time, we knew only about dysplasia, trauma, and idiopathic etiologies. Ganz and his colleagues introduced the role of femoroacetabular impingement (FAI) as a primary hip disorder in 2003, and shortly thereafter, Trousdale and colleagues scientifically observed that labral tears rarely occur in absence of some bony abnormality [4, 5]. Our understanding of labral pathology is improving, but this understanding clearly remains incomplete.

Three statistically relevant bits of clinical information are important when evaluating a labral tear. First, isolated labral tears are uncommon [6]. If there is a labral tear, it is highly likely that there is some amount of accompanying articular damage. Second, imaging studies including magnetic resonance imaging (MRI) and gadolinium arthrography with MRI (MRA) are reasonable at detecting labral lesions but less reliable at assessing the severity of associated articular damage [7]. Third, the results of arthroscopy are most influenced by the severity of articular problems [8]. Thus, the status of the articular surface is the "wild card" in trying to forecast for a patient the likelihood of success with arthroscopic intervention. Some of this is only determined once the severity of articular damage has been assessed at the time of arthroscopy. Thus, be cautious of the concept of "it's just a labral tear." Often, patients may be referred with the diagnosis of a labral tear and inference by the referring physician that this could be a simple problem to correct. However, most often the labral lesion is found to just be part of the overall joint problem.

Anatomy

Triangular in shape on cross section, the labrum is a fibrocartilaginous ring that rims the acetabulum (Fig. 13.1). Inferiorly, it is contiguous with the transverse acetabular ligament which bridges the inferior aspect of the acetabular fossa. The posterior labrum tends to be the most consistent in size and morphology, while the anterior and lateral labrum may be more variable in both.

There is no capsulolabral complex in the hip as there is in the shoulder. The capsule attaches directly to the bony rim of the acetabulum, separate from the labrum. There is variability in the capsulolabral reflection which may demonstrate a deep separation and sometimes appear almost contiguous (Fig. 13.2a, b).

Vascular injection studies have demonstrated that the labrum receives its blood supply from the adjoining hip capsule (Fig. 13.3) [9]. Thus, the peripheral one-third of the labrum is vascular while two-thirds of its articular side are avascular. Thus, like the meniscus in the knee, a tear of the labrum is felt to have minimal healing capacity. However, like the meniscus in the knee, there are frequent clinical examples of patients with MRI evidence of a labral tear that have gone on to be asymptomatic in absence of surgical treatment.

The labrum is described as having a transitional zone as it merges with the hyaline articular cartilage of the acetabular surface (Fig. 13.4) [10]. However, years ago, we described a normal cleft that may partly separate the labrum from the adjoining articular cartilage (Fig. 13.5) [3]. One must be careful not to confuse this normal variation with a pathological detachment. Often, MRI and MRA cannot conclusively distinguish between a cleft and a tear. Increased signal within the substance of the labrum and contrast interdigitating within the labral tissue are additional features that would substantiate a pathological tear (Fig. 13.6). Since posterior tears are uncommon, any time an MRI or MRA reports the presence of a posterior labral lesion, statistically the assumption that this is more likely a cleft will usually be correct. Posterior tears usually occur only as a consequence of

J.W.T. Byrd, M.D.
Nashville Sports Medicine Foundation,
2011 Church Street, Suite 100, Nashville, TN 37203, USA
e-mail: byrd@nsmfoundation.org

J.W.T. Byrd (ed.), *Operative Hip Arthroscopy*,
DOI 10.1007/978-1-4419-7925-4_13, © Springer Science+Business Media New York 2013

Fig. 13.1 Acetabulum and fibrocartilaginous labrum. Triangular in cross section, the labrum's morphology is most variable anterior and lateral. A cleft is sometimes present that partly separates the articular rim of the acetabulum from the labrum and is most common posteriorly. The labrum's principal blood supply enters on its capsular surface at the capsulolabral junction. Inferiorly, the labrum is contiguous with the transverse acetabular ligament. (All rights are retained by Dr. Byrd)

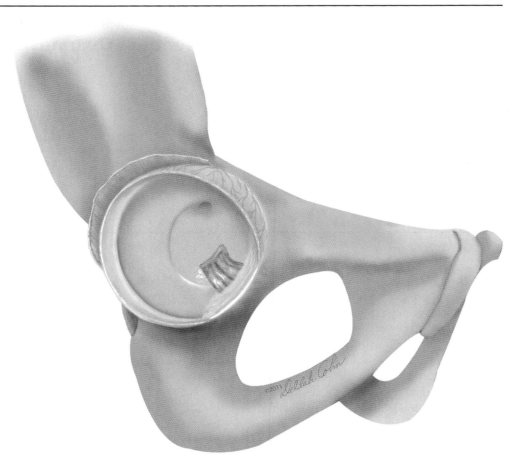

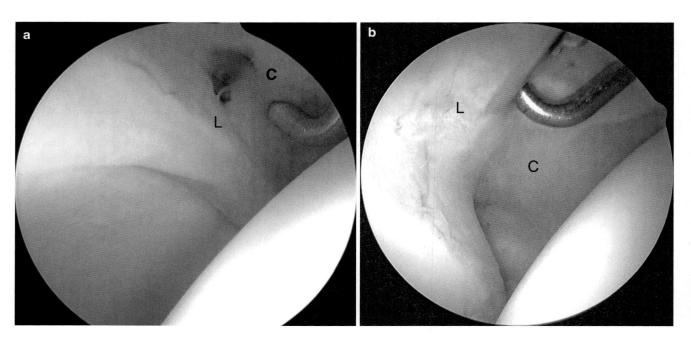

Fig. 13.2 Arthroscopic images illustrating variations on the capsulolabral reflection. (**a**) A deep reflection results in a generous divide between the capsule (*C*) and capsular side of the labrum (*L*). (**b**) The reflection is mostly absent, suggesting a continuum between the capsule (*C*) and labrum (*L*). (All rights are retained by Dr. Byrd)

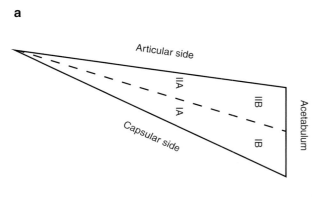

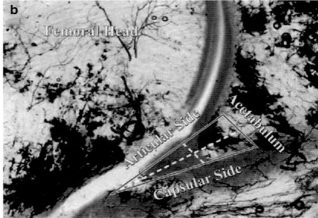

Fig. 13.3 (**a**) Zones of the hip labrum: the articular side of the labrum is adjacent to the femoral head and the capsular side of the labrum is adjacent to the periacetabular sulcus. (**b**) High-power photograph of the anterior superior labrum in a coronal Spalteholz section of a left hip (Reprinted from Kelly et al. [9]. With permission from Elsevier). (All rights are retained by Dr. Byrd)

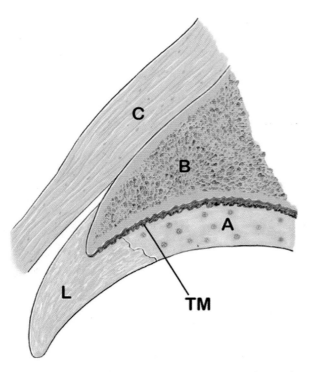

Fig. 13.4 Relationship of the acetabular labrum and capsule as described by Seldes including the bone of the acetabulum (*B*), labrum (*L*), articular cartilage (*A*), the tide mark (*TM*), and capsule (*C*). (All rights are retained by Dr. Byrd)

extension of anterior or lateral tears. While isolated posterior lesions are infrequent, they do occasionally exist.

Unlike the meniscus in the knee, the acetabular labrum possesses nociceptive nerve fibers, so it is easy to explain how a tear can be painful [11]. Receptors are present for pressure, deep sensation, and temperature, which may have regulatory functions in addition to mechanoreceptors responsible for proprioception.

Labral Function

The labrum seems to have minimal mechanical properties of importance to the hip. It has little weight-bearing function; as shown in a cadaveric study by Konrath et al. removal of the labrum did not substantially alter contact forces between the surfaces of the femoral head and the acetabulum [12]. Similarly, Ferguson et al., in a poroelastic model, showed that mechanically the labrum had only a small effect in enhancing joint stability [13].

However, the hydraulic seal effect of the labrum in the hip has great importance on joint function. Ferguson et al. have shown in both a poroelastic model as well as cadaveric studies that the labral seal maintains the fluid film within the joint, providing even distribution of contact forces across the articular surfaces (Fig. 13.7) [14–16]. This labral seal has also been shown to enhance joint stability, although it is not airtight [17].

These observations have great importance when it comes to labral repair. For example, in the shoulder where the labrum has more mechanical properties, creating a bolster of the labrum up on the face of the glenoid articular surface is helpful for added stability [18, 19]. This is not necessary in the hip where it is more principally a matter of restoring the labral anatomy and reapproximating it to the rim of the acetabulum.

Labral Management Algorithm

In the presence of a symptomatic labral tear, the prospect of preservation is always more appealing than resection but may not always be the best solution. There are numerous factors that go into the decision-making process. Sometimes, these factors contradict each other, and the surgeon may have

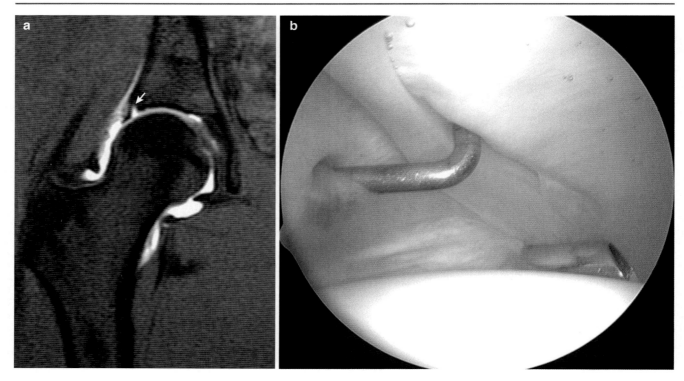

Fig. 13.5 Illustrative example of a normal cleft separating the lateral labrum from the acetabulum. (**a**) On a coronal MRA image, contrast demarcates a significant separation of the lateral labrum (*arrow*) from the lateral acetabular rim. (**b**) Arthroscopic image reveals the normal nature of the cleft. There is no evidence of trauma, secondary damage, or attempted healing. (All rights are retained by Dr. Byrd)

Fig. 13.6 (**a**) Example of a T2 coronal MRI demonstrating increased signal within the substance of the labrum (*arrow*) indicative of significant labral pathology. (**b**) Example of a coronal MRA demonstrating contrast interdigitating within the substance of the labrum indicating significant labral pathology instead of a normal labral cleft. (All rights are retained by Dr. Byrd)

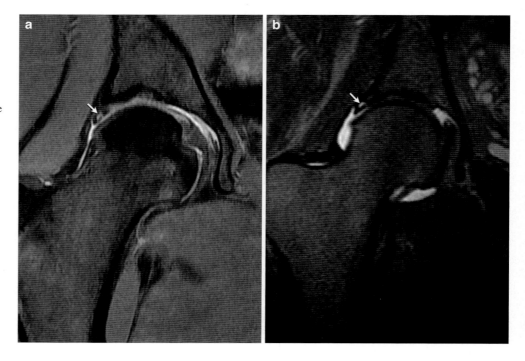

to prioritize in making the best choice. Certainly, the younger the patient, the more one is inclined to try to preserve the labrum and lessen the long-term consequences of a labral-deficient hip. However, diseased tissue is diseased tissue almost regardless of the patient's age. If the labrum is severely degenerated or destroyed, aggressive attempts at trying to repair severely compromised tissue are unlikely to be of great value to the patient. The patient must also be prepared

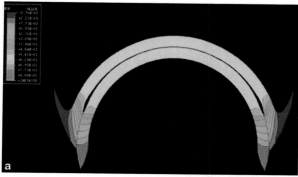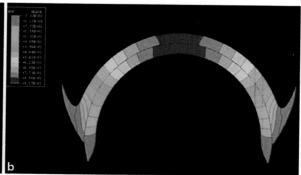

Fig. 13.7 An axisymmetric finite element model designed by Ferguson [16]. (**a**) Fluid layer sealed between the two cartilage surfaces results in uniform distribution of pressure across the joint. (**b**) Absence of the fluid layer results in direct contact between the two cartilage surfaces with less uniform distribution and higher peak pressures (Reprinted from Ferguson [16]. With permission from Stephen Ferguson). (All rights are retained by Dr. Byrd)

for the rehab process necessary in protecting a repaired labrum. If they are unable or unwilling to demonstrate compliance with the rehab strategy, then repair may not be a preferable choice. Other associated pathology may also influence this choice. For example, in a young person with dysplasia where the labrum has much greater weight-bearing responsibility, more aggressive attempts at preservation are appropriate. Of course, these are circumstances where one might first need to consider the role of a PAO as a potentially lifelong joint-preserving procedure. Conversely, if a patient has advanced articular loss, the surgeon must question whether there is any value in trying repair of the labrum. Remembering that the importance of the labrum is its protective effect on the articular surface, then if the articular loss is already extensive, it is less likely that repairing the labrum would be of any predictable long-term value.

Labral Debridement

In properly selected patients with a properly performed procedure, it is unlikely that labral debridement will accelerate degenerative hip disease. Damaged or degenerated labrum can be the source of substantial symptoms and does not have protective qualities for the joint. However, simple debridement alone does nothing to address the underlying etiology, and it is not going to positively influence the natural progression of disease. Excessive labral excision can accelerate joint degeneration. Espinosa et al. showed this when subtotal labrectomy resulted in faster progression of arthritis [20]. Our study with 10-year follow-up of labral debridement showed 83% successful outcomes after 10 years among those patients who did not have clinical findings of arthritis at the time of the index procedure [21]. However, there are two significant caveats to this observation. First, this represented early experience in arthroscopy, and these were highly vetted patients. Arthroscopy was considered only under the most

select of circumstances and probably represented a most ideal subset of patients for arthroscopic intervention. Most of these had experienced protracted symptoms, yet had not developed significant secondary wear and thus had already demonstrated very durable joints. More importantly, among those patients who had findings of arthritis at the time of labral debridement, 88% had gone on to total hip arthroplasty by 10 years and the few that had not were doing poorly but simply choosing to live with their natural joint. This small cohort is indicative of a large population that exists today and a clearly unsolved problem. We are often observing younger adults, and even adolescents, who already have significant secondary findings of damage at the time of arthroscopy. For this large group, it is evident that simple debridement procedures alone are severely insufficient.

Numerous factors go into the decision-making process of labral debridement. The quality of the tissue, accompany damage, underlying etiology, and patient expectations are just a few factors.

Debridement Techniques

(See Video 13.1: http://goo.gl/dlWTb.) The principles of labral debridement are simple: (1) Remove the damaged tissue, (2) preserve as much healthy tissue as possible, and (3) establish a stable transition zone to minimize propagation of further tearing or persistent symptoms. Mechanical shavers are efficient at debulking damaged labrum. Creation of a stable transition zone is normally the greatest challenge. This is hindered by limited angles of access and limited maneuverability of instrumentation within the joint. This is in contrast to a knee, shoulder, or elbow where the less dense surrounding soft tissues allow better maneuverability and joint position can easily be changed for angles of debridement. Radiofrequency devices provide an advantage in the hip for overcoming these limitations (Fig. 13.8). It is important to

Fig. 13.8 Arthroscopic view of a right hip from the anterior portal. (**a**) A fragmented labral tear with degeneration within its substance is identified. (**b**) Debridement is initiated with the power shaver. (**c**) A portion of the comminuted labral tear is conservatively stabilized with a radiofrequency probe. (**d**) The damaged portion has been removed, preserving the healthy substance of the labrum. (All rights are retained by Dr. Byrd)

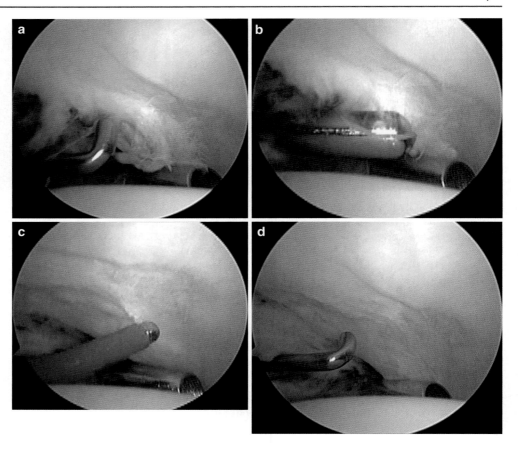

remember that tissue responds to thermal treatment by heating the water content in the cells [22]. Diseased fibrocartilage has increased water content and thus selectively responds to thermal treatment. Therefore, selective ablation of the damaged labrum can be performed at lower temperature settings, potentially resulting in less collateral thermal injury. Diseased tissue can be proportionately removed simply by observing its response to treatment. Healthy labrum demonstrates minimal response at these low temperature settings. Thus, when no response is observed, this indicates healthier labrum and repeated passes with a thermal device should be avoided because it can subsequently result in unnecessary cell death. Normally, in the course of creating an area of stable transition, if there is a small zone of cell death, this is still better than the overt excessive removal that may accompany less precise mechanical debridement. Thorough inspection, access, and then assessment of the area of resection typically require switching between various portals for completeness.

Labral Repair

Primary labral repairs are relatively uncommon. Most repairs are in the form of refixation accompanying acetabuloplasty to correct underlying pincer impingement. There

are few reports on the outcomes of such primary labral repairs [23, 24]. Our unpublished experience has been that the outcomes of primary labral repairs, while successful, are not as good as those reported with refixation. Lesser results are not due to failure of the repair site. In fact, repeat arthroscopy usually reveals a healed repair. Thus, a continued search is necessary for the underlying cause of a tear and a potential source of persistent symptoms among patients considered as candidates for primary labral repair.

There is animal model evidence to support the healing capacity of the acetabular labrum [25]. More importantly, our clinical experience has demonstrated excellent capacity of the labrum to heal. Among patients undergoing repeat arthroscopy, whether following labral repair or labral refixation, rarely is failure of the repair site a problem. However, there are two caveats about labral healing. First, the goal is not simply to repair the labrum but, more importantly, to restore its function. Thus, repair must focus on restoring the anatomy and not simply successfully reapproximating the labrum somewhere on the acetabular rim. Second, a healed labrum still does not have the appearance of normal, native labral tissue. This is in contrast to the meniscus in the knee where a healed meniscus often looks essentially normal.

Labral Repair Technique

(See Video 13.2: http://goo.gl/8JbTV.) The goal of primary labral repair is to reapproximate the labrum as closely as possible to the normal edge of the articular surface of the acetabulum. It is not necessary to create a bolster effect such as popularly performed with the glenoid labrum in the shoulder [19]. The acetabular labrum does not share the mechanical properties of the glenoid labrum as a bumper for deepening the socket [18]. It is its hydraulic effect from the labral seal that is important. Thus, reconstituting this with an anatomic reapproximation is important.

Restoration of the labrum is determined by (1) placement of the anchors and (2) how the sutures are used to secure the labrum.

It is important for the anchors to be placed close to the edge of the articular surface, but they do not need to be placed onto the face of the articular surface as is performed in the shoulder. More importantly, the surgeon must be certain that the anchor does not perforate the articular surface as it is placed into the acetabular bone (Video 13.3: http://goo.gl/uwc1d). This could potentially result in accelerated breakdown of the articular cartilage and progressive arthritis that would be much worse than having simply removed the damaged labrum. The most common error that is made to avoid this complication is to just place the anchors further away from the articular surface. However, in this circumstance, the surgeon then has a false sense of satisfaction that the labrum has been reapproximated with a good likelihood of healing, but it does not restore the normal labral anatomy and is unlikely to result in restoration of the labrum's function.

There are several techniques to assist in placing the anchors adequately close to the acetabular rim while avoiding perforation. The modified anterior portal is popular because of its slightly more distal position, allowing more divergence of the anchor from the face of the acetabulum [24]. However, sometimes, this site is still insufficiently distant for adequate divergence, and the surgeon can still be forced to place the anchors further away from the rim. A more extreme distal position of this portal compromises its utility for carrying out other aspects of arthroscopy of the central compartment. Our preference is to place the anterior portal wherever it provides the greatest utility for access and instrumentation within the joint and not rely on it for anchor placement [26]. We utilize a percutaneous anchor system that can be placed as distally as necessary to assure divergence from the face of the acetabulum (Fig. 13.9a, b) [27]. Typically, it is placed distally midway between the anterior and anterolateral portals. This allows anchor placement anywhere between the three o'clock and twelve o'clock positions of a right hip. Far medial anchors can be placed from the anterior portal, and more lateral anchors can be placed from the anterolateral portal. If a

percutaneous anchor system is not available, a small distally based portal can suffice for passage of an anchor delivery system. Also of note, fluoroscopy does little to aid in assuring proper anchor placement in this zone because the direction of placement comes closer to paralleling the x-ray beam than being perpendicular (Fig. 13.10). However, for anchors placed laterally such as from the anterolateral portal, fluoroscopy can be quite helpful in making sure that the anchor clears the subchondral acetabular surface (Fig. 13.11).

A recent innovation is the curved anchor delivery system (Fig. 13.12). This can be especially advantageous with the modified anterior portal, providing a greater angle of divergence.

As with any technique, preparation and exposure are critical to performing the procedure well. Small capsulotomies around an anterior and anterolateral portal aid in maneuverability and access for the repair (Fig. 13.13). These can be enlarged as necessary for complete exposure. As long as a small bridge of capsule is left between the two so that they are not completely connected, the capsulotomies should not be a concern with instability or require formal closure.

Typically, for primary labral repair, the rim of the acetabulum is exposed between the articular surface and the articular edge of the labrum (Fig. 13.14a, b). A bone-cutting-type synovial resector can be useful for freshening the rim without damaging the labrum that is destined for repair. A burr is more likely to harm some of this tissue. Sufficient bony preparation is necessary to assure a good healing response with the approximated labrum. Anchors are then placed against the rim on the articular side of the labrum (Fig. 13.14c, d). A spacing of 8–10 mm between anchors is usually sufficient to assure secure fixation of the labrum.

How the sutures are passed through the labrum is equally important for restoring the labral anatomy. The paramount feature of suture management is to assure that good quality tissue is being reapproximated. Philosophically, our preference is to avoid having suture interposed between the labrum and the articular surface of the femoral head because of concern that this exposed foreign material can be harmful to the joint, especially the femoral surface. Thus, simple looped sutures around the labrum are not our first choice but can be necessary to secure sufficient tissue. In clinical practice, we have had the opportunity to rescope a number of cases in which the looped suture technique has been used and have not actually observed any evidence of secondary damage due to this method. However, for primary repair, our preferred technique is passing both limbs of the suture through the labrum in a mattress fashion, providing a more anatomic reapproximation. The suture limbs can simply be grasped with a tissue-penetrating device and pulled out to the capsular side of the labrum (Fig. 13.14e, f). If the labrum is small or the tissue friable, alternatively, we will use a monofilament

Fig. 13.9 (**a**) For this right hip, three standard portals are utilized for routine arthroscopy, including the anterior (*A*), anterolateral (*AL*), and posterolateral (*PL*). A large diameter disposable cannula has been placed anteriorly for suture management. The anchor delivery system (*arrow*) has been placed distally midway between the anterior and anterolateral portals. (**b**) Schematic illustrates the drill sleeve placed against the acetabular rim. (All rights are retained by Dr. Byrd)

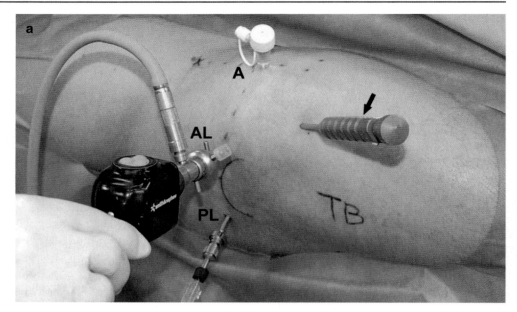

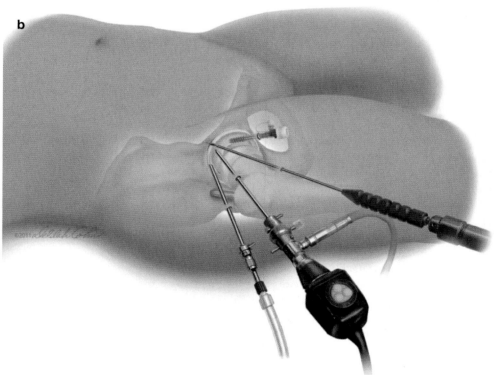

suture shuttle technique which provides the smallest perforation through the tissue (Fig. 13.14g, h).

With this method, all anchors are placed and the sutures are passed, before they are tied (Fig. 13.14i, j). Tying a suture before placing the next anchor can block access for seating the anchor against the acetabular rim.

If the labrum is robust, such as commonly seen in the presence of borderline dysplasia, then reapproximation with

anchors placed on the articular side of the labrum may not be the best choice (Fig. 13.15a, b). It can be difficult to instrument around the labral tissue without damaging it, and repairing a robust labrum in this fashion can inordinately distort its shape. For this circumstance, it may be better to expose the bony rim from the capsular side of the labrum. The anchors are then placed on the capsular side, and the sutures can be passed in a modified single-limb mattress

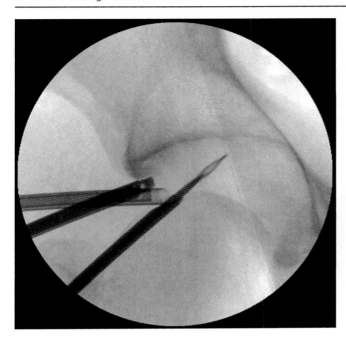

Fig. 13.10 Fluoroscopic image of a right hip as drilling is performed for an anteriorly based anchor. Since the direction of placement is partly in the plane of the image, it is not helpful for assuring proper placement. (All rights are retained by Dr. Byrd)

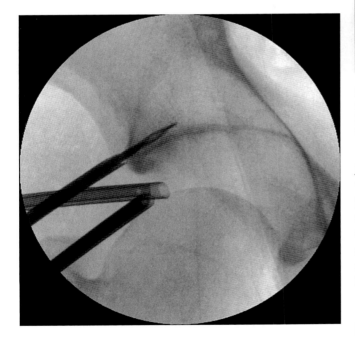

Fig. 13.11 AP fluoroscopic image of a right hip with the anchor drill hole being placed laterally. Since this is perpendicular to the x-ray beam, the image is helpful in assuring that the anchor will diverge from the articular surface. (All rights are retained by Dr. Byrd)

fashion providing better restoration of its anatomy and approximation of the labrum against the articular edge (Fig. 13.15c–f). This is accomplished with a soft-tissue-penetrating device where a limb of the suture is passed into the

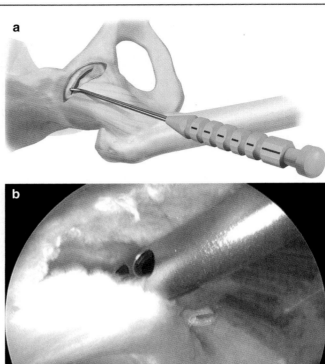

Fig. 13.12 (**a**) A curved delivery system can aid in assuring divergence of the anchor from the surface of the acetabulum. (**b**) Right hip arthroscopic image illustrates positioning of the curved guide for anchor placement against the anterolateral rim. (All rights are retained by Dr. Byrd)

joint at the articular margin of the labrum and then grasped with a second pass through the substance of the labrum and pulled out to the capsular side. Typically, it is best to have a slightly larger bite of tissue within the suture than you would estimate to be necessary. As the suture is tied, the tissue always compresses. This technique is comparable to the method commonly employed with labral refixation following acetabular rim trimming.

Labral Reconstruction

There have been several reports on labral reconstruction, mostly with a variety of autologous graft sources [28, 29]. Most popular among these is a tubularized strip of iliotibial band formed to reconstitute an absent labrum. Presently, this procedure remains limited to tertiary referral centers. Refinements continue in both the techniques and the indications for performing this procedure. The clearest current

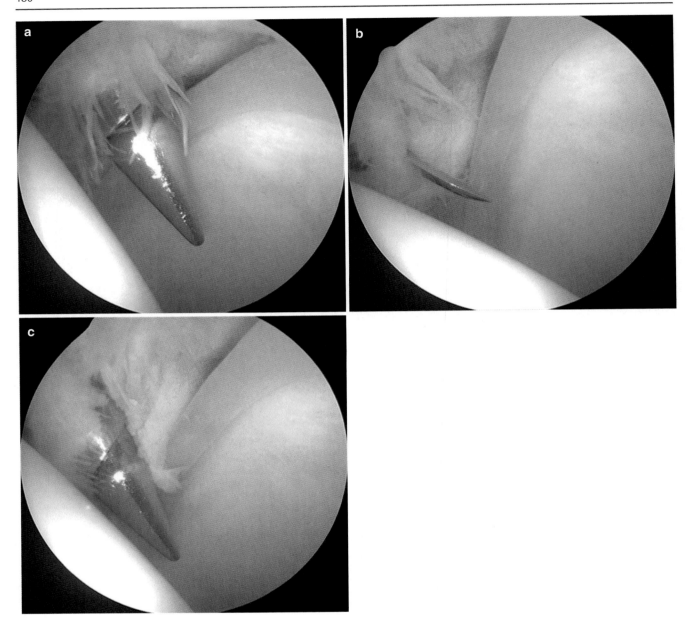

Fig. 13.13 Viewing the anterior portal from the anterolateral portal of a left hip. (**a**) Initial cannula placement is seen through the anterior capsule. (**b**) A transverse capsulotomy is made with an arthroscopic knife to provide better maneuverability and access to the labral tear. (**c**) The cannula has been returned with greater maneuverability. (All rights are retained by Dr. Byrd)

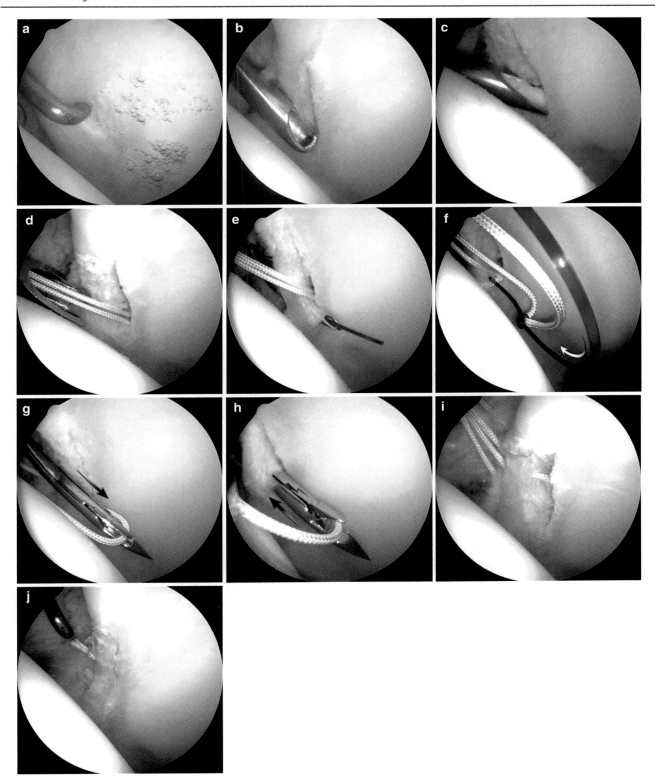

Fig. 13.14 An anterior labral repair is performed in this left hip. (**a**) The tear is probed from the anterior portal. (**b**) Preparation of the bony rim is performed with a bone-cutter blade. (**c**) An anchor is being placed adjacent to the rim from a distally based portal site assuring that it will diverge from the acetabular surface. (**d**) Suture limbs from the anchor are on the articular side of the labrum. (**e**) A suture shuttling device passes a monofilament suture through the labrum for a suture shuttle technique. (**f**) The braided suture from the anchor is tied to the monofilament and is being pulled through the labrum. (**g**) Another limb of the suture is pushed further into the joint. (**h**) The tissue-penetrating device then grasps the suture through the substance of the labrum for the second limb of a mattress technique. (**i**) Two anchors have been placed with all four suture limbs passed through the labrum in a mattress pattern. (**j**) The sutures have been tied, securing the labrum back to the rim of the acetabulum in its anatomic position. (All rights are retained by Dr. Byrd)

Fig. 13.15 Viewing anteriorly from the anterolateral portal of this left hip. (**a**) The labrum is hypertrophic with tearing at the chondrolabral junction identified with the probe. (**b**) An anchor has been placed with the sutures on the capsular side of the labrum. (**c**) A soft-tissue-penetrating device pushes one limb of the suture into the joint at the chondrolabral junction. (**d**) With the suture in the joint, the penetrator is repositioned within the midsubstance of the labral tissue. (**e**) The limb of suture is grasped. (**f**) The suture limb is then retrieved outside the joint creating a single-limb-modified suture pattern. (**g**) Repair has been completed with two suture anchors, securing the labrum, reconstituting the chondrolabral junction without distorting the labral morphology. (All rights are retained by Dr. Byrd)

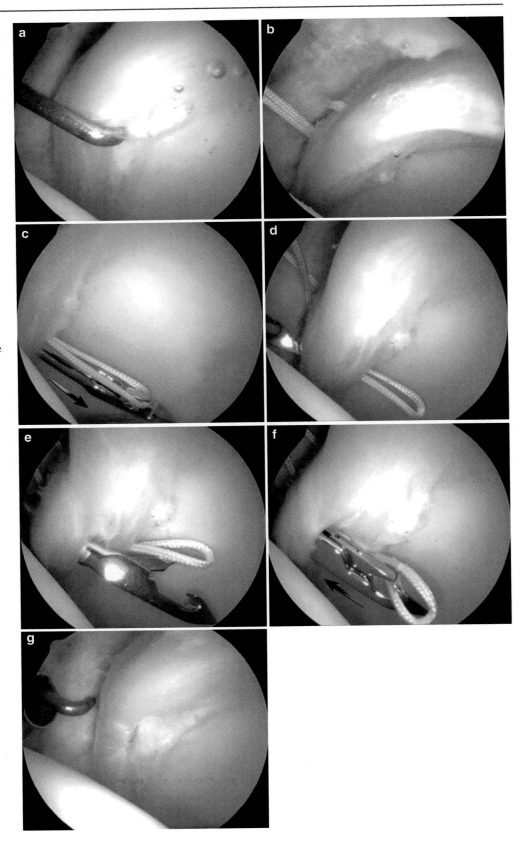

indication is among patients who are symptomatic due to a deficient labrum. Because of the sometimes multifactorial sources of pain, the causal relationship with labral deficiency can be difficult to confirm. Presently, labral reconstruction is not indicated as a primary procedure among patients who have not yet demonstrated problems due to an absent labrum.

Summary

The results of labral management will improve with better understanding of the labral enigma. This enigma includes an understanding of labral function; the ability of restoration techniques to restore the labrum's function, which is more than simply an assessment of labral healing; and whether restoration results in improved long-term outcomes.

References

1. Byrd JWT. Hip arthroscopy utilizing the supine position. Arthroscopy. 1994;10(3):275–80.
2. Byrd JWT. Hip arthroscopy: surgical indications. Arthroscopy. 2006;22(12):1260–2.
3. Byrd JWT. Labral lesions, an elusive source of hip pain: case reports and review of the literature. Arthroscopy. 1996;12(5):603–12.
4. Ganz R, Parvizi J, Beck M, et al. Femoroacetabular impingement: a cause for osteoarthritis of the hip. Clin Orthop Relat Res. 2003; 417:112–20.
5. Wenger DE, Kendell KR, Miner MR, et al. Acetabular labral tears rarely occur in the absence of bony abnormalities. Clin Orthop Relat Res. 2004;426:145–50.
6. Byrd JWT, Jones KS. Prospective analysis of hip arthroscopy with two year follow up. Arthroscopy. 2000;16(6):578–87.
7. Byrd JWT, Jones KS. Diagnostic accuracy of clinical assessment. MRI, gadolinium MRI, and intraarticular injection in hip arthroscopy patients. Am J Sports Med. 2004;32(7):1668–74.
8. Sampson TG. Complications of hip arthroscopy. Clin Sports Med. 2001;20(4):831–5.
9. Kelly BT, Shapiro GS, Digiovanni CW, et al. Vascularity of the hip labrum, a cadaveric investigation. Arthroscopy. 2005;21(1):3–11.
10. Seldes RM, Tan V, Hunt J, et al. Anatomy, histologic features, and vascularity of the adult acetabular labrum. Clin Orthop Relat Res. 2001;382:232–40.
11. Kim YT, Azuma H. The nerve endings of the acetabular labrum. Clin Orthop Relat Res. 1995;320:175–81.
12. Konrath GA, Hamel AJ, Olson SA, et al. The role of the acetabular labrum and the transverse acetabular ligament in load transmission in the hip. J Bone Joint Surg Am. 1998;80(12):1781–8.
13. Ferguson SJ, Bryant JT, Ganz R, et al. The influence of the acetabular labrum on hip joint cartilage consolidation: a poroelastic finite element model. J Biomech. 2000;33(8):953–60.
14. Ferguson SJ, Bryant JT, Ganz R, et al. The acetabular labrum seal: a poroelastic finite element model. Clin Biomech. 2000; 15(6):463–8.
15. Ferguson SJ, Bryant JT, Ganz R, et al. An in vitro investigation of the acetabular labral seal in hip joint mechanics. J Biomech. 2003;36(2):171–8.
16. Ferguson SJ. Biomechanics of the acetabular labrum, Ph.D. Thesis. Queen's University, Kingston; 2000: ISBN 3–905363–00–3.
17. Takechi H, Nagashima H, Ito S. Intra-articular pressure of the hip joint outside and inside the limbus. J Jpn Orthop Assoc. 1982; 56(6):529–36.
18. Lippitt S, Matsen F. Mechanisms of glenohumeral joint stability. Clin Orthop Relat Res. 1993;291:20–8.
19. Cole BJ, Millett PJ, Romeo AA, et al. Arthroscopic treatment of anterior glenohumeral instability: indications and techniques. Instr Course Lect. 2004;53:545–58.
20. Espinosa N, Rothenfluh DA, Beck M, et al. Treatment of femoroacetabular impingement: preliminary results of labral refixation. J Bone Joint Surg Am. 2006;88(5):925–35.
21. Byrd JWT, Jones KS. Hip arthroscopy for labral pathology: prospective analysis with 10-year follow-up. Arthroscopy. 2009;25(4): 365–8.
22. Edwards III RB, Yu L, Markel M. The basic science of thermally assisted chondroplasty. Clin Sports Med. 2002;21(4): 619–47, viii.
23. Murphy KP, Ross AE, Javernick MA, et al. Repair of the adult acetabular labrum. Arthroscopy. 2006;22(5):567.el–3.
24. Kelly BT, Weiland DE, Schenker ML, et al. Arthroscopic labral repair in the hip: surgical technique and review of the literature. Arthroscopy. 2005;21(12):1496–504.
25. Philippon MJ, Arnoczky SP, Torrie A. Arthroscopic repair of the acetabular labrum: a histologic assessment of healing in an ovine model. Arthroscopy. 2007;23(4):376–80.
26. Byrd JWT. Routine arthroscopy and access: central and peripheral compartments/iliopsoas bursa/peritrochanteric space. In: Byrd JWT, editor. Operative hip arthroscopy. 3rd ed. New York: Springer; 2012.
27. Byrd JWT. Utility of the modified anterior portal. AAOS Multimedia Education Center, 2012 Annual Meeting. San Francisco; 2012.
28. Philippon MJ, Briggs KK, Hay CJ, et al. Arthroscopic labral reconstruction in the hip using iliotibial band autograft: technique and early outcomes. Arthroscopy. 2010;26(6):750–6.
29. Sierra RJ, Trousdale RT. Labral reconstruction using the ligamentum teres capitis: report of a new technique. Clin Orthop Relat Res. 2009;467(3):753–9.

Hip Arthroscopy: Management of Chondral Injuries

14

Christopher M. Larson, Rebecca M. Stone, and Corey A. Wulf

Introduction

Articular cartilage pathology is a frequent finding at the time of hip arthroscopy. Hip joint chondral injuries can be the result of acute trauma, the result of underlying hip joint developmental pathomorphology, or less frequently the result of avascular necrosis. Traumatic chondral injuries include hip subluxation, dislocation, and "lateral impact syndrome." Hip joint developmental pathomorphology that can result in chondral pathology includes femoroacetabular impingement (FAI), dysplasia, Legg-Calve-Perthes, and slipped capital femoral epiphysis. Chondroplasty and microfracture have traditionally been employed as first-line treatment for arthroscopic management of chondral disorders. As our understanding of intra-articular hip disorders advances and arthroscopic techniques improve, alternative treatment options are beginning to emerge and the indications for such procedures are evolving.

Anatomy

The articular cartilage surfaces of the femoral head, head-neck junction, and acetabulum are made up of hyaline cartilage which is composed of primarily type II hyaline cartilage. This is similar to articular cartilage in other joints. The structure of hyaline cartilage can be divided into layers: superficial (tangential), middle (transitional), deep (radial), and calcified layers. In addition, the acetabular labrum provides a seal between the acetabulum and femoral head that maintains a film of synovial fluid that functions to distribute contact forces within the hip [1]. The femoral head and head-neck junction is normally spherical, and the acetabulum is normally anteverted and covers roughly 75% of the femoral head superiorly. Many encountered chondral abnormalities are seen in the setting of hip pathomorphology. Structural impingement can be the result of an aspherical femoral head-neck junction, acetabular overcoverage, or alternatively extra-articular hip impingement. Dysplasia, on the other hand, is typically associated with areas of acetabular undercoverage, increased acetabular inclination, femoral head and head-neck dysplastic deformities, excessive femoral neck anteversion, and coxa valga.

Pathomechanics and Chondral Injury

A disruption of articular cartilage in the hip and or the labrum can result in pain and disability but more importantly may lead to progressive degenerative changes. A finite element model revealed that labral dysfunction/pathology results in loss of the normal sealing function with a 92% increase in joint reactive forces that may predispose the hip to premature degenerative changes [1]. Therefore, intact articular cartilage and an intact acetabular labrum may be critical for the long-term health of the hip.

The calcified cartilage layer plays an important role in the development of chondral injuries that can result from shear forces seen in the setting of FAI. As the chondral surface of the acetabulum sees increased shear forces during impingement, the force is transmitted to the calcified layer, which is relatively weak and ultimately the sight of failure. An aspherical head-neck junction or cam-type impingement can lead to a labral-chondral separation with varying degrees of chondral delamination typically present at the anterosuperior acetabulum (Fig. 14.1). Pincer-type impingement can be focal (typically anterior) or global as seen in profunda, protrusio, and in the presence of an ossified labrum [2]. Pincer-type impingement typically leads to labral degeneration with associated

C.M. Larson, M.D. (✉) • R.M. Stone, M.S., ATC • C.A. Wulf, M.D.
Minnesota Orthopedic Sports Medicine Institute,
Twin Cities Orthopedics,
4010 West 65th Street, Edina, MN 55435, USA
e-mail: chrislarson@tcomn.com

J.W.T. Byrd (ed.), *Operative Hip Arthroscopy*,
DOI 10.1007/978-1-4419-7925-4_14, © Springer Science+Business Media New York 2013

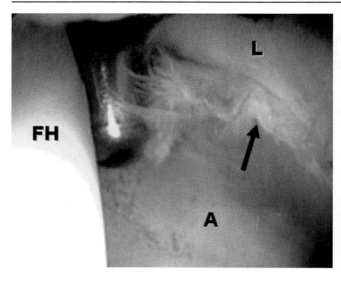

Fig. 14.1 Labral-chondral disruption (*black arrow*) in a left hip viewed through the anterolateral portal with the shaver in the mid-anterior portal. *FH* (femoral head), *A* (acetabulum), *L* (labrum)

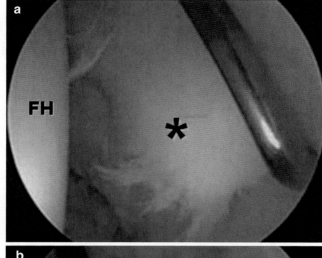

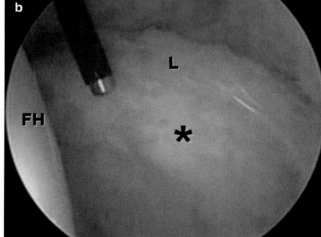

Fig. 14.3 Arthroscopy of a left hip with the arthroscope in the antero-lateral portal reveals (**a**) medial disruption of the acetabular articular cartilage (*asterisks*). (**b**) Chondral and articular-sided labral debride-ment revealed a partial thickness chondral injury, and microfracture was not required. *A* (acetabulum), *FH* (femoral head), *L* (labrum)

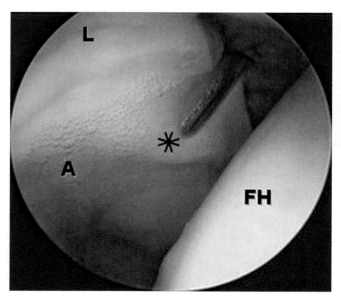

Fig. 14.2 "Wave sign/carpet delamination" in a right hip as viewed through the anterolateral portal with an arthroscopic knife in the mid-anterior portal reveals pathologic buckling or chondral-debonding (*asterisks*)-type lesion. *FH* (femoral head), *A* (acetabulum), *L* (labrum)

linear chondral wear to the posterior acetabular rim or "con-trecoupe" lesions [2]. Occasionally, however, a debonding injury or "carpet delamination" is seen which presents as a "wave sign" without a disruption at the labral-chondral junc-tion (Fig. 14.2). Chondral lesions can also be seen that involve detachment of the acetabular articular cartilage away from (towards the lunate fossa) the labral-chondral junction (Fig. 14.3a, b). In more advanced cases, full-thickness chon-dral lesions with exposed subchondral bone are seen

(Fig. 14.4). Chondral injuries associated with dysplasia predominantly involve both the anterosuperior acetabulum and femoral head [3]. Lesions involving the femoral head in the setting of dysplasia typically involve the superior weight-bearing portion of the head as opposed to involvement of the lateral, non-weight-bearing head-neck junction seen in FAI. These different patterns of chondral injury seen in the setting of structural impingement (FAI) and structural instability (dysplasia) relate to the variability in patterns and degree of pathomorphology combined with specific types and level of activity for these patients.

Chondral injuries can also be the result of a traumatic epi-sode. In a series of hips that sustained lateral impact injuries, chondral lesions were located medially, with three patients demonstrating lesions on the medial weight-bearing region just superior to the cotyloid fossa and one patient with a

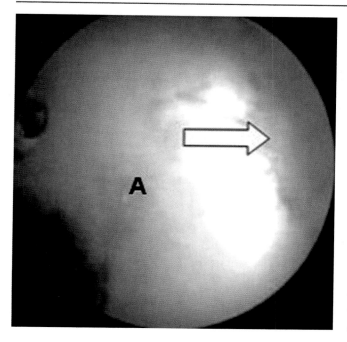

Fig. 14.4 Full-thickness chondral defect in the anterosuperior acetabulum (*arrow*) in a left hip viewed through the anterolateral portal. *A* (acetabulum)

lesion of the medial femoral head [4]. Traumatic subluxation of the hip or dislocation may also result in osseous and chondral injuries. Philippon et al. reported on 14 professional athletes who were treated after traumatic dislocations of the hip, and each patient was reported to have an associated chondral lesion [5]. Two had isolated femoral head chondral defects, six had isolated acetabular chondral defects, and six had chondral defects on both surfaces. Moorman et al. described an MRI triad for patients who sustained traumatic hip subluxations [6]. The triad included a lesion located at the acetabular rim, based on the direction of injury, with a posterior osteochondral and labral avulsion from the acetabulum being most common. Researchers have suggested that hips with FAI may be at risk for hip subluxation/dislocation with resultant levering of an aspherical femoral neck out of the acetabulum. Traumatic subluxation or dislocation may also result in avascular necrosis (AVN) of the femoral head. Nontraumatic etiologies of AVN are also common. Regardless of the etiology, AVN most commonly results in osteochondral lesions of the anterosuperior femoral head. If subchondral collapse occurs, this typically leads to further degenerative changes throughout the hip.

Our observations are similar to those reported by McCarthy et al. [7]. They reviewed their findings of 457 hip arthroscopies and found the anterior and superior acetabulum to be most prevalent, accounting for 73% of the cartilage lesions. They also found the majority of the anterior lesions to be Outerbridge III or IV [7]. Each of the previously mentioned patterns of chondral injury has specific management options which will be outlined in this chapter.

History

A complete history is the first step in determining the etiology and a suspicion for potential hip chondral injuries. Clinicians should inquire about traumatic etiologies such as hip subluxations, dislocations, and direct falls onto the lateral hip "lateral impact syndrome." It is more common to elicit an insidious onset of groin or deep lateral hip pain rather than a single traumatic episode. Occasionally, symptoms are referred to the posterior/buttock region or a combination of anterior and posterior pain as indicated by the "C sign" [8]. Presenting complaints of pain are often exacerbated by activities such as running, cutting and pivoting, getting in and out of a car, arising from a seated position, and prolonged sitting. Although unstable chondral flaps can lead to mechanical symptoms, it is more common for these patients to present with intermittent groin and deep lateral hip-related pain. In the author's experience, "clunking" is more often associated with a coxa saltans and not labral or chondral pathology. It is difficult on exam alone to differentiate between labral pathology, chondral pathology, and other intra-articular pathology. In fact, in the majority of cases, labral, chondral, and other intra-articular hip disorders often coexist.

Physical Examination

A comprehensive physical examination is important when evaluating patients with any suspected intra-articular and extra-articular hip pathology. Most chondral lesions are associated with underlying structural hip impingement or instability. An examination that includes range of motion (ROM) assessment, impingement testing and other provocative maneuvers, and pain elicited with varying hip positions can help determine whether underlying intra-articular pathology and associated hip pathomorphology is present. Examination begins with an evaluation of gait which is typically normal or mildly antalgic in the presence of chondral injuries. Severely antalgic gait patterns are more typical of acute traumatic injury such as hip subluxation, dislocation, and "lateral impact syndrome" or alternatively can be seen in the presence of more advanced degenerative changes and AVN. In the setting of acute trauma associated with a hip effusion/hemarthrosis, the patient may hold their leg in slight flexion, external rotation, and abduction. This position places the joint capsule at maximal volume and is a more comfortable position.

Specific tests may be consistent with intra-articular hip pathology and can give clues with respect to location of the pathology. Anterior pain with anterior impingement testing (hip flexion, adduction, internal rotation) is consistent with anterior hip pathology. Anterior or deep lateral pain with flexion, abduction, internal rotation, and FABER's (flexion, abduction, external rotation) test is consistent with more superior and superoposterior hip pathology. Posteriorly based pain with posterior impingement testing (hip extension, external rotation) is consistent with posteriorly based hip pathology. Significantly increased internal rotation or generalized hypermobility may be consistent with excessive femoral neck anteversion or dysplasia. Decreased flexion and internal rotation may be consistent with femoral neck retroversion or underlying structural impingement. Motion may be limited by guarding in either the traumatic or chronic setting due to synovitis of the hip. The supine log roll test may be consistent with hip irritability and is suggestive of an intra-articular process [8]. Palpation of the involved hip should include the following areas: groin, trochanteric and peritrochanteric regions, anterior and inferior iliac spines, buttocks, lumbar spine, pubic rami and symphysis, insertion of the rectus abdominis, external oblique, and adductor origins. Extra-articular pain often accompanies intra-articular pathology, and the clinician should ascertain the pain generators that best reproduce the patients presenting complaints [9].

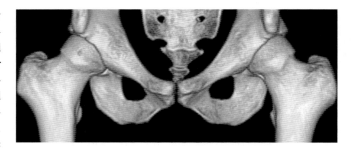

Fig. 14.5 A three-dimensional CT reconstruction of a patient with bilateral anterosuperior cam lesions of the proximal femurs

Imaging

Imaging is the first step to identify the potential pathomorphology at work. Plain radiographs that are typically obtained include a well-centered anteroposterior (AP) pelvis radiograph of both hips with symmetric obturator foraminae and approximately 0–3 cm between the tip of the coccyx and pubic symphysis. A lateral view of the proximal femur (modified 45° Dunn), a cross-table lateral, and false-profile radiograph are routinely ordered by the current author. Plain radiographs may reveal rim fractures in the setting of hip dislocation or subluxation and can identify structural abnormalities such as FAI, dysplasia, AVN, LCP or loose bodies. Any joint space narrowing should be noted on plain radiographs as this may significantly impact the success of any hip joint preservation procedure [10]. In the setting of hip subluxation or dislocation, Judet views may allow for better assessment of the acetabulum and more specifically the acetabular rim. Various radiographic measurements are routinely performed in order to better understand the etiology of the intra-articular pathology. Our routine measurements include the lateral center-edge angle, anterior center-edge angle, Tonnis angle, presence of femoral head lateralization, AP and lateral alpha angles, presence of a crossover sign, prominent ischial spines, coxa profunda or protrusio, os acetabuli or rim fractures, neck shaft angle, as well as Tonnis grading for degenerative changes.

Computerized tomography (CT) scans are frequently obtained in the setting of hip subluxation and dislocation and may reveal osteochondral loose bodies and posterior or less frequently anterior rim fractures. The current authors find that 3-dimensional CT scans provide a more global understanding of the hip and may be invaluable when planning potential arthroscopic hip procedures (Fig. 14.5). 3-dimensional CT scans can accurately define acetabular version, anterior/superior/posterior acetabular coverage, the location of rim fractures or os acetabuli, and pattern and extent of cam lesions, and slices through the femoral condyles allow for an additional evaluation of femoral neck version. Ultimately, newer magnetic resonance imaging (MRI) techniques will likely allow for an accurate 3-dimensional evaluation of the proximal femur and pelvis with comparable bony detail and superior soft tissue detail compared to CT scans without the risk of radiation exposure.

Magnetic resonance imaging and MR arthrogram provide a better assessment of soft tissues than CT. Non-arthrogram MRI is noninvasive but has been reported to have less accuracy in identifying labral and chondral pathology [11]. MR arthrography, however, is less sensitive for diagnosing chondral lesions in comparison to labral pathology. Keeney et al. published their results comparing MR arthrography to hip arthroscopy and found MR arthrography to have a sensitivity of 47%, specificity of 89%, positive predictive value of 84%, negative predictive value of 59%, and accuracy of 67% [12]. The addition of a "diagnostic anesthetic injection" is helpful to better confirm the hip joint proper as the source of pain [13]. In the future, newer MRI techniques may allow for improved detection of subtle chondral lesions as well as predelamination and debonding injuries [10].

Indications

In most cases, surgery is considered for patients with suspected intra-articular chondral injury when appropriate conservative regimens have failed. More urgent management is considered for hip subluxations/dislocations with nonconcentric reductions secondary to osteochondral fragments and/or soft tissue interposition. Intra-articular mechanical symptoms such as locking and catching may be indicative of loose bodies or unstable cartilage lesions which can be associated with AVN, Perthes, FAI, or prior hip dislocation/subluxation. Removal of symptomatic loose bodies is one of the clearest indications for hip arthroscopy. Patients with hip impingement can be expected to have some degree of chondral damage, and concomitant management of impingement, labral pathology, and chondral lesions should be performed to optimize outcomes. Arthroscopy for significant hip dysplasia should be entertained with extreme caution as arthroscopy alone will not correct the underlying pathomechanics at work. In a patient with very mild dysplasia/instability, arthroscopy can be considered with every attempt made to preserve the labrum, avoid rim resection, and perform capsular repair or capsular plication.

Contraindications

Contraindications to arthroscopic treatment of chondral injuries must be kept in perspective in order to optimize outcomes. The strongest contraindication when managing hip chondral injuries may be advanced arthritic changes. One study reported that bipolar MRI grades 3 and 4 chondral changes, greater than 50% joint space narrowing compared to a normal contralateral hip or prior radiographs, or <2 mm joint space remaining on radiographs resulted in no improvement at any time point postoperatively [10]. The inability to restore normal biomechanics can lead to failure of any cartilage restoration procedure regardless of the joint.

Therefore, significant structural instability/dysplasia is a relative contraindication, and hips with associated superior and or lateral subluxation should not be considered candidates for hip arthroscopy in the current author's opinion. Patients with severe acetabular retroversion and a severely deficient posterior rim might be better served with a reverse peri-acetabular osteotomy, at which time any chondral defects may be addressed open or arthroscopically. Structural impingement not accessible with hip arthroscopy, such as posteriorly based cam lesions, may be better addressed with an open surgical dislocation with chondral pathology managed at the same setting.

Surgical Technique

When conservative measures have failed, the hip joint proper is deemed to be the source of disability, and appropriate indications are met, surgery can be entertained.

Patient Positioning

Although hip arthroscopy can be performed in either the supine or lateral position, the current author uses the supine position. The patient is placed on a fracture table or operating room table with a distractor attachment (Fig. 14.6). The involved hip is positioned in 5–10° of flexion, neutral or

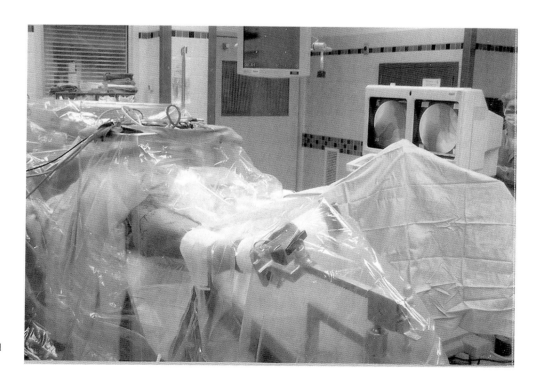

Fig. 14.6 Supine setup for a right hip arthroscopy performed using a standard fracture table

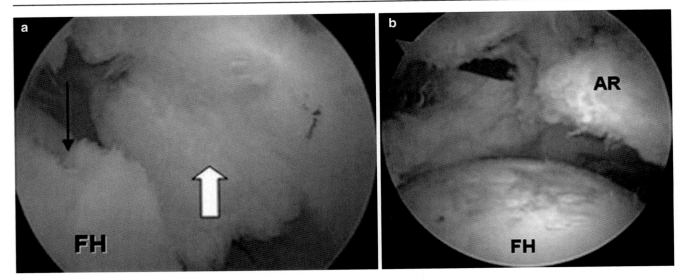

Fig. 14.7 Cartilage defects. (**a**) Loose cartilage flap (*block arrow*) from the right femoral head (*arrow*) viewed through the anterolateral portal. (**b**) Full-thickness cartilage loss in the presence of some general-ized osteoarthritis of a right femoral head as viewed through the ante-rior peritrochanteric portal with an ablation probe in the anterior portal. *FH* (femoral head), *AR* (acetabular rim)

slight abduction/adduction, and maximal internal rotation. The contralateral hip is abducted and externally rotated. A thorough fluoroscopic evaluation of the hip is then performed. The bed is rotated, aligning the anterior superior iliac spines parallel to the floor, in an attempt to recreate a well-centered preoperative AP pelvis radiograph for further evaluation of bony resections when indicated [14]. The femoral head-neck junction is evaluated with the hip in varying degrees of hip flexion, extension, internal, neutral, and external rotation. Distraction is then applied to verify that adequate distraction is achieved and the distraction is then released prior to prepping and draping.

Portal Placement

A standard anterolateral portal is made under fluoroscopic guidance. Saline is then flushed into the joint, and backflow may reveal varying degrees of chondral debris which may be more consistent with greater degenerative changes. A spinal needle is placed in the standard posterolateral position for outflow under direct arthroscopic visualization. We do not routinely complete a posterolateral portal unless chondral lesions or loose bodies are located posteriorly or posterior rim resection with or without labral refixation is required. A mid-anterior portal is established in line with or lateral to the anterior superior iliac spine and approximately 45° distal to the anterolateral portal under direct arthroscopic visualization. Further distal placement of portals allows for a better angle when placing suture anchors and performing microfracture to the acetabulum.

Inspection

Initial arthroscopic evaluation includes an evaluation of the anterior, superior, and posterior labrum, labral-chondral junction, and acetabulum. The femoral head, lunate fossa, and ligamentum teres are inspected. Chondral injuries can be quite obvious in the case of exposed full-thickness chondral defects and obviously displaced chondral flaps (Figs. 14.7 and 14.8). Chondral injuries, however, can be quite elusive, and although initial inspection may appear normal, thorough probing can reveal subtle labral-chondral disruptions and deep debonding or "carpet delaminations" (Fig. 14.2).

Specific Management Techniques

Different management techniques can be employed based on the pattern of chondral injury and associated pathomorphology. Microfracture is still the first-line treatment for exposed full-thickness chondral defects (Video 14.1: http://goo.gl/GM2Sg). Initially, any loose chondral fragments and flaps are debrided with a combination of an angled punch, ring curette, and or shaver taking care to leave a stable chondral edge (Fig. 14.9a–i). It is important to verify that the surrounding chondral surface and opposing chondral surface (femur or acetabulum) have relatively healthy cartilage to ensure a contained lesion. Chondral repair techniques may not be appropriate in lesions that are not contained and when bipolar grades 3 and 4 chondral lesions are present. Failure of containment occurs when the articular cartilage of the femoral head contacts the subchondral bone of an acetabular defect or when the articular cartilage of the acetabulum contacts subchondral bone of a femoral head defect after debridement and release of traction. A ring curette is then used to remove the calcified cartilage layer, and microfracture awls are used to penetrate the subchondral plate with visualization of fat droplets and or marrow elements.

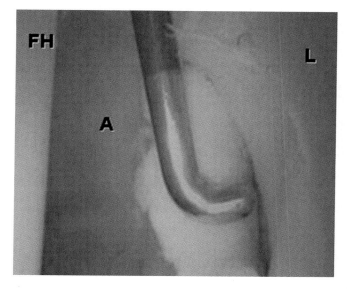

Fig. 14.8 Full-thickness cleavage delamination of the articular cartilage from the anterosuperior acetabulum in a left hip as viewed through the anterolateral portal with a probe introduced via the mid-anterior portal. *FH* (femoral head), *A* (acetabulum), *L* (labrum)

Microfracture begins at the periphery and ends at the center of the lesion placing perforations 3–4 mm apart. Performing microfracture often requires use of varying angled awls which provides access to the majority of lesions on both the acetabular and femoral head with the exception of lesions located on the most central portion of the femoral head. When the microfracture is complete, fluid flow is stopped and subchondral bleeding is assessed to insure an adequate depth of penetration. In the presence of AVN, chondral flaps are removed to a stable edge (Fig. 14.10a, b) (Video 14.2: http://goo.gl/eMVxD). Although the underlying bone is generally avascular, microfracture or deeper penetration with a drill or K-wire can be performed if an appropriate angle can be achieved in an attempt to reach the deeper vascular bone. In addition, core decompression can be performed concomitantly.

There are specific chondral injury patterns that deserve special mention with respect to management techniques. As previously mentioned, the underlying pathomechanics should be addressed when possible when treating the following injury patterns which may be amenable to arthroscopy or in some situations require an open surgical approach. A labral-chondral separation with adjacent partial-thickness or full-thickness acetabular chondral delamination is frequently encountered in the setting of cam-type FAI (Video 14.3: http://goo.gl/XYVrh). If there is only partial-thickness chondral delamination, this can be simply debrided followed by FAI correction. If there is a full-thickness chondral

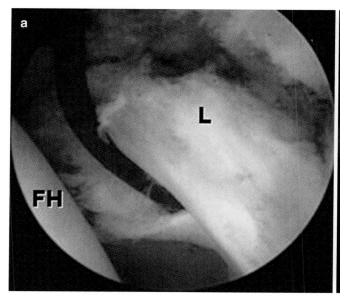

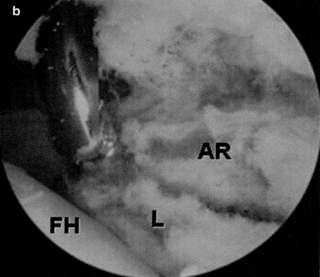

Fig. 14.9 A left hip in a patient with combined pincer- and cam-type FAI. (**a**) Typical labral-chondral disruption with delamination of the articular cartilage as viewed through the anterolateral portal. (**b**) A burr is introduced through the mid-anterior portal, and a rim resection is performed; (**c**) a punch is used to debride the unstable chondral flap; (**d**) a ring curette is used to debride the articular cartilage back to a stable rim; and (**e**) a 90° microfracture awl is used to perform microfracture.

(**f**) A further distal and lateral accessory anterior portal established with a spinal needle allows for better angle for microfracture, and (**g**) a 45° awl is placed through this accessory anterior portal to complete the microfracture. (**h**) Reduction in fluid pressure reveals bleeding from the microfracture site. (**i**) Final image after rim resection, microfracture, and labral refixation

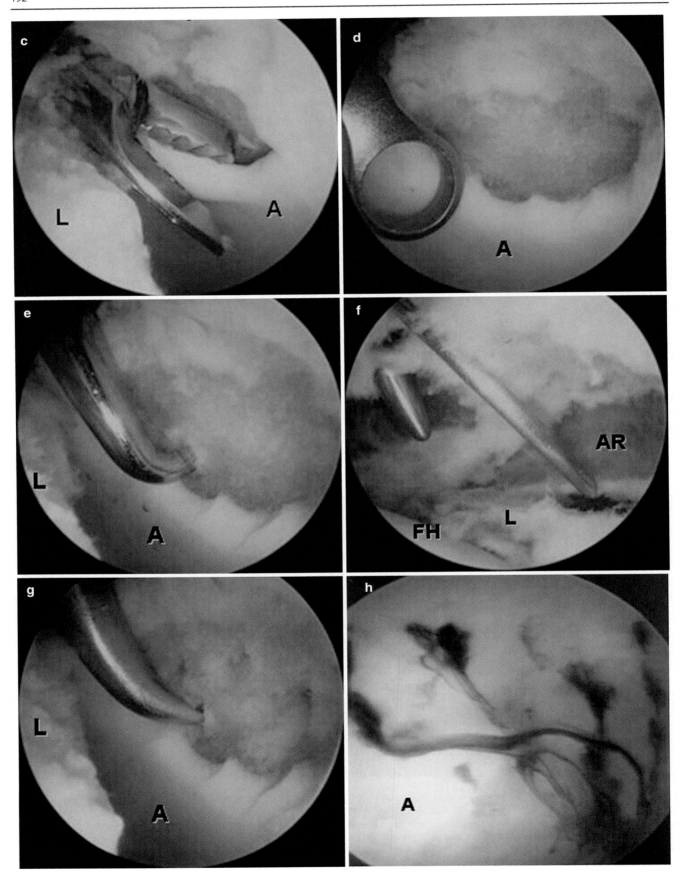

Fig. 14.9 (continued)

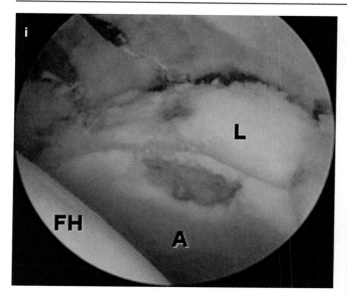

Fig. 14.9 (continued)

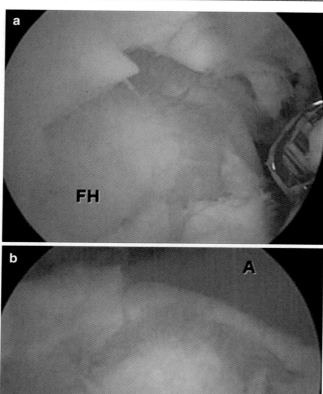

Fig. 14.10 Right femoral head with AVN, subchondral collapse, and full-thickness cartilage lesions viewed through the anterolateral portal and instrumentation introduced via the mid-anterior portal. (**a**) Removal of unstable chondral flaps is performed with various biters/punches. (**b**) After removal of unstable chondral flaps. *A* (acetabulum), *FH* (femoral head)

delamination, various treatment options are available. The traditional treatment consists of excision of the unstable chondral delamination, followed by microfracture and FAI correction as outlined previously. Newer techniques, however, are emerging, but published outcomes are limited or not available at this time. Some surgeons are performing microfracture deep to large chondral delaminations followed by refixation of the delamination with fibrin glue. If there is an exposed full-thickness defect or the chondral delamination is excised, some surgeons have recommended enhanced microfracture technique with mesenchymal stem cells or platelet-rich plasma (PRP). Alternatively, some surgeons have recommended implantation of a scaffold or matrix into larger full-thickness defects incorporating mesenchymal stem cells or autologous chondrocytes into the scaffold. Clinical outcomes, however, are necessary to evaluate these newer techniques and their respective outcomes in comparison to traditional microfracture technique.

Deep chondral delamination involving the labral-chondral junction without intra-articular extension "carpet delamination" is another characteristic finding that can be encountered (Fig. 14.11a–e) (Video 14.4: http://goo.gl/cKQ2g). In this situation, the labrum can be detached from the acetabular rim, or alternatively from the acetabular articular cartilage in order to access the deep delamination. We prefer to detach the labrum from the rim and adjacent unstable articular cartilage with a beaver blade. The chondral wave or deep delamination is then removed with a punch and shaver, and rim resection is performed when indicated. Microfracture is then

performed as previously described, and the labrum is refixed with suture anchors placed 1 cm apart (typically 3–4 anchors). Labral refixation can be performed with either looped suture or labral-base refixation techniques. Passing the suture through the labrum creates a mattress stitch which may better preserve the labral sealing function, but clinical outcomes are not available to support one technique over the other (Fig. 14.12). Alternatively, some surgeons have recommended detachment of the labral-chondral injury off the acetabular rim, leaving the labral-chondral junction intact. Microfracture is then performed deep to the injury, and the labral-chondral injury is then secured with labral refixation and or fibrin glue between the chondral delamination and subchondral bone. Again, published clinical outcomes are

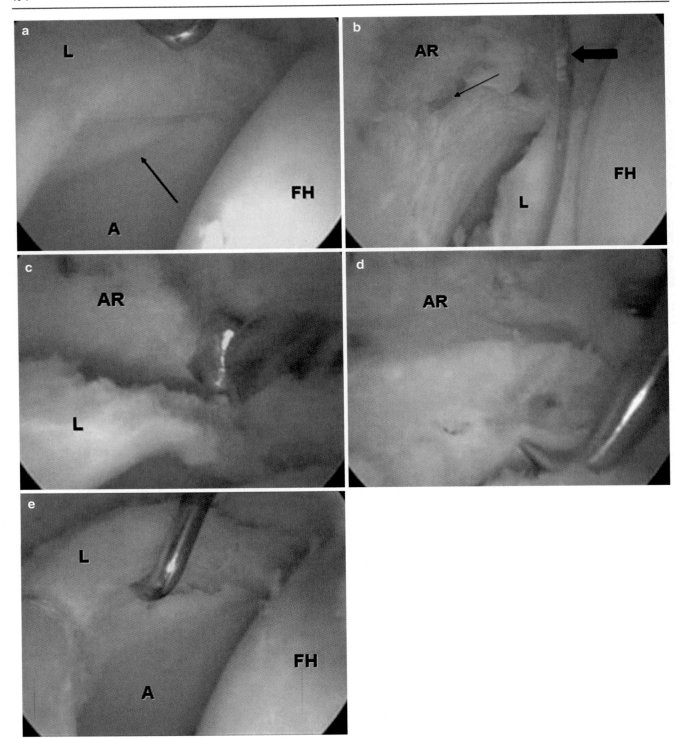

Fig. 14.11 An example of a deep chondral delamination without labral-chondral disruption "carpet delamination" in a patient with combined-type FAI of the right hip. All views are through the anterolateral portal with instrumentation introduced via the anterior portal. (**a**) A wave sign or carpet delamination (*black line arrow*) is noted during probing. (**b**) A delamination of the articular cartilage (*line arrow*) from the acetabular rim (*AR*) is evident after the labrum (*L*) has been taken down with an arthroscopic knife (*block arrow*) and displaced towards the femoral head (*FH*). (**c**) Rim resection is performed with a motorized burr, (**d**) and microfracture was performed with a 90° awl. (**e**) Significant decrease in the size of the lesion after rim resection and labral refixation

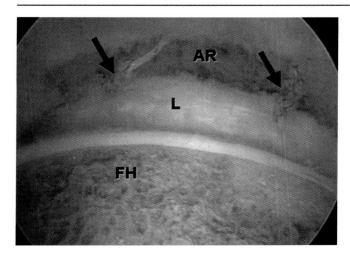

Fig. 14.12 Passing the suture through the labrum (*arrows*) creates a mattress stitch which may better restore the sealing function of the labrum in certain situations. *AR* (acetabular rim), *FH* (femoral head), *L* (labrum)

currently lacking with respect to this technique, and it is unclear whether the articular cartilage can firmly heal back to the underlying acetabular subchondral bone.

Another pattern of injury involves chondral detachment/delamination away from (closer to the lunate fossa) the labral-chondral junction (Fig. 14.3) (Video 14.5: http://goo.gl/DAohA). In this case, the articular cartilage is excised with a shaver and biter to the edge of the labrum. In the absence of pincer impingement, the labrum can be debrided on the articular side if the periphery is stable. When the labrum is torn to or through the periphery or is associated with pincer-type FAI, labral repair or takedown and refixation is performed. For any of the above described lesions, if delaminations or disruptions are partial thickness, the remaining stable cartilage is left in place and microfracture is not typically performed. The final portion of the procedure involves an evaluation of the peripheral compartment, and cam-type FAI correction is performed when indicated. As previously mentioned, in the setting of mild structural instability/dysplasia, rim resection should be avoided or minimal and every attempt should be made to preserve or repair the acetabular labrum and capsule.

Postoperative Rehabilitation

Postoperative rehabilitation begins the day of surgery. Early ROM is instituted with well-leg stationary cycling and or continuous passive motion machines. Foot flat or 30-lb weight-bearing restrictions are recommended for 2 weeks postoperatively when microfracture is not performed and continued for 4–8 weeks after microfracture procedure. Core strengthening is initiated postoperatively, with care to avoid any exercises that do not comply with the weight-bearing restrictions. At 6–8 weeks, progressive unrestricted strength-

ening is allowed along with the addition of aerobic training and sport-specific drills beginning at 2–3 months if microfracture is not performed. When microfracture is performed, we typically delay higher impact activities for 3–6 months which is based on the size of the lesion.

Outcomes

Microfracture remains the first-line treatment for grade IV chondral defects regardless of location [15]. Several authors have reported the results of microfracture in the hip within small subsets of larger case series or as case reports [16–19]. Byrd et al. reported on 21 patients with a mean follow-up of 2 years who underwent microfracture for grade IV chondral defects [20]. The average size of the lesion was 122 mm^2, and the mean improvement was 23.9 points (preoperative 51.4; postoperative 75.2). Philippon et al. reported on nine patients during revision hip arthroscopy that previously underwent microfracture [21]. The time from index arthroscopy to revision arthroscopy ranged from 10 to 36 months, and the original lesion size averaged 163 mm^2. Eight of nine patients had 95–100% coverage of an isolated acetabular chondral lesion, and one patient with an acetabular lesion was associated with a femoral head lesion, with grade 1 or 2 appearance of the repair product at an average of 20 months follow-up. One patient with diffuse osteoarthritis failed, with only 25% coverage 10 months after index arthroscopy. Although the number of studies and patient numbers are limited in these reports, the findings are encouraging.

There has been recent interest and preliminary reports looking at alternative techniques for arthroscopic hip cartilage restoration techniques. Surgeons are beginning to look at enhanced microfracture with PRP and mesenchymal stem cells for full-thickness chondral defects, but published clinical results are forthcoming. Villar recently reported his experience in 102 patients that underwent arthroscopic fibrin glue refixation of chondral lesions in the hip [22]. They microfractured the base of the chondral lesion and refixed the unstable articular cartilage to subchondral bone with fibrin glue. At up to 3-year follow-up, they had only three revisions, but further outcome evaluation and follow-up is necessary. Surgeons are beginning to explore the use of autologous chondrocytes and mesenchymal stem cells implanted into biological scaffolds for full-thickness chondral defects. Fontana reported non-peer-reviewed results of arthroscopic autologous chondrocytes implanted into a scaffold versus debridement [23]. The BioSeed-C scaffold was used for delivery of the cultured chondrocytes in a staged method. The average postoperative HHS improved in both groups. However, a greater increase was seen in the ACT group when compared to debridement alone with the scores being 86 and 65, respectively [23]. Osteochondral autograft transplantation (OATS) and osteochondral allografts can be technically done arthroscopically for femoral chondral lesions. Medial lesions do not allow for appropriate angles of implantation, but in other locations, an appropriate angle can be achieved and treated with 8–10-mm grafts taken from the anterolateral femoral head-neck junction with the hip out of traction. The grafts can then be implanted with or without traction depending on the location of the lesion. This has been performed, but clinical data and outcomes are lacking. Although the use of osteochondral grafting for arthroscopic management of acetabular-sided chondral lesions has not been reported, researchers are currently looking at the feasibility of implanting these graft in a retrograde fashion under direct arthroscopic visualization.

Conclusions

Chondral lesions are frequently encountered at the time of hip arthroscopy and remain a challenge. It is imperative to understand and treat the underlying pathomechanics when treating these lesions in order to optimize the potential for healing. Although alternative methods are being explored for arthroscopic management of hip chondral lesions, microfracture remains the first-line treatment until further clinical data becomes available. In the future, a combination of arthroscopic and open surgical approaches and the use of newer techniques and materials may improve our ability to treat and optimize outcomes for various hip chondral lesions.

References

1. Ferguson SJ, Bryant JT, Ganz R, Ito K. The acetabular labrum seal: a poroelastic finite element model. Clin Biomech (Bristol, Avon). 2000;15:463–8.
2. Larson CM. Management of pincer-type impingement. Sports Med Arthrosc. 2010;18(2):100–7.
3. Noguchi Y, Miura H, Takasugi S, Iwamoto Y. Cartilage and labrum degeneration in the dysplastic hip generally originates in the anterosuperior weight-bearing area: an arthroscopic observation. Arthroscopy. 1999;15(5):496–506.
4. Byrd JWT. Lateral impact injury a source of occult hip pathology. Clin Sports Med. 2001;20(4):801–15.
5. Philippon MJ, Kuppersmith DA, Wolff AB, Briggs KK. Arthroscopic findings following traumatic hip dislocation in 14 professional athletes. Arthroscopy. 2009;25(2):169–74.
6. Moorman III CT, Warren RF, Hershman EB, Crowe JF, Potter HG, Barnes R, O'Brien SJ, Guettler JH. Traumatic posterior hip subluxation in American football. J Bone Joint Surg Am. 2003;85-A(7):1190–6.
7. McCarthy JC, Lee JA. Arthroscopic intervention in early hip disease. Clin Orthop Relat Res. 2004;429:157–62.
8. Byrd JWT. Operative hip arthroscopy. 2nd ed. New York: Springer; 2005. p. 43.
9. Larson CM, Pierce BR, Giveans MR. Treatment of athletes with symptomatic intra-articular hip pathology and athletic pubalgia/sports hernia: a case series. Arthroscopy. 2011;27(6):768–75.
10. Larson CM, Giveans MR, Taylor M. Does arthroscopic correction improve function with radiographic arthritis? Clin Orthop Relat Res. 2010;468:555–64.
11. Czerny C, Hofmann S, Neuhold A, Tschauner C, Engel A, Recht MP, Kramer J. Lesions of the acetabular labrum: accuracy of MR imaging and MR arthrography in detection and staging. Radiology. 1996;200(1):225–30.
12. Keeney JA, Peell MW, Jackson J, Rubin D, Maloney WJ, Clohisy JC. Magnetic resonance arthrography versus arthroscopy in the evaluation of articular hip pathology. Clin Orthop Relat Res. 2004;429:163–9.
13. Byrd JWT, Jones KS. Diagnostic accuracy of clinical assessment, magnetic resonance imaging, magnetic resonance arthrography, intra-articular injection in hip arthroscopy patients. Am J Sports Med. 2004;32(7):1668–74.
14. Larson CM, Wulf CA. Intraoperative fluoroscopy for evaluation of bony resection during arthroscopic management of femoroacetabular impingement in the supine position. Arthroscopy. 2009;25:1183–92.
15. Steadman JR, Briggs KK, Rodrigo JJ, et al. Outcomes of microfracture for traumatic chondral defects of the knee: average 11-year follow-up. Arthroscopy. 2003;19:477–84.
16. Kelly BT, Williams 3rd RJ, Philippon MJ. Hip arthroscopy: current indications, treatment options, and management issues. Am J Sports Med. 2003;31:1020–37.
17. Hardy P, Hinojosa JF, Coudane H. Osteochondritis dissecans of the acetabulum. Apropos of a case. Rev Chir Orthop Reparatrice Appar Mot. 1992;78:134–7.
18. Roy DR. Arthroscopic findings of the hip in new onset hip pain in adolescents with previous Legg-Calve-Perthes disease. J Pediatr Orthop. 2005;14:151–5.
19. McCarthy J, Barsoum W, Puri L, et al. The role of hip arthroscopy in the elite athlete. Clin Orthop Relat Res. 2003;406:71–4.
20. Byrd JWT, Jones KS. Microfracture for grade IV chondral lesions of the hip (SS-89). Arthroscopy. 2004;20 Suppl 1:e41.
21. Philippon MJ, Schenker ML, Briggs KK, Maxwell RB. Can microfracture produce repair tissue in acetabular chondral defects? Arthroscopy. 2008;24:46–50.
22. Villar RN. Arthroscopic fibrin fixation of chondral lesions. In: Vail hip arthroscopy symposium, Vail; 17 Mar 2011.
23. Fontana A. Arthroscopic approach in hip defects. In: Zanasi S, Brittberg M, Marcacci M, editors. Basic science, clinical repair and reconstruction of articular cartilage defects: current status and prospects. Bologna: TIMEO Editore; 2006. p. 419–22.

Lesions of the Acetabular Fossa (Ligamentum Teres and Pulvinar)

15

G. Peter Maiers II

Introduction

The acetabular fossa has a cloverleaf shape with three lobes (anterior, superior, and posterior) present in all patients, but vary in prominence, that disrupt the inner edge of the lunate surface of the acetabulum [1] (see Fig. 15.1) (Video 15.1: http://goo.gl/ikSmq). The inferior aspect of the acetabular fossa is bordered by the transverse acetabular ligament, which arises from the periosteum of posterior-inferior acetabulum and attaches to the anterior inferior labrum [2]. This ligament divides acetabulum from the inferior capsular recess, and during weight bearing, it sees an increase in tension as the acetabulum expands in volume due to the natural incongruity of the joint [2]. The normal contents of the fossa include the ligamentum teres, a mobile fat pad in the lower portion, and dense fibroconnective tissue, which often anchors the fat pad to the superior aspect of the acetabular fossa (see Fig. 15.1). In addition to the normal contents of the acetabular fossa, loose bodies and synovial disease such as focal or diffuse pigmented villonodular synovitis can be identified in the acetabular fossa. Tears of the ligamentum teres, fibrosis of the fibroconnective tissue, plicae (1), and synovitis of the fat pad have all been seen and are thought to contribute to pain coming from the hip joint.

Ligamentum Teres: Anatomy and Physiology

The ligamentum teres is a collagenous structure that originates from the transverse acetabular ligament and inserts into the fovea on the femoral head, slightly posterior and inferior to

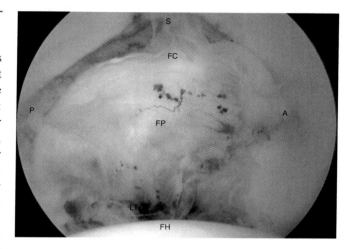

Fig. 15.1 The acetabular fossa of a right hip viewed with a 70-degree arthroscope from the anterior portal. The superior (*S*) and posterior (*P*) lobes are well visualized; the anterior lobe (*A*) is obscured by some of the fatty tissue of the pulvinar. *FP* the mobile fat pad of the acetabular fossa, *FC* fibroconnective tissue which anchors the fat pad to the superior aspect of the fossa, *LT* ligamentum teres, just the midportion of the ligamentum is seen from this view

the center [3, 4]. It is composed of types I, III, and V collagen and is triangular in structure (11). The medial epiphyseal artery is a continuation of the artery of the ligamentum teres, which is a branch of the posterior division of the obturator artery [3, 5, 6]. The medial epiphyseal artery plays an important role in blood supply of the capital femoral epiphysis, providing up to 80% of the blood supply of the femoral head in children [5]. In the skeletally mature hip, this artery often provides negligible blood flow to the femoral head [6].

Other than the role the artery of the ligamentum teres plays in children, the function of the ligamentum itself is relatively unknown. In cadaveric studies, the ligament becomes taught in adduction, flexion, and external rotation, and arthroscopically, the ligamentum is seen to tighten in external rotation and relax in internal rotation [3]. This suggests that the ligament can be damaged in extremes of adduction and external rotation. This conflicts with many

G.P. Maiers II, M.D.
Methodist Sports Medicine – The Orthopedic Specialists,
Indianapolis, IN, USA

Department of Orthopaedic Surgery, Indiana University,
201 N. Pennsylvania PKWY, Suite 100, Indianapolis, IN 46032, USA
e-mail: pmaiers@methodistsports.com

J.W.T. Byrd (ed.), *Operative Hip Arthroscopy*,
DOI 10.1007/978-1-4419-7925-4_15, © Springer Science+Business Media New York 2013

197

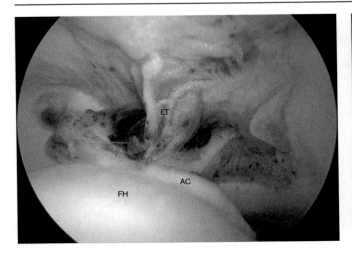

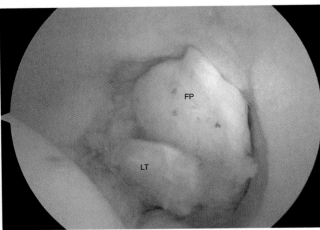

Fig. 15.2 A type I ligamentum teres tear, occurred as a result of a hyperabduction injury. The ligamentum *LT* is seen scarred into the acetabular fossa, and the avulsed cartilage *AC* demonstrates the location on the femoral head *FH* where ligamentum originally attached

Fig. 15.3 This is a 19-year-old elite ballerina with a 6-month history of popping and catching in her hip. The partially torn (type II) ligamentum teres *LT* is seen as well as fibrotic pulvinar tissue *FP*

clinical reports of injury to the ligamentum teres secondary to a traumatic hyperabduction injury [3, 7, 8]. One porcine study examined the mechanical properties of the ligamentum teres and found the load to failure of the ligamentum teres to be similar to that of the human anterior cruciate ligament [9]. Beck and colleagues excised the ligamentum teres in 18 patients undergoing open hip surgery and performed histologic analyses of the excised tissue. They found free nerve endings (type IVa) in all 18 ligamenta. Based on these findings, they concluded that the ligamentum teres may play a role in proprioception and joint protection by limiting excessive motion that may be harmful to the joint [10].

Tearing of the ligamentum teres has been described by several authors [3, 4, 7, 11–15]. Gray and Villar [15] have classified ligamentum teres tears into three types, based on arthroscopic findings. Type 1 is a complete tear and often a result of major trauma (see Fig. 15.2). Five of the seven patients in their series had significant hip trauma, and the other two patients had a history of hip dysplasia. Type 2 tears are partial tears of the ligamentum and were not associated with trauma (see Fig. 15.3). These patients typically reported a long history of hip pain and multiple prior tests to evaluate the source of their hip pain. Type 3 tears are degenerative tears (see Fig. 15.4). All patients with type 3 tears had significant osteoarthritis, and patients in this group frequently had other comorbid conditions of their hip including Perthes disease, developmental dysplasia, and slipped capital femoral epiphysis. The pattern of degeneration of the ligamentum teres is similar to that of tendons beginning with mucoid degeneration and progressing to fatty infiltration and fibromatous degeneration. Degenerative tearing of the ligamentum teres appears to be related to excessive loading with focal hypoxia and impaired

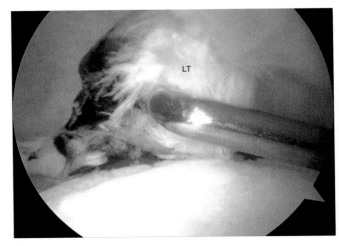

Fig. 15.4 A type III ligamentum teres tear in a patient with mild osteoarthritis

metabolic activity, which leads to collagen damage. Tearing and degeneration of the ligamentum teres can be detected by MR arthrogram; however, this is a diagnosis typically made at the time of surgery [16].

Ligamentum Teres Tear: Clinical Presentation

Patients with traumatic rupture of the ligamentum teres most frequently present with mechanical symptoms including catching, popping, and locking and occasionally limitation of motion [4, 7, 17]. Delcamp and colleagues reported on two patients with tears of the ligamentum teres as a result of forceful wide abduction of the hip without hip dislocation.

Both of these patients presented with hip pain, limited motion, and an antalgic gait. They were both found to have avulsions of the ligamentum teres from the fovea with large bony fragments attached to the torn ligament. Byrd reported on 23 patients with a traumatic tear of the ligamentum teres, all patients reported pain deep in the groin, and the majority of these patients (19 of 23) had mechanical-type symptoms [4]. All patients experienced pain with maximal flexion and internal rotation, and 15 of the 23 had pain with log rolling of the hip [4]. Pain that is elicited with log rolling of the hip and with flexion and internal rotation is very sensitive for detecting pathology related to the hip joint, but is not specific for detecting tears of ligamentum teres. Eight of the patients had an isolated injury, while in 15 of the 23 patients, there were other intra-articular findings at the time of arthroscopy. It is not uncommon for patients with a tear of the ligamentum teres to go undiagnosed for long periods of time prior to treatment [4, 7]. Kusma and colleagues reported on a horse rider with a history of several episodes of minor traumatic hyperabduction injuries who presented with limited motion, pain, and locking in the hip for 2 years. At the time of surgery, she was found to have a torn ligamentum teres and several osteochondral fragments adherent to the femoral attachment of the ligament. She was successfully treated with arthroscopic excision of the bony fragments and the torn portion of the ligament [7].

Elongation and hypertrophy of the ligamentum teres has been reported in patients with hip dysplasia 14. In one study [13], ligamentum teres tear was the third most common finding among patients with dysplasia treated arthroscopically. Treatment of a torn ligamentum teres or removal of loose bodies resulted in the most favorable outcomes in patients with hip dysplasia undergoing arthroscopy. In a study of patients with a history of Legg-Calve-Perthes disease treated with arthroscopic hip surgery, a torn ligamentum teres was the most common arthroscopic finding [18]. They were treated with debridement, and the average pain-free interval after debridement was 5 years.

Degenerative rupture of the ligamentum teres has been associated with acute onset of pain. In a case report, Yamamoto reported on a 78-year-old female with moderate degenerative disease who presented with an acute onset of lumbar and gluteal pain and limited external rotation [12]. A MRI demonstrated a thickened ligamentum teres compared to the contralateral side, and she obtained complete temporary relief of her symptoms with an intra-articular injection. At the time of arthroscopy, a ruptured degenerative ligament was found to be trapped in the posterior joint space. Following debridement, the patient's symptoms returned to her previous level, and her loss of external rotation resolved. Traumatic tears of the ligamentum teres do have the capacity to heal. Schaumkel and Villar report on two patients a structure that resembled an intact ligamentum teres when

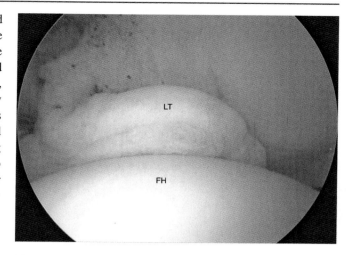

Fig. 15.5 A normal ligamentum teres *LT* inserting on the femoral head *FH* viewed with the 70-degree arthroscope from the anterior portal

they underwent arthroscopic surgery several years after a documented hip dislocation for treatment of labral and chondral damage [19].

In summary, tears of the ligamentum teres can be difficult to diagnose as there is not a specific physical exam finding or diagnostic test that is reliable in detecting a tear of the ligamentum teres. The author recommends a high clinical suspicion for patients with mechanical symptoms related to the hip joint following a traumatic injury and in patients with either congenital or acquired deformities of the hip joint (DDH, Perthes). Liberal use of diagnostic injections with long-acting local anesthetic can be very useful in isolating the hip joint as the source pathology.

Treatment of Ligamentum Teres Tears

Several authors have described successful treatment of pathology of the ligamentum teres [3, 4, 7, 8, 12–15] (Video 15.2: http://goo.gl/O39Bn). The femoral attachment of ligamentum teres is best visualized with the 70-degree arthroscope in either the anterior or the anterolateral portal (see Fig. 15.5), and the acetabular attachment is best visualized with the 30-degree arthroscope in the anterolateral portal (see Fig. 15.6). Selective debridement of the torn aspect of the femoral attachment and midsubstance of the ligament is most effectively accomplished with instruments placed through a direct anterior portal. Curved and flexible instruments can be useful in working around the femoral head (see Fig. 15.7). Debridement of the acetabular attachment is best accessed by placing instruments through the posterolateral portal, as the attachment site is along the posterior-inferior aspect of the acetabulum.

In a relatively large series of debridement of the ligamentum teres, the preoperative modified Harris Hip Score improved from 47 to 90 postoperatively, with 22 of 23

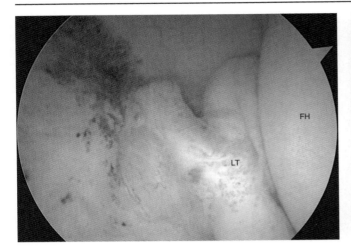

Fig. 15.6 A normal ligamentum teres *LT* viewed from the anterolateral portal with the 30-degree arthroscope. Note the acetabular attachment is well visualized, and the actual attachment site on the femoral head *FH* is not clearly identified

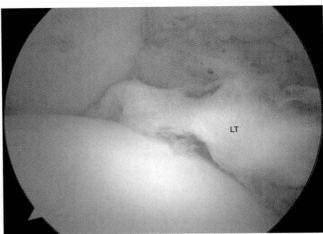

Fig. 15.8 The left hip of a 21-year-old collegiate gymnast found to have a frayed ligamentum teres *LT* viewed from the anterior portal with the 70-degree arthroscope

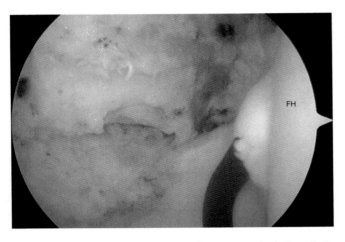

Fig. 15.7 Here, a flexible curved radiofrequency probe is brought in from the posterolateral portal to debride the loose ligamentum fibers and a chondral flap from the fovea capitis in a patient with a complete ligamentum teres tear

experiencing greater than a 20-point improvement [4]. In a study on 44 athletes treated with hip arthroscopy, 11 patients were found to have a torn ligamentum teres [14]. Those with damage to the ligamentum teres, loose bodies, and impinging osteophytes had the best results. Similarly, in patients with hip dysplasia tears treated with arthroscopy, those with ligamentum teres tears and loose bodies had better outcomes than patients with other findings [13].

Simpson, Fields, and Villar presented a case of a reconstruction of the ligamentum teres utilizing a LARS ligament [20]. The patient had prior surgery with debridement of a complete ligamentum teres tear and continued to have pain and instability. The femoral tunnel was positioned with the exit point in the center of the fovea, and the position of the acetabular tunnel was positioned in the posteroinferior aspect of the cotyloid fossa. The graft was secured on the acetabular side with an endobutton and with an interference screw on the femoral side. At 8-month follow-up, the knocking feeling she had been experiencing prior to surgery had resolved and her Non-Arthritic Hip Score was 89. The indications for this procedure have yet to be defined, but this procedure has shown to be beneficial in very carefully selected patients.

Case Presentation: Ligamentum Teres Tear

A 21-year-old collegiate gymnast presents with greater than a 1-year history of left groin pain. Two months prior to her presenting to our center, her symptoms of catching and popping had increased significantly to the point where she was no longer able to compete in, or practice gymnastics. On physical exam, she has pain in the groin with flexion and internal rotation as well as with external rotation. She has symmetric range of motion compared to her right hip. Her radiographs as well as her MRI scan are unremarkable; however, she did respond well to an intra-articular injection of ropivacaine. At the time of surgery, she was found to have a partially torn ligamentum teres (see Fig. 15.8) which was debrided with a curved shaver and a flexible radiofrequency probe (see Fig. 15.9) (Video 15.3: http://goo.gl/3M3iF). At 2 months following surgery, she was able to participate in gymnastics with only mild hip soreness, and at 1-year follow-up, she was still active in gymnastics and had no complaints with regard to her hip.

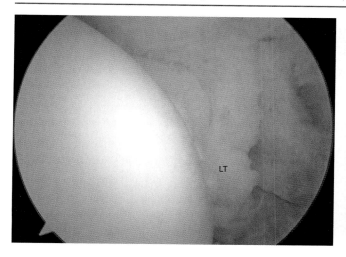

Fig. 15.9 The ligamentum has been selectively debrided leaving the remaining healthy tissue intact. The remaining ligamentum *LT* is visualized here from the anterolateral portal with a 30-degree arthroscope

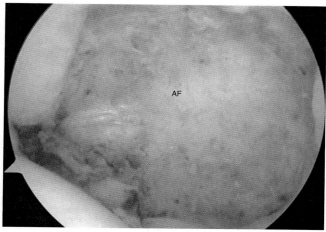

Fig. 15.11 Following debridement of the inflamed pulvinar, the acetabular fossa *AF* has been decompressed

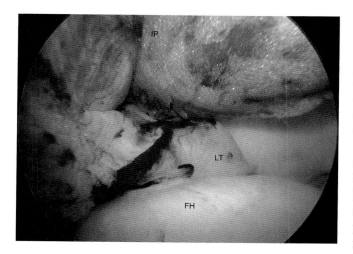

Fig. 15.10 An inflamed pulvinar *IP* is identified in a 52-year-old female with an 8-month history of left hip pain and inability to sleep

Other Lesions of the Acetabular Fossa

Much like the fat pad in the knee, the fatty tissue of the acetabular fossa (pulvinar) can become inflamed and irritated (see Fig. 15.10). In the author's experience, patients with this disorder often have a long history of symptoms related to the hip joint and minimal, if any, findings on diagnostic testing. These patients typically experience pain with provocative testing of the hip joint such as log rolling or flexion and internal rotation, and they usually have a positive response to an intra-articular injection of local anesthetic. Fibrosis of the pulvinar rarely if ever is a diagnosis made prior to surgery; rather, it is an intra-operative finding in many patients who have had a long history

of hip pain that has not responded well to conservative treatment. Irritation of the pulvinar tissue often coexists with other intra-articular pathology. Although occasionally, a patient will present with pain that is localized to the hip joint, but no obvious source can be identified. At the time of surgery, if irritation of the fibro-fatty tissue of the acetabular fossa is identified, selective debridement can provide significant and often sudden relief of the patient's symptoms (see Fig. 15.11).

Katz and colleagues reported on two cases of symptomatic hip plicae that were identified on MR arthrogram [21]. Both cases were adolescent females who had a prominent band medial to the ligamentum teres identified by MR arthrography and at the time of surgery. Both patients had a positive response to an intra-articular injection. There were no other intraoperative findings, and they were treated with arthroscopic resection of the prominent band; both patients experienced good relief of their symptoms. Pathology revealed synovial and fibroconnective tissue that was similar to a plica in the knee.

Loose bodies often accumulate in the acetabular fossa after trauma to the hip or in association with synovial disorders such as synovial chondromatosis [20]. Arthroscopic removal of these loose bodies can often provide symptomatic relief. When several loose bodies are present such as with synovial chondromatosis (see Fig. 15.12), utilizing a large cannula connected to suction tubing positioned in the posterolateral portal can facilitate removal. Similarly, use of a large diameter shaver will prevent frequent clogging of the shaver and allow the surgeon to make efficient use of their traction time. While it is sometimes impossible to remove all loose bodies from the acetabular fossa arthroscopically, the arthroscopic approach can provide significant symptomatic relief with less morbidity and a quicker recovery than an open approach.

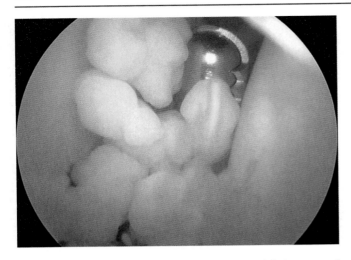

Fig. 15.12 Loose bodies from synovial chondromatosis being removed from the acetabular fossa with a large diameter shaver introduced from the posterolateral portal

Summary

The acetabular fossa can be a source of significant pathology in the hip joint. Ligamentum teres tears can occur either acutely, often as a result of a hyperabduction injury, or insidiously. Patients with ligamentum teres tears often have mechanical symptoms of catching, locking, and popping. Successful treatment of ligamentum teres tears has been reported with selective debridement alone. Reconstruction of the ligamentum teres has been reported, but the indications for this procedure are still evolving. Other lesions of the acetabular fossa include fibrosis of the pulvinar fat pad, plica, and loose bodies. All of these conditions can be successfully treated with arthroscopic surgery. Often, disorders of the acetabular fossa are not able to be diagnosed prior to surgery. A comprehensive history and physical exam that are suggestive of disorders of the hip joint, a high index of suspicion, and liberal use of diagnostic injections will help identify appropriate surgical candidates. At the time of surgery, a thorough diagnostic arthroscopy with the use of both the 30- and 70-degree arthroscopes will allow the surgeon to appropriately identify and treat pathology of the acetabular fossa.

References

1. Rissech C, Sañudo JR, Malgosa A. The acetabular point: a morphological and ontogenetic study. J Anat. 2001;198:743–8.

2. Lohe F, Eckstein F, Sauer T, Putz R. Structure, strain and function of the transverse acetabular ligament. Acta Anat. 1996;157:315–23.

3. Rao J, Zhou YX, Villar RN. Injury to the ligamentum teres: mechanisms, findings, and results of treatment. Clin Sports Med. 2001;20:791–800.

4. Byrd JWT, Jones KS. Traumatic rupture of the ligamentum teres as a source of hip pain. Arthroscopy. 2004;20:385–91.

5. Trueta J. The normal vascular anatomy of the human femoral head during growth. J Bone Joint Surg Br. 1957;39B:358–94.

6. Trueta J, Harrison MH. The normal vascular anatomy of the femoral head in adult man. J Bone Joint Surg Br. 1953;35B:442–61.

7. Kusma M, Jung J, Dienst M, Goedde S, Kohn D, Seil R. Arthroscopic treatment of an avulsion fracture of the ligamentum teres of the hip in an 18-year-old horse rider. Arthroscopy. 2004;20:64–6.

8. Kashiwagi N, Suzuki S, Seto Y. Arthroscopic treatment for traumatic hip dislocation with avulsion fracture of the ligamentum teres. Arthroscopy. 2001;17:67–9.

9. Wenger D, Miyanji F, Mahar A, Oka R. The mechanical properties of the ligamentum teres: a pilot study to assess its potential for improving stability in children's hip surgery. Pediatr Orthop. 2007;27:408–10.

10. Leunig M, Beck M, Stauffer E, Hertel R, Ganz R. Free nerve endings in the ligamentum capitis femoris. Acta Orthop Scand. 2000;71:452–4.

11. Tibor LM, Sekiya JK. Differential diagnosis of pain around the hip joint. Arthroscopy. 2008;24:1407–21.

12. Yamamoto Y, Usui I. Arthroscopic surgery for degenerative rupture of the ligamentum teres femoris. Arthroscopy. 2006;22:689.e1–e3.

13. Byrd JWT, Jones KS. Hip arthroscopy in the presence of dysplasia. Arthroscopy. 2003;19:1055–60.

14. Byrd JWT, Jones KS. Hip arthroscopy in athletes. Clin Sports Med. 2001;4:749–61.

15. Gray AJR, Villar RN. The ligamentum teres of the hip: an arthroscopic classification of its pathology. Arthroscopy. 1997;13:575–8.

16. Sampatchalit S, Barbosa D, Gentili A, Haghighi P, Trudell D, Resnick D. Degenerative changes in the ligamentum teres of the hip: cadaveric study with magnetic resonance arthrography, anatomical inspection, and histologic examination. Comput Assist Tomogr. 2009;33:927–33.

17. Delcamp DD, Klaaren HE, Pompe van Meerdervoort HF. Traumatic avulsion of the ligamentum teres without dislocation of the hip. Two case reports. J Bone Joint Surg Am. 1988;70:933–5.

18. Roy DR. Arthroscopic findings of the hip in new onset hip pain in adolescents with previous Legg-Calvé-Perthes disease. J Pediatr Orthop. 2005;14:151–5.

19. Schaumkel JV, Villar RN. Healing of the ruptured ligamentum teres after hip dislocation – an arthroscopic finding. Hip Int. 2009;19:64–6.

20. Simpson JM, Field RE, Villar RN. Arthroscopic reconstruction of the ligamentum teres. Arthroscopy. 2011;27:436–41.

21. Katz LD, Haims A, Medvecky M, McCallum J. Symptomatic hip plica: MR arthrographic and arthroscopic correlation. Skeletal Radiol. 2010;39:1255–8.

Synovial Disease and Sepsis

16

J.W. Thomas Byrd

Introduction

There is a paucity of scientific literature on the role of arthroscopy for synovial-based disorders of the hip with only two review articles on the subject [1, 2]. Generally, the indications for arthroscopic synovectomy in the hip are comparable to those reported for other joints. It is difficult to state that a complete synovectomy can be performed arthroscopically, but with meticulous techniques of the central and peripheral compartments, a sufficiently thorough synovectomy can be performed to warrant the advantage of a much less-invasive procedure. Synovial disorders of the hip may also extend into the iliopsoas bursa because of a common communication, sometimes necessitating concomitant iliopsoas bursoscopy.

Hajdu developed a classification system for soft tissue tumors based on the tissue of origin [3]. Tumors of tendosynovial tissue seem to have the greatest predilection for the hip and include synovial chondromatosis and pigmented villonodular synovitis.

This is consistent with our observations as the two most common disorders that we have treated are synovial chondromatosis ($n=38$) and pigmented villonodular synovitis ($n=13$). Additionally, we have treated a number of PVNS-like cases ($n=4$) characterized by patients with all of the clinical, imaging, and arthroscopic findings of PVNS yet lacking histologic confirmation because of absence of giant cells on histology. Rarely has arthroscopy been performed for inflammatory arthritides, the most common of which would be rheumatoid disease. As with other joints, improved pharmacological management has eliminated the need for most surgical synovectomies.

Nonspecific synovial metaplasia is often observed within the acetabular fossa in conjunction with other damage to the joint. The pulvinar tissue (fat pad lined by synovium) within the fossa is the "canary in the coal mine" among various hip disorders. This tissue demonstrates some type of reaction in conjunction with most any other hip pathology.

Chondrocalcinosis is a metabolic problem, not a synovial-based disorder. However, it is included in this chapter because of its common inflammatory component.

Synovial Chondromatosis

(See Video 16.1: http://goo.gl/EUAwj). The correct term is synovial chondromatosis (Figs. 16.1, 16.2, and 16.3). Synovial osteochondromatosis implies ossification of the loose bodies, which does not always occur and is partly responsible for why such an obvious disease is not always so evident on preliminary evaluation. McCarthy reported that half of the cases were unrecognized prior to arthroscopy [4]. While this number may be high with the current quality of imaging, the diagnosis may still not be obvious. An MRI will reveal synovial disease, but it may appear nonspecific. The synovial disorder may not be evident at all when intra-articular contrast has been used, and close attention must be given to look for the loose bodies, which sometimes measure only a few millimeters.

We have seen a number of cases of classic femoroacetabular impingement compounded by the presence of synovial chondromatosis. With the obvious impingement as an explanation for problems, closer scrutiny for the synovial disorder may be lacking. The clinical assessment will provide obvious clues. Patients with protracted synovial chondromatosis tend to be very painful, even with inactivity and painful with range of motion of the hip in all planes. This is in contrast to the more specific findings typically associated with simple impingement.

The hip is surpassed only by the knee and elbow as the site of involvement of synovial chondromatosis [5, 6]. Milgram described three phases of synovial chondromatosis based on a temporal sequence [7]. During phase I, the synovial disease is active, but no loose bodies are yet present. The second phase is transition, in which there is active synovial proliferation and loose bodies are present. In the third

J.W.T. Byrd, M.D.
Nashville Sports Medicine Foundation,
2011 Church Street, Suite 100, Nashville, TN 37203, USA
e-mail: byrd@nsmfoundation.org

J.W.T. Byrd (ed.), *Operative Hip Arthroscopy*,
DOI 10.1007/978-1-4419-7925-4_16, © Springer Science+Business Media New York 2013

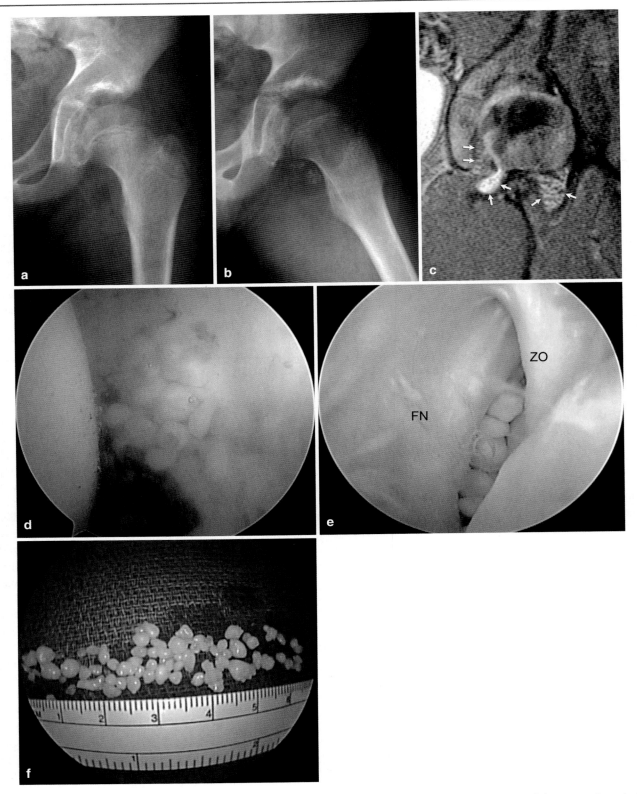

Fig. 16.1 A 10-year-old male with a two-year history of left hip pain. (**a** and **b**) AP and lateral radiographs reveal numerous densities consistent with synovial chondromatosis. (**c**) Coronal MRI reveals more numerous filling defects (*arrows*) indicative of ossified and non-ossified loose bodies. (**d**) Arthroscopic view of the central compartment reveals clusters of loose bodies. (**e**) Viewing the periphery, more loose bodies are embedded posterior to the femoral neck (*FN*) underneath the zona orbicularis (*ZO*). (**f**) Most were debrided with a shaver, but loose bodies expressed through the cannula are illustrated. (All rights are retained by Dr. Byrd)

Fig. 16.2 A 48-year-old male presented for evaluation of chronic left knee pain. Examination revealed his knee symptoms to be referred from his hip. (**a** and **b**) AP and lateral radiographs reveal evidence of synovial chondromatosis. (**c**) Loose bodies are further evident on CT scan with 3D reconstruction. (**d**) A digital subtraction image reveals significant cam morphology. (**e**) Viewing from the central compartment, loose bodies are identified (*asterisks*). (**f**) Viewing peripherally, the loose bodies were large (*asterisks*) and required removal with hand instruments. (**g**) Femoroplasty has been completed. (**h**) Some of the removed fragments are shown. (All rights are retained by Dr. Byrd)

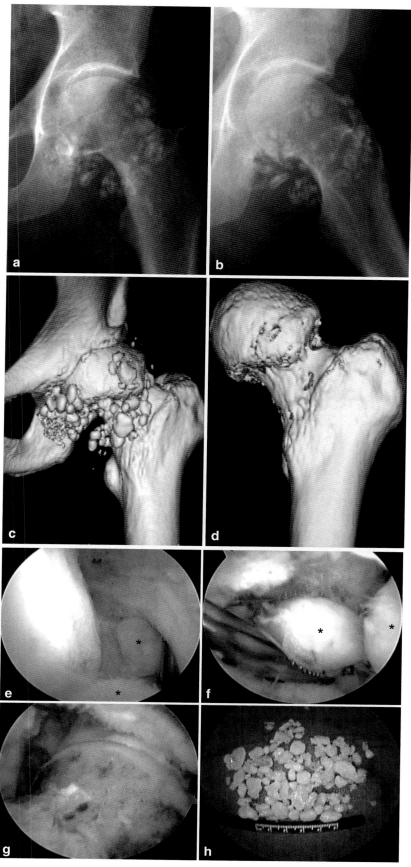

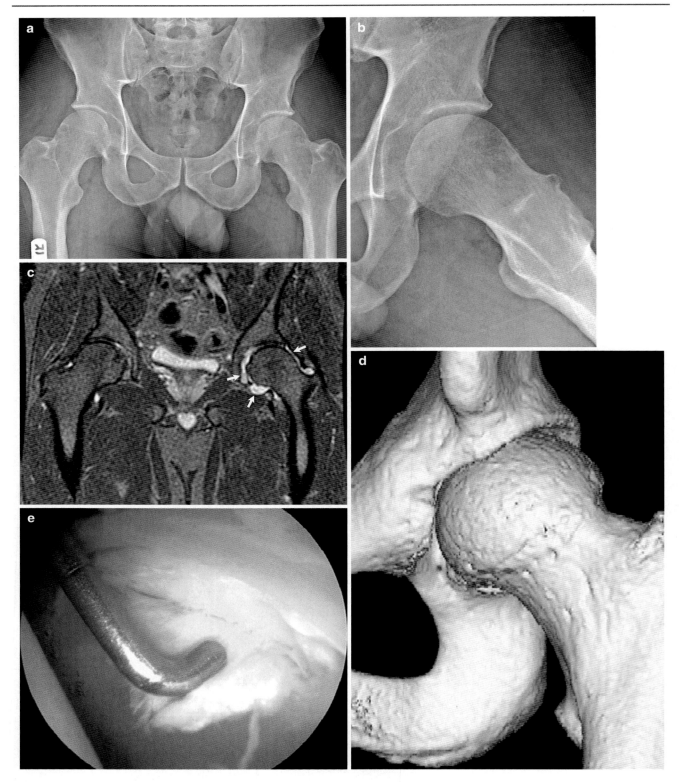

Fig. 16.3 A 36-year-old male miner with a 10-month history of left hip pain following a squatting injury. (**a**) AP pelvis reveals cam morphology with a herniation pit bilaterally and dysplasia with a CE angle of 19 on the left. (**b**) Lateral radiograph reveals loss of normal anterior femoral offset. (**c**) Coronal T2-weighted large-field-of-view MRI reveals a left hip effusion. (**d**) 3D CT scan reveals findings consistent with cam impingement and borderline dysplasia. (**e**) Arthroscopy reveals articular delamination of the anterior acetabulum being probed consistent with pathological cam impingement. (**f**) Loose bodies (*asterisks*) are identified within the acetabular fossa. (**g**) The fossa has been cleared. (**h**) Loose bodies (*asterisks*) are identified in the periphery. (**i**) After loose body removal, the cam lesion is identified (*asterisk*). (**j**) The cam lesion has been corrected. (**k**) Some of the removed debris is illustrated. (All rights are retained by Dr. Byrd)

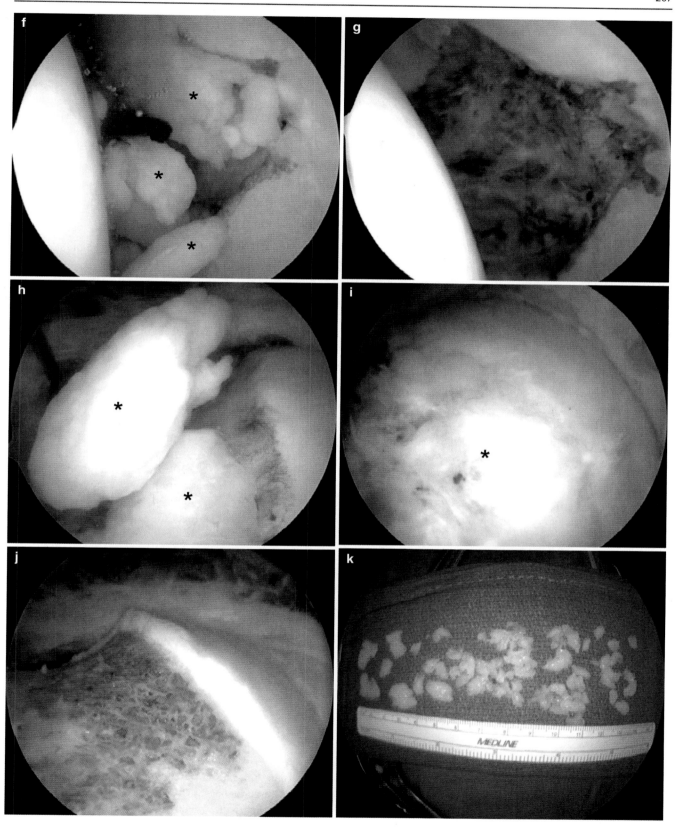

Fig. 16.3 (continued)

phase, the synovium becomes quiescent with no demonstrable disease, but the loose bodies remain. Because of the insidious nature of the disease, by the time symptoms become significant enough to incite diagnosis and surgical intervention, the synovial process has long since receded, leaving behind only the loose bodies to create symptoms. Thus, the histologic diagnosis is often in limbo unless synovium can be identified actively producing loose bodies. Recurrence of disease is possible, but recurrence of symptoms following arthroscopy is usually more accurately the result of residual disease, because it can be difficult to ensure that an absolutely thorough debridement has been performed.

Boyer and Dorfmann have reported the largest series of synovial chondromatosis treated by arthroscopy with 120 cases [8]. Twenty-three patients required repeat arthroscopy while 42 went on to open surgery and another 22 had gone on to total hip replacement. Many of these patients were treated with arthroscopy only of the peripheral compartment without traction. Current techniques would routinely incorporate traction to address the central (intra-articular) compartment as well as the periphery for more thorough management.

In our experience, we have had a 20% reoperation rate, but repeat arthroscopy can still result in successful outcomes. More than one-third of our patients had concomitant findings of FAI.

Pigmented Villonodular Synovitis

(See Video 16.2: http://goo.gl/Tp8j0) Pigmented villonodular synovitis (PVNS) has been described as having a nodular and a diffuse pattern [9] (Figs. 16.4 and 16.5). The hip is the second most frequent site of involvement with both patterns having been encountered [6, 10].

Synovectomy is the recommended treatment. Many of these patients have significant secondary joint destruction due to the disease by the time the diagnosis is made. Thus, the less-invasive nature of the arthroscopic approach can be especially appealing in this group. In our experience, the diagnosis was established preoperatively in less than half of these patients. Arthroscopic synovectomy can result in good to excellent outcomes and allows treatment of the secondary damage to the joint as well. Almost one-third had accompanying FAI. In these cases, the primary synovial disease may be overlooked on imaging studies and misinterpreted as simply a secondary synovitis.

Treatment may be as simple as removing a single or multiple nodules, or may require more extensive synovectomy of the central and peripheral compartments and possibly iliopsoas bursa in diffuse patterns. Our results have been comparable with both nodular and diffuse types, with none requiring further surgery for recurrent synovial disease. The future outlook is often dictated by the severity of secondary damage present at the time of the index arthroscopic procedure.

Thus, it is possible that some may still be facing the prospect of a future arthroplasty even with successful management of the synovial disease.

Intra-articular radioisotope injection has been described as an ionizing method of synovectomy [11, 12]. However, there is little information on its application in the hip and the success is limited. Perhaps it might be considered as adjuvant therapy with arthroscopic synovectomy, but its role is not yet defined, and thus far, we have found satisfactory results with arthroscopy alone.

Nonspecific Inflammatory Disorders of the Pulvinar

(See Video 16.3: http://goo.gl/GoU98) The pulvinar tissue has been reported as an important trigger of joint pain with a substantial pattern of nociceptive innervation [13]. It undergoes significant upregulation of these neurons in painful conditions such as osteoarthritis. We have observed that lesions in this area can be quite painful and may represent the neural equivalent of the fat pad in the knee as described by Scott Dye's neural mapping.

Metaplasia of this synovial tissue can occasionally be a primary pain generator in the hip and frequently occurs in association with numerous types of joint pathology [14]. These metaplastic changes are variable and may be characterized as typical villous synovitis, fibrous hyperplasia, or dense contracted fibrosis. As stated in the opening comments, the pulvinar tissue is the canary in the coal mine for the hip and reacts with almost any joint problem.

Primary synovial lesions in this area can be quite painful and respond very well to debridement. Thus, our tendency is to remove the abnormal tissue when present in conjunction with other disorders. It is important to preserve the ligamentum teres, if it is intact, and avoid unnecessarily violating this structure. Also, for some hips, if access to the fossa is difficult, then the surgeon should not risk damaging the joint surfaces in an effort to remove the diseased tissue. For aggressive synovial disorders such as PVNS, thermal ablation can be performed with a flexible radio frequency device.

Chondrocalcinosis

(See Video 16.4: http://goo.gl/axPvB) Chondrocalcinosis is most commonly caused by calcium pyrophosphate deposition (CPPD or pseudogout) [15] (Fig. 16.6). Gout typically attacks peripheral joints with lower temperature that promotes precipitation of calcium urate crystals and would be very uncommon in the hip [16]. In fact, there is only one reported case of monoarticular gouty arthritis of the hip [17].

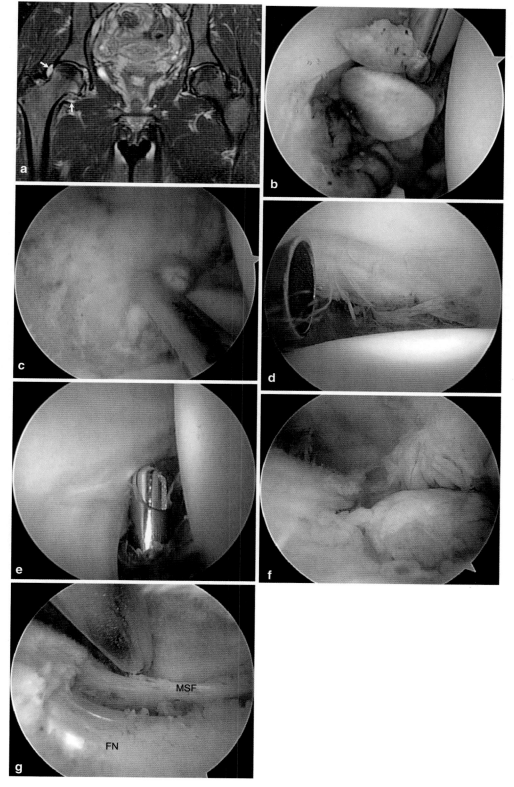

Fig. 16.4 A 23-year-old female with a two-year history of right hip pain. Radiographs were unrevealing. (**a**) Large-field-of-view T2-weighted coronal image demonstrates a right hip effusion (*arrows*). (**b**) Looking medially, synovial disease consistent with a diffuse pattern of pigmented villonodular synovitis is identified within the acetabular fossa. Debridement is begun with the shaver from the anterior portal. (**c**) Synovectomy of the fossa is completed with the shaver from the posterolateral portal. (**d**) Looking posteriorly, further synovial disease is evident behind the labrum. (**e**) Synovectomy of the posterior capsule is accomplished from the posterolateral portal. (**f**) Now viewing in the periphery, the normal anatomy is obscured by synovial disease. (**g**) The same view after synovectomy reveals the anterior neck of the femur (*FN*) and medial synovial fold (*MSF*). (All rights are retained by Dr. Byrd)

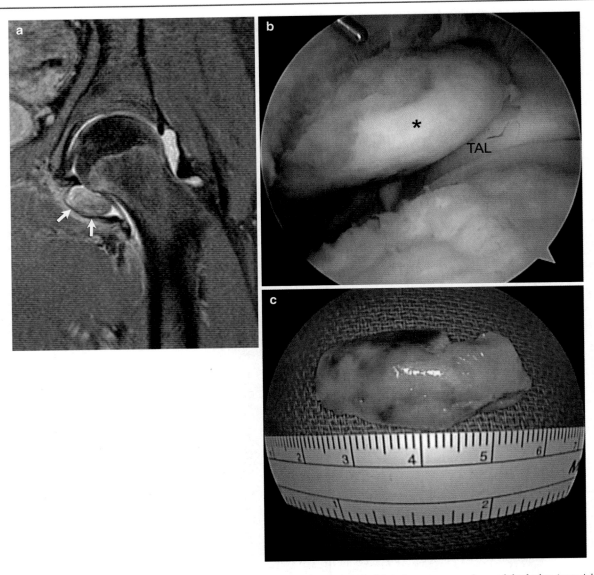

Fig. 16.5 A 14-year-old female dancer with a 3-month history of worsening left hip pain. Radiographs are unremarkable. (**a**) Coronal MRI reveals a nodular lesion (*arrows*) adjacent to the medial base of the femoral neck. (**b**) Arthroscopy reveals a nodular lesion (*asterisk*) underneath the transverse acetabular ligament (*TAL*). (**c**) The nodular PVNS lesion has been excised. (All rights are retained by Dr. Byrd)

Chondrocalcinosis is characterized by the crystallite material embedded within the hyaline cartilage and sometimes the labrum. This is different than amorphous globular calcific deposits that may develop within diseased labrum (Fig. 16.7). This occurs because the diseased labrum loses its inhibitory properties to prevent these deposits. This type of calcific deposition is more comparable to the pathophysiology of calcific deposits within a diseased rotator cuff.

Chondrocalcinosis in the hip is not as radiographically evident as it is in the knee, where the meniscus is often silhouetted by the depositions. The deposits alter the structural properties of the articular surface and labrum making them more susceptible breakdown. Treatment typically consists of addressing the damaged cartilage. Sometimes, superficial deposits can be swept off, but aggressive efforts to excise the embedded material are not necessary. In the knee, arthroscopic surgery in the presence of chondrocalcinosis is often followed by a stormy early postoperative course due to recurrent painful effusions. Fortunately, in the hip, only occasionally is this observation made. It is worthy to be aware of this scenario and warn patients so that they will be prepared in case the initial few days of recovery are difficult.

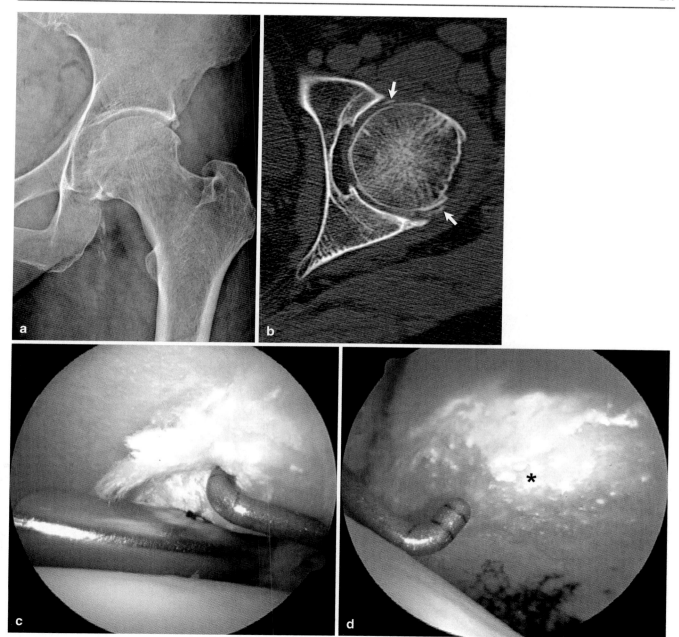

Fig. 16.6 A 59-year-old female with long-standing left hip pain. (**a**) AP radiograph of the left hip reveals some densities around the acetabulum. (**b**) Axial CT scan reveals evidence of calcification embedded within the articular surface. (**c**) Arthroscopy reveals calcific deposition is embedded within the substance of the degenerated labrum which is being probed. (**d**) A stippled pattern of calcific deposition within the articular surface of the acetabulum is revealed (*asterisk*). (All rights are retained by Dr. Byrd)

Sepsis

(See Video 16.5: http://goo.gl/7ze8I) A septic hip does not require a thorough synovectomy but simply needs prompt, thorough debridement and lavage (Fig. 16.8). There are several case series that report successful results with arthroscopic treatment of hip joint sepsis [18–22]. El-Sayed also published a prospective randomized level one study, reporting better results of arthroscopy over open methods in treating early septic arthritis among children [23]. It seems that arthroscopy would be an appropriate first line of surgical treatment for virtually any septic joint. Successful results

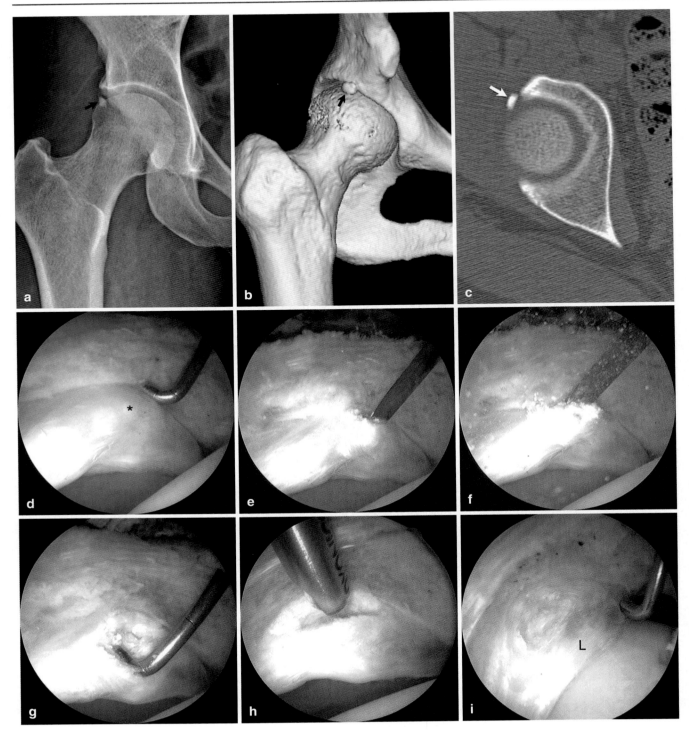

Fig. 16.7 A 41-year-old female with calcific deposition within the substance of the anterolateral labrum of her right hip. (**a**) AP radiograph reveals a small density (*arrow*). (**b**) 3D CT scan demonstrates the density geographically within the area of the anterolateral labrum (*arrow*). (**c**) Axial CT image reveals increased homogeneous density compared to bone, suggesting calcification instead of ossification (*arrow*). (**d**) Arthroscopic view from the anterolateral portal reveals the area of calcific deposition within the anterolateral labrum (*asterisk*). (**e**) An arthroscopic knife is being used to open the area of calcific deposit. (**f**) A slurry of calcific debris is expressed creating the snowfield appearance. (**g**) The pocket has been opened. (**h**) Debridement is completed with a shaver. (**i**) Viewing with the traction released, excision has been completed, preserving the structural integrity of the labrum (*L*). (All rights are retained by Dr. Byrd)

Fig. 16.8 A 59-year-old man with evidence of a septic hip. (**a**) AP radiograph is unremarkable. (**b**) Coronal MRI demonstrates a pronounced effusion (*white arrows*) and surrounding soft tissue edema (*black arrows*). (**c**) Arthroscopy revealed diffuse exudative material throughout the joint. (All rights are retained by Dr. Byrd)

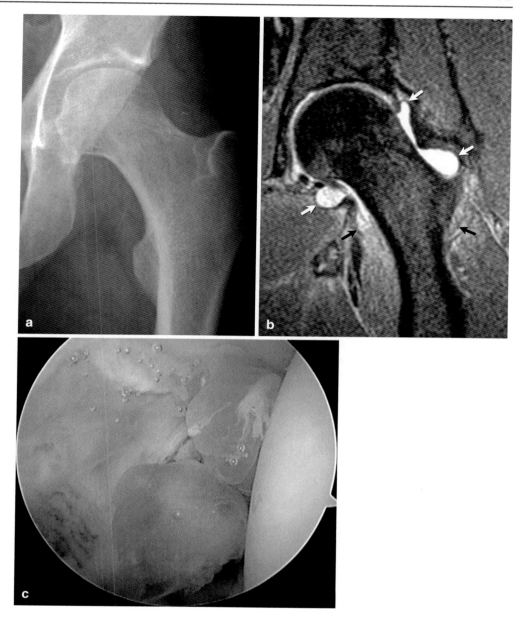

have also been reported in the arthroscopic treatment of infected total hip arthroplasties [24, 25]. This was first proposed for ill, medically compromised patients who would not tolerate a more extensive open procedure. However, it appears that arthroscopy would be appropriate for most infected total joints. McCarthy also found that occult infection, diagnosed by tissue biopsy at arthroscopy, turned out to be the source of pain following arthroplasty for a small group of patients with previous negative aspirates.

Summary

Arthroscopic synovectomy is appropriately indicated in the hip for a variety of conditions. Often, the secondary damage to the joint is significant and further emphasizes the advantage of a less-invasive arthroscopic approach for these patients who are often still facing a future arthroplasty. Arthroscopy is also appropriately indicated for many cases of hip joint sepsis.

References

1. Godde S, Kusma M, Dienst M. Synovial disorders and loose bodies in the hip joint. Arthroscopic diagnostics and treatment. Orthopade. 2006;35(1):67–76.
2. Krebs VE. The role of hip arthroscopy in the treatment of synovial disorders and loose bodies. Clin Orthop Relat Res. 2003;406:48–59.
3. Hajdu SI. Tumors of tendosynovial tissue. In: Hajdu SI, editor. Pathology of soft tissue tumors. Philadelphia: Lea & Febiger; 1979. p. 165–226.
4. McCarthy JC, Bono JV, Wardell S. Is there a treatment for synovial chondromatosis of the hip joint? Arthroscopy. 1997;13(3):409–10.
5. Villacin AB, Brigham LN, Bullough PG. Primary and secondary synovial chondrometaplasia. Hum Pathol. 1979;10(4):439–51.
6. Spjut JH, Dorfmann HD, Fechner RD, Ackerman LV, Firminger HI, editors. Tumors of bone and cartilage. In: Atlas of tumor pathology, second series. Washington, DC: Armed Forces Institute of Pathology; 1983. p. 391–410.
7. Milgram JW. Synovial osteochondromatosis. J Bone Joint Surg Br. 1977;59:792–801.
8. Boyer T, Dorfmann H. Arthroscopy in primary synovial chondromatosis of the hip: description and outcome of treatment. J Bone Joint Surg Br. 2008;90(3):314–8.
9. Enneking WF. Musculoskeletal tumor surgery. New York: Churchill Livingstone; 1983. p. 1167–74.
10. Danzig LA, Gershuni DH, Resnick D. Diagnosis and treatment of diffuse pigmented villonodular synovitis of the hip. Clin Orthop. 1982;168:42–77.
11. Shabat S, Kollender Y, Merimsky O. The use of surgery and yttrium 90 in the management of extensive and diffuse pigmented villonodular synovitis of large joints. Rheumatology. 2002;41:1113–8.
12. Zook JE, Wurtz DL, Cummings JE, et al. Intra-articular chromic phosphate (^{32}P) in the treatment of diffuse pigmented villonodular synovitis. Brachytherapy. 2011;10(3):190–4.
13. Saxler G, Loer F, Skumavc M, et al. Localization of SP- and CGRP-immunopositive nerve fibers in the hip joint of patients with painful osteoarthritis and of patients with painless failed total hip arthroplasties. Eur J Pain: Ejp. 2007;11(1):67–74.
14. Byrd JWT. Indications and contraindications. In: Byrd JWT, editor. Operative hip arthroscopy. 2nd ed. New York: Springer; 2005. p. 6–35.
15. Rosenthal AK. Update in calcium deposition diseases. Curr Opin Rheumatol. 2007;19:158–62.
16. Fitzgerald BT, Setty A, Mudgal CS. Gout affecting the hand and wrist. J Am Acad Orthop Surg. 2007;15:625–35.
17. Parhami N, Feng H. Gout in the hip joint. Arthritis Rheum. 1993;36(7):1026.
18. Blitzer CM. Arthroscopic management of septic arthritis of the hip. Arthroscopy. 1993;9(4):414–6.
19. Chung WK, Slater GL, Bates EH. Treatment of septic arthritis of the hip by arthroscopic lavage. J Pediatr Orthop. 1993;13:444–6.
20. Yamamoto Y, Ide T, Hachisuka N, et al. Arthroscopic surgery for septic arthritis of the hip joint in 4 adults. Arthroscopy. 2001;17(3):290–7.
21. Kim SJ, Choi NH, Ko SH, et al. Arthroscopic treatment of septic arthritis of the hip. Clin Orthop Relat Res. 2003;407:211–4.
22. Nusem I, Jabur MK, Playford EG. Arthroscopic treatment of septic arthritis of the hip. Arthroscopy. 2006;22(8):902.e1–3.
23. El-Sayed AMM. Treatment of early septic arthritis of the hip in children: comparison of results of open arthrotomy versus arthroscopic drainage. J Child Orthop. 2008;2(3):229–37.
24. Hyman JL, Salvati EA, Laurencin CT, Rogers DE, et al. The arthroscopic drainage, irrigation, and debridement of late, acute total hip arthroplasty infections: average 6-year follow-up. J Arthroplasty. 1999;14(8):903–10.
25. McCarthy JC, Jibodh SR, Lee JA. The role of arthroscopy in evaluation of painful hip arthroplasty. Clin Orthop Relat Res. 2009;467(1):174–80.

My Approach to Femoroacetabular Impingement

17

J.W. Thomas Byrd

Introduction

Impingement is not a new concept. As early as 1913, Vulpius and Stöffel described a bony resection procedure for the deformity created by a slipped capital femoral epiphysis [1]. In 1936, Smith-Petersen described an operation with excision of the acetabular rim sometimes combined with a wedge resection of the femoral head/neck junction for cases of protrusio, slipped epiphysis, and coxa plana [2]. Although primitive, the technique bears a striking similarity to the recent descriptions of open surgical dislocation for pincer and cam impingement. This combined approach received no further mention in the literature, but osteoplasty for the femoral deformity associated with chronic slipped capital femoral epiphysis was popularized by Heyman and Herndon and has similarly been described for the misshapen femoral head of coxa plana as a sequela of Perthes disease [3, 4].

However, it was Professor Ganz and colleagues who formulated the concept of femoroacetabular impingement (FAI). This was first described as an iatrogenic process associated with overcorrection of periacetabular osteotomy (PAO) performed for dysplasia [5]. Subsequently, they described FAI occurring in the native hip as a precursor to the development of osteoarthritis [6]. They subgrouped this into pincer, cam, and combined types and described an open surgical approach for correction [7]. Successful reports have been published with a goal of delaying the progression of osteoarthritis, but this has not been a technique advocated for the resumption of an active lifestyle [8].

It is our perspective that FAI is not a cause of hip pain. It is simply a morphologic variant that predisposes the joint to intra-articular pathology that then becomes symptomatic. Pincer impingement, caused by an overhanging of the anterolateral rim of the acetabulum, results primarily in breakdown of the acetabular labrum and secondarily, over time, a variable amount of associated articular damage to the acetabulum (Fig. 17.1). Cam impingement, created by the prominent portion of a nonspherical femoral head engaging against the articular surface of the acetabulum, results in selective delamination and failure of the articular surface of the acetabulum with relative preservation of the labrum (Fig. 17.2). These observations are important in the

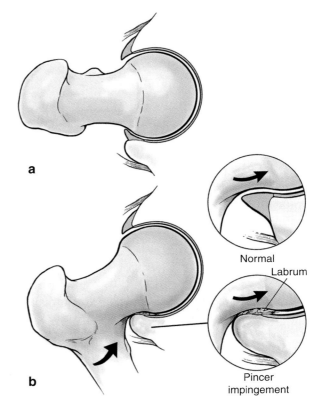

Fig. 17.1 (a) Bony over-coverage of the anterior labrum sets the stage for pincer impingement. (b) With hip flexion, the anterior labrum gets crushed by the pincer lesion against the neck of the femur. Secondary articular failure occurs over time. In the normal circumstance, there is adequate clearance for the labrum during hip flexion. (All rights are retained by Dr. Byrd)

J.W.T. Byrd, M.D.
Nashville Sports Medicine Foundation,
2011 Church Street, Suite 100, Nashville, TN 37203, USA
e-mail: byrd@nsmfoundation.org

J.W.T. Byrd (ed.), *Operative Hip Arthroscopy*,
DOI 10.1007/978-1-4419-7925-4_17, © Springer Science+Business Media New York 2013

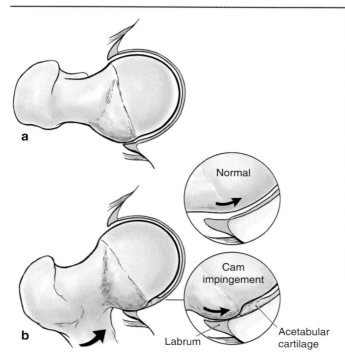

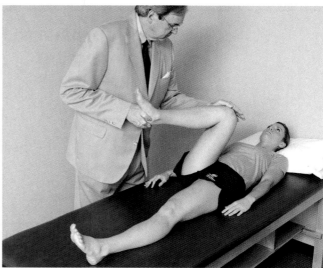

Fig. 17.3 The impingement test is performed by provoking pain with flexion, adduction, and internal rotation of the symptomatic hip. (All rights are retained by Dr. Byrd)

Fig. 17.2 (**a**) The cam lesion is characterized by the bony prominence centered on the anterolateral femoral head/neck junction. (**b**) Cam impingement occurs with hip flexion as the nonspherical portion of the femoral head (cam lesion) glides under the labrum engaging the edge of the articular cartilage and results in progressive delamination. Initially, the labrum is relatively preserved, but secondary failure occurs over time. (All rights are retained by Dr. Byrd)

proposed arthroscopic management of FAI. Hips may possess the morphologic features of FAI without developing the cartilage failure associated with pathological impingement. Thus, the arthroscopic findings are a determinant in the course of management for patients who possess radiographic features of FAI. Impingement is not the sole cause of intra-articular pathology and hip joint symptoms in active adults.

Patient Evaluation

The onset of symptoms associated with FAI is variable, but the damage results from the cumulative effect of cyclical abnormal wear associated with the altered joint morphology. Examination will usually demonstrate diminished internal rotation caused by the altered bony architecture of the joint. However, many patients may have reduced internal rotation and still not suffer from pathological impingement. Also, while uncommon, pathological impingement is occasionally observed in individuals with normal or even increased internal rotation. Forced flexion, adduction and internal rotation, is called the impingement test in reference to eliciting symptoms associated with impingement (Fig. 17.3).

However, virtually any irritable hip, regardless of the etiology, will be uncomfortable with this maneuver. Thus, while it is quite sensitive, it is not necessarily specific for impingement. Athletic pubalgia may mimic or coexist with FAI and necessitates careful evaluation of the lower abdominal and adductor region (Fig. 17.4). Tenderness with resisted sit-ups, hip flexion, or adduction should raise an index of suspicion for athletic pubalgia. Pain with passive flexion and internal rotation is more indicative of an intra-articular source.

Imaging

Radiographs should include a well-centered AP pelvis view and a lateral view of the affected hip (Fig. 17.5) [9, 10]. Overcoverage of the anterior acetabulum, characteristic of pincer impingement, is evaluated by the presence of a crossover sign (Fig. 17.6). This can be due to acetabular retroversion, indicated by the posterior wall sign (Fig. 17.7). The lateral center edge (CE) angle of Wiberg was described to quantify dysplasia which is variously defined as less than 20–25° among different reports. No true measure for impingement has been defined, but it is generally associated with higher CE angles. Dysplasia can sometimes coexist with acetabular retroversion, and trimming the acetabular rim would be contraindicated (Fig. 17.8). For some cases, a false profile view can be helpful to further assess acetabular over- or undercoverage. The sphericity of the femoral head is assessed on both the AP and the lateral views (Fig. 17.9). We tend to rely on a frog lateral view as a routine screening radiograph. It is easy to obtain in a reproducible fashion.

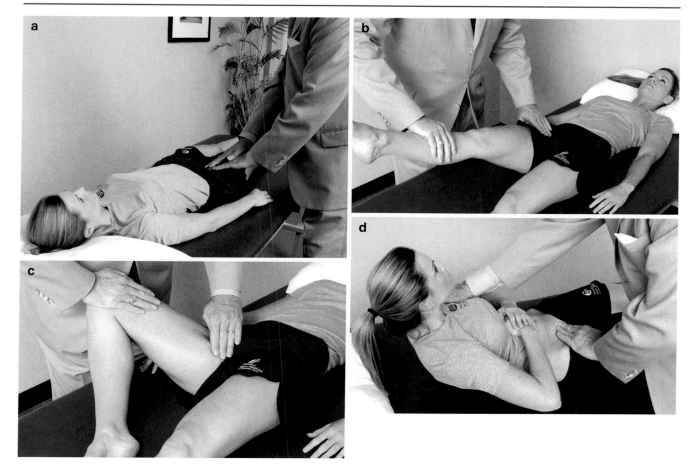

Fig. 17.4 (**a**) Careful palpation aids in assessing for the presence of soft tissue pelvic pathology. (**b**) Hip flexor soreness is elicited by palpation during resisted contraction. (**c**) Tenderness is elicited at the origin of the adductors by palpation during resisted contraction.

(**d**) The insertion of the rectus abdominis is palpated for tenderness during resisted contraction. Counterpressure is applied to the contralateral shoulder causing selective recruitment and contraction of the involved side. (All rights are retained by Dr. Byrd)

One study showed that the 40° Dunn view most predictably demonstrates the cam lesion [11]. However, because of the variable shape and location of the lesion, no radiograph is consistently reliable. Magnetic resonance imaging (MRI) and gadolinium arthrography with MRI (MRA) can both be helpful at detecting the intra-articular damage accompanying FAI. These studies are best at defining labral pathology but are less reliable in assessing the associated articular damage [12]. In the presence of a cam lesion, anticipate that the articular damage will be more extensive than the labral pathology. Also, subchondral edema in the anterior acetabulum is usually a harbinger of subjacent articular failure. With MRAs, the injection of long-acting anesthetic along with the contrast is important to substantiate whether the hip disease is the source of the patient's symptoms. This distinction may not always be clear on clinical examination alone. Computed tomography (CT) is much better at showing bone architecture and structure. Three-dimensional reconstructions provide the clearest image of the impingement

morphology. These images are especially helpful in the arthroscopic management, providing a clear interpretation of the exact shape of the abnormal bone that must be exposed and then resected.

Arthroscopic Procedure

(See Video 17.1: http://goo.gl/n2RMq) Arthroscopic management of FAI begins with arthroscopy of the central compartment. This is where the intra-articular damage, indicative of pathological impingement, is identified. The patient is positioned supine with traction applied, and three standard portals provide optimal access for surveying and accessing intra-articular pathology (Fig. 17.10a, b) [13, 14]. Portal placement is usually routine. However, severe impingement cases with a tight capsule and altered bony architecture can introduce significant challenges. It is important that the surgeon be prepared for these challenges in order to perform the

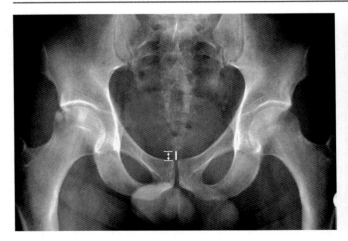

Fig. 17.5 A properly centered AP radiograph must be controlled for rotation and tilt. Proper rotation is confirmed by alignment of the coccyx over the symphysis pubic (*vertical line*). Proper tilt is controlled by maintaining the distance between the tip of the coccyx and the superior border of the symphysis pubis at 1–2 cm. (All rights are retained by Dr. Byrd)

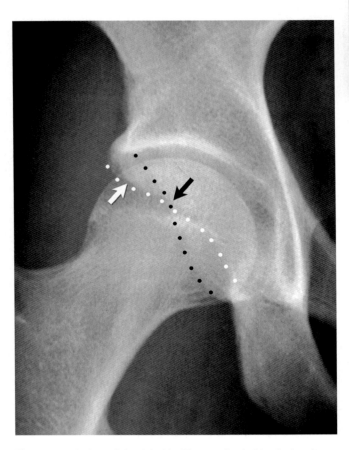

Fig. 17.6 AP view of the right hip. The anterior (*white dots*) and posterior (*black dots*) rim of the acetabulum are marked. The superior portion of the anterior rim lies lateral to the posterior rim (*white arrow*) indicating overcoverage of the acetabulum. Anteriorly, it assumes a more normal medial position, creating the crossover sign (*black arrow*) as a positive indicator of pincer impingement. (All rights are retained by Dr. Byrd)

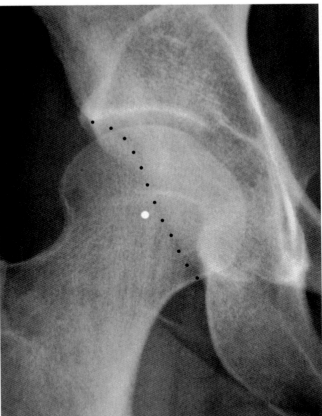

Fig. 17.7 AP view of the right hip. Acetabular retroversion as a cause of pincer impingement is indicated by a shallow posterior wall in which the posterior rim of the acetabulum (*black dots*) lies medial to the center of rotation of the femoral head (*white dot*). (All rights are retained by Dr. Byrd)

procedure as atraumatically as possible. Unique challenges of the stiff and arthrofibrosed hip are discussed in Chap. 27.

There are three arthroscopic parameters of pincer impingement. First is the presence of anterior labral pathology that must be present in order to have pathological pincer impingement. Second, positioning of the anterior portal may be difficult despite adequate distraction, and this is due to the bony prominence of the anterolateral acetabulum. Third is the presence of bone overhanging the labrum where normally there would just be a capsular reflection when pincer impingement is not present. The amount of bone to be removed is determined in conjunction with the radiographic and arthroscopic findings. In determining whether to excise bone, the radiographs should be carefully assessed for evidence of dysplasia. Retroversion in a dysplastic hip can give a false sense of pincer impingement. Recontouring the acetabulum in this setting can result in iatrogenic instability.

If the labrum appears normal, we would be hesitant to violate healthy tissue to correct a pincer lesion because of the theory that it could be a problem (Video 17.2: http:// goo.gl/dxws7). A normal labrum will never look the same

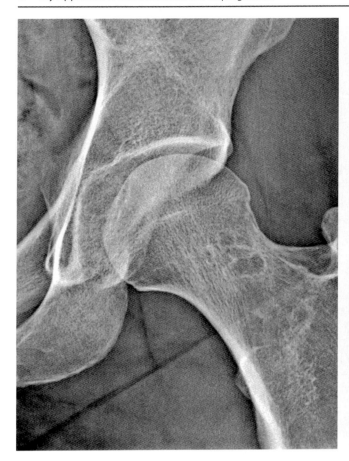

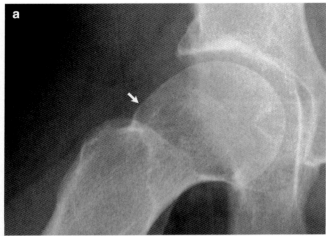

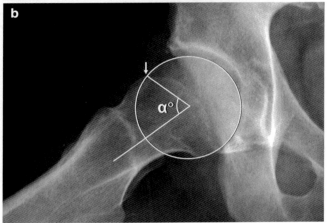

Fig. 17.8 AP radiograph of the left hip of a 24-year-old female demonstrates acetabular retroversion (crossover sign) in conjunction with dysplasia (CE angle 19°). Misinterpreting this as an impingement problem and trimming the acetabulum would place the patient at high risk of instability. (All rights are retained by Dr. Byrd)

Fig. 17.9 A frog lateral view of the right hip. (**a**) The cam lesion (*arrow*) is evident as the convex abnormality at the head/neck junction where there should normally be a concave slope of the femoral neck. (**b**) The alpha angle is used to quantitate the severity of the cam lesion. A *circle* is placed over the femoral head. The alpha angle is formed by a line along the axis of the femoral neck (1) and a line (2) from the center of the femoral head to the point where the head diverges outside of the *circle* (*arrow*). (All rights are retained by Dr. Byrd)

when it is restored. Assessing a damaged labrum is usually straightforward. However, assessing impending labral failure can be more subjective. This is especially important in younger patients. If the labrum is starting to appear crushed and draped across a bony prominence of the acetabular rim, then it is preferable not to wait until it is severely damaged to make the choice of correcting the accompanying pincer impingement (Video 17.3: http://goo.gl/EQtIA). Deciding how abnormal is abnormal enough to make this decision can sometimes be challenging.

If labral degeneration is extensive, as is often seen in middle age, then it may be managed with simple debridement (Video 17.4: http://goo.gl/r9dxf). The labral damage may not be salvaged, but recontouring the acetabulum opens the joint and may substantially improve mobility and symptoms. After completely inspecting the joint, attention is turned to the labral lesion. Selective debridement of the damaged portion will reveal the overhanging lip of bone instead of the normal capsular reflection from the labrum (Fig. 17.11a–e). Once the damaged tissue has been removed,

exposing the pincer lesion, the bone is then recontoured with a spherical burr. Generous capsulotomies around the portals facilitate maneuverability and access. The pincer lesion is addressed switching the arthroscope and instrumentation between the anterior and anterolateral portals. Resection is typically carried to the articular edge of the acetabulum. The amount of bone to be removed is dictated by the severity of the pincer lesion. Proximally, the bone is resected flush with the anterior column of the acetabulum. The anteromedial and lateral extent of the bony resection is dictated by the margin of healthy labrum. The bone is recontoured to create a smooth transition with the healthy portion of the labrum, which is preserved. A variable amount of associated secondary articular damage may be present which is addressed with a chondroplasty or microfracture for grade IV lesions.

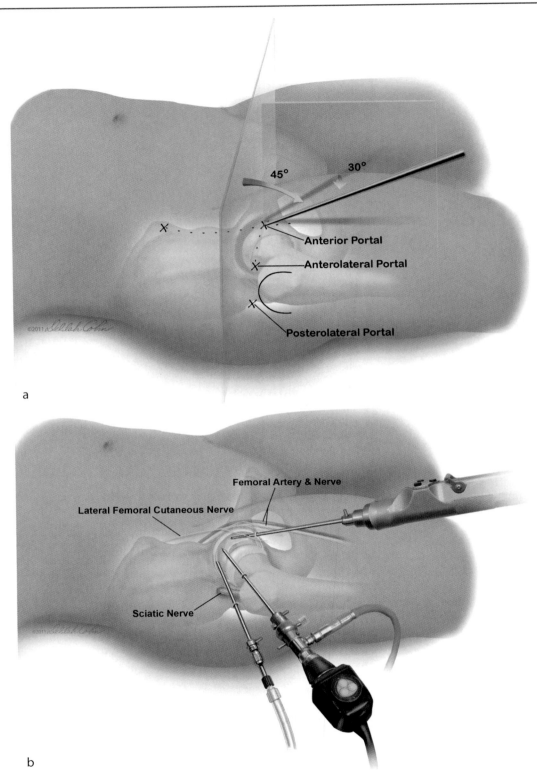

Fig. 17.10 (**a**) The site of the anterior portal coincides with the intersection of a sagittal line drawn distally from the anterior superior iliac spine and a transverse line across the superior margin of the greater trochanter. The direction of this portal courses approximately 45° cephalad and 30° toward the midline. The anterolateral and posterolateral portals are positioned directly over the superior aspect of the trochanter at its anterior and posterior borders. (**b**) The relationship of the major neurovascular structures to the three standard portals is illustrated. The femoral artery and nerve lie well medial to the anterior portal. The sciatic nerve lies posterior to the posterolateral portal. The lateral femoral cutaneous nerve lies close to the anterior portal. Injury to this structure is avoided by using proper portal placement. The anterolateral portal is established first because it lies most centrally in the safe zone for arthroscopy. (All rights are retained by Dr. Byrd)

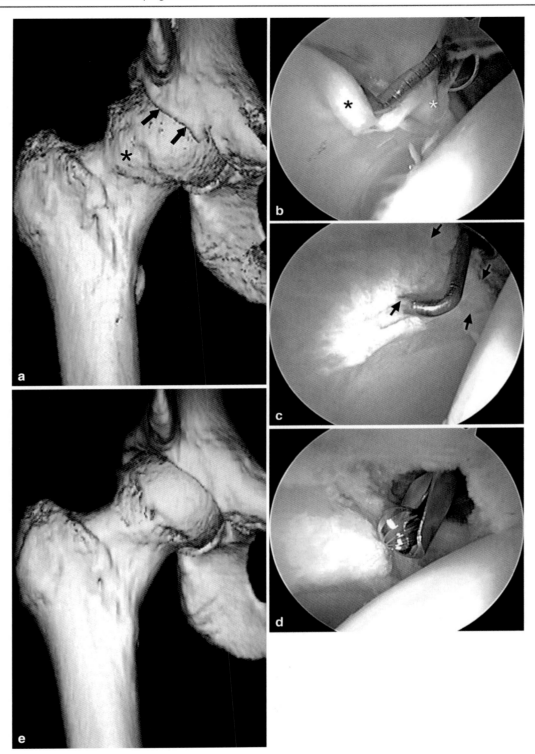

Fig. 17.11 A 38-year-old female with progressive pain and loss of motion of the right hip. (**a**) A 3D CT scan illustrates pincer impingement (*arrows*) as well as a kissing lesion characterized by osteophyte formation on the femoral head (*asterisk*). (**b**) Viewing anteriorly from the anterolateral portal, there is maceration of the anterior labrum (*white asterisk*) and some associated articular delamination (*black asterisk*). (**c**) Debridement of the degenerate labrum exposes the pincer lesion (*arrows*). (**d**) The pincer lesion is recontoured with a burr. (**e**) A postoperative 3D CT scan demonstrates the extent of bony recontouring of the acetabulum and the femoral head. (All rights are retained by Dr. Byrd)

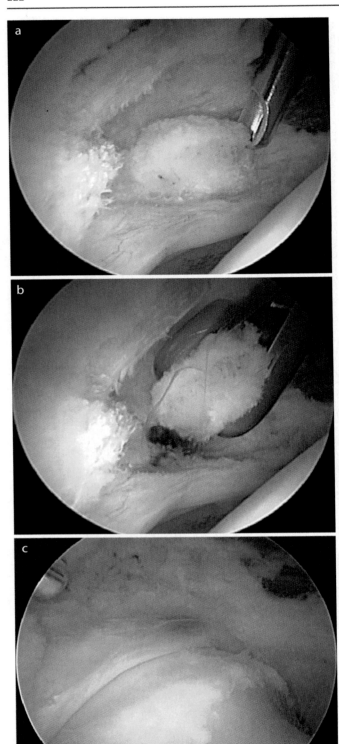

Fig. 17.12 A pincer lesion created by an os acetabulum along the anterolateral rim of a right hip. (**a**) The fragment is exposed. (**b**) The fragment is being removed. (**c**) The integrity of the labrum has been preserved. (All rights are retained by Dr. Byrd)

In the presence of good quality labral tissue and especially in younger patients, preservation of the labrum is preferred. In a few cases, the bony lesion can be exposed on the capsular side of the labrum and recontoured without compromising the labrum's structural integrity (Fig. 17.12) (Video 17.5: http://goo.gl/2bUcp). More often, when the labrum is failing due to pincer impingement, it is mobilized to resect the pincer lesion and then refixed (Fig. 17.13). The portion of the labrum to be mobilized must be exposed at its bony attachment on the capsular side. The labrum is sharply dissected from the overlying bone to reveal the pincer lesion. The acetabulum is then recontoured with a high-speed burr, taking care to preserve the mobilized labrum. With this technique, adequate mobilization of the labrum is necessary to visualize the bony margins of the pincer lesion for recontouring. Inadequate exposure results in simply a small scalloped defect in the acetabular rim with incomplete correction. The depth of resection is typically 3–5 mm but is determined by the dimensions of the pincer lesion. Resection of the bony rim requires good arthroscopic visualization. Do not rely solely on fluoroscopy because it will cause you to underestimate the amount of bone being removed anterior to the 12 o'clock position. After reshaping the rim, the labrum is then refixed with suture anchors. The anchors are placed in the rim of the acetabulum on the capsular side of the labrum. The anchor placement is consistent from one case to the next. The anchors are spaced approximately 8–10 mm and as close to the rim as possible while assuring that they do not perforate the surface of the acetabulum. For this purpose, we use a percutaneous delivery system that allows the skin entry site of the drill sleeve to be placed as distally as necessary to make sure that the anchor diverges from the acetabular surface. This is placed distally, halfway between the anterior and anterolateral portals (Fig. 17.14). The modified anterior portal, that is sometimes popular, may not always be distal enough to assure the correct amount of diversion [15]. However, there is also a curved drill guide system that can give a better angle for this portal (Fig. 17.15). Either way, it is imperative that the articular surface is visualized while drilling. Any evidence of rippling of the cartilage indicates that the drill is too close, and it must be repositioned (Video 17.6: http://goo.gl/4LKKp). The most common error is not allowing enough divergence, which forces the drill hole to be placed further away from the rim of the acetabulum in order to avoid perforation. Then, when the labrum is tied down, it is not properly reapproximated to the rim, and its function has not been restored. With the distal percutaneous site halfway between the anterior and anterolateral portals, or with the use of the modified anterior portal, anchors can be placed along the anterior acetabulum up to the 12 o'clock position. Note that fluoroscopy is not very helpful because the direction of entry is more in

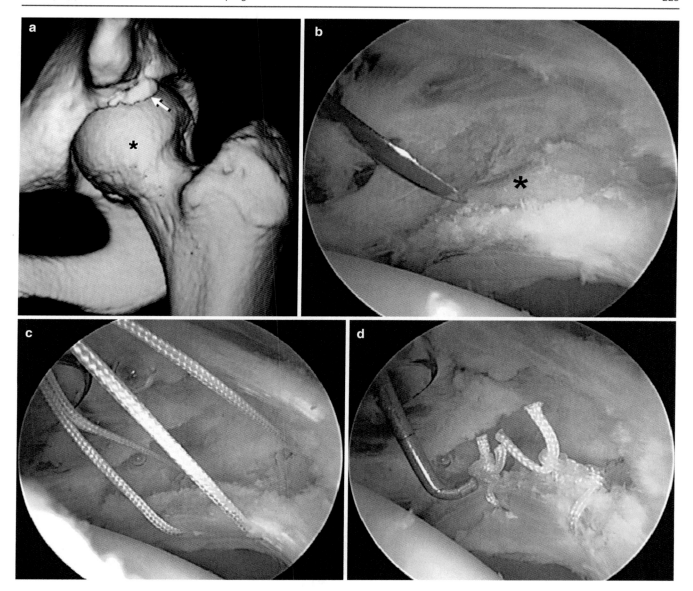

Fig. 17.13 A 15-year-old female gymnast with pain and reduced internal rotation of the left hip. (**a**) A 3D CT scan defines a pincer lesion with accompanying os acetabulum (*arrow*) and cam lesion (*asterisk*). (**b**) Viewing from the anterolateral portal, the pincer lesion and os acetabulum (*asterisk*) are exposed with the labrum being sharply released with an arthroscopic knife. (**c**) The acetabular fragment has been removed and the rim trimmed with anchors placed to repair the labrum. (**d**) The labrum has been refixed. (All rights are retained by Dr. Byrd)

the plane of the x-ray beam (Fig. 17.16). Far lateral anchors are best placed from the anterolateral portal, and for these, fluoroscopy can be helpful in seeing that the drill is diverging from the subchondral surface (Fig. 17.17).

While anchor placement is consistent, the pattern and method of suture passage is variable depending on the damage and morphology of the labrum. If the chondrolabral junction is intact, then a simple suture passage is used through the midsubstance of the labrum and tied against the capsular side. This reconstitutes the labrum against the rim well. The suture can be passed through the labrum with a tissue-penetrating device, or if the labrum is small, then a suture shuttle technique allows the smallest possible hole in the labral tissue (Fig. 17.18). If the labrum is robust, then a simple suture technique may distort its configuration, or if the articular edge of the labrum has been separated from the adjacent articular surface, then a different type suture must be used to reconstitute the chondrolabral junction. For this, a modified single limb mattress suture is used (Fig. 17.19) (Video 17.7: http://goo.gl/GS58c). One limb of the suture is passed into the joint at the chondrolabral junction, using a tissue-penetrating device. It is then grasped through the midportion of the labrum and pulled out for tying against the capsular edge.

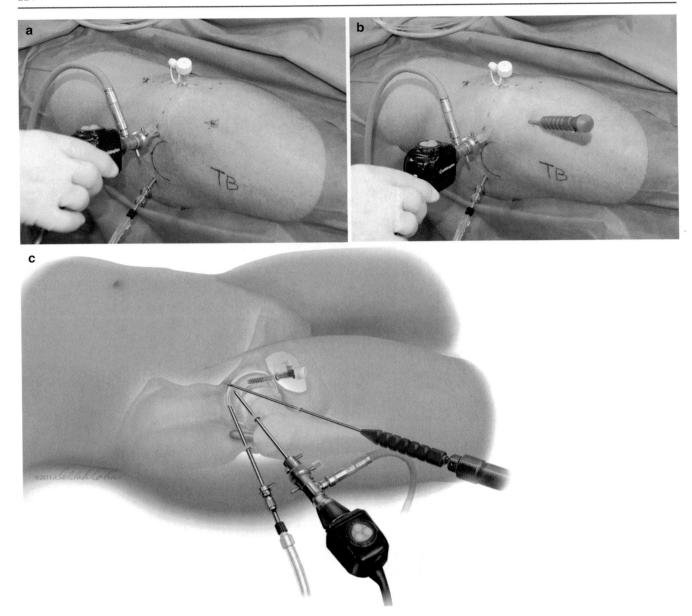

Fig. 17.14 An anchor delivery system can be placed percutaneously and thus not depend on portals. Placed midway between the anterior and anterolateral portals, it is positioned as distally as necessary to assure that the anchors will diverge from the face of the acetabulum. (**a**) Prepositioning is performed with a spinal needle. (**b**) The anchor delivery system has been percutaneously placed. (**c**) Schematic illustrates the drill sleeve placed against the acetabular rim. (All rights are retained by Dr. Byrd)

This anatomically restores the labrum to the rim of the acetabulum and avoids distortion. If the quality of the labral tissue is poor, then simply looping the suture around the labrum may be necessary in order to assure that sufficient tissue has been reapproximated.

Management of cam impingement also begins with arthroscopy of the central compartment to assess for the pathology associated with cam lesion [16]. The characteristic feature of pathological cam impingement is articular failure of the anterolateral acetabulum. The femoral head remains well preserved until late in the disease course. Early stages of the disease are characterized by closed grade I chondral blistering, which sometimes must be distinguished from normal articular softening (Video 17.8: http://goo.gl/s10Ws). Our experience has been that most already have grade III or grade IV acetabular changes by the time of surgical intervention. The articular surface is seen to separate or peel away from its attachment to the labrum (Fig. 17.20), and this is caused by the shear effect of the cam lesion (Video 17.9: http://goo.gl/Jo7hV). The labrum may be relatively

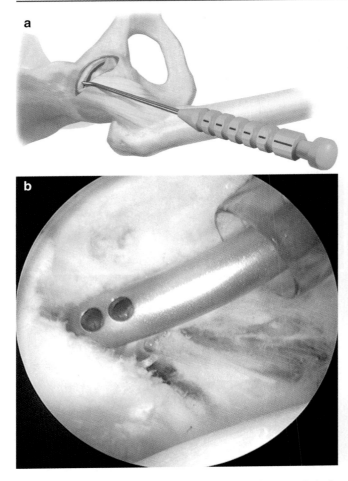

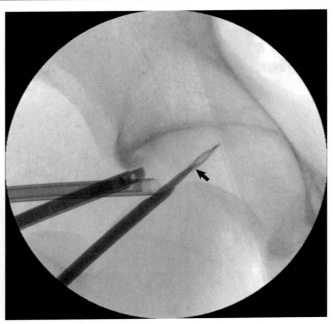

Fig. 17.16 Fluoroscopic image of a right hip drilling for placement of an anchor in the anterior rim of the acetabulum (*arrow*). Fluoroscopy does not help in assessing the anchor position. (All rights are retained by Dr. Byrd)

Fig. 17.15 (**a**) A curved anchor delivery system provides more latitude for assuring divergence when the anchor is placed through a conventional portal. (**b**) The curved system is placed against the acetabular rim from the modified anterior portal in this right hip with appropriate divergence for the acetabular surface. (All rights are retained by Dr. Byrd)

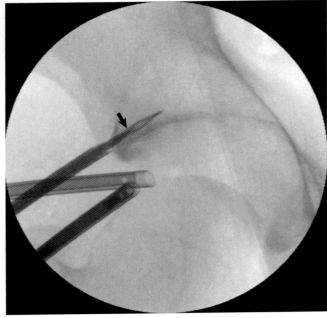

Fig. 17.17 AP fluoroscopic image of a right hip drilling for an anchor in the lateral acetabulum (*arrow*). From this angle, the image helps to assure that the drill does not violate the subchondral surface. (All rights are retained by Dr. Byrd)

well preserved but, with time, progressive fragmentation occurs. Often, the damaged articular edge of the labrum can be selectively debrided, preserving the capsular margin and potentially some of its labral seal function. If there is good quality tissue that has been detached, repair can be performed with suture anchors (Fig. 17.21). If pincer impingement is not present, the anchors can be placed adjacent to the articular surface, between the acetabulum and the labrum (Video 17.10: http://goo.gl/hDbFw). The suture limbs can be grasped through the labrum with a penetrator device and tied with the knots on the capsular side of the labrum. Passing both limbs of the suture in a mattress fashion avoids suture rubbing against the femoral head, but occasionally, looping the sutures may be necessary to assure that good substance of the tissue is secured to the rim of the acetabulum. The articular pathology is addressed with chondroplasty and microfracture as dictated by its severity.

After completing arthroscopy of the central compartment, the cam lesion is addressed from the peripheral compartment. A capsulotomy is created by connecting the anterior and anterolateral portals (Fig. 17.22). The amount of

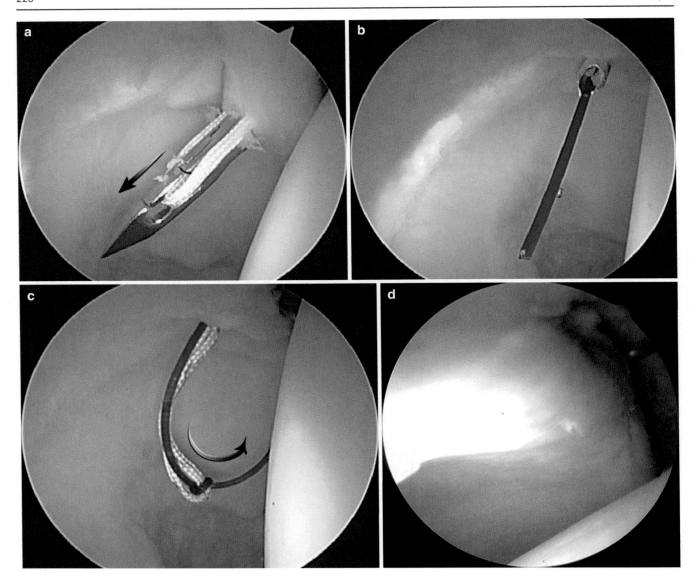

Fig. 17.18 Arthroscopic view of a right hip. Acetabuloplasty has been completed, and the anchor has been seated in the anterior acetabulum. The chondrolabral junction is preserved. (**a**) A soft tissue-penetrating device is used to push the suture limb through the labrum. (**b**) As an alternative method, a suture passing device is placed to introduce a monofilament suture. (**c**) The braided anchor suture is then shuttled through the labrum, secured to the monofilament with a single half-hitch. (**d**) Three anchors have been placed with sutures tied, reapproximating the labrum to the rim of the acetabulum. (All rights are retained by Dr. Byrd)

capsulotomy is titrated to the specifics of the case. For a tight hip with restricted rotational motion, the capsulotomy becomes more of an aggressive capsulectomy, which is partly therapeutic in helping to regain better mobility as well as pain relief. It may be extended posterolaterally and anteromedially. For hips where instability may be a concern, the capsulotomy can be limited to simply connecting the two portals with an incision of only 1.5–2 cm. This may be necessary, for example, in a hip where dysplasia coexists with a cam lesion. By titrating the capsulotomy to the needs of the

case, capsular repair has rarely been necessary in our experience. If more exposure is needed in a hip that might be susceptible to instability, then a vertical T-shaped capsulotomy can be extended distally. The flaps are preserved, and the vertical limb can be reapproximated at the completion of the procedure.

After preparing the capsulotomy, the posterolateral portal can be removed, and the anterior and anterolateral cannulas are simply backed out of the central compartment. The traction is released, and the hip flexed approximately 35°. As

Fig. 17.19 Arthroscopic view of a right hip from the anterolateral portal. (**a**) The labrum is robust with disruption of the chondrolabral junction. (**b**) Viewing peripheral to the labrum, the acetabuloplasty (*asterisk*) has been completed. (**c**) A suture anchor has been seated in the bony rim and one limb of the suture is grasped with a soft tissue-penetrating device. (**d**) With the penetrator, the suture has been passed into the joint at the chondrolabral junction. (**e**) The penetrator has been repositioned through the midsubstance of the labrum, preparing to grasp the suture limb. (**f**) The suture has been grasped and is withdrawn back out to the capsular rim. (**g**) Three anchors have been placed with sutures tied, restoring the labrum and the chondrolabral junction. (**h**) Labral restoration is further observed peripherally with reconstitution of the labral seal. (All rights are retained by Dr. Byrd)

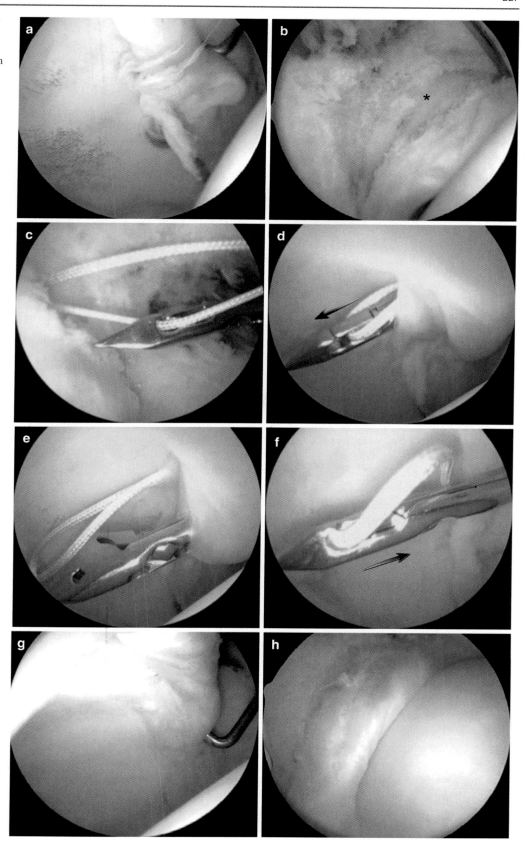

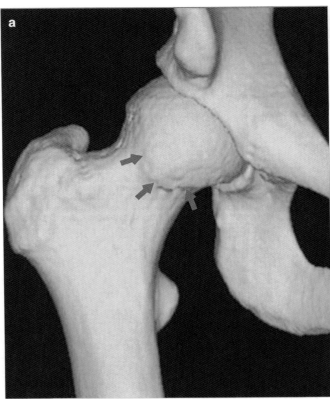
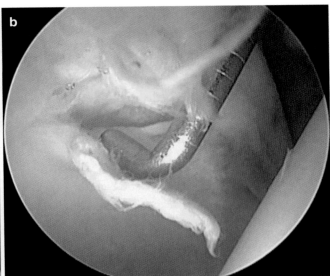

Fig. 17.20 A 20-year-old hockey player with a 4-year history of right hip pain. (**a**) A 3D CT scan defines the cam lesion (*arrows*). (**b**) Viewing from the anterolateral portal, the probe introduced anteriorly displaces an area of articular delamination from the anterolateral acetabulum characteristic of the peel-back phenomenon created by the bony lesion shearing the articular surface during hip flexion.

the hip is flexed under arthroscopic visualization, the line of demarcation between healthy femoral cartilage and abnormal fibrocartilage that covers the cam lesion can usually be identified. Flexing the hip too far can cause part of the cam lesion to disappear under the acetabulum. In general, slightly more or less flexion may be necessary, just depending on the position that best brings the cam lesion into view.

A cephalad anterolateral portal is established approximately 5 cm above the anterolateral portal, entering through the capsulotomy that has already been established. These proximal and distal anterolateral portals work well for accessing and addressing the cam lesion (Fig. 17.23). Removing the anterior portal provides an unobstructed image for the C-arm, although the portal can be maintained if it is needed for better access to the medial side of the femoral neck.

Most of the work for performing the recontouring of the cam lesion (femoroplasty) lies in the soft tissue preparation. This includes capsular resection as necessary to assure complete visualization of the lesion and then removal of the fibrocartilage and scar that covers the abnormal bone (Fig. 17.24). With the hip flexed, the proximal portal provides better access for the lateral and posterior portion, while the distal portal is more anterior relative to the joint and pro-

vides best access for the anterior part of the lesion. The lateral synovial fold is identified as the arthroscopic landmark for the retinacular vessels, and care is taken to preserve this structure during the recontouring (Fig. 17.25). Switching between the portals is important for full appreciation of the three-dimensional anatomy of the recontouring.

Once the bone has been fully exposed, recontouring is performed with a spherical burr. The goal is to remove the abnormal bone identified on the preoperative CT scan and recreate the normal concave relationship that should exist where the femoral neck meets the articular edge of the femoral head. It is best to begin by creating the line and depth of resection at the articular margin. The resection is then extended distally, tapering with the normal portion of the femoral head (Figs. 17.26a, b and 17.27a, b). We recommend beginning the resection at the lateral/posterior limit of the cam lesion with the arthroscope in the more distal portal and instrumentation in the more proximal portal. The posterior extent of the resection is usually the most difficult; the resection is also the most critical to avoid notching the tensile surface of the femoral neck, and particular attention must be given to avoid and preserve the lateral retinacular vessels. Then, switching the arthroscope to the proximal portal, the

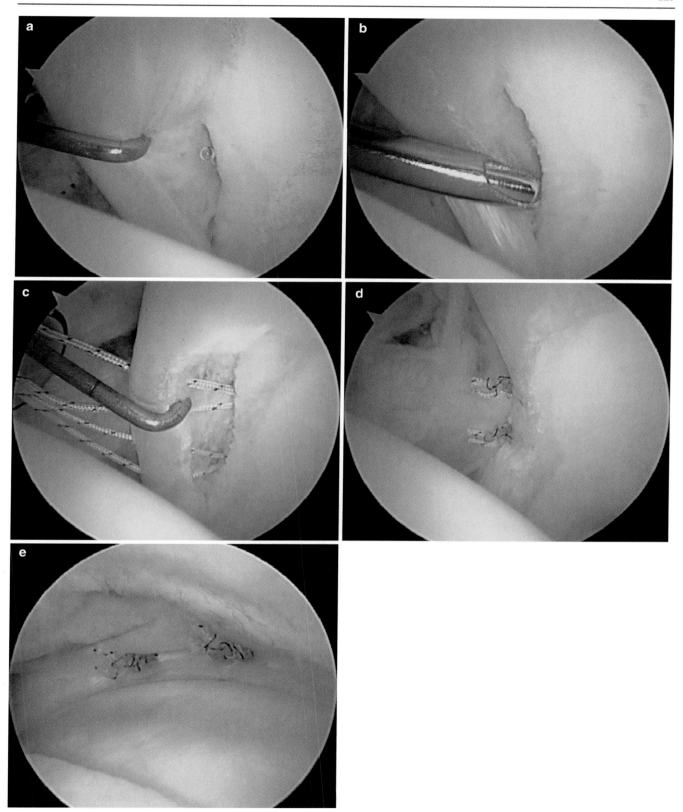

Fig. 17.21 An anterior labral tear of a right hip is being viewed from the anterolateral portal. (**a**) Pathological detachment of the labrum from the rim of the acetabulum is being probed. (**b**) Freshening the rim of the acetabulum, creating a bleeding bony surface, aids in potentiating healing of the repair. (**c**) Two anchors have been placed in the rim of the acetabulum with the sutures passed through the labrum in a mattress fashion. (**d**) The sutures have been tied securely reapproximating the labrum to the rim of the acetabulum. (**e**) Now viewing from the peripheral compartment, the repair is inspected showing approximation of the labrum against the femoral head with the sutures well removed from the articular surface. (All rights are retained by Dr. Byrd)

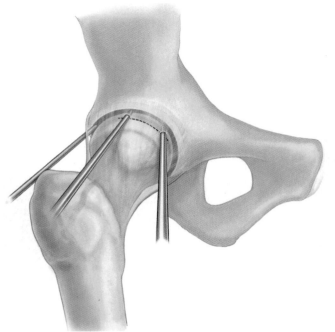

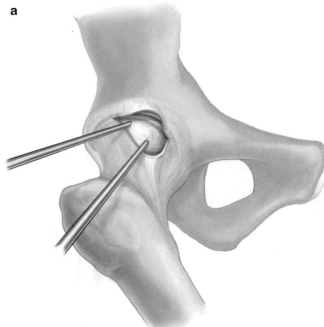

a

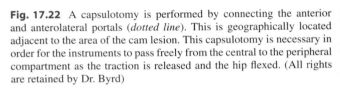

Fig. 17.22 A capsulotomy is performed by connecting the anterior and anterolateral portals (*dotted line*). This is geographically located adjacent to the area of the cam lesion. This capsulotomy is necessary in order for the instruments to pass freely from the central to the peripheral compartment as the traction is released and the hip flexed. (All rights are retained by Dr. Byrd)

burr is introduced distally, and the reshaping is completed along the anterior head and neck junction. Lastly, attention is given to make sure that all bone debris is removed as thoroughly as possible to lessen the likelihood of developing heterotopic ossification. The quality of the recontouring is assessed, and preservation of the lateral retinacular vessels is confirmed (Fig. 17.28a–c). Closure of the capsulotomy is not routinely performed. In cases where instability might be a potential concern, a T-shaped capsulotomy is used, and the vertical limb can be closed with single interrupted braided absorbable sutures (Fig. 17.29a–d).

Comments on Determining the Correct Amount of Bone to Remove

With proper exposure and meticulous technique, the entirety of the bony impingement can be identified for precise resection. What is less clear is knowing the exact amount of bone to remove. Presently, 3D CT scans provide the clearest image of the bony lesion. Thus, we use this as the principal determinant for interpreting the bone to be removed. The goal is not so much to recreate a standard-looking hip but to

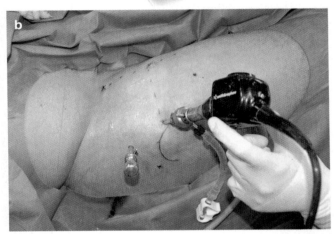

b

Fig. 17.23 (**a**) With the hip flexed, the anterolateral portal is now positioned along the neck of the femur. A cephalad (proximal) anterolateral portal has been placed. These two portals allow access to the entirety of the cam lesion in most cases. Their position also allows an unhindered view with the C-arm. (**b**) Photograph illustrates the proximal and distal anterolateral working portals for the peripheral compartment. (All rights are retained by Dr. Byrd)

remove the offending bone and, on the femoral side, recreate the normal concavity that should exist at the head/neck junction. In the near future, computer navigation will assist in accurately quantitating the amount of removal that must now be done by subjective interpretation. This will be performed with 3D MRI that will supplant computed tomography. For the present, one must be cautious about relying much on intraoperative fluoroscopy. The line of resection does not parallel the x-ray beam, and thus, it is easy to go astray relying solely on fluoroscopy. We find fluoroscopy most helpful in assessing the posterior limit of the resection. Sometimes the lateral aspect of the cam lesion starts to disappear underneath the posterior acetabular rim. Fluoroscopy can be helpful to make sure that adequate proximal resection has been performed. In some cases, briefly reapplying traction may be helpful to fully access this posterior limit. Intraoperative range of motion is not a substitute for complete visualization of the abnormal bone. Our goal is, again, to remove the abnormal bone and recreate the normal concavity. Once this has been accomplished, it is unlikely that greater resection would be of more benefit. It is also unclear how well passive range of motion of an anesthetized patient with a joint distended with fluid equates with how the patient's hip functions in vivo.

Post-op Rehabilitation

The recovery strategy depends on the extent of pathology that is encountered at the time of arthroscopy and what is done to address it. For simple labral debridement and recontouring of the acetabular rim, the patient is allowed to weight bear as tolerated, with an emphasis on range of motion and joint stabilization. If the labrum is refixed, then precautions are necessary to protect the repair site during the early healing phase. This includes protected weight bearing and avoiding extremes of flexion and external rotation for the first 4 weeks. Among patients requiring a second-look arthroscopic procedure, rarely is failure of a labral repair found to be a problem. Thus, our rehab strategy protecting the repair site may still be too conservative when we need to emphasize prevention of adhesions, but we are still careful not to be too aggressive.

Reshaping of the femoral head/neck junction necessitates some precautions. Fracture of the femoral neck is an unlikely, but potentially serious, complication. Full weight bearing is allowed, but crutches are used to avoid awkward twisting movements during the first 4 weeks. Once full motor control has been regained, the joint is adequately protected for light activities. If osteopenia is present, then these precautions become more imperative, especially in postmenopausal women and any patient over the age of 55. Full bony remodeling takes 3 months, during which time, some precautions are necessary to avoid high impact or torsional forces. If microfracture is performed, strict protected weight bearing is continued for 2 months to optimize the early maturation of the fibrocartilaginous healing response. During this time, gentle range of motion is emphasized to stimulate the healing process.

At 3 months, specific precautions are lifted, and functional progression is allowed. The rate at which the individuals advance is variable and may require another 1–3 months for full activities. Athletes are generally advised that return to sports following surgical correction of FAI can take 4–6 months.

Results

We have published two studies reporting the outcomes of our earliest experience in arthroscopic management of FAI [17, 18]. In a study of our first 100 consecutive patients with minimum 2-year follow-up, the median improvement was 21.5 points using the modified Harris hip score with 79% good and excellent results [17]. Ninety-two percent had grade III or grade IV acetabular articular damage, including 18 patients who underwent microfracture with a median improvement of 21 points. Twenty-three patients had concomitant articular damage to the femoral head demonstrating slightly lesser improvement of 17 points. No patient required conversion to total hip arthroplasty, although six underwent a subsequent arthroscopic procedure for recurrent or persistent symptoms. There were three complications: a transient neurapraxia of the pudendal nerve and the lateral femoral cutaneous nerve, both of which resolved uneventfully, and one mild case of heterotopic ossification within the capsule which did not preclude a successful outcome. In another study of our first 200 consecutive athletes with minimum 1-year follow-up, the median improvement was 24 points. Eighty-nine percent had grade III or grade IV articular damage with 49 undergoing microfracture and demonstrating a median improvement of 26 points [18]. Twenty percent had concomitant articular damage to the femoral head and demonstrated lesser improvement of 16 points. Overall, 90% returned to sport (95% professional, 85% collegiate). There were five transient neurapraxias that resolved. One athlete was converted to a total hip arthroplasty and four underwent repeat arthroscopy.

The results of our earliest experiences seem good, even though most of these included labral debridements. As we have recognized the healing capacity of the labrum and successful techniques for repair, the majority of patients now undergo labral repair or refixation. As evidenced by the work of others, it does appear that this may provide even more favorable results [19, 20]. Our observation has been that a high majority of patients have grade III or grade IV articular damage to the acetabulum by the time arthroscopic intervention is undertaken. Despite the severity of damage, our results are still good. This indicates that grade III and grade IV damage is not a contraindication to the procedure, but it also indicates that we are intervening late in the

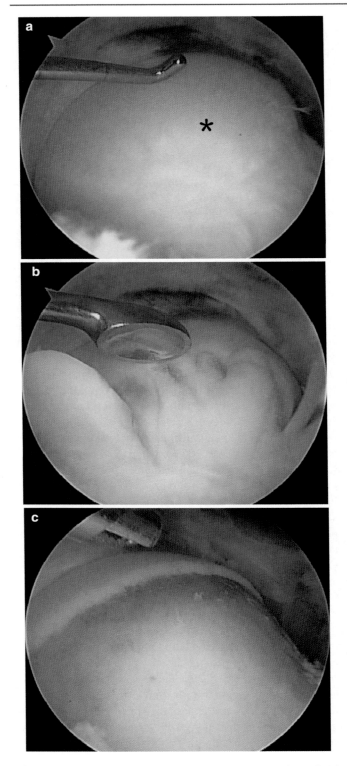

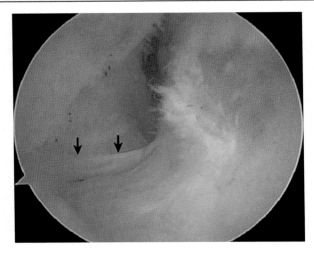

Fig. 17.25 Viewing laterally, underneath the area of the lateral capsulotomy, the lateral synovial fold (*arrows*) is identified along the lateral base of the neck, representing the arthroscopic landmarks of the lateral retinacular vessels. (All rights are retained by Dr. Byrd)

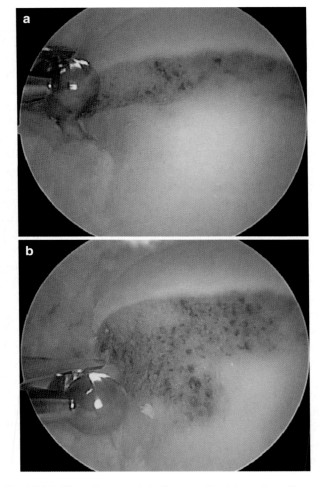

Fig. 17.24 The right hip is viewed from the anterolateral portal. (**a**) The cam lesion is identified, covered in fibrocartilage (*asterisk*). (**b**) An arthroscopic curette is used to denude the abnormal bone. (**c**) The area to be excised has been fully exposed. The soft tissue preparation aids in precisely defining the margins to be excised. (All rights are retained by Dr. Byrd)

Fig. 17.26 The arthroscope is in the more distal (anterolateral) portal with the instrumentation placed from the proximal portal. (**a**) Bony resection is begun at the articular margin. (**b**) The resection is then carried distally, recreating the normal concave relationship. (All rights are retained by Dr. Byrd)

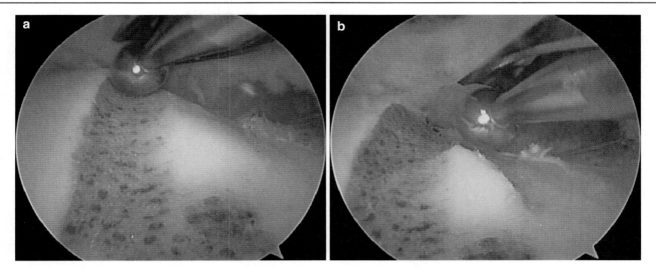

Fig. 17.27 The arthroscope is now in the proximal portal with the instrumentation introduced distally. (**a**) The line of resection is continued along the anterior articular border of the bump. (**b**) The recontouring is completed. (All rights are retained by Dr. Byrd)

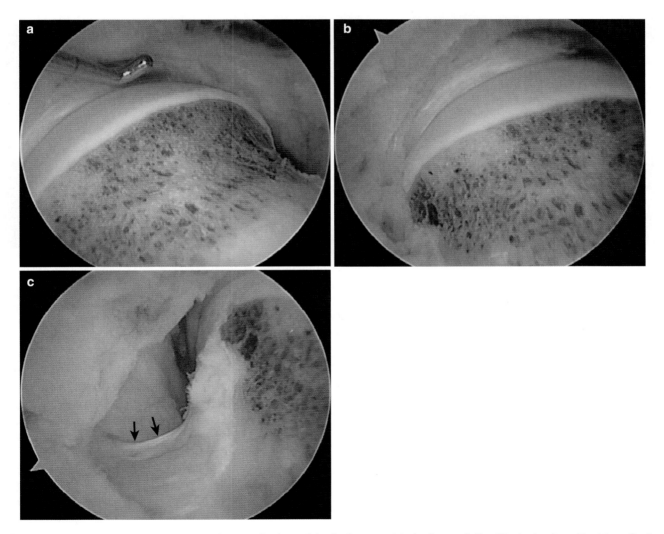

Fig. 17.28 The arthroscope has been returned to the distal portal for final survey, (**a**) viewing medially; (**b**) viewing laterally; (**c**) confirming preservation of the lateral retinacular vessels (*arrows*). (All rights are retained by Dr. Byrd)

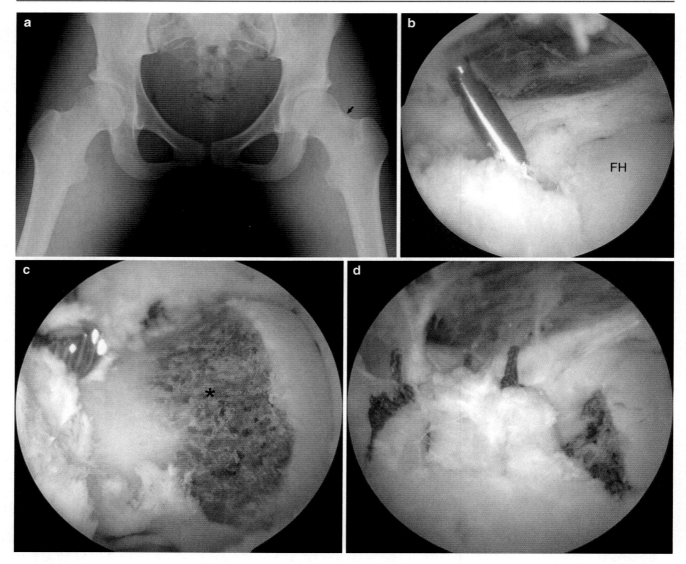

Fig. 17.29 (**a**) Dunn view of the pelvis of an elite level female hurdler with a symptomatic cam lesion (*arrow*) in her left lead leg associated with dysplasia (CD angle 20°). (**b**) Viewing the left hip from the anterolateral portal, a small capsulotomy has been made connecting the anterior and anterolateral portals, exposing the femoral head (*FH*). An arthroscopic knife is used to create a vertical T-limb to the capsulotomy to expose the cam lesion. (**c**) The cam lesion has been corrected (*asterisk*) recreating the normal concavity of the head/neck junction. (**d**) Same view with the vertical limb of the capsulotomy reapproximated with interrupted braided absorbable sutures. (All rights are retained by Dr. Byrd)

disease course. Thus, we need to learn how to detect and properly select patients for earlier intervention. Of course, we would not recommend surgery in someone who is asymptomatic, but patients who are minimally symptomatic should be educated on warning signs of progressive damage that might necessitate a proactive approach. Microfracture is perhaps an imperfect solution for full-thickness articular loss, but our results have still been quite favorable. With FAI, the articular surface of the femoral head tends to remain well preserved until very late in the disease course. Our observation is that once the femoral surface starts to fail, the results, although favorable, are not as good. In fact, for cases

with mixed findings of impingement and dysplasia, the arthroscopic findings may aid in determining the principal culprit. With impingement, the femoral surface will remain well preserved despite advanced acetabular changes while, with dysplasia, articular erosion is more equally distributed to both surfaces. Among athletes, 95% returned to sport at the professional level and 85% at the collegiate level. It is unlikely that this difference indicates that we were doing a better surgical procedure among the professional athletes but indicates the reality that there are numerous other factors beyond just the surgical procedure itself that can influence successful outcomes. Our very low rate of conversion to total hip arthroplasty seems to indicate that we are doing a good job properly selecting patients who are potentially candidates for arthroscopic correction of FAI, but our modest reoperation rate indicates that we could also be doing a better job with the technical aspects of the procedure.

We concur with others that grade III Tonnis changes are a contraindication to surgical correction of FAI. However, grade II changes are less clear. By definition, a severe cam lesion fulfills the criteria for grade II Tonnis. Many patients with grade II changes do well while others do not. In our opinion, this reflects that grade II Tonnis encompasses a broad spectrum of disease and reflects the inadequacies of plain radiography to accurately reflect the extent of intra-articular pathology.

Conclusions

Most cases of FAI can be managed with arthroscopic surgery. This can be a technically challenging procedure, but these challenges are lessened by a methodical, systematic approach to accessing the joint and addressing the pathology. Severe protrusio and cases that require a periacetabular or a proximal femoral osteotomy represent contraindications. The favorable aspect of the arthroscopic approach is its less invasive nature, avoiding the problems of open surgery, hospitalization, and rehabilitation. However, arthroscopy exposes the patient to risks not associated with the open procedure. The biggest concerns are problems associated with traction, iatrogenic injury to the joint, or less well-executed correction of the bony anatomy. These problems are accentuated in stiffer hips. There are further steps that can be taken to address these added challenges and a thoughtful, experienced approach in weighing the benefits of arthroscopy over an open procedure is required.

References

1. Vulpius O, Stöffel A. Orthopäadische Operationslehre. Stuttgart: F. Enke; 1913.
2. Smith-Petersen MN. Treatment of malum coxae senilis, old slipped upper femoral epiphysis, intrapelvic protrusion of the acetabulum, and coxa plana by means of acetabuloplasty. J Bone Joint Surg Am. 1936;18:869–80.
3. Heyman CH, Herndon CH. Slipped femoral epiphysis with severe displacement: a conservative operative treatment. J Bone Joint Surg Am. 1957;39:293–413.
4. Garceau GJ. Surgical treatment of coxa plana. J Bone Joint Surg Br. 1964;46:779–80.
5. Myers SR, Eijer H, Ganz R. Anterior femoroacetabular impingement after periacetabular osteotomy. Clin Orthop. 1999;363:81–92.
6. Ganz R, Parvizi J, Beck M, Leunig M, Notzli H, Siebenrock KA. Femoroacetabular impingement: a cause for osteoarthritis of the hip. Clin Orthop. 2003;417:112–20.
7. Lavigne M, Parvizi J, Beck M, Siebenrock KA, Ganz R, Leunig M. Anterior femoroacetabular impingement: part I. Techniques of joint preserving surgery. Clin Orthop. 2004;418:61–6.
8. Beck M, Leunig M, Parvizi J, Boutier V, Wyss D, Ganz R. Anterior femoroacetabular impingement: part II. Midterm results of surgical treatment. Clin Orthop. 2004;418:67–73.
9. Parvizi J, Leunig M, Ganz R. Femoroacetabular impingement. J Am Acad Orthop Surg. 2007;15(9):561–70.
10. Clohisy JC, Carlisle JC, Trousdale R, et al. Radiographic evaluation of the hip has limited reliability. Clin Orthop Relat Res. 2009;467:666–75.
11. Meyer DC, Beck M, Ellis T, Ganz R, Leunig M. Comparison of six radiographic projections to assess femoral head/neck asphericity. Clin Orthop. 2006;445:181–5.
12. Byrd JWT, Jones KS. Diagnostic accuracy of clinical assessment, MRI, gadolinium MRI, and intraarticular injection in hip arthroscopy patients. Am J Sports Med. 2004;32(7):1668–74.
13. Byrd JWT. The supine approach. In: Byrd JWT, editor. Operative hip arthroscopy. 2nd ed. New York: Springer; 2005. p. 145–69.
14. Byrd JWT. Hip arthroscopy by the supine approach. Instr Course Lect. 2006;55:325–36.
15. Kelly BT, Weiland DE, Schenker ML, et al. Arthroscopic labral repair in the hip: surgical technique and review of the literature. Arthroscopy. 2005;21(12):1496–504.
16. Byrd JWT, Jones KS. Arthroscopic "femoroplasty" in the management of cam-type femoroacetabular impingement. Clin Orthop Relat Res. 2009;467:739–46. Epub 2008 Dec 19.
17. Byrd JWT, Jones KS. Arthroscopic management of femoroacetabular impingement with minimum two-year follow-up. Arthroscopy. 2011;27(10):1379–88. Epub 2011 Aug 20.
18. Byrd JWT, Jones KS. Arthroscopic management of femoroacetabular impingement (FAI) in athletes. Am J Sports Med. 2011;39: 7–13.
19. Larson CM, Giveans MR. Arthroscopic debridement versus refixation of the acetabular labrum associated with femoroacetabular impingement. Arthroscopy. 2009;25(4):369–76.
20. Philippon MJ, Briggs KK, Yen Y-M, Kuppersmith DA. Outcomes following hip arthroscopy for femoroacetabular impingement with associated chondrolabral dysfunction. J Bone Joint Surg Br. 2008; 91-B:16–23.

My Approach to Femoroacetabular Impingement

18

Trevor R. Gaskill and Marc J. Philippon

Introduction

Since its earliest description, femoroacetabular impingement (FAI) is increasingly being recognized as a frequent cause of hip pain in young patients. Similarly, our understanding of and ability to diagnose and treat FAI is also rapidly evolving [1–3]. To this end, mounting evidence suggests that FAI is responsible for mechanical damage to chondrolabral tissue within the hip. For this reason, some authors have suggested that FAI may contribute to early arthritic degeneration in young adult patients [1, 2].

Two mechanisms of femoroacetabular impingement were traditionally described based on characteristic cartilage and labral injury patterns [1]. Cam impingement occurs when a prominence of the femoral neck is forced under the acetabular rim with hip motion. This results in a shearing force on acetabular cartilage and labral tissue. If of sufficient magnitude and duration, cartilage delamination and labral tearing occur. By contrast, pincer impingement is caused by relative or actual acetabular overcoverage of the femoral head. With sufficient hip motion, this area of overcoverage may impact the femoral neck, resulting in a crush-type injury to the labrum. If this conflict is recurrent, this impingement pattern results in intra-substance labral degeneration or tearing and contrecoup chondral injuries [1].

Research performed at the Steadman Philippon Research Institute, Vail, CO, USA.

T.R. Gaskill, M.D.
Bone and Joint Sports Medicine Institute,
Naval Medical Center Portsmouth,
620 John Paul Jones Circle, Portsmouth, VA 23708, USA

Steadman Philippon Research Institute,
The Steadman Clinic, Vail, CO, USA
e-mail: gaski011@gmail.com

M.J. Philippon, M.D. (✉)
Department of Hip Arthroscopy, Steadman Philippon Research Institute and Steadman Clinic, 181 West Meadow Dr., Suite 1000, Vail, CO 81657, USA
e-mail: karen.briggs@sprivail.org, mjp@sprivail.org, drphilippon@sprivail.org

It is critical to understand, however, that FAI is a dynamic disorder. Impingement is ultimately the summation of an individual's specific osseous anatomy and habitual hip motion. Therefore, even normal osseous anatomy may result in symptomatic impingement if hip motion is extreme. Conversely, abnormal acetabular or femoral anatomy is not sufficient to result in impingement unless adequate motion is present. Therefore, abnormal osseous morphology may place a hip at risk and, when coupled with motion beyond a certain threshold, result in symptomatic conflict.

These concepts emphasize that FAI should not be diagnosed based solely on radiologic criteria. Its proper diagnosis and treatment must be based on multiple clinical and subjective factors. This can be difficult considering the array of extra-articular and intra-articular sources of hip pain. To this end, we present our approach to the diagnosis and treatment of femoroacetabular impingement.

Presentation

Femoroacetabular impingement comprises a spectrum of injury patterns and clinical presentations. Moreover, the diagnosis of FAI is complicated by the fact that disorders both intrinsic and extrinsic to the hip can be responsible for eliciting hip symptoms. Despite these complexities, some characteristic findings do exist (Table 18.1).

The majority of patients with symptomatic FAI present secondary to progressive hip pain that is moderate or severe in as many as 85% of this population [4]. Pain located in the anterior groin is a characteristic finding, yet considerable symptomatic overlap does exist. It is our experience that lateral hip, deep posterior hip, and sacroiliac discomfort is experienced by 61%, 52%, and 23% of FAI patients, respectively, upon initial presentation [4]. Others may describe stiffness, weakness, or functional loss as primary complaints, and as many as 92% of patients with FAI will report moderate difficulty or the inability to participate in desired sporting activities [4].

J.W.T. Byrd (ed.), *Operative Hip Arthroscopy*,
DOI 10.1007/978-1-4419-7925-4_18, © Springer Science+Business Media New York 2013

Table 18.1 Common presenting symptoms

Insidious onset of anterior groin pain
Difficulty putting on socks or shoes
Pain when seated for long periods of time or in deep-seated chairs
Hip stiffness or functional loss with sporting activities

Walking greater than 15 min, difficulty getting in or out of cars, and sitting for long periods in deep-seated chairs are activities that are commonly difficult for those with FAI. Others may describe difficulty putting on shoes or socks because of the deep hip flexion required to perform these activities. Less commonly, lumbar, pubis, or lower leg pain is reported. Many of these symptoms likely represent the sequela of compensatory routines developed in response to intra-articular pathology. To this end, many of these symptoms resolve after addressing the femoroacetabular conflict as gait patterns normalize.

More than half of patients report an insidious onset of symptoms without a specific traumatic event [5, 6]. It is not uncommon for patients to initially ignore these symptoms and present only when functional limitations are more significant. In our practice, we have found the time from symptom onset to arthroscopy to be nearly 30 months [5]. As might be expected, longer symptomatic duration has been associated with older patients and arthritic degeneration of the hip [5]. Onset variability does exist, however, and approximately one-quarter of patients will experience symptoms after a traumatic injury, and an additional one-quarter of patients present with acute onset of pain without an associated traumatic event [5]. It is our experience that patients with traumatic etiologies are on average younger and less likely to have osteoarthritis than those with other presentations. More than half of our patients associate symptomatic onset with some type of sporting activity [5].

Potential sources of referred pain to the hip should be thoroughly discussed including degeneration of the lumbar spine, sacroiliac joint, and sciatic nerve involvement. Radicular symptoms are more likely the result of peripheral or central nerve entrapment and may indicate the need for more detailed imaging. Hip flexor- or adductor-related injuries are capable of closely emulating intra-articular symptoms and may be more difficult to differentiate from intra-articular disorders by history alone. Pain localized to the lateral aspect of the hip is often the result of trochanteric bursitis or abductor injury. Patients with these symptoms may complain of difficulty sleeping on the affected side or with activities that load the abductor tendon.

It is apparent, therefore, that patients with FAI encompass a spectrum of disease states and consequently, varied clinical presentations. Groin pain with activity, however, should be recognized as a common complaint for those with symptomatic FAI. Though other presentations are not uncommon,

experience combining multiple facets of the history, physical, and radiographic evaluation will provide an appropriate diagnosis in most circumstances.

Physical Examination

An improved understanding of FAI has resulted in a more effective clinical examination of the hip over the past decade. A comprehensive examination provides the opportunity to evaluate both dynamic and static etiologies of hip pain and to differentiate intra-articular from extra-articular sources of pain. Therefore, the history obtained facilitates an appropriately directed physical examination that is in turn, a critical foundation for further evaluation, imaging, and surgical recommendations.

Our physical examination typically begins with an assessment of the patient's gait and stance. A Trendelenburg gait or sign indicates poor abductor function that is usually the result of chronic deconditioning or advanced arthritic change. An antalgic gait is also frequently seen in the setting of degenerative changes. It is our anecdotal experience that inadequate abductor function is a poor prognostic indicator with respect to surgical outcome. If patients are otherwise good candidates for arthroscopic intervention, they are first referred to physical therapy for rehabilitation. Evidence of global hyperlaxity is also assessed as these patients may be more likely to experience postsurgical instability and may require anterior capsular plication.

It is our practice to next palpate all bony protuberances of the hip. Though this is admittedly unrevealing with regard to intra-articular pain etiologies, it often facilitates identification of extra-articular referred pain sources and concomitant secondary pain generators. Exquisite point tenderness just posterior to the greater trochanter is characteristic of trochanteric bursitis. Though this frequently improves with nonsurgical management postarthroscopy, it may be necessary to release the iliotibial band in chronic or recalcitrant cases. More proximal and anterior greater trochanteric tenderness is characteristic of degeneration or partial tearing of the gluteus medius insertion [7]. Abductor injuries can be mistaken for trochanteric bursitis and should therefore be considered when trochanteric injections do not relieve discomfort [8]. Anterior thigh tenderness may reflect psoas irritation or chronic coxa saltans. Less commonly, tenderness of the hamstrings, quadratus lumborum, piriformis, sacroiliac joint, pubis, or ischium may suggest potential sources of referred pain.

Hip range of motion is assessed and is commonly decreased as compared to the uninvolved extremity [5]. For this reason, bilateral hip motion is routinely assessed and recorded with the use of a goniometer. Supine hip flexion, abduction, adduction, and extension and prone internal and external rotation are customarily recorded. We have found the prone position to provide a reproducible and accurate measurement of hip internal and external rotation. It is also occasionally helpful to measure internal and external rotation with the hip flexed to 90° if postsurgical adhesions are suspected. This position relaxes the iliofemoral ligament, which may become entrapped in the presence of anterior capsular adhesions. Regardless of technique, it is important to stabilize the pelvis with each measurement to avoid axial skeleton compensation of decreased femoroacetabular motion. Pain at end ranges of motion is also recorded as these areas may indicate areas of irritability or conflict.

Specialized Tests

FABER

As in the knee and shoulder, we have found a number of specialized maneuvers helpful in the assessment of patients with femoroacetabular impingement. The FABER test is performed by placing the heal of 1 ft just above the patella of the contralateral extremity [5, 9]. The vertical distance between the lateral femoral epicondyle and the examination table is measured while stabilizing the pelvis. This distance is compared to the contralateral extremity and is almost uniformly greater in the symptomatic hip (see Fig. 18.1). We regard this measurement as an indication of articular irritability and apprehension, as examination under anesthesia

typically reveals nearly symmetric measurements. An abnormal examination has been reported to be present in as many as 97% of patients with FAI [5].

Impingement Signs

As described by Klaue et al., the anterior impingement sign is performed by flexing the hip to 90° and maneuvering the hip into adduction and internal rotation [10]. This position reproduces femoroacetabular conflict in the anterosuperior quadrant of the acetabulum and results in pain when positive. We regard this as the most sensitive test for traditional FAI, and it is reported to be present in 99% of this population [5]. Conversely, the posterior impingement test is performed by positioning the patient near the end of the examination table with both legs flexed to the chest, thereby eliminating lumbar lordosis. The affected extremity is then abducted and externally rotated into an extended position. This maneuver reproduces posterior rim conflict and will result in pain if positive. Martin et al. recently reported this test has high interobserver agreement but is infrequently performed by many surgeons [4].

Capsular Laxity Tests

Hip instability is assessed using the external rotation dial test and axial traction apprehension test [11]. The examiner assesses the resting external rotation of the knee. An abnormal examination is present if the extremity rests in some

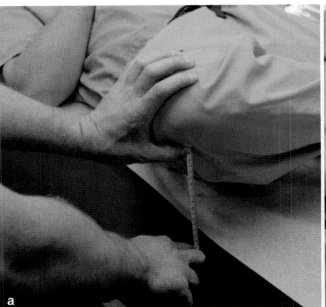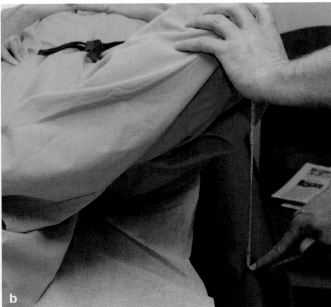

Fig. 18.1 Clinical image depicting a FABER test for hip apprehension and capsular irritability. The asymptomatic side (**a**) demonstrates a shorter measured distance from the lateral epicondyle to the examining table as compared to the symptomatic side (**b**)

degree of external rotation and a firm endpoint is not encountered with additional manual external rotation [11] (see Fig. 18.2). By contrast, the examination is normal if the extremity rests in a neutral position or a firm endpoint is encountered with external rotation. The axial traction apprehension test is performed by stabilizing the pelvis of the involved extremity with one hand while applying axial traction with the other (see Fig. 18.3). If apprehension or a "pop" is experienced, this may indicate generalized capsular laxity that is analogous to the sulcus sign of the shoulder. We believe these tests indicate iliofemoral or generalized capsular laxity that may require a capsular plication for management.

Psoas Irritation

Psoas irritation or labral damage can be assessed using the resisted straight leg raise or Stinchfield test [12]. This maneuver should reproduce anterior groin or thigh pain when positive. Maslowski et al. recently found this test to be the most specific test for intra-articular hip pain [12]. A positive test may indicate psoas irritation or compression of a damaged acetabular labrum [4]. If confirmed at arthroscopy, a fractional psoas lengthening may be required, especially if in the context of increased femoral anteversion (see Fig. 18.4). We no longer perform psoas releases at its insertion on the lesser trochanter because of the prolonged weakness associated with this release. Under the appropriate circumstances, iliotibial band, hip flexor, and abductor flexibility is also assessed.

Pain Test

We will also frequently perform a pain test using 1% lidocaine without epinephrine as a diagnostic measure to confirm an intra-articular etiology of pain in complicated cases [13]. This can be performed in the clinic or under fluoroscopic guidance. Although varied reports exist, the reliability of pain relief after an intra-articular injection of local anesthetic is as high as 90% in some series [13].

As with most orthopedic disorders, the combination of a comprehensive history and physical examination reveals a diagnosis in the majority of patients. Furthermore, it provides a foundation for which to base imaging studies, nonsurgical management, or appropriate subspecialty referral.

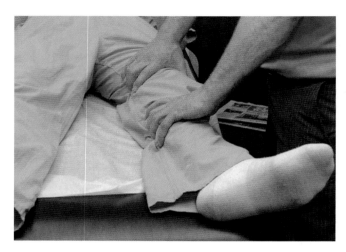

Fig. 18.2 Clinical image demonstrating the external rotation dial test for anterior capsular laxity. The extremity must rest in external rotation and no firm endpoint met with passive external rotation for the test to be considered abnormal

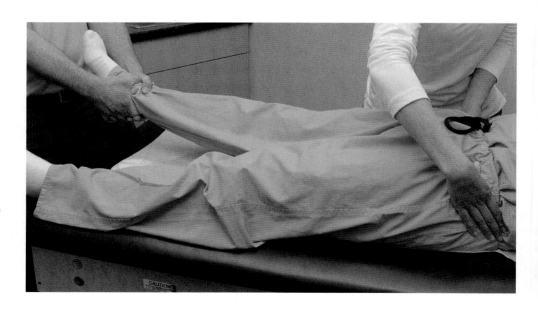

Fig. 18.3 Clinical image depicting the axial traction apprehension test. The pelvis is stabilized and axial traction is applied to the symptomatic extremity. If apprehension or discomfort is experienced, the possibility of hip instability should be considered

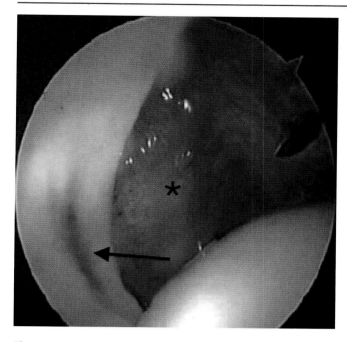

Fig. 18.4 Intraoperative image of a right hip viewing from the antero-lateral portal in the supine position. Capsular (*asterisk*) and labral irritation (*arrow*) are common in the setting of psoas dysfunction

Imaging

Plain Radiographs

Radiographic evaluation of the young adult hip has evolved considerably over the past decade as our understanding of structural hip disorders has improved. Hip imaging is presently a critical element of understanding the pathoanatomical causes of hip pain and, in some cases, can be predictive of surgical outcome. To this end, many radiographic measurements and signs have been described as markers of structural disease. While it is outside the scope of this chapter to discuss each of these markers, we will discuss the ones we utilize frequently in clinical practice.

Plain radiographs are the foundation upon which more sophisticated techniques are built and are obtained on all patients being evaluated for FAI. We prefer an anteroposterior (AP) view of the pelvis and a cross-table lateral. Radiographs are highly technique dependent, and to ensure accurate and reproducible diagnosis of structural abnormalities, it is important that standardized imaging protocols be used [14].

The AP pelvic radiograph is used primarily to assess the bony morphology of the acetabulum. We routinely calculate the lateral center edge angle, sharps angle, and weight-bearing surface (WBS) inclination as indicators of acetabular coverage. Though normal values vary, we generally use center edge angles >40°, WBS inclination <0°, and sharps angles <30° as indicators of acetabular overcoverage [15]. By contrast, values of <25°, >10°, and >42° for center edge, WBS inclination, and sharps angles, respectively, are indicators of inadequate acetabular coverage [15]. Femoroacetabular joint space is measured at the fovea, lateral, and medial sourcil. We have found that any measurement less than 2 mm is a significant indicator of poor surgical outcome after hip arthroscopy [3]. A foveal measurement of >10 mm indicates a lateralized femoral hip center and is frequently seen in patients with acetabular dysplasia [14]. By contrast, measurements significantly less than 10 mm can indicate relative acetabular overcoverage by way of a medialized hip center [14]. Measurements are used in combination to assess morphology and preoperatively estimate the magnitude of correction necessary to correct the deformity. Recommending hip arthroscopy in patients with even subtle dysplasia should be undertaken cautiously. Recent evidence suggests many of these patients will not benefit from hip arthroscopy for isolated labral treatment and, in some cases, may actually accelerate arthritic progression [16].

Although these measurements provide an objective assessment of acetabular morphology, an appraisal of relative acetabular overcoverage is also important. Relative acetabular overcoverage occurs with the acetabular orientation, or depth is abnormal enough to result in impingement despite normal bony morphology. Evidence of either acetabular protrusion or coxa profunda or the presence of a crossover sign is an indicator of relative overcoverage. The crossover sign is described as a radiographic indicator of acetabular retroversion [17]. If true acetabular retroversion results in a relative overcoverage anteriorly and acetabular morphology is normal, it must consequently produce a relative undercoverage posteriorly. Therefore, true acetabular retroversion is accompanied by an abnormal posterior wall sign (center of femoral head is lateral to posterior wall) (see Fig. 18.5). By contrast, isolated anterior overcoverage is recognized by the presence of a crossover sign without posterior wall deficiency (normal posterior wall sign). These subtleties are important when determining appropriate rim resection in cases of pincer impingement.

The cross-table lateral radiograph is used to calculate an alpha angle as an indicator of abnormal femoral neck morphology [18]. We typically consider angles greater than 45–50° abnormal; however, it is important to realize that lesser deformity may still contribute to symptomatic impingement. Though conflicting evidence exists, we have found that an increased alpha angle is correlated with decreased hip range of motion and increased chondral and labral injury [19].

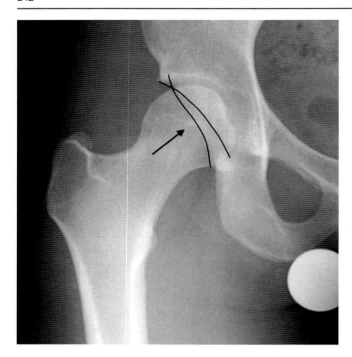

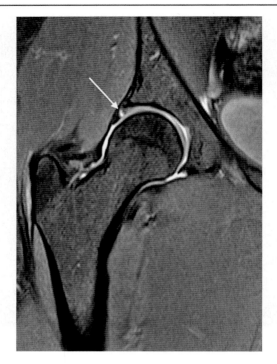

Fig. 18.5 Anteroposterior radiograph of right hip demonstrating a crossover sign consistent with acetabular retroversion. Note the anterior and posterior rim "crossover" (*lines*) prior to meeting at the lateral acetabular edge. A posterior wall sign is also visualized, as the posterior acetabular wall does not pass lateral to the center of the femoral head (*arrow*). This is consistent with true acetabular retroversion and not isolated anterior overcoverage

Fig. 18.6 Representative sagittal T2-weighted MRI image of the right hip. Evidence of chondrolabral injury consistent with femoroacetabular impingement is apparent (*arrow*)

Magnetic Resonance Imaging

Perhaps some of the most fundamental advances in the diagnosis and treatment of young adult hip pain have emerged from MRI technology. It has the unique ability to precisely define soft tissue abnormalities that are not appreciable by plain radiograph or CT. For this reason all patients with suspected FAI undergo MRI imaging. MR arthrograms have been traditionally recommended for evaluation of FAI. Many authors have suggested that an MR arthrogram is more sensitive in detecting labral tears and chondral defects as compared to non-contrasted studies [20–22]. Currently, we do not routinely obtain arthrogram images because our clinical experience has been good using higher resolution 3-T images. Regardless of the images obtained, the hip should be evaluated for labral tears and chondral defects characteristic of FAI (see Fig. 18.6). The tear magnitude and residual labral tissue available for repair should be estimated, as some degenerative labral tears may not be repairable. When diminutive labral tissue is present, we frequently recommend an iliotibial band labral reconstruction in an attempt to restore the anatomic labral seal [23, 24]. Finally, evidence of ligamentum teres injury, capsular laxity, and femoral anteversion is sought. Ligamentum teres injury can contribute to intra-articular hip pain and may be important to hip stability in

patients such as ballet dancers who display extreme motion ranges [25–30]. To date, the ability of MRI and MRA imaging to diagnose ligamentum injuries has been modest at best. Therefore, it is important to carefully evaluate this structure at the time of arthroscopy.

Surgical Technique

Surgical Setup and Traction

(See Video 18.1: http://goo.gl/Vxww3) All arthroscopic hip procedures are performed on a standard fracture table in a modified supine position. We commonly place patients under a general anesthetic although spinal anesthesia can also be used. Regardless of the surgical anesthetic, it is necessary to maintain complete skeletal muscle relaxation at all times to ensure the minimum amount of traction is used to maintain hip distraction (Table 18.2).

After carefully padding both feet, distraction of the operative hip is accomplished by first placing the extremity in a position of 10° of hip flexion, 15° of internal rotation, and neutral abduction (see Fig. 18.7). A large perineal post is used to avoid excessive perineal pressure and to apply a lateralizing force on the proximal femur. Traction is applied to break the hip suction seal. The extremity is then slightly adducted across the perineal post, acting to lever the femoral

Table 18.2 Key surgical technique points

Supine positioning with large perineal post
Complete muscle paralysis ensured prior to application of traction
Confirm femoroacetabular distraction of 1 cm radiographically
Establish anterolateral and mid-anterior portals
Capsulotomy made >1 cm distal to labrum avoiding the iliofemoral ligament
Diagnostic arthroscopy performed
Synovectomy and debridement of unrepairable labral tissue completed
Traction removed to perform CAM resection, thereby minimizing duration of traction time
Traction applied for pincer resection, labral repair, and completion of intra-articular work
Dynamic examination performed ensuring no residual impingement exists and that the labral seal is reproduced
Fine adjustments of labral repair and osteoplasty made as needed

head slightly laterally. After applying countertraction to the contralateral limb, additional traction is applied to produce a minimum of 10-mm distraction as confirmed by fluoroscopy. Usually, approximately 50 lb of traction is needed to produce this amount of distraction [31].

Portal Placement

As with all arthroscopic procedures, accurate portal placement is essential to avoid neurovascular structures, provide optimal visualization, and facilitate anchor placement. We utilize two portals for arthroscopic hip procedures including the anterolateral and mid-anterior portals (see Fig. 18.8). The anterolateral portal is placed 1 cm superior and 1 cm anterior to the tip of the greater trochanter. The mid-anterior portal is localized in the soft area between the sartorius and tensor musculature approximately 7 cm distal and medial to the anterolateral portal on a 45° plane. The anterolateral portal is localized using a spinal needle, which is advanced at an angle of approximately 20° cranially and 20° posteriorly (toward the floor) to enter the joint. Fluoroscopy can be utilized if difficulty is encountered placing the needle within the acetabulum. The joint is then insufflated, and retrograde flow should be noted, thereby confirming intra-articular placement. Efflux of particulate matter confirms intra-articular damage.

Once the anterolateral portal is established, the arthroscope is introduced and the anterior triangle formed by the capsule, labrum, and femoral head is visualized. A spinal needle is placed under direct visualization to avoid injury to the labrum and articular cartilage. The arthroscope is switched into the mid-anterior portal to confirm the anterolateral portal does not pass through the lateral labrum. A beaver blade is used to perform a capsulotomy 1 cm distal to the labrum,

connecting the two arthroscopic portals. Once this is accomplished, a thorough diagnostic arthroscopy is performed.

The pathology identified preoperatively and confirmed during the diagnostic arthroscopy dictates the operative arthroscopic procedure. It is critical to carefully examine the ligamentum teres for damage as it is elusive to current imaging techniques, can contribute to hip pain, and may be critical to stability in some highly flexible patients [11, 29, 30, 32]. Typically a synovectomy and ligamentum teres debridement is performed using a radio-frequency (RF) probe when capsular synovitis or ligamentum hypertrophy is present (see Fig. 18.9). Any degenerative, unrepairable labral tissue is carefully debrided using the oscillating shaver or RF probe. Next, any intra-articular chondral damage is addressed by performing chondroplasty or microfracture for partial or full thickness injuries, respectively [33, 34].

Traction is removed, and the hip is flexed in neutral rotation to approximately 45°. An oscillating shaver is used to debride soft tissue exposing the peripheral compartment. A femoral neck osteoplasty is then completed using a shielded round burr from the medial to lateral synovial fold (see Fig. 18.10). This should recreate a normal anatomic femoral neck contour. Failure to extend the femoral neck osteoplasty far enough distally is, in our experience, a common cause of failure of FAI procedures. Therefore, it is critical to be conscious of this during dynamic hip examination.

If a rim resection is required, traction is reapplied, and the central compartment is entered again. To decrease the incidence of adhesions between the capsule and labrum, we have begun performing labral detachment and rim resection extracapsularly while viewing from the central compartment (see Fig. 18.11). A curved banana blade is used extracapsularly to separate the labrum from the bony acetabulum. Next, a shielded arthroscopic burr is used to correct acetabular overcoverage. It is critical to avoid excessive bony resection as this can lead to iatrogenic hip instability [11, 35, 36]. The labrum is then repaired back to the acetabular rim by sequentially placing anchors to secure detached labral tissue [37, 38] (see Fig. 18.12). We believe it to be biomechanically important for the suture from at least one of these anchors to be placed circumferentially around the labrum to facilitate early hip mobilization. The remainder of the stitches is selectively placed around or through the labrum to appropriately evert the labrum to anatomically conform to the femoral head. We believe this is critical in an attempt to restore the labral seal (see Fig. 18.13). We will frequently take the extremity in and out of traction to perform dynamic examinations to ensure appropriate suture tension and labral eversion.

Once the labrum is reattached, the hip is taken out of traction, and dynamic examinations are performed to ensure

Fig. 18.7 Preoperative image illustrating patient positioning and the standard operative setup for a right hip arthroscopy in the supine position (**a**). Note the operative extremity is flexed approximately 15° and internally rotated. The standard preparation and draping is completed using a shower curtain (**b**)

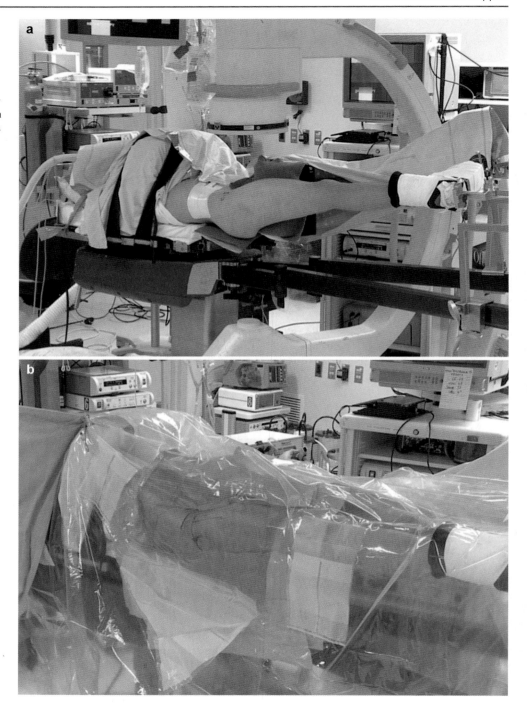

impingement is no longer possible considering the activities they desire to return to. We also meticulously evaluate the conformity of the labrum to the femoral head. If the labrum lifts away from the femoral head or is lifted by abnormal bony morphology, labral fixation is revisited or fine femoral neck contouring is performed. This is continued until a smooth transition is noted through all motion planes. Athletes are taken out of traction boots and placed through sport-specific motions to ensure no impingement occurs during these activities.

Prior to procedure completion, specific releases are performed as clinically indicated. Often, an erythematous capsule is noted when significant psoas irritation is present (see Fig. 18.4). We perform a fractional lengthening by releasing only the tendinous fibers of the psoas. Again, in an effort to prevent capsular adhesions, we perform this lengthening

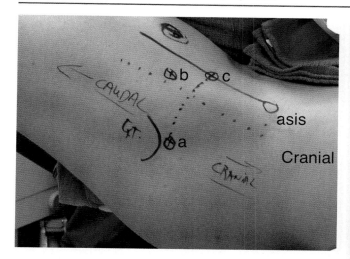

Fig. 18.8 Intraoperative image illustrating a left hip in the supine position. Standard lateral peritrochanteric (*a*) mid-anterior portals (*b*) are visualized. An anterior arthroscopic portal is also marked (*c*) for illustrative purposes but is not routinely used by the senior author

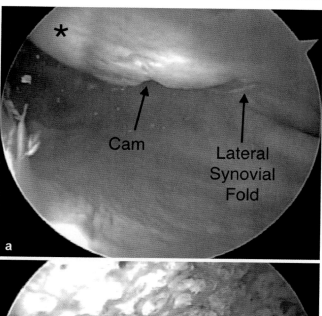

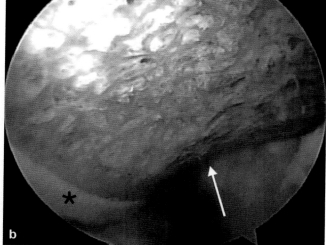

Fig. 18.10 Intraoperative image of a right hip viewing from the anterolateral peritrochanteric portal in the supine position. A CAM lesion is visualized along the lateral femoral neck (**a**). The distal femoral head (*asterisk*) and lateral epiphyseal vessels are also visualized (*arrow*). A completed femoral neck osteoplasty after recontouring of the CAM deformity (*arrow*) is visualized (**b**)

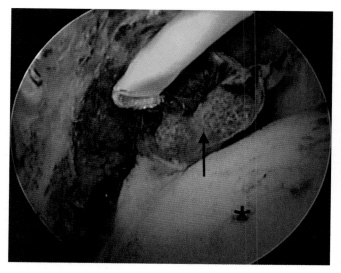

Fig. 18.9 Intraoperative image of a left hip viewing from the anterolateral peritrochanteric portal in the supine position. A synovitic and partially torn ligamentum teres (*arrow*) and cotyloid fossa are illustrated prior to radiofrequency debridement. The femoral head is also visualized (*asterisk*)

extracapsularly by viewing through a small capsular window rather than extend our capsulotomy medially to visualize the psoas tendon. We feel a more extensive medial release can lead to anterior hip instability by releasing the entire iliofemoral ligament. Peritrochanteric arthroscopy is performed as necessary at this point after traction has been released.

We believe the iliofemoral ligament is critical to postoperative anterior hip stability [11]. For this reason, we avoid performing an extensive capsulotomy and routinely repair or plicate the anterior capsule at the completion of each case (see Fig. 18.14). In patients with redundant capsule or an abnormal preoperative external rotation dial test, a capsular plication is performed. Alternatively, the capsular edges are simply reapproximated using a heavy absorbable rack-and-hitch-type stitch. It is also our practice to supplement arthroscopic surgical repairs using a platelet-rich plasma injection. Routine portal closure is performed and sterile dressings applied. Anti-rotational boots designed to avoid external rotation are applied to prevent tensioning the anterior capsular repair in the immediate postoperative period.

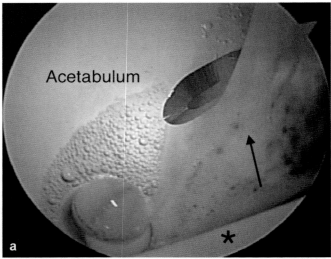

Fig. 18.11 Intraoperative image of the anterolateral acetabular rim of a right hip, viewing from the anterolateral peritrochanteric portal in the supine position. A beaver blade is used to separate the capsulolabral interface using an extracapsular approach to minimize capsulolabral adhesions (**a**). A hemorrhagic labrum (*arrow*) and the femoral head (*asterisk*) are also seen. A burr (*arrow*) is used extracapsularly to resect the pincer lesion prior to labral repair (**b**). The acetabular labrum is also visualized (*asterisk*)

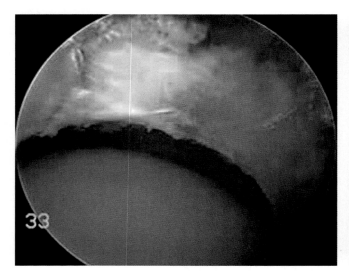

Fig. 18.12 Intraoperative image of a right hip viewing from the mid-anterior portal in the supine position. The repaired labrum is seen prior to releasing traction and testing the labral seal

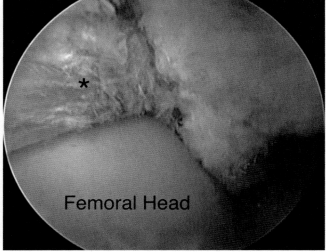

Fig. 18.13 Intraoperative image of a left hip viewing from the antero-lateral peritrochanteric portal in the supine position. The repaired labrum (*asterisk*) is visualized, reapproximated, and appropriately everted against the femoral head. We believe this is important to help restore the normal labral seal

Rehabilitation

Though recommended rehabilitation protocols will vary based on the specific procedure performed, 10–12 weeks of supervised therapy is generally sufficient for most arthroscopic hip procedures. Immediate postsurgical goals include inflammation control, restoration of motion, and protection of repaired tissues. Therapy routinely begins the morning of postoperative day 1, although it may begin the same day as

surgery in some circumstances. A postoperative hip brace is worn to limit abduction and axial rotation. Depending on the procedure performed, weight bearing is restricted to 20 lb for 3–8 weeks postoperatively. Anti-rotation bands are used for the first few weeks to avoid excessive tension on the repaired anterior capsular structures. This initial phase is typically 4–6 weeks in duration and incorporates early continuous passive motion (CPM), stationary bicycle, and circumduction. Extreme flexion or abduction is restricted to avoid irritation of the capsulolabral complex. Full passive range of motion is

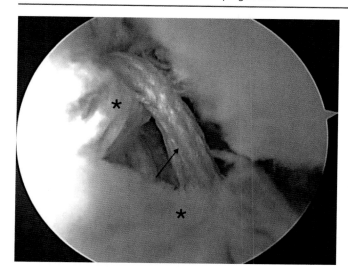

Fig. 18.14 Intraoperative image of a left hip viewing from the antero-lateral peritrochanteric portal in the supine position. Capsular edges (*asterisks*) can be seen being reapproximated by a large absorbable suture (*arrow*) prior to final tensioning

usually allowed beginning 2 weeks after surgery as dictated by the patient's comfort. Activity progression though this phase integrates active motion, isometric exercises targeting the gluteus medius muscle, an aquatic program, and upper body exercises. An emphasis on circumduction (passive motion) has resulted in a dramatic decrease in the incidence of adhesion formation in our patients.

The second phase of rehabilitation begins 4–6 weeks postsurgically with the goals of improving lumbopelvic stability and beginning early strengthening exercises. Weight bearing is slowly advanced over the first 7–10 days as tolerated by the patient. Gentle stretching exercises focusing on hip flexors, quadriceps, hamstrings, and iliotibial band are also initiated. Hip rotation is also started during this phase of rehabilitation. A specific focus on hip abductor strengthening is also beneficial during this phase of recovery. A sport-specific program is instituted, and, based on the procedure performed and patient progress, return to sport is typically possible between 10 and 16 weeks postsurgically.

Results

Evidence documenting satisfactory outcomes after arthroscopic management of femoroacetabular impingement continues to accumulate. Two-year follow-up of a cohort of 112 patients revealed a significant improvement in modified Harris hip score and an overall patient satisfaction score of 9 out of 10 [3]. Byrd et al. also reported a series of patients with two year follow-up and found favorable results [39]. Despite these encouraging reports, outcomes are not uniform

and patient selection remains important. Patients who exhibit considerable arthritic change or less than 2 mm of acetabular joint space are associated with poor surgical outcomes [3]. It is also our experience that patients with lower preoperative modified Harris hip scores or abductor deconditioning are at high risk for less optimal surgical results [3]. Although treatment plans are individualized to the patient, these cohorts represent relative contraindications to arthroscopic intervention in our practice.

Caution should also be used in cases of mild acetabular dysplasia. These patients tend to be highly dependent on the labrum for hip stability but may also demonstrate focal retroversion, subspinous impingement, or large CAM lesions. If arthroscopy is recommended, it is our experience that minimal acetabular resection, capsular plication, and labral repair, augmentation, or reconstruction are critical to maximize surgical improvement. Therefore, while interest in arthroscopic management of femoroacetabular impingement is high, it is apparent that patient selection and realistic postoperative expectations remain critical to maximize patient satisfaction.

Acknowledgments   No financial support in the form of grants, equipment, or other items was received in relation to the completion of this work.

Vail Valley Medical Center IRB approval (PRO# 2002-03) was received for completion of this manuscript.

References

1. Ganz R, Parvizi J, Beck M, et al. Femoroacetabular impingement: a cause for osteoarthritis of the hip. Clin Orthop Relat Res. 2003;(417):112–20.
2. McCarthy JC, Noble PC, Schuck MR, et al. The Otto E. Aufranc Award: the role of labral lesions to development of early degenerative hip disease. Clin Orthop Relat Res. 2001;(393):25–37.
3. Philippon MJ, Briggs KK, Yen YM, et al. Outcomes following hip arthroscopy for femoroacetabular impingement with associated chondrolabral dysfunction: minimum two-year follow-up. J Bone Joint Surg Br. 2009;91:16–23.
4. Martin HD, Kelly BT, Leunig M, et al. The pattern and technique in the clinical evaluation of the adult hip: the common physical examination tests of hip specialists. Arthroscopy. 2010;26:161–72.
5. Philippon MJ, Maxwell RB, Johnston TL, et al. Clinical presentation of femoroacetabular impingement. Knee Surg Sports Traumatol Arthrosc. 2007;15:1041–7.
6. Clohisy JC, Knaus ER, Hunt DM, et al. Clinical presentation of patients with symptomatic anterior hip impingement. Clin Orthop Relat Res. 2009;467:638–44.
7. Tibor LM, Sekiya JK. Differential diagnosis of pain around the hip joint. Arthroscopy. 2008;24:1407–21.
8. Domb BG, Nasser RM, Botser IB. Partial-thickness tears of the gluteus medius: rationale and technique for trans-tendinous endoscopic repair. Arthroscopy. 2010;26:1697–705.
9. Vad VB, Bhat AL, Basrai D, et al. Low back pain in professional golfers: the role of associated hip and low back range-of-motion deficits. Am J Sports Med. 2004;32:494–7.

10. Klaue K, Durnin CW, Ganz R. The acetabular rim syndrome. A clinical presentation of dysplasia of the hip. J Bone Joint Surg Br. 1991;73:423–9.
11. Philippon MJ, Zehms CT, Briggs KK, et al. Hip instability in the athlete. Oper Tech Sports Med. 2007;15:189–94.
12. Maslowski E, Sullivan W, Forster Harwood J. The diagnostic validity of hip provocation maneuvers to detect intra-articular hip pathology. PM R. 2010;2:174–81.
13. Byrd JW, Jones KS. Diagnostic accuracy of clinical assessment, magnetic resonance imaging, magnetic resonance arthrography, and intra-articular injection in hip arthroscopy patients. Am J Sports Med. 2004;32:1668–74.
14. Clohisy JC, Carlisle JC, Trousdale R, et al. Radiographic evaluation of the hip has limited reliability. Clin Orthop Relat Res. 2009;467: 666–75.
15. Sharp IK. Acetabular dysplasia: the acetabular angle. J Bone Joint Surg Br. 1961;43-B:268–72.
16. Parvizi J, Bican O, Bender B, et al. Arthroscopy for labral tears in patients with developmental dysplasia of the hip: a cautionary note. J Arthroplasty. 2009;24:110–3.
17. Reynolds D, Lucas J, Klaue K. Retroversion of the acetabulum. A cause of hip pain. J Bone Joint Surg Br. 1999;81:281–8.
18. Notzli HP, Wyss TF, Stoecklin CH, et al. The contour of the femoral head-neck junction as a predictor for the risk of anterior impingement. J Bone Joint Surg Br. 2002;84:556–60.
19. Johnston TL, Schenker ML, Briggs KK, et al. Relationship between offset angle alpha and hip chondral injury in femoroacetabular impingement. Arthroscopy. 2008;24:669–75.
20. Burgess RM, Rushton A, Wright C. The validity and accuracy of clinical diagnostic tests used to detect labral pathology of the hip: a systematic review. Man Ther. 2011;16(4):318–26. Epub 2011 Feb 10.
21. Keeney JA, Peelle MW, Jackson J, et al. Magnetic resonance arthrography versus arthroscopy in the evaluation of articular hip pathology. Clin Orthop Relat Res. 2004;(429):163–9.
22. Smith TO, Hilton G, Toms AP, et al. The diagnostic accuracy of acetabular labral tears using magnetic resonance imaging and magnetic resonance arthrography: a meta-analysis. Eur Radiol. 2011;21:863–74.
23. Philippon MJ, Briggs KK, Hay CJ, et al. Arthroscopic labral reconstruction in the hip using iliotibial band autograft: technique and early outcomes. Arthroscopy. 2010;26:750–6.
24. Philippon MJ, Schroder e Souza BG, Briggs KK. Labrum: resection, repair and reconstruction sports medicine and arthroscopy review. Sports Med Arthrosc. 2010;18:76–82.
25. Haviv B, O'Donnell J. Arthroscopic debridement of the isolated Ligamentum Teres rupture. Knee Surg Sports Traumatol Arthrosc. 2011;19(9):1510–3. Epub 2010 Nov 13.
26. Bardakos NV, Villar RN. The ligamentum teres of the adult hip. J Bone Joint Surg Br. 2009;91:8–15.
27. Cerezal L, Kassarjian A, Canga A, et al. Anatomy, biomechanics, imaging, and management of ligamentum teres injuries. Radiographics. 2010;30:1637–51.
28. Wenger D, Miyanji F, Mahar A, et al. The mechanical properties of the ligamentum teres: a pilot study to assess its potential for improving stability in children's hip surgery. J Pediatr Orthop. 2007;27:408–10.
29. Wenger DR, Mubarak SJ, Henderson PC, et al. Ligamentum teres maintenance and transfer as a stabilizer in open reduction for pediatric hip dislocation: surgical technique and early clinical results. J Child Orthop. 2008;2:177–85.
30. Wettstein M, Garofalo R, Borens O, et al. Traumatic rupture of the ligamentum teres as a source of hip pain. Arthroscopy. 2005;21:382; author reply 383.
31. Byrd JW. Hip arthroscopy. The supine position. Clin Sports Med. 2001;20:703–31.
32. Byrd JW, Jones KS. Traumatic rupture of the ligamentum teres as a source of hip pain. Arthroscopy. 2004;20:385–91.
33. Philippon MJ, Schenker ML, Briggs KK, et al. Can microfracture produce repair tissue in acetabular chondral defects? Arthroscopy. 2008;24:46–50.
34. Crawford K, Philippon MJ, Sekiya JK. Microfracture of the hip in athletes. Clin Sports Med. 2006;25:327–35, x.
35. Matsuda DK. Acute iatrogenic dislocation following hip impingement arthroscopic surgery. Arthroscopy. 2009;25:400–4.
36. Ranawat AS, McClincy M, Sekiya JK. Anterior dislocation of the hip after arthroscopy in a patient with capsular laxity of the hip. A case report. J Bone Joint Surg Am. 2009;91:192–7.
37. Philippon MJ, Wolff AB, Briggs KK, et al. Acetabular rim reduction for the treatment of femoroacetabular impingement correlates with preoperative and postoperative center-edge angle. Arthroscopy. 2010;26:757–61.
38. Philippon MJ, Schenker ML. A new method for acetabular rim trimming and labral repair. Clin Sports Med. 2006;25:293–7, ix.
39. Byrd JWT, Jones KS. Arthroscopic management of femoroacetabular impingement with minimum two-year follow-up, Arthroscopy 2011;27(10):1379–1388.

Computer Navigation in Hip Arthroscopy

19

Michael Knesek, Jack G. Skendzel, and Asheesh Bedi

Introduction

The term femoroacetabular impingement (FAI) was first described by Ganz et al. [1, 2] as an anatomic abnormality whereby there is a loss of femoral head-neck offset and prominence at the head-neck junction. The pathomechanics of hip impingement has been implicated as a significant cause of hip pain, and there is evidence to suggest that these changes are associated with the premature development of hip osteoarthritis [1–6]. In addition, focal rim impingement of the acetabular labrum with subsequent damage and tearing has been suggested as an important step in the pathway of hip degeneration [4, 6]. Recently, arthroscopic surgical techniques have evolved to treat a spectrum of pathologic conditions associated with femoroacetabular impingement. Despite these advances, however, hip arthroscopy remains a technically challenging procedure with a steep learning curve. As a result, computer-assisted navigation and modeling have emerged as a potential solution to improve both the preoperative planning for FAI lesions, including determination of the location and size of cam and rim lesions, as well as increasing the accuracy of intraoperative correction of the osseous deformity. The goal of these technologies is to improve efficiency, reproducibility, and long-term clinical outcomes by minimizing the potential for incomplete correction of the osseous deformities.

Computer-Assisted Surgery in Orthopedics

The goal of computer- and navigation-based systems in orthopedic surgery is to provide patient-specific tools that improve accuracy and allow for reliable execution of focused, preoperative surgical plans in the operating room [7]. Ideal application of these systems would integrate the display of a preoperative plan based on prior imaging studies (CT or MRI) with surgical treatment workflows for various procedures that correlate with intraoperative anatomy, allowing for precise placement of tools with instant quantitative feedback to assess the execution of the operative plan. As described by Specht and Koval [8], computers augment orthopedic care through five fundamental characteristics: geometric precision, reproducibility, perfect "memory," lack of fatigue, and insensitivity to radiation. Currently, applications of computer-assisted devices in orthopedic surgery include navigated total knee and hip replacement, navigated ACL reconstruction, and robotic unicondylar knee replacement [9–11].

Data to support improved outcomes after computer-navigated orthopedic surgery are still lacking. Although navigated total knee arthroplasty is one of the most popular applications of computer-assisted orthopedic surgery, no studies are available to validate these technologies and to prove a short- or long-term benefit. While navigation has been shown to improve the acetabular cup position in total hip arthroplasty and the position of unicondylar total knee replacements, the purported benefits of technical precision and reproducibility have yet to be correlated with superior clinical outcomes [10, 12]. As elements of navigation technology currently utilized in the field of joint arthroplasty are applied to hip arthroscopy, critical examination of its limitations and potential for improvement is of paramount importance. There remain significant obstacles in the integration of computer-assisted surgery, including but not limited to the cost of these systems,

M. Knesek, M.D. • J.G. Skendzel, M.D.
Department of Orthopaedic Surgery,
University of Michigan,
1500 East Medical Center Drive,
Ann Arbor 48109, MI, USA
e-mail: mknesek@gmail.com; jacksken@med.umich.edu

A. Bedi, M.D. (✉)
Sports Medicine and Shoulder Surgery,
Department of Orthopaedic Surgery,
Hospital for Special Surgery,
24 Frank Lloyd Wright Drive, Lobby A,
Ann Arbor, MI 48106, USA

MedSport,
Ann Arbor, MI, USA
e-mail: abedi@umich.edu

J.W.T. Byrd (ed.), *Operative Hip Arthroscopy*,
DOI 10.1007/978-1-4419-7925-4_19, © Springer Science+Business Media New York 2013

the learning curve associated with new devices, and a lack of documented improvements on long-term clinical outcome and patient satisfaction.

As our understanding of FAI continues to improve, however, there is increased interest regarding computer-assisted planning and navigation to treat pathologic abnormalities associated with FAI. The challenges of preoperative characterization of the mechanical deformities combined with the difficulties of reliable intraoperative exposure and correction of impingement lesions may make computer-assisted surgical systems particularly useful in this setting. While the long-term clinical outcome may be multifactorial, a reproducible and accurate surgical correction of the deformity may be one of the few surgeon-controlled variables with FAI to maximize the likelihood of a successful clinical outcome.

Pathoanatomy of Femoroacetabular Impingement

The hip joint is a constrained articulation between the femoral head and the acetabulum. It acts as a multiaxial ball-and-socket joint that transfers forces from the upper body to the lower extremity, in addition to allowing for motion throughout the gait cycle. In fact, nearly all hip motion is rotational with very little translation [13]. For the purpose of discussion and for the computer software that models hip motion, the center of rotation is assumed to be a fixed point on the femoral head.

Femoroacetabular impingement is a distinct pathological entity that occurs as a result of abnormal contact between the proximal femur and the acetabular rim [2, 14] (Fig. 19.1). FAI is recognized as an early cause of hip dysfunction, including pain generation, degeneration, and tearing of the labrum, and is the most common cause for degenerative changes in the nondysplastic hip [1, 2, 15–17]. Although two distinct types of FAI are recognized ("cam" and "pincer"), most often patients present with clinical and radiographic findings suggestive of both deformities [5]. Cam impingement refers to a decrease in the femoral head-neck offset and/or asphericity of the femoral head-neck junction, causing a prominent osseous lesion that impinges on the acetabulum. While most anterior "cam" lesions impinge with flexion, adduction, and internal rotation of the hip joint, the location of impingement is unique and defined by the medial-lateral, proximal-distal, and circumferential margins of the loss of offset. Pincer or focal rim impingement lesions cause abnormal edge loading of the acetabular rim and can be attributed to focal or global acetabular retroversion, coxa profunda, or protrusio acetabuli [1, 18].

Characteristic injury to the labrum and chondral surfaces has also been observed with FAI and reflects repetitive microtrauma from the abnormal osseous morphology. The labrum has multiple functions, including augmentation of femoral head coverage, hip stability, cartilage nutrition, and a "joint-sealing" effect [19, 20]. The patterns of injury to the

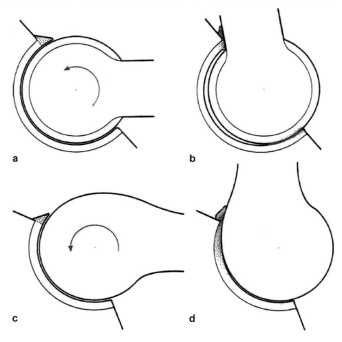

Fig. 19.1 Femoroacetabular impingement. (**a**) In pincer impingement, there is acetabular overcoverage which leads to mechanical "pinching" of the labrum anteriorly between the femur and acetabular rim (**b**). In cam impingement, there is a loss of femoral head-neck offset with a prominent "bump" (**c**) that causes damage to the articular cartilage and labrum during hip flexion and internal rotation (**d**) (Reprinted from Ganz [1]. With permission from Springer Science+Business Media)

labrum and articular cartilage are a unique "fingerprint" that reflects the specific rim and head-neck offset deformity. In typical cam impingement, there is early delamination of the cartilage with labral degeneration and detachment over time as a result of chronic repetitive stresses. In contrast, the labrum is often the first structure to be affected by rim impingement due to mechanical impingement between the bony femur and acetabulum with subsequent degeneration, ossification, and eventual failure [5].

Both open and arthroscopic approaches can be effectively employed in the surgical management of FAI. Ganz et al. [21] described a technique of open surgical dislocation of the hip joint to minimize iatrogenic injury to the articular surfaces and obtain a safe, 360° view of the hip joint. The risks of open dislocation include avascular necrosis due to disruption of femoral head blood supply, nonunion after trochanteric osteotomy, and increased morbidity with soft tissue dissection [22]. Other open techniques have been described, including the Hueter anterior approach, which provides direct visualization of the femoral head-neck junction without dislocation, although lateral and posterior femoral and rim pathology may not be addressed [23]. Hip arthroscopy has evolved to treat both labral and chondral lesions as well as correct osseous impingement lesions, allowing for a minimally invasive approach to the central and peripheral compartments [24–26]. Arthroscopic treatments for FAI-associated pathology (labral tears, chondral damage, synovitis, and loose bodies) have been reported with favorable short- and midterm clinical outcomes [24, 27–29]. Furthermore, Bedi et al. [26] and Ng et al. [30] performed systematic reviews to assess differences in outcomes between open and arthroscopic treatment of FAI. The authors concluded that, despite limited data, open techniques to address FAI and labral tears are not superior to arthroscopic techniques.

Computer-Aided Surgery in Femoroacetabular Impingement

Computer-aided navigation in hip arthroscopy was developed to overcome the limitations and technical difficulties inherent to arthroscopic treatment of FAI. The procedure has a "steep" learning curve and incomplete exposure, and correction of the pathologic mechanical factors is not an uncommon cause for surgical failure [31, 32]. Specifically, the hip joint is located deeper within the body and surrounded by numerous muscles, ligaments, and critical neurovascular structures. In addition, its constrained osseous geometry and enveloping capsule result in a limited working area, making visualization difficult [33]. These anatomic factors may prevent the surgeon from appreciating the size and location of focal rim lesions and/or abnormal femoral offset, resulting in either an inadequate resection or overzealous resection, precipitating an increased risk of femoral neck fracture [34, 35].

The theoretical goals of computer-assisted navigation include improved objective kinematics and clinical outcomes through resection of the entire impingement zone in an accurate, reproducible, and efficient way that is less dependent upon surgical experience. In addition, it can allow for identification of neurovascular structures at risk and anatomical variants, improving the level of safety. While further research is required to improve the integration of computer navigation with current surgical techniques, it is an emerging field that has many potential benefits in the treatment of prearthritic hip disease and femoroacetabular impingement.

Preoperative CT scans can be used by navigation software to create a 3D model of the area of interest. This allows for definition of the impingement location and quantification of the size and morphology of the cam and focal rim lesions. As a result, the surgeon can plan and "template" the amount and location of osteoplasty preoperatively and compare the intraoperative fluoroscopic images to the templated, ideal correction. The previously obtained CT or MRI imaging data may also be linked to the patient's position through identification of anatomic landmarks that allow for accurate tracking of the acetabulum and femur in real time. The mechanical axis of the femur, as defined by the center of the femoral head and the midpoint between the femoral condyles, in addition to the anatomic axis of the femur is defined. The position of the pelvis is also entered based on specific landmarks. The areas of pathologic bone can be highlighted and complete removal ensured through the use of navigation software. By registration of the tools as well, their

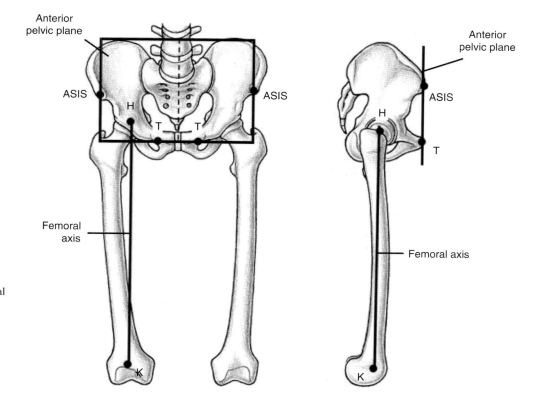

Fig. 19.2 The computer software utilizes various reference points both on the pelvis and femur to define spatial orientation. *ASIS* anterior superior iliac spine, *T* pubic tubercle, *H* hip center, *K* knee center (Reprinted from Tannast et al. [36, p. 125]. With permission from John Wiley & Sons, Inc.)

position in real time can be tracked relative to the femur and pelvis to help guide the surgeon to resect the impingement lesions in the anatomically correct regions.

Several authors have described specific computer-aided systems for the arthroscopic treatment of FAI [36–39]. Tannast et al. [36] described a noninvasive, three-dimensional CT-based method to evaluate the accuracy and reliability of a computer-assisted system in the assessment and treatment of FAI. The authors developed and validated a software program called HipMotion prior to testing in a clinical pilot study. This software creates a 3D model of the pelvis and femur based on preoperative CT scans of the pelvis and femoral condyles, utilizing various reference points including the anterior superior iliac spines and the pubic tubercles to define the so-called anterior pelvic plane (APP). Femoral reference points including the center of the femoral head and knee are used to set the mechanical axis, and the plane of the posterior aspect of the femoral condyles sets the coronal femoral reference (Fig. 19.2). Validation using cadaveric hips and sawbones was performed by comparing the virtual predicted hip ROM to the real hip motion. In a pilot study involving 150 normal hips in the control group, and 31 hips with clinical and radiographic signs of FAI in the study group, those with FAI had significantly decreased flexion, internal rotation at 90° of flexion, and abduction ($p < 0.001$); there was a trend toward decreased flexion in hips with pincer-type impingement when compared to those with cam-type impingement, although it was not statistically significant ($p = 0.08$). The authors demonstrated that hips with FAI have significantly decreased motion in flexion and internal rotation and that the HipMotion software provides reliable kinematic analysis of hip range of motion for the evaluation of hip impingement, both preoperatively and after femoral and acetabular reshaping procedures (Fig. 19.3). This model was further validated by Kubiak-Langer et al. [37] with surgically simulated femoroacetabular osteoplasty, showing predictable decreases in flexion, internal rotation at 90° of flexion, and abduction in those with FAI and significant improvements in these motions after virtual resection of the osseous lesions. These models, however, are not without limitations. They currently do not model for soft tissues and their effect on joint motion. Furthermore, they cannot be applied to dysplastic and severely osteoarthritic hips where a nonconcentric joint allows rotational and translational motion that makes reliable determination of the femoral head center of rotation difficult. Although the authors' computer software (HipMotion) was not directly linked to a surgical navigation system, it is nevertheless a useful tool for the development of future computer-navigated technologies in hip arthroscopy.

Brunner et al. [38] developed a computer-navigated system based on CT imaging to assess offset correction after resection of cam-type FAI lesions. Fifty patients with cam FAI were prospectively evaluated and treated, with 25 patients randomly assigned to a navigated treatment group and 25 to a

non-navigated treatment. Preoperative CT scans of the pelvis were compared to postoperative MRI imaging to determine if there was a significant reduction in the alpha angle after arthroscopic treatment. An alpha angle less than 50° or an absolute reduction in the alpha angle greater than 20° was considered effective treatment. The navigation software utilized (modified version of Brainlab Hip CT, Brainlab AG, Feldkirchen, Germany) generated 3D imaging of the hip-based preoperative CT scans and allowed for cross-referencing with intraoperative fluoroscopy. This allowed for real-time visualization of instrument position in relation to the head-neck junction and cam lesion during the procedure (Fig. 19.4). Overall, the mean alpha angle improved from 76.6° to 54.2° after hip arthroscopy with computer-navigated guidance. Despite this improvement, six patients in each group failed to show sufficient femoral head-neck restoration of offset (12/50 = 24%). The authors concluded that the magnitude of alpha angle correction was not reliably improved with a computer-based navigation system. There was no, however, significant difference in clinical outcomes between those with adequate and inadequate correction of the alpha angle after a mean follow-up of 26.5 months. In addition to a short follow-up period, a significant limitation of this study was the initial evaluation and 3D modeling of the deformity based on preoperative CT scans with subsequent postoperative comparison made on 2D MRI studies to measure the alpha angle.

Monahan and Shimada [40] tested the effectiveness of a computer-aided navigation system using an encoder linkage

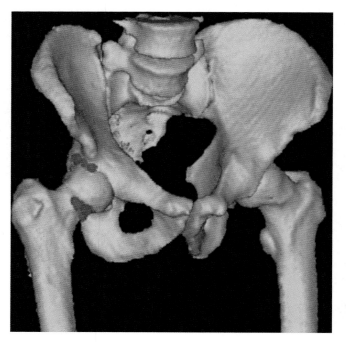

Fig. 19.3 The HipMotion software is able to predict the impingement sites on both the femur and acetabulum, as indicated by *red dots* (Reprinted from Tannast et al. [36, p. 125]. With permission from John Wiley & Sons, Inc.)

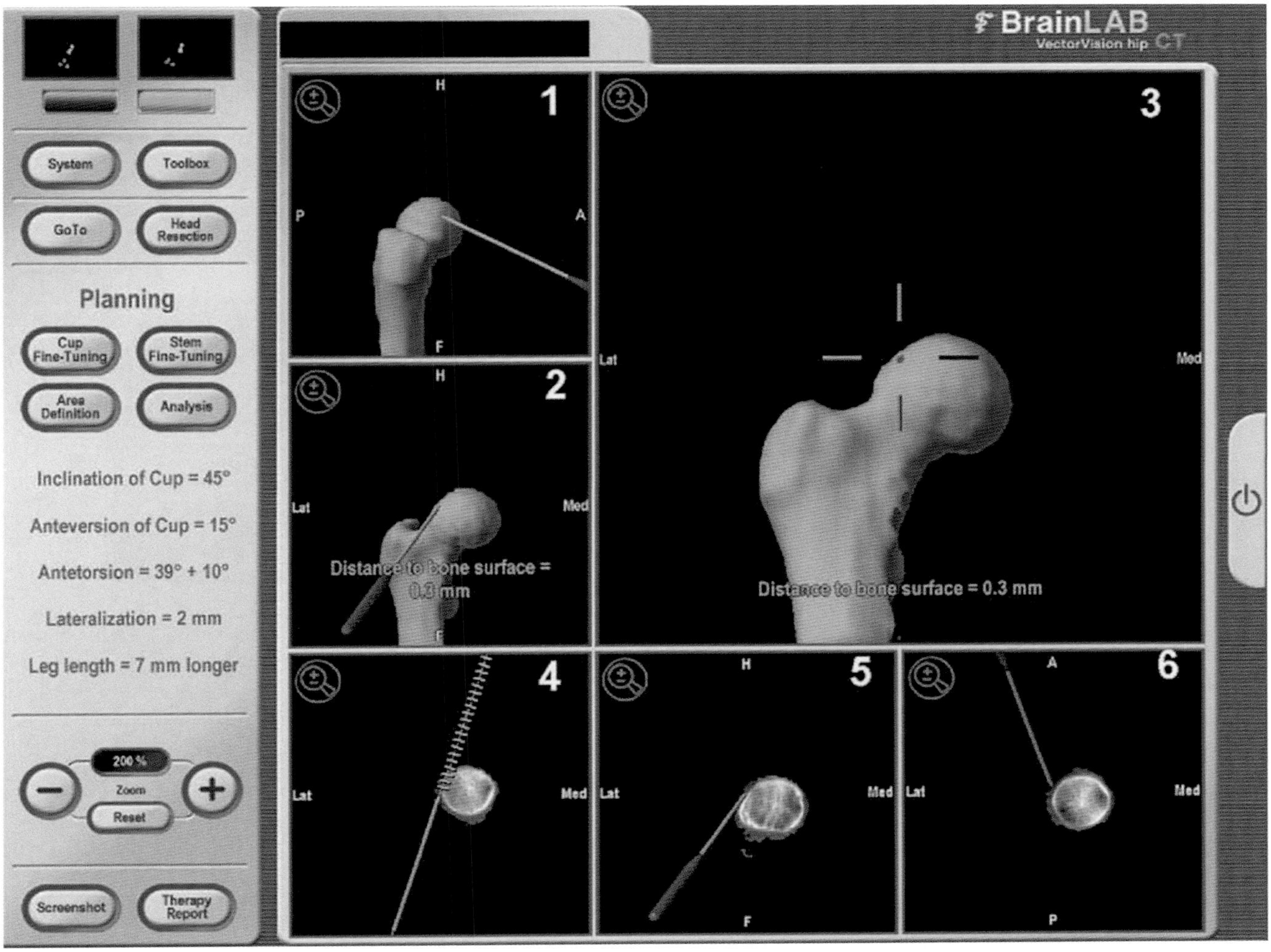

Fig. 19.4 Screen shot demonstrates the ability to visualize the position of the surgical instrument in real time in relation to the femoral head and neck (Reprinted from Brunner et al. [38, p. 386]. With permission from Elsevier)

to determine arthroscopic tool position in relation to the patient's anatomic structures. The authors developed a computer system to increase visual feedback to the surgeon in real time through a set of linkage encoders that are attached both to the surgical instrument and to a base pin for reference [33, 40] (Fig. 19.5). The base pin is placed in the patient's hip and serves as the connector between the linkage system and the patient. Preoperative 3D imaging data (CT or MRI) is used to create a model of the patient's anatomy, including critical neurovascular structures that must be avoided during arthroscopic surgery. Using a simulated hip joint model, including a plastic cover to mimic skin and cotton filling to simulate soft tissues, ten participants were instructed to find two targets on the femur by using the arthroscopic camera and encoder linkage system. The time for task completion was recorded from the beginning of the simulation until the targets were identified with the camera. The tool path length was also collected based on the 3D coordinates of the tool

throughout the study. After completing the simulation both with and without the computer-aided navigation encoder linkage system, there was an average 38% reduction in the time to task completion and an average 71.8% decrease in tool path length with the navigation system.

While there are clear benefits to decreasing tool motion during a hip arthroscopy procedure, such as a decreased risk of damage to soft tissues and neurovascular structures, the authors acknowledge there is much room for improvement in computer-aided hip navigation, including better visual display of the tool position alongside the camera display, and obtaining input and feedback regarding the system from experienced, adept hip arthroscopists.

Lastly, a novel in vitro hip joint simulation algorithm termed "the equidistant method" was developed by Puls et al. [39] to detect the location and size of FAI lesions. Using sawbone model (Pacific Research Laboratories, Vashon, WA) of pelvises and femora, modifications were made to the head-neck

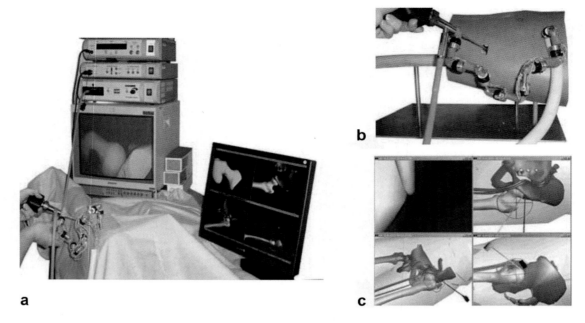

Fig. 19.5 Setup during computer-aided hip arthroscopy. (**a**) Computer system; (**b**) camera with attached encoder linkage system; (**c**) screenshots showing visual representation of the surgical tools and patient's anatomy during the procedure (Reprinted from Monahan and Shimada [40, p. 304]. With permission from IOS Press)

junction of the proximal femur and to the acetabulum to simulate the pathoanatomy of cam and focal rim impingement lesions. Three-dimensional models were then created based on these models. The pelvi were subsequently fixed in space to a table, and specific anatomic landmarks (i.e., anterior superior iliac spine, anterior inferior iliac spine, etc.) were identified to create a coordinate system and to register the sawbones with their respective 3D digital models. The models were then taken through various paths of motions that were recorded through a navigation system. Areas of impingement were identified, and four simulation algorithms (equidistant, simple, constrained, and translated) were applied to the motion paths and 3D modeling data to detect impingement (Fig. 19.6). The results demonstrated that the equidistant method was the most accurate hip joint simulation algorithm tested in the study ($p < 0.05$) and that the size of the impingement zone with the equidistant method was smaller when compared to the other methods. The authors attributed the improved accuracy of their method to the ability of the software to calculate a dynamic hip center of rotation instead of a predefined, fixed center of rotation as used in the other algorithms. Nevertheless, there were several limitations to this study, including the use of sawbones and the absence of load-bearing and dynamic muscular contribution to the kinematic analysis. In addition, the algorithm only models areas of osseous impingement and does not account from impingement from both the static (i.e., labrum, capsule) and dynamic (i.e.,

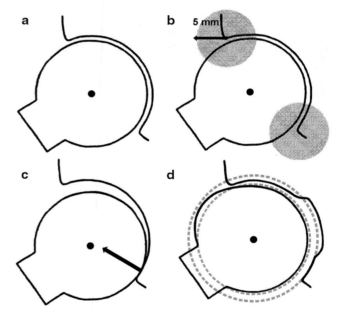

Fig. 19.6 Schematic depiction of the four different hip joint simulation methods: (**a**) Simple method has a fixed center of rotation. (**b**) Constrained method uses a 5-mm detection perimeter at the acetabular rim. (**c**) Translated method has an additional translation vector which is perpendicular to areas of intra-articular impingement. (**d**) Equidistant method uses a computer femoral and acetabular sphere to compute a dynamic hip center of rotation (Reprinted from Puls et al. [39, p. 76]. With permission from Taylor & Francis, Inc.)

muscle, tendon). Further investigation is required to determine the clinical utility of this model and its ability to achieve efficient and reproducible resection of impingement pathology.

Case Example of Preoperative Planning for FAI

Case examples of combined FAI (Video 19.1: http://goo.gl/3c1aV) and subspinous impingement (Video 19.2: http://goo.gl/peYLu) are illustrated. The authors' preferred system (*A2 Surgical*) for preoperative planning of FAI surgery is demonstrated. This tool is the only available system that incorporates the complex anatomical parameters on both the femoral and acetabular side and dynamically determines all potential sources of mechanical conflict (including femoral version, neck-shaft angle, acetabular version, three-dimensional head-neck offset, etc.). In this regard, the system is unique in that it provides insight into (i) whether an arthroscopic, open, or combined approach is necessary to address intra-articular and extra-articular pathology, (ii) whether acetabular, femoral, or combined deformity must be addressed, (iii) where the specific location of mechanical conflict is occurring with dynamic maneuvers of the hip, and (iv) how much must be resected to eliminate mechanical conflict and achieve a target improvement in hip kinematics and motion.

A high-resolution computed tomography (CT) scan of the involved hip is loaded into the system. The sequences must include thin cut images of the iliac spines, hip, and knee to allow for development of an accurate three-dimensional model (left screen). The model is built to allow for synchronized evaluation of structures on the standard two-dimensional sequences (right) to correlate with the location on the three-dimensional model (left) (Fig. 19.7).

The software will then automatically calculate and determine the center of the femoral head (Fig. 19.8). This position can be manually adjusted by the user if necessary to adjust to preferable location.

A three-dimensional model of the femur is generated. The neck-shaft angle and anteversion is determined. A three-dimensional map of the head-neck junction is also generated (Fig. 19.9).

Similarly, a three-dimensional model of the pelvis and acetabulum is generated. A virtual fluoroscopic image is also created (right). This is of tremendous value, as it can be matched with the preoperative radiographs or intraoperative fluoroscopic image to correct for pelvic tilt or rotation. The three-dimensional

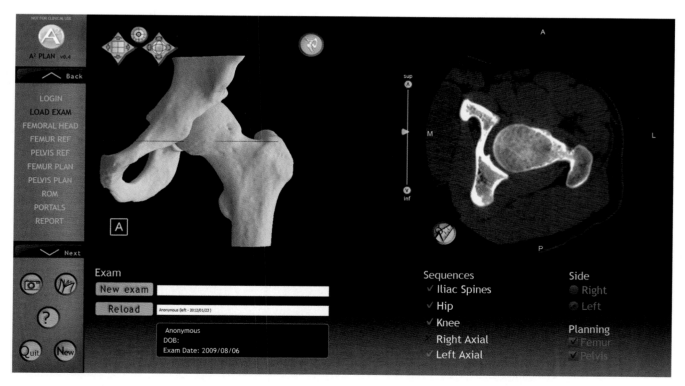

Fig. 19.7 High-resolution computed tomography (CT) scan of the involved hip is loaded into the system. The sequences must include thin cut images of the iliac spines, hip, and knee to allow for development of an accurate three-dimensional model (*left screen*). The model is built to allow for synchronized evaluation of structures on the standard two-dimensional sequences (*right*) to correlate with the location on the three-dimensional model (*left*)

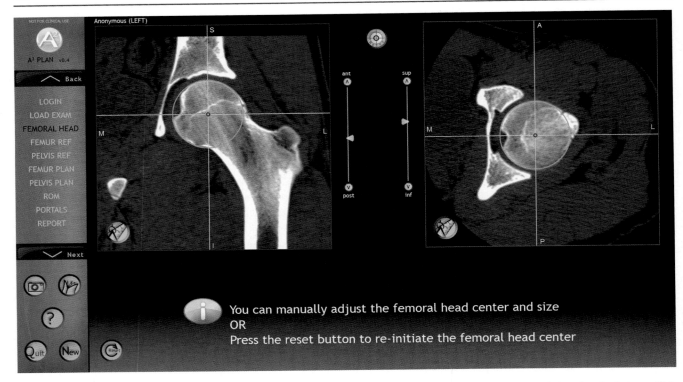

Fig. 19.8 The software will automatically calculate and determine the center of the femoral head in the coronal, axial, and sagittal planes. This position can be manually adjusted by the user if necessary to adjust to preferable location

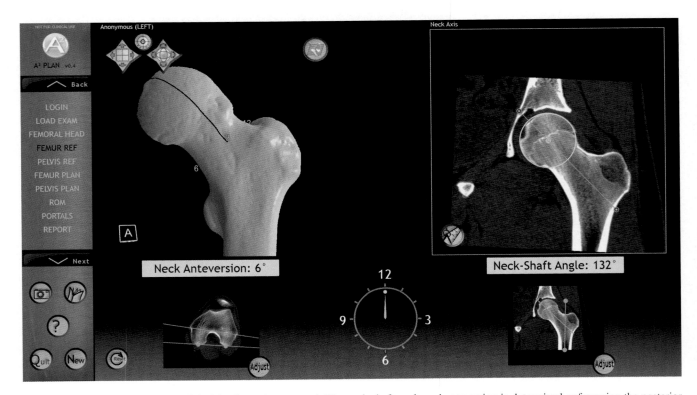

Fig. 19.9 A three-dimensional model of the femur is generated. The neck-shaft angle and anteversion is determined, referencing the posterior condylar axis at the knee. A three-dimensional map of the head-neck junction is also generated

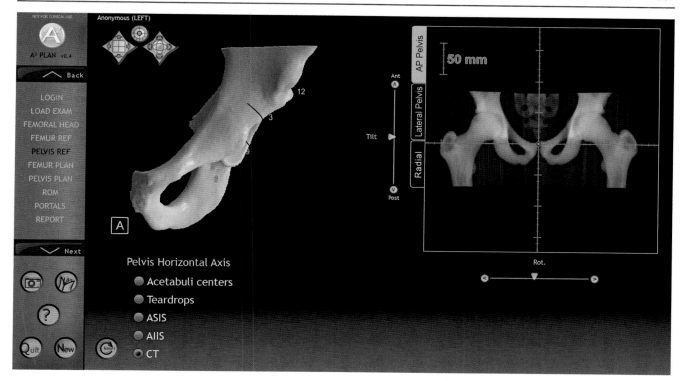

Fig. 19.10 A three-dimensional model of the pelvis and acetabulum is generated. A virtual fluoroscopic image is also created (*right*). This is of tremendous value, as it can be matched with the preoperative radio-graphs or intraoperative fluoroscopic image to correct for pelvic tilt or rotation. The three-dimensional model (*left*) will correspondingly adjust with the fluoroscopic image to reflect these changes in tilt and obliquity

model (left) will correspondingly adjust with the fluoroscopic image to reflect these changes in tilt and obliquity (Fig. 19.10).

The femoral-sided correction can now be defined and templated (Fig. 19.11). The target alpha angle to restore desired sphericity can be adjusted (in this example, a target of 47° has been selected). The software then determines the three-dimensional region of asphericity and delineates a topographic map of the cam lesion. The peak zone of loss of offset is also defined along the clockface of the head-neck junction and is of significant utility in defining the optimal intraoperative fluoroscopic position necessary to identify and resect bone at the location of maximum deformity. The volume of the necessary resection is also defined.

The desired correction on the acetabular side can also be templated (Fig. 19.12). The desired correction can be determined via several methods. This includes by defining a "global" target version for the entire socket or "focal" target versions for each different location along the circumference of the acetabulum (i.e., 0° at 12 o'clock, 5° at 1 o'clock, 10° at 2 o'clock, and 15° at 3 o'clock). The correction can also be simply defined by the area of mechanical conflict that observed after dynamization of the hip to positions that are reproductive of the patient's symptoms.

The templating software can also generate a virtual fluoroscopic image (right) demonstrating changes that occur pre- and post-correction of the acetabulum (Fig. 19.13). This feature is of great utility in correlating the template resection with anticipated changes in the crossover sign (right) or other radiographic landmarks that can be appreciated intraoperatively.

The combined model can be dynamized to determine the precise locations of mechanical conflict (Fig. 19.14). The dynamization can simulate physical examination maneuvers that were reproductive of clinical symptoms, but may also include dynamic, sport-specific motions (i.e., throwing a baseball, kicking a football, etc.) that are specific athletic complaints secondary to the hip impingement. In this regard, the A2 software is remarkably powerful in generating a patient-specific, individualized treatment plan that is unique to their specific demands and expectations.

After dynamization, the pelvis and/or acetabulum can be variably subtracted from the image to allow for direct definition and inspection of the zone of mechanical impingement on the rim and/or head-neck junction (Fig. 19.15). Zones of extra-articular impingement (i.e., ischiofemoral impingement, sub-spine impingement, etc.) may also be apparent that may alter the treatment plan or indicate the need for a combined surgical approach.

The computer software system also allows for direct comparison of the femoral deformity before and after surgical

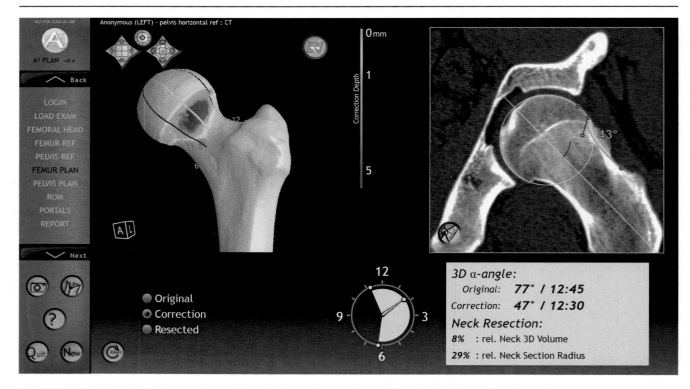

Fig. 19.11 The femoral-sided correction is defined and templated. The target alpha angle to restore desired sphericity can be adjusted. The software then determines the three-dimensional region of asphericity and delineates a topographic map of the cam lesion. The peak zone of loss of offset is also defined along the clockface of the head-neck junction and is of significant utility in defining the optimal intraoperative fluoroscopic position necessary to identify and resect bone at the location of maximum deformity

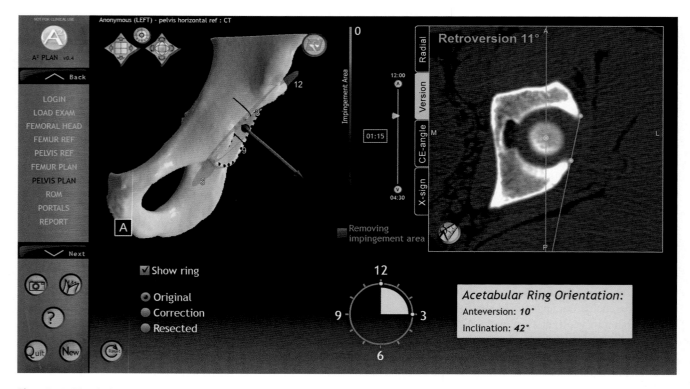

Fig. 19.12 The desired correction on the acetabular side can be templated. In this example, it is defined relative to a "global" target version for the entire socket. The program also allows for "focal" target versions for each different location along the circumference of the acetabulum (i.e., 0° at 12 o'clock, 5° at 1 o'clock, 10° at 2 o'clock, and 15° at 3 o'clock)

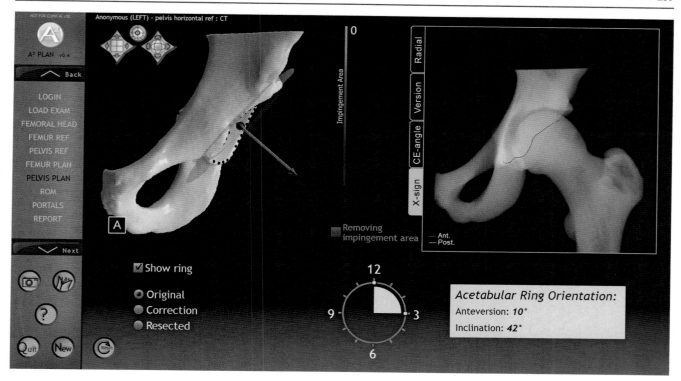

Fig. 19.13 The templating software can generate a virtual fluoroscopic image (*right*) demonstrating changes that occur pre- and post-correction of the acetabulum. This feature is of great utility in correlating the template resection with anticipated changes in the crossover sign (*right*) or other radiographic landmarks that can be appreciated intraoperatively

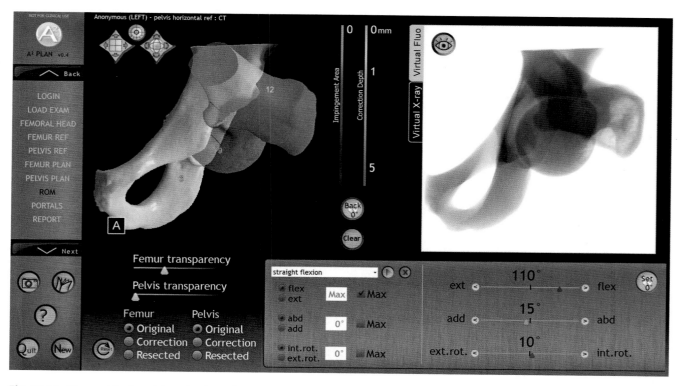

Fig. 19.14 The combined model can be dynamized to determine the precise locations of mechanical conflict. The dynamization can simulate physical examination maneuvers that were reproductive of clinical symptoms, but may also include dynamic, sport-specific motions that are specific athletic complaints secondary to the hip impingement

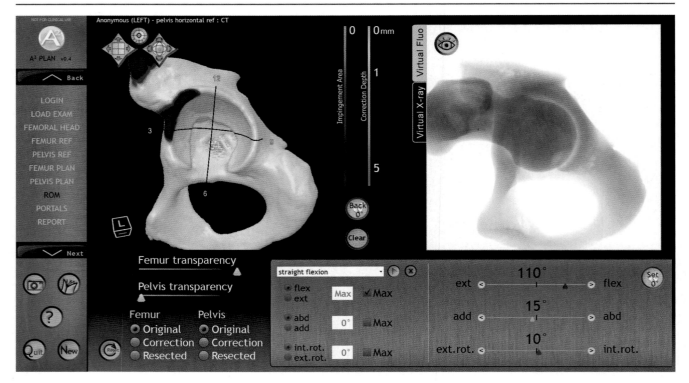

Fig. 19.15 Zones of extra-articular impingement (i.e., ischiofemoral impingement, sub-spine impingement) may also be apparent that may alter the treatment plan or indicate the need for a combined surgical approach. The femur can be subtracted to help in the direct visualization and identification of these areas of potential conflict

correction (Fig. 19.16a, b) It provides not only a three-dimensional image of the femoral head-neck junction but also a corresponding extended neck lateral fluoroscopic image with the precise coordinates of leg flexion/extension, adduction/abduction, and internal/external rotation to achieve this optimal view intraoperatively. The software will generate a three-dimensional model and fluoroscopic image that correlates to the specified, "templated" correction. In this regard, the surgeon can truly use these images as a guide to assure that the intraoperative correction is complete and recapitulates the templated plan in thoroughly addressing the mechanical sources of impingement.

In the current system, high-resolution CT scans are utilized to generate models for dynamization and preoperative templating. Because of the recent concerns in the media regarding radiation exposure from diagnostic studies, we looked into reducing the doses of all our CT scans and altered our scan parameters with our applications team. In consultation with our medical physicist, we looked at our CT hip exposure dose which ranged between 6.8 and 8.2 rad, compared to 3 view x-rays of the hip/pelvis which is 3.4 rad (skin exposure). We have subsequently developed a new protocol decreasing our mAs to a dose of 1.6 rad which is about half of the dose received from 3 plain radiographic views of the hip/pelvis. This protocol has not compromised the quality or diagnostic value of the CT scan.

In the future, improvements in three-dimensional magnetic resonance imaging (MRI) will likely supplant the need for a CT scan for computer-based templating systems. Furthermore, the MRI will also account for potential soft tissue impingement and, in this capacity, offer an even more accurate assessment of range-of-motion and potential pain generators.

Conclusion

Computer-navigation has many potential applications in the diagnosis and treatment of FAI. An ideal system would allow for an accurate dynamic, preoperative assessment of hip impingement based on CT imaging studies and subsequently link this data to the intraoperative anatomy to facilitate an accurate and complete osseous resection. The challenges are numerous, including the financial burden of software development and maintenance, as well as the learning curve associated with these advanced technologies. Currently, no studies are available to show improved clinical outcomes as a result

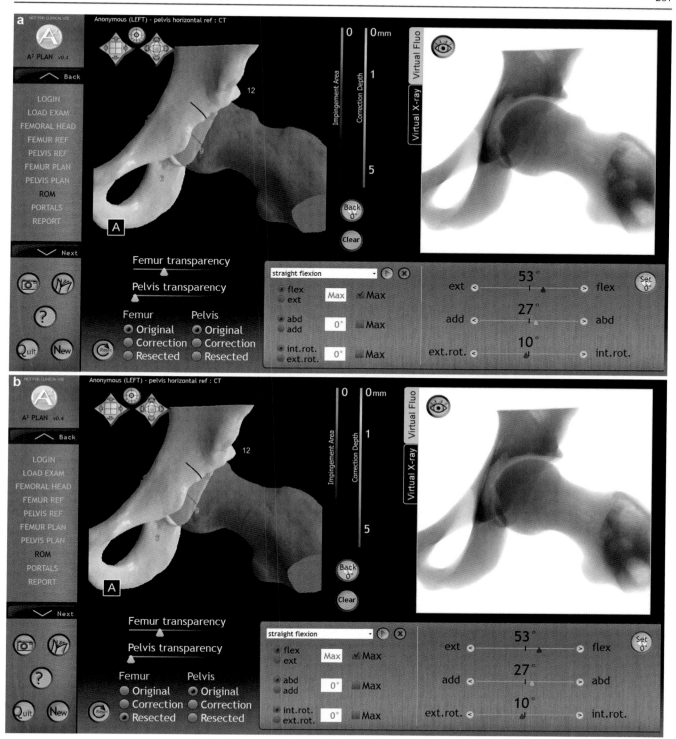

Fig. 19.16 The computer software system also allows for direct comparison of the femoral deformity (**a**) before and (**b**) after surgical correction. It provides not only a three-dimensional image of the femoral head-neck junction but also a corresponding extended neck lateral fluoroscopic image with the precise coordinates of leg flexion/ extension, adduction/abduction, and internal/external rotation to achieve this optimal view intraoperatively. The software will generate a three-dimensional model and fluoroscopic image that correlates to the specified, "templated" correction

of computer navigation in hip arthroscopy. Nevertheless, preliminary work has been encouraging, with the development of software applications that have improved safety and accuracy of tool motion paths and orientation for surgeons relatively new to the practice of hip arthroscopy.

References

1. Ganz R, Leunig M, Leunig-Ganz K, Harris WH. The etiology of osteoarthritis of the hip – an integrated mechanical concept. Clin Orthop. 2008;466(2):264–72.

2. Ganz R, Parvizi J, Beck M, Leunig M, Notzli H, Siebenrock KA. Femoroacetabular impingement: a cause for osteoarthritis of the hip. Clin Orthop. 2003;417:112–20.

3. Murray RO. The aetiology of primary osteoarthritis of the hip. Br J Radiol. 1965;38:810–24.

4. Leunig M, Beck M, Woo A, Dora C, Kerboull M, Ganz R. Acetabular rim degeneration: a constant finding in the aged hip. Clin Orthop. 2003;413:201–7.

5. Beck M, Kalhor M, Leunig M, Ganz R. Hip morphology influences the pattern of damage to the acetabular cartilage – Femoroacetabular impingement as a cause of early osteoarthritis of the hip. J Bone Joint Surg Br. 2005;87B:1012–8.

6. McCarthy JC, Noble PC, Schuck MR, Wright J, Lee J. The Otto E. Aufranc award: the role of labral lesions to development of early degenerative hip disease. Clin Orthop. 2001;393:25–37.

7. Pearle AD, Kendoff D, Musahl V. Perspectives on computer-assisted orthopaedic surgery: movement toward quantitative orthopaedic surgery. J Bone Joint Surg Am. 2009;91 Suppl 1:7–12.

8. Specht LM, Koval KJ. Robotics and computer-assisted orthopaedic surgery. Bull Hosp Jt Dis. 2001;60:168–72.

9. Seon JK, Song EK. Navigation-assisted less invasive total knee arthroplasty compared with conventional total knee arthroplasty – a randomized prospective trial. J Arthroplasty. 2006;21:777–82.

10. Cobb J, Henckel J, Gomes P, et al. Hands-on robotic unicompartmental knee replacement: a prospective, randomised controlled study of the acrobot system. J Bone Joint Surg Br. 2006;88:188–97.

11. Voos JE, Musahl V, Maak TG, Wickiewicz TL, Pearle AD. Comparison of tunnel positions in single-bundle anterior cruciate ligament reconstructions using computer navigation. Knee Surg Sports Traumatol Arthrosc. 2010;18:1282–9.

12. Beckmann J, Stengel D, Tingart M, Gotz J, Grifka J, Luring C. Navigated cup implantation in hip arthroplasty. Acta Orthop. 2009;80:538–44.

13. Bowman Jr KF, Fox J, Sekiya JK. A clinically relevant review of hip biomechanics. Arthroscopy. 2010;26:1118–29.

14. Lavigne M, Parvizi J, Beck M, Siebenrock KA, Ganz R, Leunig M. Anterior femoroacetabular impingement: part I. Techniques of joint preserving surgery. Clin Orthop. 2004;418:61–6.

15. Harris WH. Etiology of osteoarthritis of the hip. Clin Orthop. 1986;213:20–33.

16. Burnett RS, Della Rocca GJ, Prather H, Curry M, Maloney WJ, Clohisy JC. Clinical presentation of patients with tears of the acetabular labrum. J Bone Joint Surg Am. 2006;88:1448–57.

17. Philippon MJ, Schenker ML. Arthroscopy for the treatment of femoroacetabular impingement in the athlete. Clin Sports Med. 2006;25:299–308, ix.

18. Laude F, Boyer T, Nogier A. Anterior femoroacetabular impingement. Joint Bone Spine. 2007;74:127–32.

19. Ferguson SJ, Bryant JT, Ganz R, Ito K. An in vitro investigation of the acetabular labral seal in hip joint mechanics. J Biomech. 2003;36:171–8.

20. Ferguson SJ, Bryant JT, Ganz R, Ito K. The influence of the acetabular labrum on hip joint cartilage consolidation: a poroelastic finite element model. J Biomech. 2000;33:953–60.

21. Ganz R, Gill TJ, Gautier E, Ganz K, Krugel N, Berlemann U. Surgical dislocation of the adult hip a technique with full access to the femoral head and acetabulum without the risk of avascular necrosis. J Bone Joint Surg Br. 2001;83:1119–24.

22. Botser IB, Smith Jr TW, Nasser R, Domb BG. Open surgical dislocation versus arthroscopy for femoroacetabular impingement: a comparison of clinical outcomes. Arthroscopy. 2011;27:270–8.

23. Laude F, Sariali E. Treatment of FAI via a minimally invasive ventral approach with arthroscopic assistance. Technique and midterm results. Orthopade. 2009;38:419–28.

24. Byrd JW, Jones KS. Hip arthroscopy in athletes: 10-year follow-up. Am J Sports Med. 2009;37:2140–3.

25. Stevens MS, Legay DA, Glazebrook MA, Amirault D. The evidence for hip arthroscopy: grading the current indications. Arthroscopy. 2010;26:1370–83.

26. Bedi A, Chen N, Robertson W, Kelly BT. The management of labral tears and Femoroacetabular impingement of the hip in the young, active patient. Arthroscopy. 2008;24:1135–45.

27. Byrd JW, Jones KS. Prospective analysis of hip arthroscopy with 10-year followup. Clin Orthop. 2010;468:741–6.

28. Byrd JW, Jones KS. Prospective analysis of hip arthroscopy with 2-year follow-up. Arthroscopy. 2000;16:578–87.

29. Larson CM, Giveans MR. Arthroscopic management of femoroacetabular impingement: early outcomes measures. Arthroscopy. 2008;24:540–6.

30. Ng VY, Arora N, Best TM, Pan XL, Ellis TJ. Efficacy of surgery for Femoroacetabular impingement a systematic review. Am J Sports Med. 2010;38:2337–45.

31. Heyworth BE, Shindle MK, Voos JE, Rudzki JR, Kelly BT. Radiologic and intraoperative findings in revision hip arthroscopy. Arthroscopy. 2007;23:1295–302.

32. Philippon MJ, Schenker ML, Briggs KK, Kuppersmith DA, Maxwell RB, Stubbs AJ. Revision hip arthroscopy. Am J Sports Med. 2007;35:1918–21.

33. Monahan E, Shimada K. Computer-aided navigation for arthroscopic hip surgery using encoder linkages for position tracking. Int J Med Robot. 2006;2:271–8.

34. Stahelin L, Stahelin T, Jolles BM, Herzog RF. Arthroscopic offset restoration in femoroacetabular cam impingement: accuracy and early clinical outcome. Arthroscopy. 2008;24:51–7.

35. McCarthy JC, Lee J. Hip arthroscopy: indications and technical pearls. Clin Orthop. 2005;441:180–7.

36. Tannast M, Kubiak-Langer M, Langlotz F, Puls M, Murphy SB, Siebenrock KA. Noninvasive three-dimensional assessment of femoroacetabular impingement. J Orthop Res. 2007;25:122–31.

37. Kubiak-Langer M, Tannast M, Murphy SB, Siebenrock KA, Langlotz F. Range of motion in anterior femoroacetabular impingement. Clin Orthop. 2007;458:117–24.

38. Brunner A, Horisberger M, Herzog RF. Evaluation of a computed tomography-based navigation system prototype for hip arthroscopy in the treatment of Femoroacetabular cam impingement. Arthroscopy. 2009;25:382–91.

39. Puls M, Ecker TM, Tannast M, Steppacher SD, Siebenrock KA, Kowal JH. The Equidistant method – a novel hip joint simulation algorithm for detection of femoroacetabular impingement. Comput Aided Surg. 2010;15:75–82.

40. Monahan E, Shimada K. Verifying the effectiveness of a computer-aided navigation system for arthroscopic hip surgery. Westwood JD, Haluck RS, Hoffman HM, et al. Medicine meets virtual reality 16 – parallel, combinatorial, convergent: Nextmed by design. Stud Health Technol Informl. 2008;132:302–7.

Decision Making with Osteoarthritis

20

Thomas G. Sampson

Arthroscopic treatment of hip arthritis is both undefined and controversial. The treatment of advanced hip arthritis is universally accepted to be a total joint replacement (THR), although it too has its own controversies involving approaches and the type of implants to be used. Non-arthroplasty methods to preserve the hip joint, such as open arthrotomy with debridement, osteotomy, and denervation procedures, were historically used with less than ideal results and eventually abandoned after the development of modern THR [1]. Many orthopedic surgeons may have worked through training and their practice careers unaware or rarely considering any alternatives to joint replacement.

With the problems of joint replacements such as early failure, dislocations and infection in a young and active patient population, as well as the numerous recalls of implants due to manufacturing defects, the public is more aware that THR should only be considered if all other alternatives fail. Information on the internet has also provided the public with both reliable and unfiltered information making them weary to throw away their natural hip joint before researching alternatives.

Hip arthroscopy has been utilized as a palliative procedure to bridge the gap for providing pain relief in those too young or with little damage from hip arthritis to justify THR.

Very little has been written on the arthroscopic treatment for hip arthritis in the past 30 years, and what has been published has described it as either not useful or having long-term benefits. To date, there cannot be any credible claims that arthroscopic hip surgery will prevent nor cure arthritis and thus eliminate the need for THR. The problem lies in the decision process as to who is an appropriate candidate for arthroscopic treatment of osteoarthritis of the hip.

T.G. Sampson, M.D.
Department of Hip Arthroscopy, Post Street Surgery,
2299 Post St, Suite 107, San Francisco, CA 94115, USA
e-mail: tgsampsonmd@gmail.com, tgsampsonmd@hotmail.com

Review of the Literature

The use of hip arthroscopy to treat osteoarthritis of the hip dates back to the early 1980s with many of the early pioneers of the procedure reporting on it as an indication and its usefulness for an early diagnosis [2–6]. We found in a study of 290 patients reported in 1999 that partial labrectomy in the presence of osteoarthritis led to poor results when treated with arthroscopic surgery [7]. At the time we almost completely abandoned treating OA arthroscopically and did not resume until we learned of the relationship of FAI as a cause of labral tears and OA [8]. From then on, we have attempted to treat OA and are constantly advancing the technique and assessing who are ideal candidates for optimal results.

Santori and Villar reported on 234 hip arthroscopies in 1999, comparing preoperative conventional radiographs to arthroscopic findings. They found 32% of the hips with arthroscopic findings of osteoarthritis had normal X-rays in a younger age group (average 36 years old) and predominantly women (71%).

Joe McCarthy described the "watershed lesion" in 2001 to be an association between a labral lesion and adjacent articular cartilage damage of the acetabulum. He stated that arthroscopic and anatomic observations in cadaver hips supported the concept that labral disruption and degenerative joint disease are frequently part of a continuum of degenerative joint disease [9, 10].

Thomas Byrd reported that osteoarthritis has a poor prognosis when treated with hip arthroscopy; however, this was based on a small cohort (eight patients), and he did buy those (seven of eight patients) a lot of time (mean time to THR 63 months) from the index procedure to THR [1]. He also found that hip arthroscopy was a valuable tool for diagnosing more advanced hip disease when the X-rays were less revealing and thereby justifying THR despite not having the typical arthritic findings seen on imaging studies.

J.W.T. Byrd (ed.), *Operative Hip Arthroscopy*,
DOI 10.1007/978-1-4419-7925-4_20, © Springer Science+Business Media New York 2013

Haviv and O'Donnell looked at the incidence of total hip arthroplasty after hip arthroscopy in osteoarthritic patients in a large retrospective study of 564 patients in a 7-year period. Sixteen percent eventually required THR, and interestingly, patients that experienced repeated hip arthroscopies had a longer time to THR than those with only a single procedure. Factors that influenced the better outcomes and longer time to THR were younger age (<55 years old), milder forms of OA, and repeat procedures [11].

Recently, Brown looked at the literature for the mature athlete with hip arthritis. He found overall the presence of OA correlated with a poor outcome and cited Philippon's work stating that better results correlated with a >2-mm joint space seen on X-rays [12].

Patient Selection

The key to good outcomes and satisfaction is patient selection and patient education. In our practice, our typical patient seeking hip arthroscopy has searched the Internet, participated in chat groups, has looked at literature through a Google search, and may have had several orthopedic consultations prior to making appointment. The public's expectations are that we may be able to cure arthritis with hip arthroscopic surgery and that they may be able to get back to all forms of recreation and sports. As a rule, they need to be educated that we are not magicians or miracle workers and that the body's natural tendencies to degrade with arthritis and or aging may be modified and not eliminated. As hip arthroscopists, we can change and repair most abnormal morphology and pathology; however, the physiologic response and local biology will determine the outcome.

Who Is a Good Candidate?

As a general rule, if the patient understands the procedure is palliative and not curative and may be a bridge to later procedures, whether it is revision arthroscopy or THR, they have the right attitude.

Signs and Symptoms of Mild Osteoarthritis

Symptomatically, the hip pain may not be as severe as with more advanced arthritis. It should be localized to the groin and hip area. Occasionally, symptoms may radiate to the low back and thigh not crossing the knee joint. Many may have mechanical complaints such as catching, unpredictable snapping, or buckling. Pain may be intermittent or associated with activities. Sitting may be painful and getting out of a deep chair or couch may be difficult and painful. In the early stages of hip arthritis, range of motion is not obviously impaired, and therefore, putting on shoes and socks poses no problems. Walking stairs or hills may be painful. Seldom is there rest pain and the hip pain may only be associated with activities.

Table 20.1 Tönnis classification of osteoarthritis by radiographic changes

Grade 0	No signs of OA
Grade 1	Increased sclerosis, slight joint space narrowing, no or slight loss of head sphericity
Grade 2	Small cysts, moderate joint space narrowing, moderate loss of head sphericity
Grade 3	Large cysts, severe joint space narrowing, severe deformity of the head

The physical findings on exam may essentially be normal, with the exception of some loss of rotational movement with the hip flexed at 90° and pain on the extremes of internal and or external rotation. Rarely is there a limp and the patient almost never requires the use of external walking aids.

Patients may present with a normal to mild Trendelenburg gait. We have found better results if the arc of hip rotation while flexed to 90° is greater than 50% compared to their normal opposite hip.

Resisted straight leg raising causes groin pain in those with areas of complete or patchy cartilage loss. A negative test has a better prognosis and indicates areas of intact articular cartilage may still exist.

Who Is a Poor Candidate?

It is obvious that any individual with advanced hip arthritis should not be considered for hip arthroscopy. If under certain circumstances individuals are prohibited from THR, however, a simple debridement may have some benefit.

Results are very poor with major joint space loss with severe osteophytes, cysts (Tonnis Grade 3) and a stiff hip. Lastly, if the patient's expectations are unreasonable and consider the procedure as a cure allowing them to return to normalcy and all sports, both the patient and the surgeon will be very disappointed.

Radiographic analysis should always include a comparison X-ray with the unaffected hip (low AP pelvis) and at least one rotational view (frog-leg or cross table view) of the hip. We have found better results if radiographs show Tönnis grade ≤1 or if they have at Tönnis grade ≤2 and the joint space is ≥50% of the opposite normal side (Table 20.1, Fig. 20.1).

An MRI or MRA may outline soft tissue lesions not appreciated on conventional X-rays such as perilabral cysts, articular delaminations or erosions, supra-acetabular cysts, fibro-osseous cysts, and loose bodies and synovial reaction (Fig. 20.2).

There must be an understanding by the patient and the surgeon that the recovery time from arthroscopic treatment for osteoarthritis may be lengthier than from a THR. Considering recovery may take from 3 months to 2 years, patients require reassurance and surgeons should not rush into early intervention or revision surgery in response reasonable ongoing patient complaints.

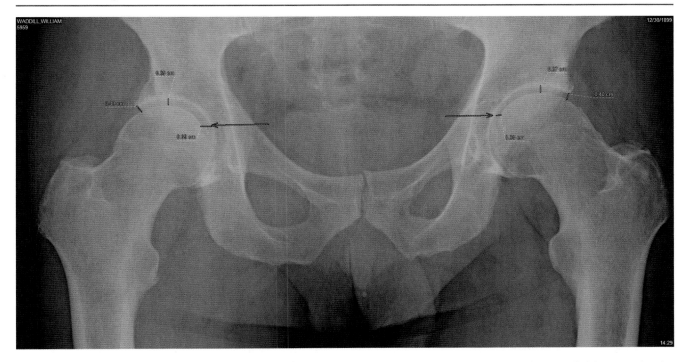

Fig. 20.1 AP X-ray hips Tönnis grade 2 in a 42-year-old man with bilateral hip pains and 25% loss of motion. Note the measurements of the joint spaces are not congruous within each hip and the left hip over-all has a narrower joint. The *arrows* point to medial the narrowing due to notch osteophytes

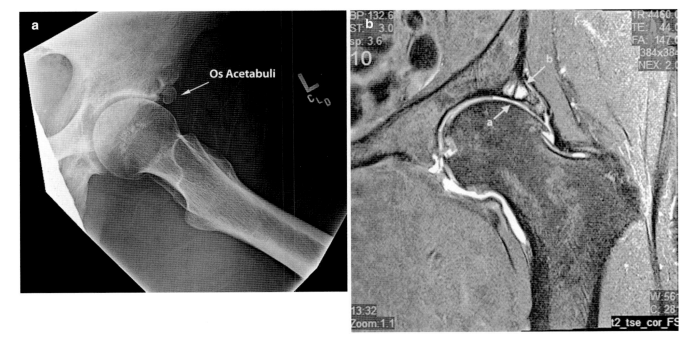

Fig. 20.2 (**a**) Frog lateral of the left hip in a 43-year-old man with 3 months duration of hip pain showing Tönnis grade 3 with an os acetabulum; (**b**) MRI demonstrating articular cartilage loss (*a*), supra-acetabular cyst and degenerative labrum (*b*)

What Pathology of Mild Hip Osteoarthritis Is Correctable?

Historically, arthroscopic treatment for mild osteoarthritis consisted of labral debridement, removal of loose bodies, and synovectomy with chondroplasty. Very little attention was paid to defining the pathology of both the central and peripheral compartments (Fig. 20.3). Table 20.2 defines the damage that requires treatment in the intra-articular and extra-articular spaces. We believe it is imperative to attempt correction of all the pathology seen to obtain the best possible result.

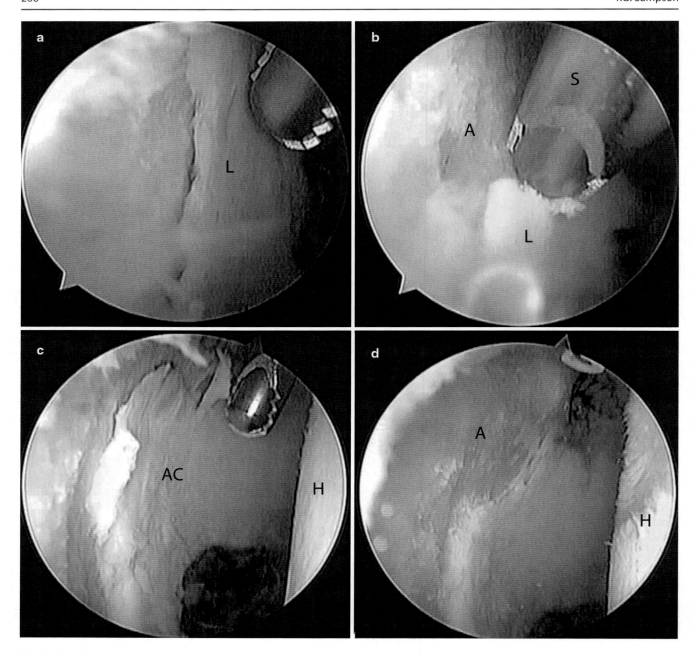

Fig. 20.3 Labral debridement and abrasion chondroplasty. Left hip, 30° arthroscope, left hip, (**a**) degenerative labrum (*L*); (**b**) shaver (*S*) debriding labrum; (**c**) shaver abrading acetabular cartilage (*AC*); (**d**) after cleanup of acetabulum (*A*) and head (*H*)

Table 20.2 Intra-articular and extra-articular findings that necessitate arthroscopic treatment

Central compartment	Peripheral compartment
Labral tears	Perilabral cysts
Labrocartilage defects	Head-neck osteophytes (bumps)
Articular cartilage defects	Fibro-osseous cysts
Notch osteophytes	Acetabular osteophytes
Supra-acetabular cysts	Synovitis
Loose bodies	Psoas impingement

Technique

Arthroscopic treatment for hip osteoarthritis involves both the central and peripheral compartments. The goal is to restore normal bone morphology, remove bone spurs and metaplastic bumps, loose bodies, and debris, preserve articular cartilage and the labrum, and remove reactive synovium. Results will be dictated by amount of articular cartilage damage, the restoration of normal morphology and joint

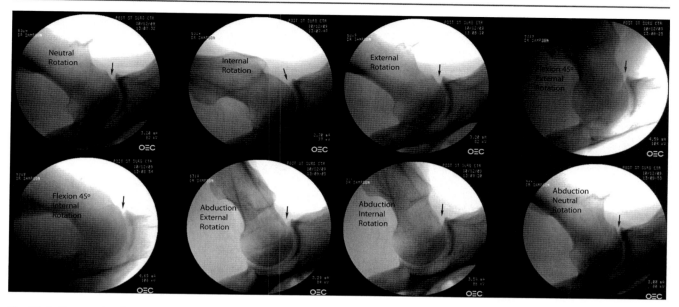

Fig. 20.4 Preoperative fluoroscopic study. Note the abnormal morphology and conflicts between the head-neck junctions and acetabular rims (*arrows*)

mechanics, and to what end the surgeon has reached his goals. The surgeon must be committed to the procedure and complete all tasks despite discouraging damage encountered during the procedure.

Approach

The procedure can be done in either the lateral or supine positions.

Preoperative Fluoroscopy

After the patient has been positioned and anesthetized, multiple fluoroscopic images are obtained rotating and flexing the femoral head to appreciate the relationship of the head-neck junction's conflicts with the acetabular rim. The range of motion may be assessed and restrictions noted for a postoperative comparison. Osteophytes or CAM bumps may exhibit a vacuum sign in external rotation and reflect the leverage of the head out of the socket by impinging bone (Fig. 20.4).

We consider two methods to approach the hip at the onset of surgery. The choice depends on the degree of restriction or capture of the femoral head by the acetabulum:
1. Distraction first to enter the central compartment
2. Approach through a capsulotomy

Other chapters discuss "distraction first" to enter the central compartment; therefore, only the approach through a capsulotomy will be presented in this chapter.

All examples will be referenced to a right hip.

Using fluoroscopic control, a spinal needle is placed through the anterolateral portal and positioned over the lateral capsule near the lateral superior rim of the acetabulum. It is checked to ensure that it repositioned to the base of the neck before leaving it at a desired position for the scope or instruments to be placed both central and peripherally in the hip joint. Using any cannulated technique, the muscle is swept away from the capsule, and the 30° arthroscope (lateral approach) or the 70° arthroscope (supine approach) is placed submuscular for viewing the reflected head of the rectus femoris near its junction with the capsule and anterior fat pad. The anterior portal is created in the same fashion through which some of the fat pad is removed with a shaver. An RF cutting wand or blade is used to incise the capsule from its base near the intertrochanteric line to a position proximal on the acetabular rim, taking care not to damage the labrum. The capsule is then released from the rim anterior to the 5 o'clock position and lateral as far as necessary for exposure of rim osteophytes. A partial capsulectomy may be necessary for diseased capsules which are often thickened and gritty. The extent of the capsulotomy is determined to provide an ideal view of the entire hip joint, both central and peripherally. Care should be taken to preserve the capsule if it is thin or for any concern of postoperative instability (Fig. 20.5).

An attempt to distract is then done; however, if the head is captured and cannot be mobilized without excessive force, rim trimming to remove the acetabular osteophytes and overcoverage of the head will facilitate entry to the central compartment. In acetabular rims with excessive overcoverage, rim trimming prior to entering the center compartment removes the blockades to instruments. The scope may then be driven into the central compartment without scuffing the cartilage (Fig. 20.6).

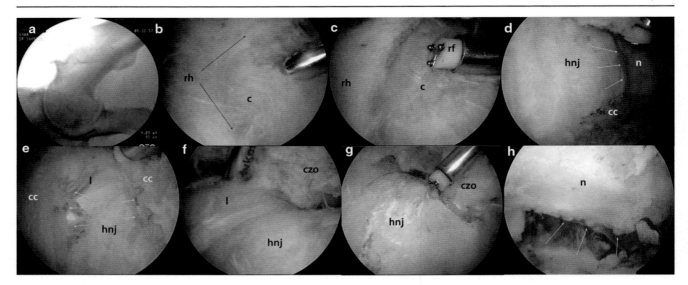

Fig. 20.5 Approach to the left hip through a capsulotomy in a 51-year-old male orthopedic surgeon. (**a**) Preoperative AP fluoroscopic image in the lateral decubitus position; (**b**) initial view of the anterior hip capsule (*c*) with a 30° arthroscope, and reflected head rectus femoris (*rh*), note edge pointed to by *arrows*; (**c**) radiofrequency probe (*rf*) separating the reflected head from the capsule; (**d**) view of head-neck junction (*hnj*) through capsulotomy along the neck of the femur (*n*). Note the edge of the CAM bump (*arrows*) and the cut capsule edge (*cc*); (**e**) exposure of the labrum (*l*), note the synovitis (*arrows*); (**f**) view of the labrum, head-neck junction through capsulotomy, not the cut edge of the zona orbicularis (*czo*); (**g**) radiofrequency probe is used to clean of the soft tissue on the head-neck junction and for synovectomy; (**h**) view of the neck with barnacle like osteophytes (*arrows*)

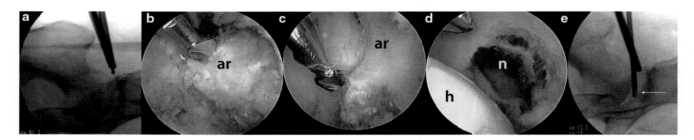

Fig. 20.6 Rim trimming of a right hip viewing through the anterior portal with a 30° arthroscope in a 53-year-old female facilitating entry into the central compartment. (**a**) Fluoroscopic view of the position of the scope and burr; (**b**) 4-mm burr trimming the lateral acetabular rim (*ar*); (**c**) the lateral rim removed with burr coursing anteriorly; (**d**) distracted hip exposing the central compartment and the notch (*n*); (**e**) fluoroscopic view of the scope at the edge of the central compartment with the shaver near the notch (*arrow*)

Once the pathology in the central and peripheral compartments is identified, a final plan should be implemented to achieve all of the goals of surgery in an efficient and timely manner. We have found leaving the central compartment treatment for last, allows for easier entry because of bone removal and soft tissue releases.

The "capsulotomy first technique" provides an overall global view similar to that seen in an open arthrotomy, and the arthroscope and instruments may easily be passed between the central and peripheral compartments.

The Surgical Plan

The order of procedures to treat arthritis of the hip are designed to create a rational sequence of events to facilitate the next part of the operation. We first encounter the head-neck junction of the femur and view it from the base of the neck to the acetabular rim proximal to the labrum. A quick distraction is done to evaluate the central compartment and to generate the plan.

Operating from external to internal, we typically trim the acetabular rim from behind the labrum to preserve the maximum amount of labral tissue as well as the labral cartilage junction. This is followed by elevation of viable appearing articular cartilage. The face of the bony surface of the acetabulum is curetted and then microfractured. We believe this procedure stimulates bonding to the backside of the preserved articular cartilage with fibrocartilage.

Fig. 20.7 Hip zones of the acetabulum

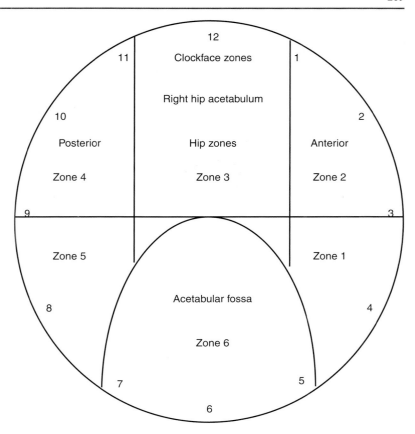

The labrum and labrocartilage junction is refixed to the trimmed acetabular rim with suture anchors. Fibrillated cartilage and labrum are removed with a shaver and RF wand.

At this point, a decision is made either to complete the acetabular work or to remove osteophytes and metaplastic bone of the head-neck junction of the femur. That decision is based on the ease of access to the central compartment and if reduction in bone volume of the head-neck junction would further loosen the joint and remove obstacles for entry.

The remaining work in the central compartment consists of further removal of fibrillated articular cartilage and labrum, microfracture, notch osteophytectomy, synovectomy, and removal of loose material and loose bodies.

Once complete with the central compartment, the final work is accomplished in the peripheral compartment with removal of metaplastic bone and contouring and shaping the head-neck junction. Often, small bony excrescences and osteophytes as well as hypertrophic synovium must be excised.

The Acetabular Rim

Most of the correctable pathology involving the acetabulum is located in zones 1–3 or 11–6 o'clock clockwise [13] (Fig. 20.7). The center edge angle (CEA) is measured preoperatively to determine the amount of rim resection that can safely be accomplished on the preoperative X-rays or directly on the fluoroscopic monitor [14]. The procedure involves acetabular rim trimming for pincer lesions and rim osteophytes without labral takedown. By viewing from the anterolateral portal, using an RF device, the capsular labral junction is detached from the rim of the acetabulum peripheral to zones 1, 2, and 3. A small amount of distraction of the head from the acetabulum is done to prevent contact of the burr on the head in areas where the labrocartilage junction is detached and the backside acetabular cartilage cannot protect the head from the burr. The arthroscopic burr is brought through the anterior or anteroinferior portal to remove the rim. The entire area of rim involvement should be trimmed. Occasionally, a posterolateral portal may be needed to trim peripheral zones 4 and 5 (the posterior rim). Decisions are necessary at this juncture: (1) to what depth the rim is trimmed and (2) how far circumferentially the rim is trimmed.

1. The depth of rim trimming should contour the rim with the ilium. Care should be taken to avoid creating a dysplastic hip with a CEA<25°. Reduction of exposed bone from cartilage loss on the face of the acetabulum should be considered as well as the ability to relocate the labrum.
2. The circumference of the rim trimming should be based on appearance of damaged adjacent articular cartilage of the acetabulum. In most cases, there is a natural demarcation zone in which the osteophyte drops off to normal rim adjacent to zone 3 or approximately 11–12 o'clock (Fig. 20.8).

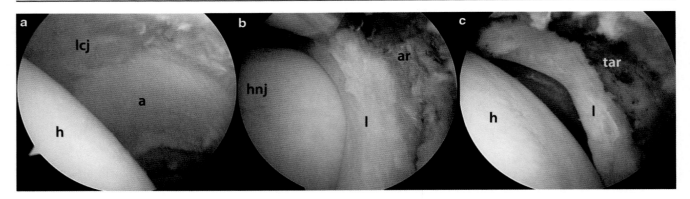

Fig. 20.8 Right hip central compartment viewing through the anterior portal with a 30° arthroscope showing (**a**) the extent of articular damage in zone 3 of the labrocartilage junction, (**b**) the extent of the rim osteophyte transitioning to normal rim (*ar*) adjacent to the articular damage, and (**c**) a view of the central and peripheral compartments after acetabular rim trimming (*art*)

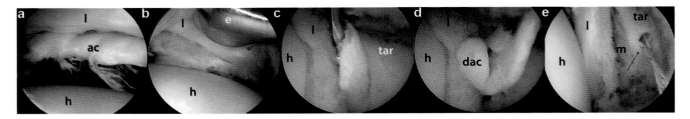

Fig. 20.9 Labral cartilage junction defect in a right hip of a 23-year-old male sailor viewed through an anterolateral portal with a 30° arthroscope; (**a**) showing a tear between the labrum (*l*) and the articular cartilage of the acetabulum (*ac*); (**b**) probing with elevator (*e*); (**c**) probing between labrum and degenerated articular cartilage (*dac*) of the acetabulum after trimmed acetabular rim (*tar*); (**d**) the articular cartilage extruded between the rim and the labrum; (**e**) leaving preserved labrum for reattachment to the new position on the trimmed acetabular rim after microfracture of the bony face (*m*) with a bone anchor (*arrow*)

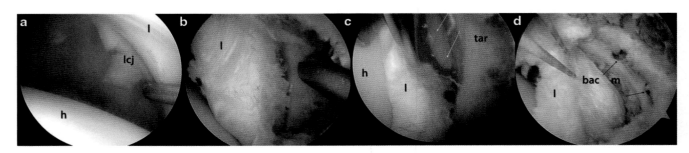

Fig. 20.10 Preservation of delaminated labral cartilage junction of a right hip in the 39-year-old female by rim trimming, elevation of the flap, microfracture, and refixation. (**a**) View from the anterolateral portal with a 30° arthroscope showing the labrum (*I*), femoral head (*h*) and the torn labrocartilage junction (*lcj*); (**b**) note the burr trimming the rim of the acetabulum behind and proximal to the labrum (*l*); (**c**) the backside of the acetabular cartilage (*arrows*) is elevated from the bony face of the acetabulum where it is delaminated after trimming of the rim (*tar*). The femoral head (*h*) and labrum (*I*) are also shown. (**d**) the whole construct of intact labrocartilage junction is repaired back to the acetabular rim (*arrows*) after microfracture (*m*) which is believed to stimulate bonding of the backside of the acetabular cartilage (*bac*)

Since the labral attachment to the capsule has been disrupted by the capsulotomy, the labrum will separate from the rim in areas where labral cartilage junction is torn or degenerated. This technique preserves the labrum whether it is healthy or not (Fig. 20.9).

Once the rim has been trimmed, the areas of the cartilage loss have been reduced in volume. Those areas of complete cartilage loss on the acetabular face behind labrocartilage flaps are curetted and microfractured. We believe there is rebonding of the cartilage flap to the acetabular bone with this technique.

The detached labrum and labrocartilage flaps are secured to their new position on the resected rim with bone anchors.

In the areas where delaminated labrum and articular cartilage of the acetabulum are intact at the junction, an attempt is made to preserve them as a flap for a repair back to the rim (Fig. 20.10).

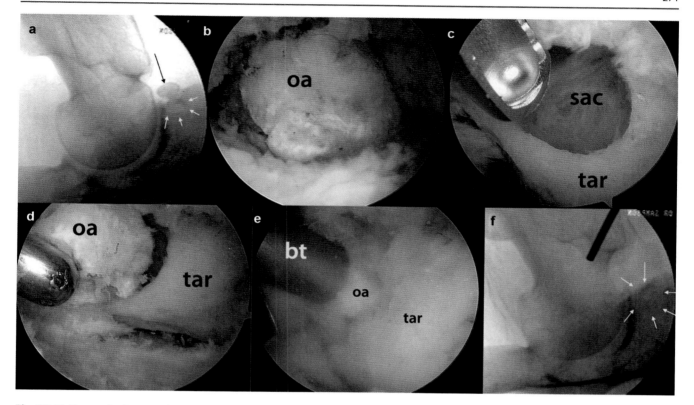

Fig. 20.11 Removal of os acetabuli, curettage supra-acetabular bone cyst and bone graft with removed os acetabuli bone. (**a**) Fluoroscopic view of a right hip showing an os acetabuli adjacent to a supra-acetabular cyst (*arrows*); (**b**) exposure of the os acetabuli (*oa*); (**c**) cleaned supra-acetabular cyst (*sac*) after removal of the os acetabuli and trimmed acetabular rim (*tar*); (**d**) bone graft using the removed os acetabuli being introduced by a grasper; (**e**) bone tamp (*bt*) impacting graft; (**f**) final fluoroscopic image after rim trimming and bone graft in place (*arrows*)

The Acetabulum

The entirety of the acetabulum is inspected for loose bodies, articular cartilage damage, and cysts. Loose bodies are removed, areas of fibrillation are gently shaved, and reactive synovium debrided. Microfracture is used in small areas of grade 4 chondromalacia, typically seen to be less than 1 cm^2 in zones 1–3. Encountered cysts are curetted. Large cysts are bone grafted (Fig. 20.11).

The Notch

Most hips with arthritis develop notch osteophytes. Notch osteophytes prevent the femoral head from proper contact with the acetabular cartilage and cause further erosion of the femoral head due to increase contact forces and mechanical abrasion [15]. It is for that reason resection of the osteophytes is necessary. The amount of osteophyte removal can be measured on a routine AP X-ray of the hip when compared with the normal hip.

Removal of the notch osteophytes adjacent to zones 1, 2, and 3 is accomplished with a long hip burr. The posterior osteophytes adjacent to zones 4 and 5 are more difficult to remove. Microfracture picks and back-cutting curettes or the addition of a posterior portal will facilitate their excision (Fig. 20.12).

The Head

Most of the work on the femoral head is done at the head-neck junction, which may extend to the base of the neck because of small osteophytes, metaplastic bone, surrounding loose bodies, and reactive synovitis. It is difficult to view the entirety of the femoral head in the central compartment and essentially impossible to reach all aspects of the femoral head with cutting instruments. Zones 1–5 L and M may be treated; however, zones 1–6 M and zones 5 and 6 L, which may have osteophytes, present a challenge to remove them (Fig. 20.13).

Gentle abrasion of cartilage defects of the femoral head is accomplished with curved shavers and RF devices. We rarely microfracture the head, as it has not found to be beneficial in our hands. The more femoral head involvement bodes for a poor prognosis (Fig. 20.14).

The Head-Neck Junction and Neck of the Femur

The recognition and arthroscopic treatment of femoroacetabular impingement (FAI), which involves the removal of metaplastic bone from the head-neck junction, has improved our overall results from arthroscopically treating osteoarthritis of the hip. Since the techniques inception in 2001, the amount of head-neck bone removal has evolved to reshaping and contouring to the level of the

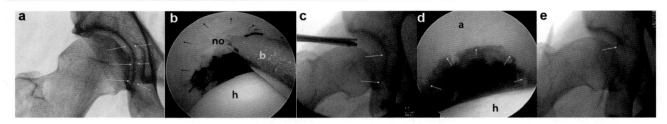

Fig. 20.12 Notch osteophytectomy in a right hip. (**a**) Fluoroscopic view with *arrows* indicating the most lateral and medial extent of the notch osteophyte; (**b**) view through anterolateral portal with burr (*b*) in anterior portal, *arrows* showing extent of the notch osteophytectomy (*no*) planned; (**c**) fluoroscopic view of the trajectory of the instruments to the notch (*arrows*); (**d**) acetabulum (*a*) showing removal of notch osteophyte (*arrows*); removed notch osteophyte (*arrows*); (**e**) fluoroscopic view of removed of notch osteophyte (*arrow*)

Fig. 20.13 Femoral head zones

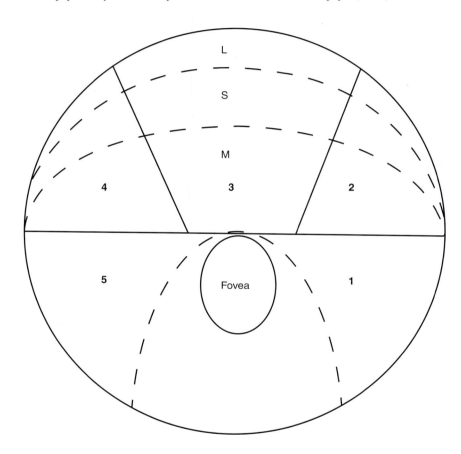

femoral neck, leaving the femoral head as spherical as possible. This is accomplished by using a 4- to 6-mm round or barrel-shaped burr.

By viewing from the anterolateral portal with the hip slightly flexed, the shaver and RF device is brought through the anterior portal to remove the soft tissue over the area of resection. The area of resection is outlined with the burr to define its borders. Care is taken not to create a flat surface on the head-neck junction by contouring and shaping with curved sweeping motion and by rotating the arthroscope to obtain different perspectives on the working area. Typically, the anterior synovial fold is the anterior boundary of resection. Contouring and shaping is carried anterolateral and then posterolateral taking care not to damage the lateral epiphyseal vessels beneath the lateral synovial fold.

It will be necessary to exchange the arthroscope and instrument portal positions to view and complete the resection. As the work is accomplished on the lateral and posterior surfaces, some distraction may be necessary to clear the osteophytes from the labrum and acetabular rim.

Motion studies are then done under direct arthroscopic viewing as well as a comparison fluoroscopic exam to ensure adequacy of the head-neck resection of the bump. If further conflicts exist, more bone resection is necessary. Often during this process, to obtain visualization, synovectomy is often done with a shaver (Fig. 20.15).

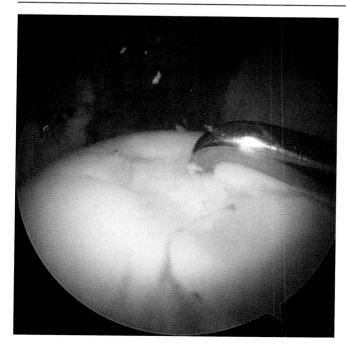

Fig. 20.14 Femoral head articular cartilage damage in zones 3LS (CM4)

A decision is necessary as to how far the resection will go on to the articular surface of the femoral head. In some cases, the lack of spherical or flattening of the head goes into the central compartment. We will visually check the resection and with fluoroscopic X-rays. Marginal osteophytes are removed when possible. It is very difficult to remove a commonly seen osteophyte posterior and inferior in zone 6 (Fig. 20.16).

Cysts

Three types of cysts are encountered in arthritis of the hip.

They include supra-acetabular cysts, perilabral cysts, and fibro-osseous cysts of the head-neck junction.

In many cases supra-acetabular cysts may be the only evidence for early hip osteoarthritis. Often, the joint space is well maintained with only small marginal osteophytes of the acetabulum and slight flattening of the head-neck junction. They are difficult to see on normal X-rays and may only be diagnosed by an MRI. The extent of the supra-acetabular cyst appears to be related to the amount of acetabular articular cartilage involvement. We have found the larger the cyst, the more destruction and delamination of the acetabular articular

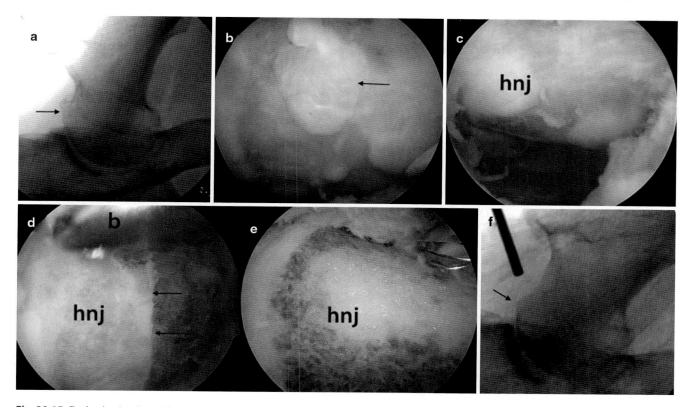

Fig. 20.15 Reshaping head-neck junction of the femur to the base of the neck and removal of neck osteophytes in a left hip. (**a**) Fluoroscopic view if the CAM bump with osteophyte (*arrow*); (**b**) view through anterior portal with a 30° arthroscope of the head-neck junction, note osteophyte (*arrow*); (**c**) viewing into anterior peripheral space of the head-neck junction (*hnj*); (**d**) burr (*b*) trimming head-neck junction (*hnj*) with *arrows* showing progress; (**e**) final view after desired bone resection; (**f**) fluoroscopic view of final resection (*arrow*)

cartilage there is. In former years, we approached the cyst through the articular cartilage with little chance to preserve functional articular cartilage. It is for that reason we changed the approach to the periphery through the capsulotomy.

Prior to refixing the labrum or the labrocartilage junction to the rim of the acetabulum, the cysts are either directly encountered through the resected rim or with elevation of the articular cartilage using a blunt instrument on the face of the acetabulum. Once encountered, the soft tissues are removed with a variety of instruments including a shaver,

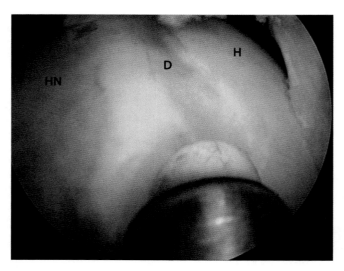

Fig. 20.16 Demarcation zone femoral head showing extent of resection onto head, (*H*) head, (*D*) demarcation zone, and (*HN*) head-neck junction

RF device, and curettes. The cyst is then contoured with a burr. The defect may be bone grafted with bone, bone substitute, or covered with the articular cartilage and labrum. See Fig. 20.11.

Fibro-osseous cysts are encountered in both FAI and hip arthritis. They may be deep to the cortex and are exposed with the head-neck osteoplasty. Their size may range from a few millimeters to 1 or 2 cm. Treatment consists of curettage and contouring and rarely bone grafted. It is not necessary to remove bone to the level of the base of the cyst as it may compromise the strength of the neck of the femur (Fig. 20.17).

Much larger cysts may need more extensive treatment, such as curettage, contouring, microfracture, and bone grafting (Fig. 20.18).

Labral Reconstruction

Although there is no clear indication in the literature for labral reconstruction, we believe it may be of benefit in rare cases when the deficient labrum no longer functions due to degeneration, previous labrectomy, or cystic changes, such as seen with paralabral cysts and with ossification combined with ongoing clinical signs of pain. Labral reconstruction usually involves intercalary grafting. Tissues that have been used include the fascia lata, hamstring tendons, hip capsule, and the reflected head of the rectus femoris [16].

The first two involve free grafting and the latter two involve local grafting. We prefer to use the reflected head of the rectus femoris since it is possible to leave the most proximal tendon attached to the rim of the acetabulum allowing for some remaining blood supply. The technique involves

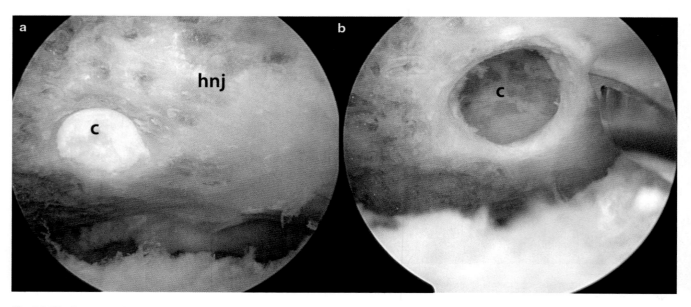

Fig. 20.17 Curettage of a small fibro-osseous cyst of the femoral neck. (**a**) View from the anterior portal with a 30° arthroscope of the cyst (*c*), head neck junction (*hnj*); (**b**) the cyst has been cleaned of its fibrous tissue

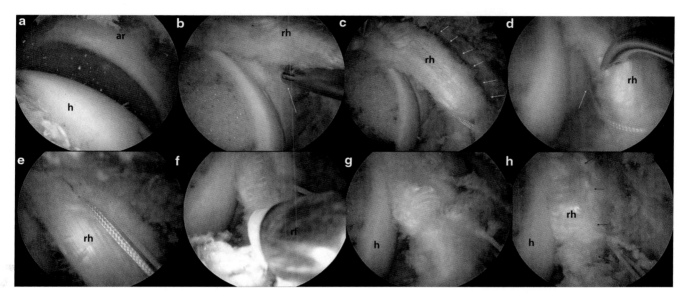

Fig. 20.18 Treatment of a large fibro-osseous cyst of a left femoral head-neck junction; (**a**) view from the anterior portal with a 30° arthroscope of the head (*h*) and head-neck junction (*arrows*); (**b**) after resection of a CAM bump exposing the large cyst (*arrows*); (**c**) removal of the contents of the cyst (*c*) with a shaver; (**d**) cyst had been contoured and microfractured with the awl (*mf*); (**e**) bone graft (*bg*) with bone putty (*arrows*)

Fig. 20.19 Rectus femoris (reflected head) graft to reconstruct degenerative labrum in a right hip. (**a**) View through anterolateral portal of a distracted head after rim trimmed (*ar*), femoral head (*h*); (**b**) placement of the 1st anchor anticipating the use of the reflected head of the rectus femoris (*rh*) for a labral graft; (**c**) release of the rectus from the rim (*arrows*); (**d**) suture relay bringing anchor suture through rectus; (**e**) base horizontal suture through rectus; (**f**) release of muscle tendon unit of rectus while tying anchor sutures; (**g**) interval tying more sutures; (**h**) final anchorage of the graft (*arrows*)

excision of the involved labrum after the rim has been trimmed followed by estimating the amount of tendon required for the repair. In most cases, the labrum is involved peripheral to zones 1, 2, and 3 and sometimes into zone 4. The proximal attachment of reflected head of the rectus femoris lies superior and adjacent the junction of the zones 3 and 4.

Leaving the proximal portion attached, an RF device is used to detach the reflected head from the area of bone just proximal to the acetabulum while still maintaining a distal muscular attachment. The partially detached tendon may be reflective down and into the defect created by the labral excision in the trimmed rim. Starting lateral and working medial to anterior, the anticipated positions of the bone anchors are drilled. Using the surgeons preferred suture passing devices, horizontal mattress sutures for a base repair are created. The suture anchors are impacted into the drill holes and the rectus tendon is secured to the anchor either with a knot or knotless

system. On approaching zone 1, the reflected head is detached from the rectus muscle for proper tensioning and prior to securing the last anchor. After securing the final anchor, a side-to-side repair is accomplished with the remaining labrum or transverse ligament in zone 1. If necessary, a side-to-side repair of the lateral attachment of the rectus femoris to the remaining lateral labrum is performed.

The integrity of the reconstruction is checked with a probe, and a motion study is performed as well as a distraction study to check for a good suction seal (Fig. 20.19).

Synovitis and Loose Bodies

An exploration and debridement of both the central peripheral compartments should be undertaken for loose debris, loose bodies, and excessive and reactive synovium. It is not necessary to do a complete synovectomy, but most highly reactive and bulky synovium should be excised. It is important to

Fig. 20.20 Removal of loose bodies and synovitis right hip. (**a**) View from anterior portal of large loose bodies in the anterior peripheral space along the head-neck junction (*hnj*); (**b**) after synovectomy and removal of loose bodies shows cleaned anterior capsule (*ac*)

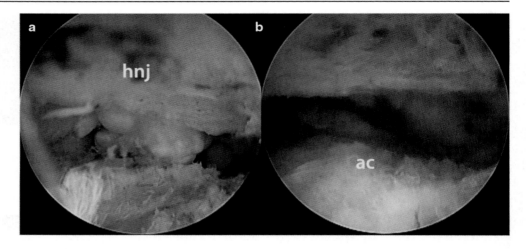

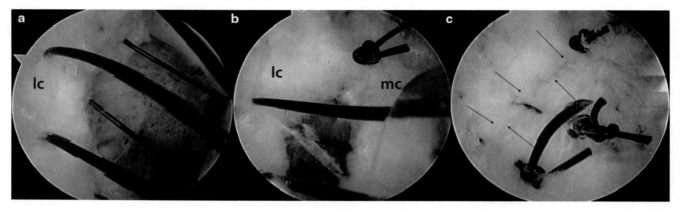

Fig. 20.21 Capsular repair re-approximates the zona orbicularis. (**a**) Sutures placed through opened capsule; (**b**) tying the suture bringing the lateral capsule (*lc*) to the medial capsule (*mc*); (**c**) closed capsule (*arrows*)

remove all bone and soft tissue debris to reduce postoperative synovitis (Fig. 20.20).

The Capsule

The involvement of the capsule varies from individual to individual and from men to women. As stated before, at the capsule may be thickened and gritty. In the presence of a stiff hip, it should be excised in areas of involvement. However, in the presence of a thin flexible capsule in which the rim excised to a near dysplastic appearance, we tend to do a partial repair of the zona orbicularis. Usually two or three sutures using a suture passer and bird beak grasper are passed between two portals and tied down (Fig. 20.21).

Postoperative Care and Rehabilitation

Protected weight bearing with two crutches is important in hips with large areas of cartilage loss or concern for instability. We tend to quickly advance patients to full weight bearing based on their reduction of symptoms, increased range of motion, and increased abductor strength. Some will come off crutches within 1–2 weeks and others may take 6 weeks or more.

During the initial postoperative recovery, we believe hip motion is paramount to the healing process. It is for that reason the use of a stationary bicycle, elliptical trainer, and swimming is employed. Once normal range of motion is nearly established, stabilization exercises and strengthening are added. Because we are dealing with a "repaired degenerative" joint, pain relief may progress slowly. The healing process is unpredictable and has its variations, with the hope that there will be overall improvements. Reports of increasing pain may require backing off or curtailing the rehabilitation process when necessary.

Physical therapy is used in certain patients who cannot attain functional restoration on their own. All patients are asked to take from 1 to 3 weeks to rest while restoring motion to allow for reduction in swelling and to obtain range of motion on their own with gentle stretching.

We evaluate the patient's progress at 1 week, 6 weeks, 3 months, 6 months, 1 year, and then as needed until a steady state has been reached. Those who exhibit signs of progressively worsening will be studied with routine hip X-rays and an MRI. Those who exhibit progressive narrowing on their

X-rays and further loss of motion are advised to undergo a hip replacement when pain becomes intolerable. If the joint space is well maintained in the face of worsening symptoms, we consider revision hip arthroscopy.

Results

We evaluated hips treated arthroscopically for osteoarthritis since January 1, 2002, who had concurrent FAI. Evolution of the procedure from prior years of simple partially labrectomy, debridement, and abrasion chondroplasty advanced by adding the more complex procedures associated with FAI. Our control group arose from the previous study in which partial labrectomy in the presence of moderate arthritis of the hip only achieved 21% good to excellent results. FAI was not treated in that group [7].

One thousand thirty-four hips were studied to March 1, 2011 (110 months) with an average of 67 months. We identified 464 hips with osteoarthritis in which 64% were female and 36% male, and all hips had concurrent FAI mostly consisting of mixed CAM and pincer lesions. Two-hundred and sixty-eight patients were below the age of 55 years old and 196 patients were above the age of 55 years old. Fifty-three (11.4%) of the patients went onto THR. Of the 53 patients, 30 were females and 23 were males. The average age of females at the index surgery was 50.9 years and males, 55.8 years. Interestingly, females degraded sooner than males with an average time from index surgery to total hip replacement of average 20 months (range 3–57 months), and males average of 60 months (range 4–94 months).

In females, radiographs were not a predictor of the outcome, and in several patients in what appeared to be normal X-rays, yet there hip degraded more quickly than expected. Hip dysplasia was a predictor for a poor outcome with a CEA of less than 25°. The X-rays on males often looked worse with narrowed joint spaces (1–3 mm) more narrowing superior-lateral, a larger CAM effect and marginal osteophytes.

MRI showing greater cartilage loss was a good predictor of a poor outcome; however, several male patients with moderate to severe cartilage loss have done well.

Decision Making

In general, we will attempt to arthroscopically treat osteoarthritis in most any young individual as a palliative procedure. We define young as under the age of 45 years old. We will be skeptical in recommending the procedure on any female over the age of 50 years old and a male over 55 years old.

We also recommend treating hips that exhibit greater than 50% rotational range of motion compared to their opposite "normal" hip and have greater than 50% joint space on the affected hip's X-ray compared to their opposite side.

We would not recommend arthroscopically treating hip joints with X-rays that show less than 2 mm of joint space

unless they are a young male athletic individual who was involved previously in some form of an aggressive sport, such as football, rugby, soccer, basketball, ice hockey, etc. He must also have realistic expectations that arthroscopy is only a palliative procedure and to expect a THR future.

Females over the age of 50 and/or perimenopausal did not seem to do well, and they comprised the early failures. We postulated it might be due to hormonal changes or the development of osteoporosis. Their failure seemed to develop rapid chondrolysis, leading to rapid joint space narrowing and superior-lateral subluxation of the femoral head with erosion of the acetabulum.

Males seemed more often better after the index arthroscopic procedure and tended to degrade more slowly than the females. They often developed increased joint space narrowing and marginal osteophytes with gradual further loss of their rotational movement.

The Degeneration Curve

In arthroscopically treating all patients with osteoarthritis of the hip, the surgeon must have a frank discussion with the patient the concept of aging and degeneration of the hip. It must be clearly understood that the procedure is not curative, and only palliative. There must be no guarantees made as to how long the individual's hip will last after the arthroscopic procedure, nor any promises for complete pain relief or returning to their desired competitive sports.

We explain to each and every patient about the "degenerative curve" to illustrate the natural progression of arthritis. In our opinion, the early stages of degeneration progress in arithmetic manner and as it progresses towards the end stages, accelerates to geometric (hyperbolic).

The patient must understand that there is no data as yet to determine the sweet spot on the curve, the point the progression changes from arithmetic to geometric. As surgeons, we can change the morphologic appearance and treat damaged tissues of an arthritic joint; however, we cannot change the natural aging process or the biologic response to arthritis. Patients want miracles these days, and they must understand that we are surgeons and not magicians.

References

1. Byrd JW, Jones KS. Hip arthroscopy for labral pathology: prospective analysis with 10-year follow-up. Arthroscopy. 2009;25(4):365–8.
2. Parisien JS. Arthroscopy of the hip. Present status. Bull Hosp Jt Dis Orthop Inst. 1985;45(2):127–32.
3. Glick JM. Hip arthroscopy using the lateral approach. Instr Course Lect. 1988;37:223–31.
4. Hawkins RB. Arthroscopy of the hip. Clin Orthop Relat Res. 1989;249:44–7.
5. Villar RN. Hip arthroscopy. Br J Hosp Med. 1992;47(10):763–6.
6. McCarthy JC, Busconi B. The role of hip arthroscopy in the diagnosis and treatment of hip disease. Orthopedics. 1995;18(8):753–6.

7. Farjo LA, Glick JM, Sampson TG. Hip arthroscopy for acetabular labral tears. Arthroscopy. 1999;15(2):132–7.

8. Ganz R, Parvizi J, Beck M, Leunig M, Notzli H, Siebenrock KA. Femoroacetabular impingement: a cause for osteoarthritis of the hip. Clin Orthop Relat Res. 2003;417:112–20.

9. McCarthy JC, Noble PC, Schuck MR, Wright J, Lee J. The Otto E. Aufranc Award: the role of labral lesions to development of early degenerative hip disease. Clin Orthop Relat Res. 2001;393:25–37.

10. McCarthy JC, Noble PC, Schuck MR, Wright J, Lee J. The watershed labral lesion: its relationship to early arthritis of the hip. J Arthroplasty. 2001;16(8 Suppl 1):81–7.

11. Haviv B, O'Donnell J. The incidence of total hip arthroplasty after hip arthroscopy in osteoarthritic patients. Sports Med Arthrosc Rehabil Ther Technol. 2010;2:18.

12. Browne JA. The mature athlete with hip arthritis. Clin Sports Med. 2011;30(2):453–62.

13. Ilizaliturri Jr VM, Byrd JW, Sampson TG, et al. A geographic zone method to describe intra-articular pathology in hip arthroscopy: cadaveric study and preliminary report. Arthroscopy. 2008;24(5): 534–9.

14. Matsuda DK. Fluoroscopic templating technique for precision arthroscopic rim trimming. Arthroscopy. 2009;25(10):1175–82.

15. Daniel M, Iglic A, Kralj-Iglic V. The shape of acetabular cartilage optimizes hip contact stress distribution. J Anat. 2005;207(1):85–91.

16. Philippon MJ, Briggs KK, Hay CJ, Kuppersmith DA, Dewing CB, Huang MJ. Arthroscopic labral reconstruction in the hip using iliotibial band autograft: technique and early outcomes. Arthroscopy. 2010;26(6):750–6.

Iliopsoas Tendon Release

21

Victor M. Ilizaliturri Jr., Humberto Gonzalez Ugalde, and Javier Camacho-Galindo

Introduction

Iliopsoas tendon release is one the most frequently performed endoscopic procedures around the hip joint [1]. The clearest indication for endoscopic iliopsoas tendon release is the internal snapping hip syndrome [1, 2]. More recently, it has been suggested that pathologic changes within the iliopsoas tendon may produce labral tears due to its close relationship to the anterior labrum [3]. Painful iliopsoas tendinitis may also be present after total hip replacement [4]. Iliopsoas tendinitis with or without total hip replacement may also be managed with an endoscopic iliopsoas tendon release [1]. Different endoscopic techniques have been developed for iliopsoas tendon release, which will be described in this chapter.

Indications for Iliopsoas Tendon Release

Internal Snapping Hip Syndrome

The internal snapping hip syndrome is produced by the iliopsoas tendon snapping over the iliopectineal eminence or the femoral head (Figs. 21.1 and 21.2). The iliopsoas tendon is located lateral to the iliopectineal eminence when the hip is in full flexion, with hip extension the tendon is displaced medially until it positions medial to the iliopectineal eminence when the hip is in neutral position [2] (Fig. 21.3). The snapping phenomenon can occur without pain in up to 10% of the general population and should be considered a normal occurrence [5]. The symptomatic internal snapping hip syndrome always presents pain in the groin associated with the snapping phenomenon. Some patients may describe accompanying flank discomfort which comes from the origin of the psoas and iliacus. The snapping phenomenon is reproduced when

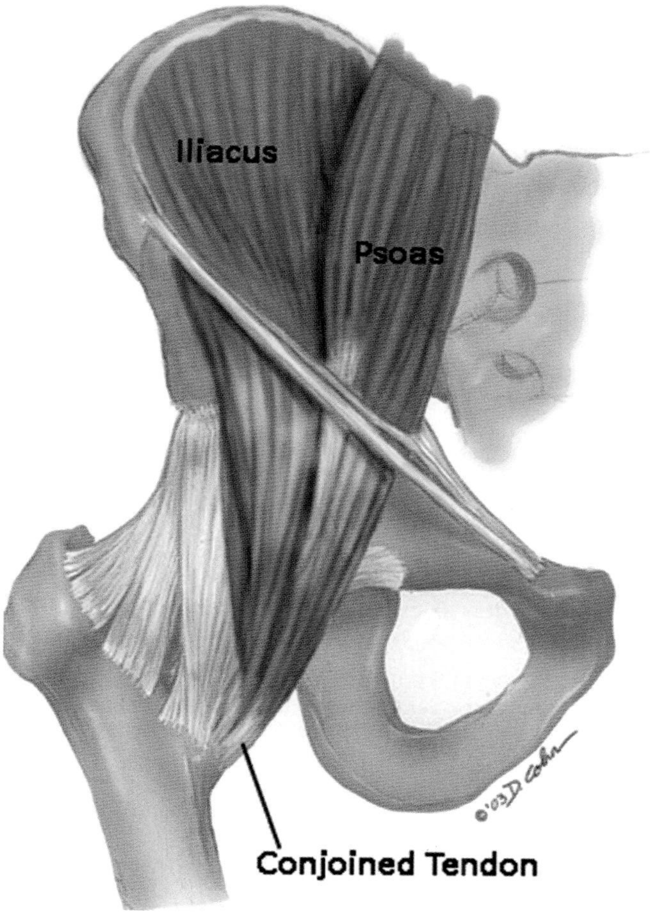

Fig. 21.1 The iliacus and psoas muscles form a conjoined tendon that inserts onto the lesser trochanter. (Courtesy, J.W. Thomas Byrd, M.D.)

V.M. Ilizaliturri Jr., M.D. (✉) • H.G. Ugalde, M.D.
J. Camacho-Galindo, M.D.
Adult Joint Reconstruction Service, Hip and Knee, National Rehabilitation Institute of Mexico, Avenida México-Xochimilco No. 289, Colonia Arenal de Guadalupe, Mexico City, DF 14389, Mexico

Department of Hip and Knee Surgery, Universidad Nacional Autónoma de México, Mexico City, DF, Mexico
e-mail: vichip2002@yahoo.com.mx; humbertogonzalezmd@gmail.com; jvrcamacho@hotmail.com

J.W.T. Byrd (ed.), *Operative Hip Arthroscopy*,
DOI 10.1007/978-1-4419-7925-4_21, © Springer Science+Business Media New York 2013

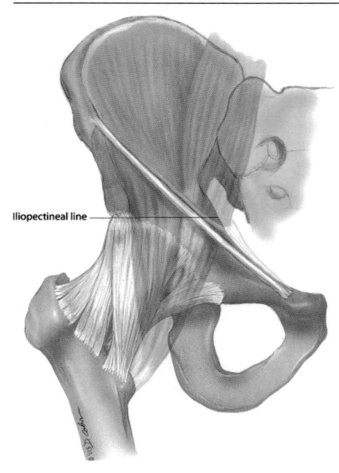

Fig. 21.2 The iliopsoas courses over the iliopectineal line. (Courtesy, J.W. Thomas Byrd, M.D.)

bringing the hip to extension from a flexed position. The patients report snapping while stair climbing or standing from a chair. The snapping phenomenon is almost always voluntary and reproducible and helps to differentiate this from an intra-articular problem [6].

Physical Examination of the Internal Snapping Hip Syndrome

Physical examination of the internal snapping phenomenon is done with the patient supine by flexing the affected hip more than 90° and extending to neutral position. This maneuver will reproduce the snapping phenomenon at the front of the groin which will be mentioned to the examiner by the patient when it occurs. The snapping phenomenon cannot be observed through the skin but frequently produces an audible snap. This may be accentuated with abduction and external rotation in flexion and adducting and internally rotating while extending (Fig. 21.4). The snapping phenomenon may be palpated by placing the hand over the affected groin. When the snapping is symptomatic, there is always an apprehension response

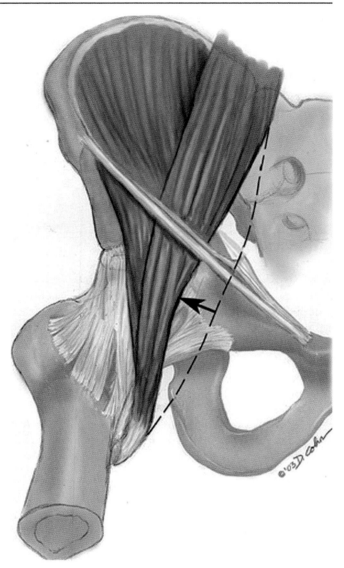

Fig. 21.3 The iliopsoas lies anterior to the hip capsule (*dotted line*) and moves lateral with hip flexion, abduction, and external rotation (*arrow*). As the hip is extended, adducted, and internally rotated, the tendon moves in a medial direction. (Courtesy, J.W. Thomas Byrd, M.D.)

from the patient when it occurs. Other positive findings in physical examination such as the presence of a C-sign, a positive log roll test, or a positive impingement test may be related to the presence of intra-articular hip pathology. More than half of the patients with internal snapping hip syndrome have associated intra-articular hip pathology [1, 5, 6].

Imaging of the Internal Snapping Hip Syndrome

Plain radiographs are usually normal; in some cases, a cam femoroacetabular impingement deformity may be documented. Psoas bursography may outline the tendon and, if combined with fluoroscopy, may document the snapping phenomenon

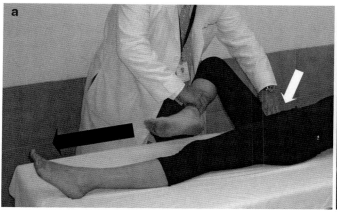 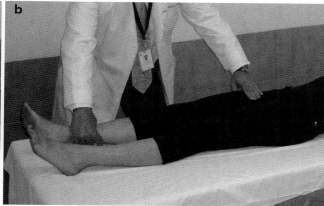

Fig. 21.4 Physical examination for internal snapping hip syndrome. The patient is supine as the right hip is examined. The examiner flexes the hip more than 90° and abducts and externally rotates (**a**). Extending the hip while bringing it to neutral abduction and adduction (*black arrow*) will reproduce the snapping phenomenon. The snapping may be audible or described by the patient. The hand of the examiner may be placed in the groin to feel the snapping phenomenon as the hip is extended (*white arrow*). (**b**) The hip is brought to neutral extension, abduction, and rotation

dynamically. The main problem is that it depends on the ability of the technician to reproduce the snapping while examining hip motion within the range of view of the C-arm [7]. Ultrasonography of the iliopsoas tendon is a dynamic noninvasive study that may document the snapping phenomenon as well as pathologic changes of the iliopsoas tendon and its bursa. Psoas ultrasonography also depends on the ability and experience of the examiner [8]. More recently, ultrasonography has also been used to describe new mechanisms of iliopsoas snapping, like the bifid iliopsoas tendon or snapping of the iliopsoas over the iliacus muscle and snapping of the iliopsoas tendon over paralabral cysts [9]. Because almost half of the patients with internal snapping hip syndrome have associated intra-articular hip pathology [5, 6, 10], magnetic resonance arthrography is the diagnostic study we prefer. It may demonstrate intra-articular pathology and report changes related to the iliopsoas tendon and bursa. The snapping phenomenon cannot be documented using magnetic resonance arthrography (Fig. 21.5).

Iliopsoas Impingement

Iliopsoas impingement may be present in both natural and artificial hips. In the case of a natural hip, it has been theorized that because of its close relationship to the anterior hip, a tight iliopsoas tendon may be a cause of anterior labral lesions (Fig. 21.6) [3]. The clinical presentation of this form of iliopsoas impingement may not be accompanied by a snapping phenomenon and have positive impingement tests, log roll, and mechanical hip symptoms more in accordance with symptoms related to a labral tear [11].

When iliopsoas impingement occurs in presence of total hip replacement, affected patients typically report persisting

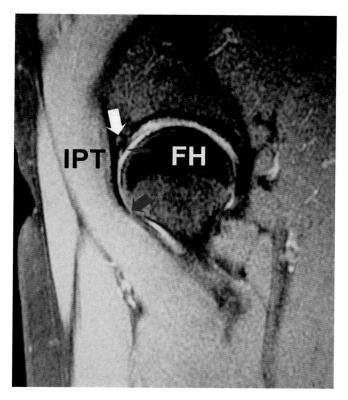

Fig. 21.5 Proton density image of a right hip. The *white arrow* points to a paralabral cyst at the perilabral sulcus behind the hip capsule and the iliopsoas muscle–tendon unit (*IPT*). The *red arrow* points to the anterior labrum. There is some contrast between the articular cartilage and the labrum corresponding to a small labral detachment. The *gray arrow* points to the contact area between the nonspherical portion of the anterior femoral head (*FH*)–neck junction and the iliopsoas muscle–tendon unit (*IPT*)

groin pain that is exacerbated by stair climbing, getting into or out of bed or a chair, and entering and exiting an automobile. A snapping phenomenon or a clunk is usually not present.

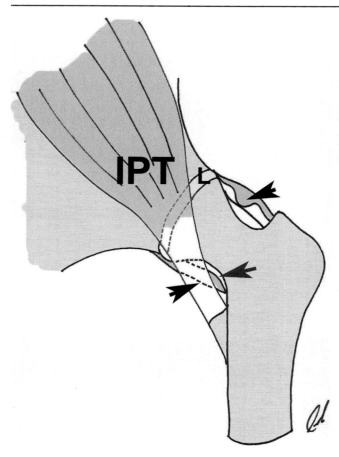

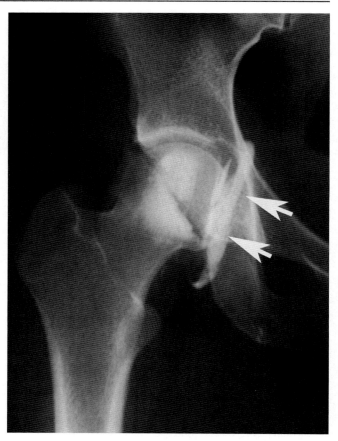

Fig. 21.6 The drawing represents the relation between the iliopsoas tendon (*IPT*) and the anterior hip joint (left hip). The anterior labrum is immediately behind the iliopsoas muscle–tendon unit. The *black arrows* point to the zona orbicularis and the hip capsule. The *red arrow* points to the medial synovial fold (Courtesy, Javier Camacho-Galindo, M.D.)

Fig. 21.7 Iliopsoas bursography in a right hip, the *white arrows* point to the contrast inside the iliopsoas bursa, the fill defect inside the iliopsoas bursa is the iliopsoas tendon itself. In this case, there is a communication between the iliopsoas bursa and the hip capsule (normal finding). Local anesthetics are always infiltrated; improvement of painful symptoms in the front of the hip is a positive diagnostic test

Gait may be affected with the patient presenting a slight limp. It is important to remember that the patients must first be evaluated for more common causes of groin pain after total hip replacement like infection, component loosening, and occult periprosthetic fractures [4, 12]. A typical finding on radiographs or computed tomography is a protruding anterior implant rim uncovered by the bony anterior acetabular wall.

Conservative treatment for both conditions (iliopsoas impingement in natural and artificial hip joints) is the same, including rest, nonsteroidal anti-inflammatory drugs, and physical therapy. Iliopsoas injections are of limited therapeutic value, but they represent a very reliable diagnostic test (Fig. 21.7). After failure of conservative treatment, surgical release of the iliopsoas tendon may be indicated.

In the case of iliopsoas impingement with a natural hip joint, hip arthroscopy will provide access for treatment of the associated lesions such as labral tears or underlying bony impingement [3, 13].

When iliopsoas impingement is present in an artificial total hip joint, acetabular component revision for reorientation

and open iliopsoas release have been reported. Both techniques seem to be effective in the treatment of iliopsoas impingement with the open release of the iliopsoas tendon presenting less morbidity [12]. It is also possible to perform endoscopic release of the iliopsoas tendon in a total hip replacement but reported results in the peer-reviewed literature is limited [1].

Endoscopic Release of the Iliopsoas Tendon

Endoscopic release of the iliopsoas tendon has evolved over the past decade. A variety of surgical techniques is available for release of the iliopsoas tendon at different anatomical regions.

As described from proximal to distal, endoscopic release of the iliopsoas tendon may be transcapsular at two different sites: [1] from the central compartment and [2] from the hip periphery. It can also be performed within the iliopsoas bursa

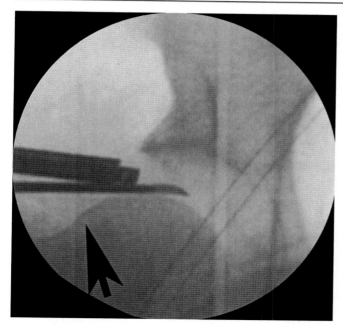

Fig. 21.8 Fluoroscopy photograph of a right hip. The hip is in traction. A 70° arthroscope through the anterolateral portal is viewing the anterior hip capsule. An anterior capsulotomy is performed using an arthroscopy knife introduced through the direct anterior portal. The *black arrow* points to a very evident cam deformity

at its insertion on the lesser trochanter. For either one of these techniques, the patient is positioned for hip arthroscopy in supine or lateral decubitus [14, 15].

Transcapsular Iliopsoas Tendon Release

Central Compartment Release

(See Video 21.1: http://goo.gl/4t3r7) Iliopsoas tendon from the central compartment is performed with the hip joint in traction [16]. The anterolateral portal [17] (as described by Dr. Byrd at the anterior superior corner of the greater trochanter) is used as the viewing portal. With a 70° arthroscope, the anterior capsule is identified. From the direct anterior portal, a radiofrequency hook probe or an arthroscopic banana knife is introduced to create an anterior hip capsulotomy relative to the 2 and 3 o'clock position of the labrum in a right hip or geographic zone 1 [18] (Figs. 21.8 and 21.9). Fibers of the iliopsoas tendon are visualized through the capsulotomy. The tendon is further exposed using a mechanical shaver. A radiofrequency hook probe is used to release the tendon in a retrograde fashion leaving the iliacus muscle intact (Fig. 21.10).

Release from the Hip Periphery

(See Video 19.2: http://goo.gl/DCHaC) Iliopsoas tendon release from the hip periphery is performed without traction.

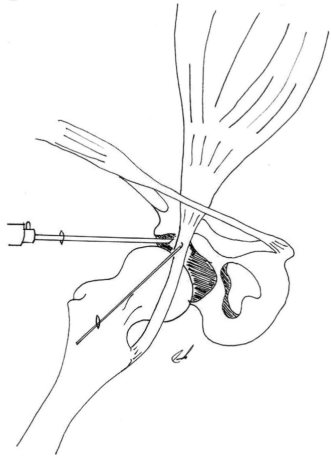

Fig. 21.9 The drawing represents a transcapsular iliopsoas tendon release in a right hip. Note that the hip is in traction. The arthroscope is in position through the anterolateral portal. The field of view is directed to the anterior hip capsule. A radiofrequency hook probe is used to perform the anterior hip capsulotomy and release the tendinous portion of the iliopsoas muscle–tendon unit in a retrograde fashion (Courtesy, Javier Camacho-Galindo, M.D.)

A 70° or a 30° arthroscope is positioned into the peripheral compartment anterior and inferior to the femoral neck through the anterolateral portal (Figs. 21.11 and 21.12). Landmarks at the hip periphery must be identified [19]. The medial synovial fold serves as the best landmark to identify the inferior aspect of the head and neck (6 o'clock position). The proximal origin of the medial synovial fold at the inferior head–neck junction is visualized. The field of view is rotated to the anterior hip capsule. The midanterior portal [20] is used to introduce instruments into the peripheral compartment. A capsulotomy is performed between the zona orbicularis and the labrum, directly above the medial synovial fold, which exposes the iliopsoas tendon fibers. In some cases, a natural communication between the anterior hip capsule and the iliopsoas bursa is already present at this level. The tendon is further exposed using a mechanical shaver.

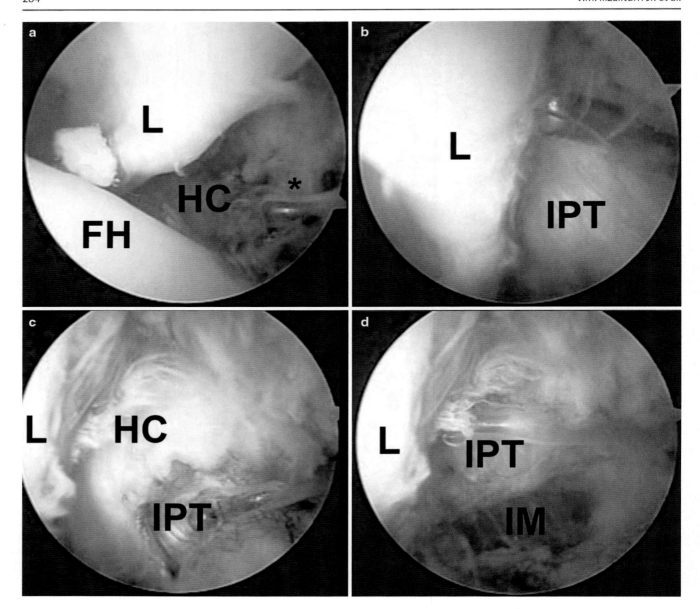

Fig. 21.10 Sequence of arthroscopic photographs demonstrating a central compartment transcapsular iliopsoas tendon release in a right hip. (**a**) A radiofrequency hook probe is used to perform a capsulotomy on the anterior hip capsule (*HC*). The anterior labrum (*L*) is at the *top* and the femoral head (*FH*) is at the *bottom*. The iliopsoas tendon (*) is coming into view through the capsulotomy. (**b**) With the capsulotomy completed, the iliopsoas tendon (*IPT*) is further exposed using a mechanical shaver. The intimate relationship between the iliopsoas ten-don (IPT) and the anterior labrum (*L*) is demonstrated. (**c**) The iliopsoas tendon (*IPT*) is released using a radiofrequency hook probe using a in a retrograde fashion. The window in the hip capsule (*HC*) used to access the iliopsoas tendon is clearly visible. The anterior labrum (*L*) is to the *left*. (**d**) A full release of the tendinous portion of the iliopsoas tendon is completed leaving the iliacus muscle (*IM*) intact. The radiofrequency hook probe is pointing to the released portion of the iliopsoas tendon (*IPT*). The anterior labrum (*L*) is to the *left*

Finally, the iliopsoas tendon is released in a retrograde fashion using a radiofrequency hook probe. The iliacus muscle is left intact behind the released iliopsoas tendon (Fig. 21.13).

Release in the Iliopsoas Bursa

(See Video 21.3: http://goo.gl/oJCcX) Using an accessory portal, a spinal needle is introduced into the iliopsoas immediately proximal to the lesser trochanter [5, 6]. The anterior aspect of the proximal femur may be palpated to navigate the needle in the sagittal plane and an image intensifier is used to navigate the needle in the coronal plane (Figs. 21.14 and 21.15). With the needle in position directly proximal to the lesser trochanter, the stylus is removed and a guidewire introduced; the cannulated hip arthroscopy instruments are used to establish a viewing portal. A 30° arthroscope is introduced and the fibers of the iliopsoas tendon at its insertion on the lesser

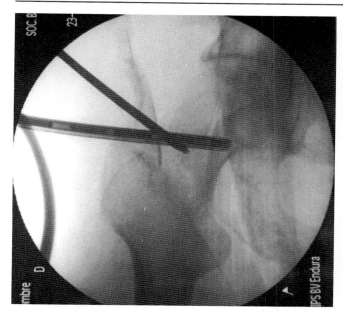

Fig. 21.11 Fluoroscopy photograph of a right hip. The arthroscope is in position at the anterior inferior aspect of the hip periphery using the anterolateral portal. Note that the hip is externally rotated (prominent lesser trochanter) and without traction. A cannulated switching stick is being introduced into the hip periphery through the midanterior portal triangulating toward the tip of the arthroscope

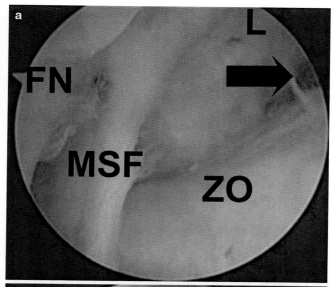

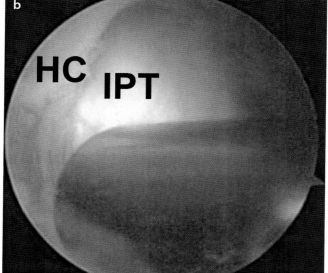

Fig. 21.13 Arthroscopic sequence of photographs demonstrating a transcapsular iliopsoas tendon release from the hip periphery. A right hip is demonstrated. (**a**) Landmarks are demonstrated at the anterior inferior hip periphery. The femoral neck (*FN*) is to the *left*. The medial synovial fold (*MSF*) and zona orbicularis (*ZO*) are to the *center* of the photograph. The anterior inferior labrum (*L*) is at the *top*. The *arrow* points to the site where the capsulotomy is performed to access the iliopsoas tendon. (**b**) A shaver is used to further expose the iliopsoas tendon (*IPT*) through the window created at the anterior inferior hip capsule (*HC*). (**c**) The iliopsoas tendon (*IPT*) is clearly identified through the window at the anterior inferior hip capsule (*HC*). (**d**) The iliopsoas tendon (*IPT*) is fully released leaving the iliacus muscle (*IM*) intact

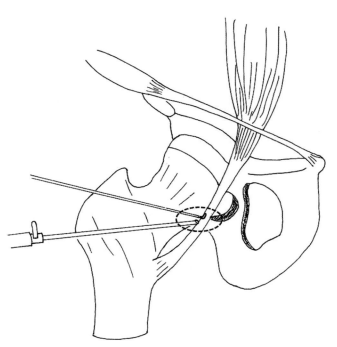

Fig. 21.12 The drawing represents a transcapsular release from the hip periphery in a right hip. Note that the hip is without traction. The arthroscope and the radiofrequency probe are in position at the anterior inferior hip periphery. A capsulotomy is performed between the zona orbicularis and the labrum directly above the medial synovial fold to expose the iliopsoas tendon (Courtesy, Javier Camacho-Galindo, M.D.)

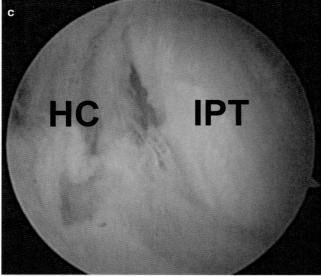

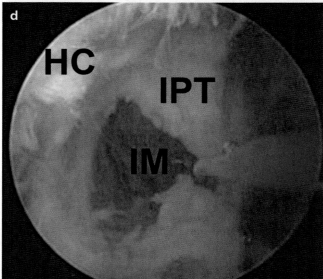

Fig. 21.13 (continued)

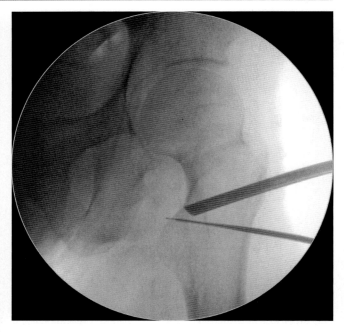

Fig. 21.14 Fluoroscopy photograph of a left hip. Instruments are in position inside the iliopsoas bursa at the insertion of the iliopsoas tendon on the lesser trochanter. Note that the hip is without traction and in external rotation to expose the lesser trochanter

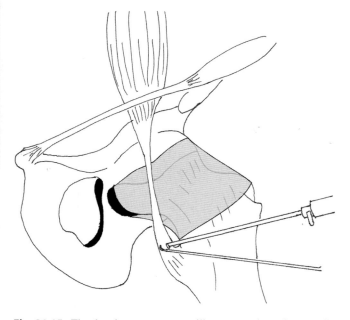

Fig. 21.15 The drawing represents an iliopsoas tendon release at the lesser trochanter in a left hip. Note that instruments are extracapsular (Courtesy, Javier Camacho-Galindo, M.D.)

trochanter identified. A second accessory portal is established triangulating a spinal needle to the tip of the arthroscope. Once the needle is observed inside the iliopsoas bursa, a guidewire and cannulated hip arthroscopy instruments are used to establish a working portal. The iliopsoas tendon is further exposed using a mechanical shaver and released in a retrograde fashion using a radiofrequency hook probe (Fig. 21.16).

Surgical anatomy of the iliopsoas tendon is important when doing an endoscopic release. The level of the release will determine the volume of the tendon that is cut and the resulting volume of the muscle fibers that are kept unreleased. In a cross-sectional anatomic study of the iliopsoas tendon, Zellner et al. [21] reported the average diameter and percentage of tendon and muscle at different levels. Using 20 embalmed cadavers, they measured the diameter of the muscle–tendon unit of the iliopsoas at the level of the labrum, the hip periph-

ery and its insertion on the lesser trochanter. At each one of the described levels, they looked at the percentage of tendon and muscle. They reported that the average circumference of the iliopsoas muscle–tendon unit at the level of the labrum was 68.3 mm in diameter, at the level of the hip periphery 58 mm in diameter, and at the lesser trochanter 45.7 mm in

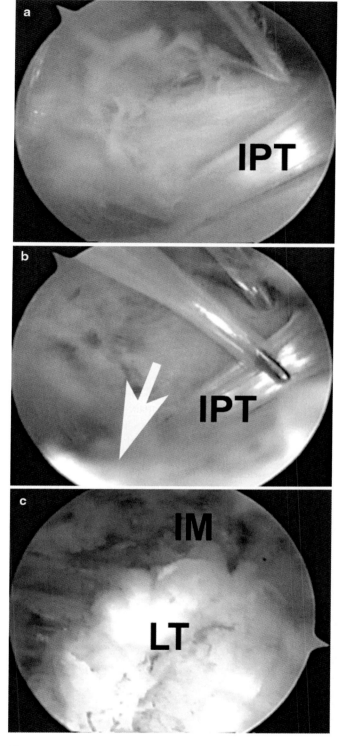

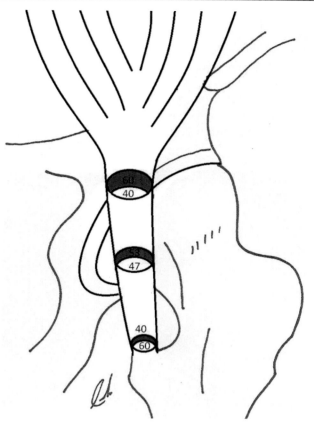

Fig. 21.17 The drawing represents a left hip. The volume of tendon and muscle of the iliopsoas tendon unit at the level of the anterior labrum, the hip periphery, and the lesser trochanter is represented (Courtesy, Javier Camacho-Galindo, M.D.)

diameter. At the level of the labrum, the muscle–tendon unit consisted of 40% tendon and 60% muscle, at the level of the hip periphery it consisted of 53% tendon and 47% muscle, and at the level of the lesser trochanter insertion it consisted of 60% tendon and 40% muscle. Based on this information, a more proximal release will leave more muscle tissue left intact and affect less the overall volume of the muscle–tendon unit (Fig. 21.17). This in theory may produce less functional compromise but could also be related to more frequency of recurrence of the snapping phenomenon after release. Our current protocol for release of the iliopsoas tendon in a primary case is at the level of the labrum. In the case of iliopsoas tendinitis in the presence of total hip replacement, our preferred technique is to release the tendon at its insertion on the lesser trochanter due to the large amount of scar tissue that may be present at the front of the prosthetic joint (Fig. 21.18).

Fig. 21.16 Endoscopic sequence of photographs demonstrating an iliopsoas tendon release at the lesser trochanter in a left hip. (**a**) The iliopsoas tendon (*IPT*) is identified inside the iliopsoas bursa at its insertion on the lesser trochanter. The arthroscope is introduced using an inferior accessory portal. (**b**) Using a second accessory portal, the radiofrequency hook probe is introduced into the bursa directed to the insertion of the iliopsoas tendon (*IPT*) on the lesser trochanter. The iliopsoas tendon is released in a retrograde fashion (the *white arrow* points to the insertion of the iliopsoas tendon on the lesser trochanter). (**c**) After the iliopsoas tendon is released from the lesser trochanter (*LT*), some fibers of the iliacus muscle (*IM*) remain intact

Results

Encouraging results have been reported with endoscopic release of the iliopsoas tendon in the treatment of the internal snapping hip syndrome. The most common technique reported has been release at the lesser trochanter [5, 6, 10]. Endoscopic release at the lesser trochanter has also been successful in the treatment of athletic population with internal snapping hip syndrome [22]. In general, there are higher success rates and less recurrence when the endoscopic technique is compared with the open procedures [23–26]; this may be because in the endoscopic studies that are published, arthroscopic treatment of intra-articular associated pathology has been performed. Frequent procedures reported in the literature to treat associated injuries are remodeling of femoroacetabular impingement deformities, labral repair, or partial labral resection and cartilage lesions repair (removal of unstable cartilage and microfractures) [5, 6, 10, 22]. A comparative analysis of endoscopic versus open release of the iliopsoas tendon for the treatment of internal snapping hip syndrome is presented in Table 21.1.

There is less literature regarding the success of endoscopic transcapsular release of the iliopsoas tendon at the level of the labrum [16] or at the hip periphery [19]. The author has reported a comparative prospective randomized study of the technique for release of the iliopsoas tendon at the lesser trochanter and transcapsular at the hip periphery and found no difference statistically significant difference between both techniques [13].

Heterotopic bone formation has been reported associated with release of the iliopsoas tendon. This complication may be associated with the need for further surgical procedures and compromise treatment outcome. This has been reported for both open and endoscopic release at the level of the lesser trochanter [27, 28]. Prophylaxis with 400 mg/day of celecoxib seems to be effective in preventing this complication, but more evidence is needed [13]. In the case of internal snapping hip, recurrence may be secondary to incomplete release or inadequate management of associated bony deformities. More recently, the presence of a bifid iliopsoas tendon has been reported as a cause of recurrence of snapping after endoscopic iliopsoas tendon release. To avoid this complication, the presence of the bifid tendon should be identified before surgery with adequate imaging if possible. Also a finding that must alert the surgeon is the presence of an unusually thin

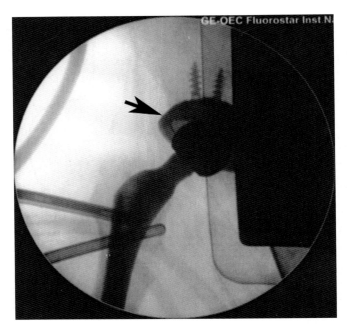

Fig. 21.18 Fluoroscopy photograph demonstrating iliopsoas tendon release at the level of the lesser trochanter in a right hip with a total hip prosthesis. The *black arrow* points to a large implant overhang relative to the patient's acetabulum

Table 21.1 Results of endoscopic iliopsoas tendon release

Author	Number of hips	Technique	Follow-up	Pain	Re-snapping
Taylor [23]	17	Open release	17 months	0	5
Jacobson [24]	20	Open Z-plasty	20 months	2 (reoperated)	6
Dobbs [25]	11	Open Z-plasty	4 years	0	1
Gruen [26]	11	Open Z-plasty	3 years	0	0
Byrd [5]	9	Endoscopic release at lesser trochanter	20 months	0	0
Ilizaliturri [6]	7	Endoscopic release at the lesser trochanter	21 months	0	0
Dienst [19]	9	Endoscopic release (preserving iliacus muscle) transcapsular	3 months (technique report)	0	0
Flanum [10]	6	Endoscopic release at the lesser trochanter	12 months	0	0
Anderson [22]	15	Endoscopic release at lesser trochanter (athletes)	9 months	0	0
Ilizaliturri [13]	19	Endoscopic release at lesser trochanter [10] and endoscopic transcapsular [9] (randomized)	20 months	0	0
Contreras [16]	7	Endoscopic transcapsular from the central compartment	24	0	0

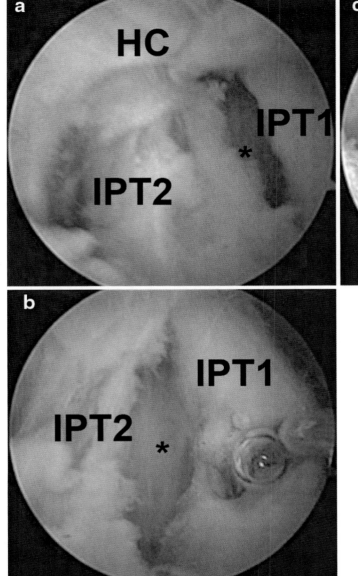

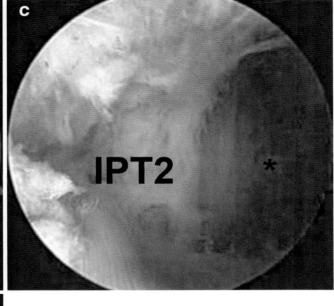

Fig. 21.19 Sequence of arthroscopic photographs during a transcapsular iliopsoas tendon release in a right hip. This case has a bifid iliopsoas tendon. (**a**) A window at the anterior hip capsule (*HC*) was performed at the anterior inferior hip periphery. Two iliopsoas tendons are observed through the capsulotomy (*IPT1* and *IPT2*). The secondary iliopsoas tendon (IPT2) is more medial. The iliacus muscle (*) can be observed behind both tendons. (**b**) The first iliopsoas tendon (*IPT1*) is released using a radiofrequency hook probe in a retrograde fashion. The iliacus muscle (*) is at the *center* and the secondary iliopsoas tendon (*IPT2*) to the *left* of the photograph. (**c**) The secondary iliopsoas tendon (*IPT2*) is released using a radiofrequency hook probe in a retrograde fashion. The iliacus muscle (*) is to the *right* of the photograph

tendon that may suggest that there is a more medial secondary tendon. It is better visualized with a long medial capsulotomy from the hip periphery (Fig. 21.19) [29].

References

1. Ilizaliturri Jr VM, Camacho-Galindo J, Evia Ramirez AN, Gonzalez Ibarra YL, Millan SM, Busconi BD. Soft tissue pathology around the hip. Clin Sports Med. 2011;30:391–415.

2. Allen WC, Cope R. Coxa saltans: the snapping hip revisited. J Am Acad Orthop Surg. 1995;3:303–8.

3. Alpert JM, Kozanek M, Li G, Kelly BT, Asnis PD. Cross sectional analysis of the iliopsoas tendon and its relationship to the acetabular labrum: an anatomic study. Am J Sports Med. 2009;37:1594–8.

4. Lachiewicz PF, Kauk JR. Anterior iliopsoas impingement and tendinitis after total hip arthroplasty. J Am Acad Orthop Surg. 2009;17:337–44.

5. Byrd JWT. Evaluation and management of the snapping iliopsoas tendon. Tech Orthop. 2005;20:45–51.

6. Ilizaliturri Jr VM, Villalobos FE, Chaidez PA, Valero FS, Aguilera JM. Internal snapping hip syndrome: treatment by endoscopic release of the iliopsoas tendon. Arthroscopy. 2005;21:1375–80.

7. Harper MC, Schaberg JE, Allen WC. Primary iliopsoas bursography in the diagnosis of disorders of the hip. Clin Orthop Relat Res. 1987;221:238–41.

8. Cardinal E, Buckwalter KA, Capello WN, Duval N. US of the snapping iliopsoas tendon. Radiology. 1996;198:521–2.

9. Deslandes M, Guillin R, Cardinal E, Hobden R, Bureau NJ. The snapping iliopsoas tendon: new mechanisms using dynamic sonography. AJR Am J Roentgenol. 2008;190(3):576–81.

10. Flanum ME, Keene JS, Blankenbaker DG, Desmet AA. Arthroscopic treatment of the painful "internal" snapping hip: results of a new endoscopic technique and imaging protocol. Am J Sports Med. 2007;35:770–9.

11. McCarthy J, Noble P, Aluisio FV, Schuck M, Wright J, Lee JA. Anatomy, pathologic features, and treatment of acetabular labral tears. Clin Orthop Relat Res. 2003;406:38–47.

12. Dora C, Houweling M, Koch P, Sierra RJ. Iliopsoas impingement after total hip replacement: results of non operative management, tenotomy or acetabular revision. J Bone Joint Surg Br. 2007;89:1031–5.

13. Ilizaliturri Jr VM, Chaidez C, Villegas P, Briseño A, Camacho-Galindo J. Prospective randomized study of 2 different techniques for endoscopic iliopsoas tendon release in the treatment of internal snapping hip syndrome. Arthroscopy. 2009;25:159–63.

14. Byrd JWT. Hip arthroscopy utilizing the supine position. Arthroscopy. 1994;10:275–80.

15. Ilizaliturri Jr VM, Mangino G, Valero FS, Camacho-Galindo J. Hip arthroscopy of the central and peripheral compartment by the lateral approach. Tech Orthop. 2005;20:32–6.

16. Contreras MEK, Dani WS, Endges WK, De Araujo LCT, Berral FJ. Arthroscopic treatment of the snapping iliopsoas tendon trough the central compartment of the hip. A pilot study. J Bone Joint Surg Br. 2010;92(B):777–80.

17. Byrd JWT, Pappas JN, Pedley MJ. Hip arthroscopy: an anatomic study of portal placement and relationship to the extraarticular structures. Arthroscopy. 1995;11:418–23.

18. Ilizaliturri Jr VM, Byrd JW, Sampson TG, Guanche CA, Philippon MJ, Kelly BT, Dienst M, Mardones R, Shonnard P, Larson CM. A geographic zone method to describe intra-articular pathology in hip arthroscopy: cadaveric study and preliminary report. Arthroscopy. 2008;24:534–9.

19. Wettstein M, Jung J, Dienst M. Arthroscopic psoas tenotomy. Arthroscopy. 2006;22:907.e1–4.

20. Robertson WJ, Kelly BT. The safe zone for hip arthroscopy: a cadaveric assessment of central, peripheral and lateral compartment portal placement. Arthroscopy. 2008;24:1019–26.

21. Zellner BS, Blomberg JR, Keene JA. Cross-sectional analysis of iliopsoas muscle tendon units at the three sites of arthroscopic tenotomies: an anatomic study. Arthroscopy. 2011;27(Suppl):e4–5.

22. Anderson SA, Keene JS. Results of arthroscopic iliopsoas tendon release in competitive and recreational athletes. Am J Sports Med. 2008;36:2363–71.

23. Taylor GR, Clarke NM. Surgical release of the "snapping iliopsoas tendon". J Bone Joint Surg Br. 1995;77:881–3.

24. Jacobson T, Allen WC. Surgical correction of the snapping iliopsoas tendon. Am J Sports Med. 1990;18:470–4.

25. Dobbs MB, Gordon JE, Luhmann SJ, Szymanzki DA, Schoenecker PL. Surgical correction of the snapping iliopsoas tendon in adolescents. J Bone Joint Surg Am. 2002;84:420–4.

26. Gruen GS, Scioscia TN, Lowenstein JE. The surgical treatment of internal snapping hip. Am J Sports Med. 2002;30:607–13.

27. McCulloch PC, Bush-Joseph CA. Massive heterotopic ossification complicating iliopsoas tendon lengthening. A case report. Am J Sports Med. 2008;34:2022–5.

28. Byrd JWT, Polkowski G, Jones KS. Endoscopic management of the snapping iliopsoas tendon. In: Presented at the 28th annual meeting of the Arthroscopy Association of North America, San Diego; 2009.

29. Shu B, Safran MR. Case report: bifid iliopsoas tendon causing refractory internal snapping hip. Clin Orthop Relat Res. 2001;469:289–93.

Iliotibial Band Release

22

Allston J. Stubbs and Phillip Mason

I have found this procedure to be safe and reproducible.

—*Victor Ilizaliturri, M.D.*

Introduction

Greater trochanteric pain syndrome comprises a variety of disorders about the lateral hip region [1]. Common complaints may include pain, weakness, numbness, and mechanical symptoms. The clinician's role is to differentiate the source of the complaint between intra-articular and extra-articular sources. One's history and physical examination will clarify the etiology in a significant number of cases. Additionally, radiology resources such as plain film, magnetic resonance imaging, bone scintigraphy, and ultrasound will define specific pathoanatomy such as calcific tendonitis, abductor muscle tears, and insidious fracture patterns. Despite modern imaging resources, a diagnostic challenge arises when one attempts to differentiate pain originating from the iliotibial band versus other sources.

The purpose of this chapter is to clarify the role of iliotibial band release in cases of symptomatic hip pain. More specifically, we will define the role of endoscopic iliotibial band release in the context of historical open surgical methods and modern hip pathomechanics. The goals for the reader are to appreciate the anatomy of the lateral hip, to understand the transition from normal iliotibial band mechanics to abnormal iliotibial band mechanics, and to develop an approach to the use of the hip endoscope in treating iliotibial band pathology.

A.J. Stubbs, M.D. (✉)
Department of Orthopaedic Surgery, Wake Forest University, 131 Miller Street, Winston-Salem, NC 27103, USA
e-mail: astubbs@wakehealth.edu

P. Mason, M.D.
Department of Orthopaedic Surgery, Wake Forest University, Medical Centre Boulevard, Winston-Salem, NC 27517, USA
e-mail: pmason@wfubmc.edu

Lateral Hip Anatomy and Pathomechanics

The iliotibial band is formed by the joining of the fascia of tensor fascia lata and the gluteus maximus and an indirect attachment to gluteus medius. It extends from the anterior ilium to Gerdy's tubercle on the lateral tibia with some additional fibers inserting on the lateral patella. At the hip, the ITB acts as a flexor, abductor, and medial rotator. It provides knee stability laterally when standing. The proximal attachments of the ITB tighten when the hip is either flexed or extended.

The abductor muscle compartment as it inserts along the greater trochanter from anterior to posterior is composed of the gluteus minimus and gluteus medius. The gluteus maximus inserts onto the linea aspera in the region of the proximal posterior femur. The iliotibial band proximally is separated from the abductor muscle compartment by the greater trochanteric bursa. Within the greater trochanter, bursal compartment originates the vastus lateralis from the proximal lateral femur.

The emergence of peritrochanteric symptoms may be a result of primary pathology of the local anatomy or may be secondary to intra-articular pathology according to the dictum of Hilton's Law [2]. Hilton's Law basically states that joints and their surrounding soft tissues share the same innervation. Effectively, Hilton's Law accounts for much of the peritrochanteric soft tissue symptomatology seen in the setting of intra-articular hip pathology such as labral tears, loose bodies, and osteoarthritis. As an example, greater trochanteric bursitis is a common diagnosis for hip pain that may have a relationship to central compartment disorders.

In greater trochanteric pain conditions, the differential diagnoses can involve chronic bursitis, abductor muscle tears, nerve entrapments, and snapping syndromes. In the situation of a chronically symptomatic snapping hip, the orthopedic surgeon may find it beneficial to recommend endoscopic evaluation of the greater trochanteric bursal space and release of the proximal iliotibial band.

J.W.T. Byrd (ed.), *Operative Hip Arthroscopy*,
DOI 10.1007/978-1-4419-7925-4_22, © Springer Science+Business Media New York 2013

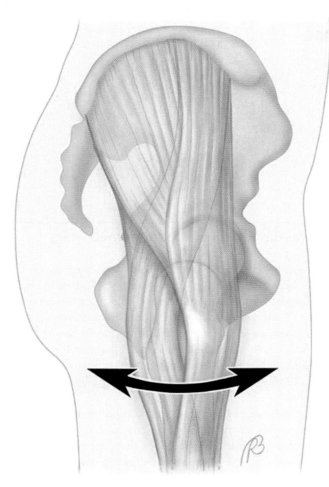

Fig. 22.1 Schematic of iliotibial band snapping: As the iliotibial band snaps back and forth across the greater trochanter, the tendinous portion may flip across the trochanter with flexion and extension, or the trochanter may move back and forth underneath the stationary tendon with internal and external rotation (Courtesy of J. W. Thomas Byrd, M.D., Nashville, TN)

Coxa Saltans Externa (The External Snapping Hip)

Coxa saltans externa is painful mechanical condition caused by the iliotibial band (ITB) or potentially the gluteus maximus snapping across the greater trochanter (GT) of the femur during flexion and extension. External snapping hip is caused by a thickening of the posterior portion of the ITB or the anterior border of gluteus maximus. The ITB is posterior to the hip in extension. When the hip is flexed, the thickened IT band or the gluteus maximus tendon snaps posterior to anterior over the GT [3] (Fig. 22.1).

These symptoms are typically reproducible on exam with hip flexion and extension [4, 5]. The flexion-extension may

be accentuated with external rotation of the leg in hip extension and internal rotation of the leg in hip flexion (Fig. 22.2a, b). Patients often have concomitant greater trochanteric bursitis. Painless external snapping is typically benign and should be considered normal, especially in athletes [3]. Patients may describe the painless external snapping as a "dislocating hip" that can be voluntarily "dislocated" and "relocated" to the amusement of friends and quandary of medical professionals not familiar with the condition. Ultimately, bilateral hip symptoms are common and women are affected more than men [1].

Physical Exam Findings

The nonarthritic snapping hip should be evaluated in a systematic fashion that comprises inspection, palpation, range of motion, muscle testing, provocative testing, and gait analysis. The physical examination should assist the evaluator in determining intra-articular pathology versus extra-articular pathology. Radiographic tests including plain film radiograph and MRI are typically normal.

The most reliable method to assess the snapping hip is to request the patient to reproduce the mechanical phenomenon. Most legitimate snapping syndromes can be voluntarily reproduced in the medical office. Typically, coxa saltans interna originates from the iliopsoas tendon and is more audible than visible. On the other hand, coxa saltans externa from the IT band or gluteus maximus is more visible than audible.

In coxa saltans externa, the snapping sensation occurs in the lateral upper thigh over the region of the greater trochanter. An audible snapping may occur during hip flexion and again when extending the hip from flexion. The majority of cases are palpable and some cases may be visible under the skin. Snapping may also be found during internal and external rotation of the extended and adducted hip [5]. Often, physical examination findings are best elicited with the patient in the lateral decubitus position with the IT band under tension. The amount of IT band tension is assessed side to side with the Ober test [4, 5, 7–9] (Fig. 22.3).

Indication for Surgery

Patients should have painful snapping over the greater trochanter and lateral hemipelvic that occurs in with hip range of motion – most often hip flexion and extension. Patients without pain should be treated nonoperatively. In most painful snapping hip cases, conservative management is usually successful and should be pursued before surgery [3–5, 10]. Conservative management includes activity modification

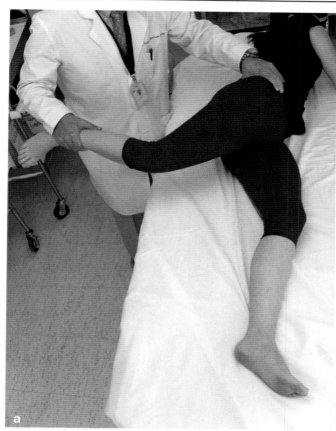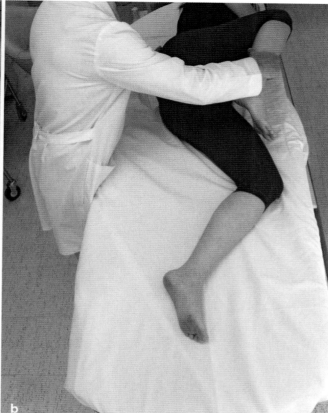

Fig. 22.2 (**a**, **b**) Physical examination of external snapping hip. (**a**) The patient is placed in a lateral position with the asymptomatic hip in the dependent position and flexed. The symptomatic hip in a position of rela- tive extension has the iliotibial band under tension. (**b**) The examiner sub- sequently can flex and extend the symptomatic hip to reproduce the external snapping (Reprinted from Ilizaliturri and Camacho-Galindo [6])

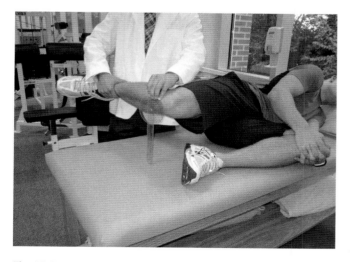

Fig. 22.3 The Ober test is obtained with the patient in a lateral posi- tion with the asymptomatic hip in the dependent position and flexed with the assistance of the hands. The symptomatic hip in a position of relative extension has the iliotibial band under tension. The distance between the medial knee and table can be measured and compared with the contralateral side

and physical therapy with modalities such as iontophoresis and phonophoresis. Nonsteroidal anti-inflammatory medica- tions and steroid injections to the greater trochanteric bursa may also be prescribed. The application of steroid prepara- tions to the greater trochanteric region should be done with care to limit the risk of local fat necrosis and atrophy.

Surgical release of the IT band should be considered when patients have failed nonoperative treatment including activ- ity modification, oral anti-inflammatories, injections, and physical therapy with modalities. In one study for open ili- otibial band release, patients were considered for surgery after failing two stretching methods [10] (Fig. 22.4a, b). Pati- ents in the first method stood on the uninvolved leg with the involved knee resting on a chair, then extended and adducted the involved leg while keeping the knee flexed. The second method offered required patients to stand perpendicular to a wall with legs crossed and the involved hip closest to the wall. Other authors considered endoscopic surgery after patients failed both physical therapy and at least one corti- costeroid injection [7].

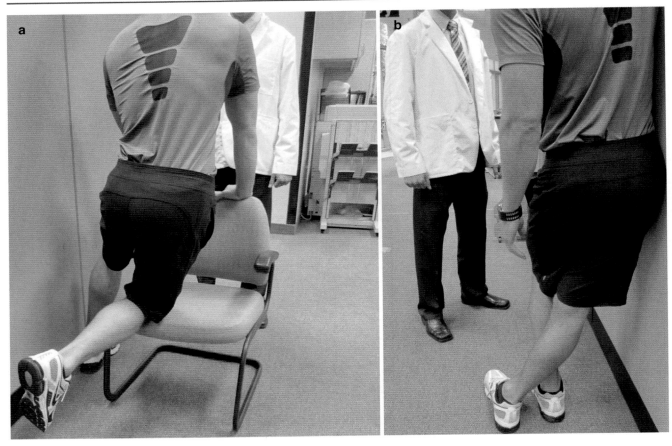

Fig. 22.4 (**a**, **b**) Stretching methods of the proximal iliotibial band. (**a**) The affected hip is positioned on a padded chair in extension and adduction. (**b**) The affected hip is positioned closer to the wall with the affected leg crossed behind the unaffected leg. The patient then leans into the wall to stretch the proximal iliotibial band

Contraindications

Contraindications for surgical management include successful conservative measures, non-painful snapping, local tissue compromise from either infection or decubitus ulceration, poor rehabilitation potential or compliance, and hip osteoarthritis that may require a total hip arthroplasty. Additionally, surgical treatment requires anesthesia and patients should undergo standard perioperative risk stratification and anesthesia preoperative evaluation and workup.

Endoscopic Iliotibial Band Release Technique

(See Video 22.1: http://goo.gl/APn1g) Historically, surgical management of the snapping hip has been open [4, 5, 10]. Endoscopic release of the iliotibial band and concomitant bursectomy has emerged as a valuable alternative to open procedures. The endoscopic technique is minimally invasive and offers patients a quicker return to activity [4, 7, 11]. Also, arthroscopic assessment and treatment of intra-articular pathology is available at the same surgical setting if preoperative evaluation supports a more comprehensive evaluation of the hip joint.

Anesthesia is induced as a general, regional, or combination anesthetic. The patient should be maintained relatively hypotensive during the case to reduce the amount of intraoperative blood loss and improve endoscopic field visualization. Euthermia should be a goal of anesthesia during the procedure and can be achieved with a fluid warmer system and intraoperative warming blanket device.

The procedural portion of surgical management should begin with a surgical timeout that confirms the patient, surgical site/side, and availability of necessary equipment. The patient is placed in the supine or lateral decubitus position on the operating table and appropriately padded along the dependent axilla, iliac crest, and dependent areas of the contralateral leg, ankle, and foot. The pelvis is stabilized by a lateral hip positioner or a beanbag, but the operative hip should remain mobile to assess the hemipelvic motion and greater trochanteric space mechanics throughout the operation. The supine position can be facilitated by positioning the affected extremity in a commercially available hip positioning and distraction system. The IT band is relaxed by placing the hip in neutral flexion, 10–20° of abduction, and, most importantly, out of any traction.

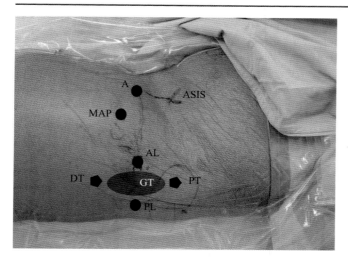

Fig. 22.5 Portal placement in supine position, left hip. *A* anterior portal, *MAP* midanterior portal, *AL* anterolateral portal, *PL* posterolateral portal, *PT* proximal trochanteric portal, *DT* distal trochanteric portal

An examination under anesthesia will occasionally evoke the external snapping hip phenomenon (Fig. 22.2a, b). The effective maneuver begins in extension and slight external rotation and progresses to flexion and mild internal rotation of the lower extremity. The purpose of the maneuver is to reproduce the iliotibial band or gluteus maximus snapping over the greater trochanteric eminence. The examination may be more likely to reproduce the snapping in chronic cases or in gynecoid type pelvises.

After sterile prep and draping, the local hip osteology is marked including the anterosuperior iliac spine and the greater trochanter. Two peritrochanteric portals are marked approximately 3 cm proximal and 3 cm distal to the greater trochanter along the axis of the femur (Fig. 22.5). Alternatively, if a hip arthroscopy central compartment examination is included in the procedure, one can utilize the anterolateral portal as one of the primary portals with an accessory portal 3 cm proximal or distal to the tip of the greater trochanter. With a two-portal approach, one portal will be for the endoscope and the other portal will be for any instrumentation. Additional portals may be needed to address tears of the gluteal muscles, concomitant exploration or treatment of the deep gluteal space, or release of the iliopsoas from the lesser trochanter.

Two different approaches are available to visualize the region of interest along the iliotibial band: one that begins within the space between the subcutaneous fascia and the iliotibial band, and a second that begins within the greater trochanteric bursa. Both approaches begin with the injection of approximately 40–60 cc of normal saline or lactated ringer's solution just distal to the tip of the greater trochanter into the tissue plane lateral to the IT Band or into the greater trochanteric bursa medial to the IT band. This application of fluid is used to define an effective space in which to deliver the endoscope.

Two arthroscopic portals are used: the infratrochanteric portal and the supratrochanteric portal, which are respectively inserted ~3 cm to the proximal and distal to the GT. The area of palpable snapping should be centered between the portals.

The inferior trochanteric portal is developed with a skin incision and the introduction of the arthroscopic cannula with a blunt obturator directed toward the tip of the greater trochanter. A 30° 4-mm arthroscopy is used with low water pressure to create a space between the iliotibial band and the subcutaneous tissue. The superior trochanteric portal is then created under direct endoscopic visualization utilizing a Seldinger-type technique. Briefly, this technique involves placing a spinal needle into the bursal space, followed by a Nitinol guidewire through the needle. The needle is removed and a cannula-obturator pair is passed over the wire. With the wire removed, the obturator-cannula system should be utilized to develop an effective space comparable to what is done in the subacromial space during shoulder arthroscopy.

A curved or straight shaving blade is inserted in the superior portal and is used to clear the subcutaneous tissue overlying the iliotibial band or the greater trochanteric bursal space. A radiofrequency probe is used through the superior portal for hemostasis and further development of the effective working space. In the subcutaneous approach lateral to the IT band, one must be careful not to overresect the subcutaneous tissue resulting in a cosmetic deformity along the lateral hip.

Once the IT band has been identified by its characteristic collagen banding and glistening surface, the surgeon can map out the release via bony landmarks, dynamic assessment, and pathologic evidence. Occasionally, we recommend the placement of spinal needles according to known external landmarks from outside the hip into the effective space as reference markers. These spinal needles can define the proximal, distal, anterior, and posterior margins of the release area.

Two endoscopic IT band release techniques have been described: the cruciform technique [6] (Fig. 22.6a–c) and the modified cruciform technique [12, 13] (Fig. 22.7a–d). The cruciform technique relies on a longitudinal cut in line with the fibers of the IT band followed by a cut transverse across the fibers of the IT band. The bisection of the cuts should be centered over the region of the IT band just lateral and slightly posterior to the greater trochanter. The second technique, the modified cruciform technique, is created from a single longitudinal cut followed by two transverse cuts spaced in thirds along the primary longitudinal cut. The central third of the modified cruciform release should be developed lateral to the greater trochanter in the area of maximal snapping.

The actual release or cutting of the IT band can be performed with either a cutting RF device or a sharp arthroscopic knife (Figs. 22.6 and 22.7). Both should be used under direct visualization. The RF has the advantage of direct hemostasis with cutting, while the arthroscopic knife may have more control with cutting. In the cruciate release, an approximately 4-cm longitudinal cut should be made along the direction of the iliotibial band fibers distal to the greater trochanter. Abducting the hip reveals the cut edges that should be developed with the shaver (Fig. 22.6c). Next, two horizontal cuts through the anterior and posterior aspects of the iliotibial band are made at the edge of the vertical cut in a cruciform pattern to create four flaps. These flaps are then resected with a shaver and ablator to generate a diamond-shaped defect over the area of suspected snapping (Fig. 22.7c). The bursa may be debrided through the defect if one is entering from

superficial to deep. In a similar fashion, the modified cruciate release is preformed, but utilizing two anterior to posterior transverse cuts. The resulting flaps are ellipsed with an arthroscopic shaver.

In both approaches, the bursa is resected until the greater trochanter is clearly seen. During the bursectomy, the

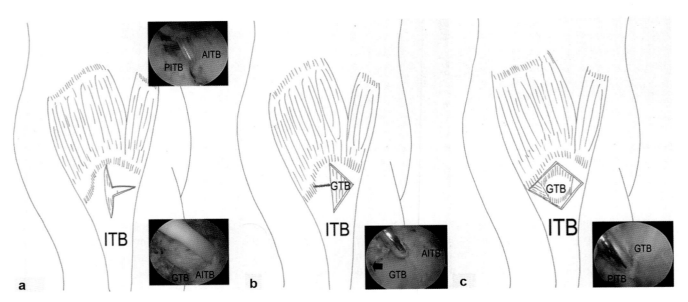

Fig. 22.6 (**a–c**) Schematic and arthroscopic imaging of IT band cruciform release technique. (**a**) Linear vertical incision and anterior horizontal incision release, (**b**) posterior horizontal incision release, (**c**) fully ellipsed release. *ITB* iliotibial band, *AITB* anterior iliotibial band, *PITB* posterior iliotibial band, *GTB* greater trochanteric bursa (Reprinted from Ilizaliturri and Camacho-Galindo [6])

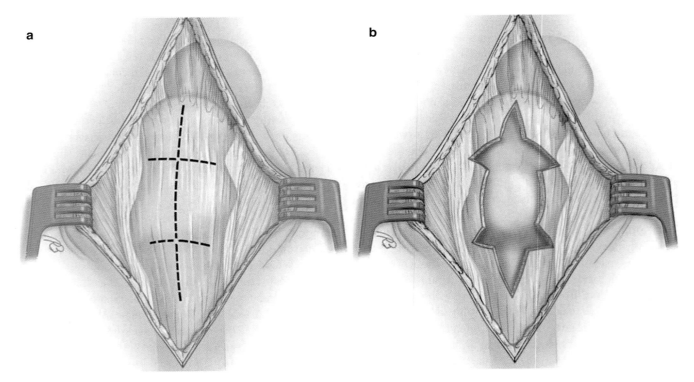

Fig. 22.7 (**a–d**) Schematic of IT band-modified cruciform release technique. (**a**) Illustration depicts the modified cruciate incision; (**b**) bi-horizontal incision release and the relaxing effect on the iliotibial band is illustrated; (**c**) viewing the peritrochanteric space of a right hip from the anterior portal, the longitudinal limb of the modified cruciate incision is being created with an arthroscopic knife; (**d**) final arthroscopic view of modified cruciate release with relaxation of the iliotibial band (Courtesy of J. W. Thomas Byrd, M.D., Nashville, TN)

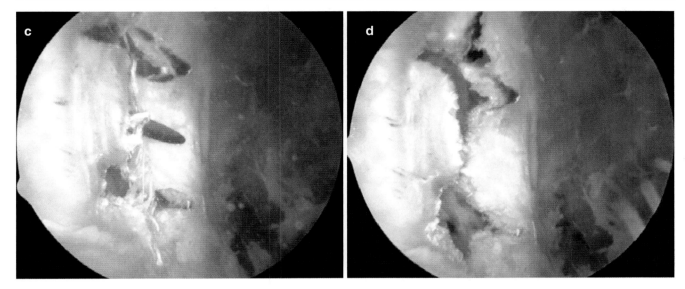

Fig. 22.7 (continued)

surgeon must respect the hip capsule, external rotators, abductor muscle envelope, and neurovascular structures that are susceptible to iatrogenic injury [4, 7, 11]. Although the snapping phenomenon is not typically observed under arthroscopic or direct visualization during anesthesia, the patient's hip should be evaluated for resolution of the snapping following bursal debridement and iliotibial band release. If no snapping is visualized directly or via the arthroscope, the release may be considered adequate. If snapping is not resolved, then debridement and release may be continued posteriorly. One must exercise care when moving posteriorly because of the close proximity of the sciatic nerve. While not extensively studied, persistent snapping may indicate a gluteal maximus etiology that should be arthroscopically evaluated. Finally, removal of hardware is recommended in cases of residual hardware about the greater trochanter such as a fixation from an intramedullary femoral nail that may upset the local soft tissue balance.

Instrumentation is removed along with excessive fluid and the portals are sutured closed. Local anesthetic may be injected about the portal sites and peritrochanteric space. Sterile compressive dressings are applied. Patients may be admitted overnight for pain control and observation. Thigh compartment syndrome is a theoretical complication of this procedure and thigh compartment status should be noted at the end of the procedure.

Postoperative Management

Patients are allowed protected flat foot weight bearing as tolerated with crutches until limping resolves. Patients usually use crutches for approximately 5–7 days based on activity level and overall peripelvic condition. While no bracing is required, an abduction orthosis may support the hip through its early stages of recovery and rehabilitation. Physical therapy may be started on postoperative day 1 with emphasis on gentle hip range of motion and gait reeducation. IT band stretching is gradually progressed according to symptoms. Range of motion optimization is followed by endurance and strengthening rehabilitation.

Results

Endoscopic release of the iliotibial band is a valuable alternative to the open procedure. The procedure allows for rapid recover with full weight bearing and range of motion within 24 h [7, 11]. Results in the literature are limited for both open and arthroscopic IT band release for external snapping hip, but initial reports are promising (Table 22.1). The outcomes appear to be at least comparable, if not superior, to open techniques. The literature reports no complications from the procedure [7, 11]. Endoscopic release may also be advantageous in obese patients when a larger incision may be subject to high tension and wound healing problems. Early physical therapy may also be started if recurrence is a concern.

While no specific complications are reported with this technique, it should be stated that one approaching the proximal IT band endoscopically should be aware of certain pitfalls. First, overresection of the IT band may predispose a patient to an obvious soft tissue defect and resulting postoperative seroma (Fig. 22.8). Next, fluid management is important and any prolonged case should be observed for compartment syndrome of the thigh. Finally, while the anatomy about the lateral hip is well understood, endoscopic visualization can be difficult and, at times, disorienting, and the surgeon should be deliberate in one's actions to avoid iatrogenic injury to normal tissue. For example, inadvertent

Table 22.1 Results of surgical treatment of external snapping hip syndrome

Study (year)	No. of hips	Technique	Follow-up	Pain	Resnapping
Fery and Sommelet (1988) [14]	35	Open, crosscut, and inverted flap suture	7 years	21 cases	10 cases
Faraj et al. (2001) [10]	11	Open, Z-plasty	12 months	3 cases	0
Provencher et al. (2004) [5]	9	Open, Z-plasty	22 months	1 case	0
White et al. (2004) [15]	17	Open vertical incision and multiple transverse cuts	32.5 months	0	2 cases (reoperated)
Ilizaliturri et al. (2006) [11]	11	Arthroscopic diamond-shaped defect	25 months	0	1 case, improved with physical therapy
Farr et al. (2007) [7]	2	Endoscopic ITB release and bursectomy	32 months 50 months	0	0

Adapted from Ilizaliturri [16]. With permission from Elsevier

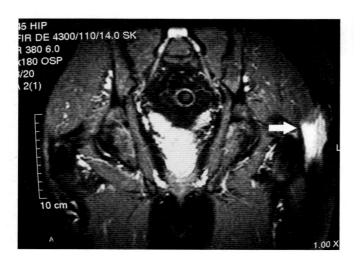

Fig. 22.8 MRI T2 coronal AP of pelvis s/p IT band release left hip. Note seroma formation as indicated by *white arrow*

surgical release of the abductor muscle insertion along the greater trochanter would be a significant complication without a reliable solution. Ultimately, conversion from an endoscopic to an open procedure would be appropriate in the setting of poor visualization or lack of anatomic orientation.

Conclusion

When painful, external snapping hip syndrome can be a significant clinical problem. Endoscopic IT band release is a reasonable treatment option in cases of failed nonoperative management. Reports of complications of the endoscopic technique are low, and return to a high level of function postoperatively is high. Endoscopic management has the distinct advantage of being a part of a global arthroscopic approach to the patient with hip pain.

References

1. Strauss EJ, Nho SJ, Kelly BT. Greater trochanteric pain syndrome. Sports Med Arthrosc. 2010;18:113–9.
2. Hilton J. Rest and pain. London: Bell; 1863.
3. Allen W, Cope R. Coxa saltans: the snapping hip revisited. J Am Acad Orthop Surg. 1995;3:303–8.
4. Ilizaliturri Jr VM, Camacho-Galindo J. Endoscopic treatment of snapping hips, iliotibial band, and iliopsoas tendon. Sports Med Arthrosc. 2010;18:120–7.
5. Provencher MT, Hofmeister EP, Muldoon MP. The surgical treatment of external coxa saltans (the snapping hip) by Z-plasty of the iliotibial band. Am J Sports Med. 2004;32:470–6.
6. Ilizaliturri VM, Camacho-Galindo J. Release of iliopsoas tendon and iliotibial band. Oper Tech Sports Med. Elsevier, Philadelphia, PA.
7. Farr D, Selesnick H, Janecki C. Arthroscopic bursectomy with concomitant iliotibial band release for the treatment of recalcitrant trochanteric bursitis. Arthroscopy. 2007;23:905.e1–5.
8. Teitz CC, Garrett Jr WE, Miniaci A. Tendon problems in athletic individuals. Instr Course Lect. 1997;46:569–82.
9. Ober FR. The role of the iliotibial band and fascia lata as a factor in the causation of low-back disabilities and sciatica. J Bone Joint Surg Am. 1936;18:105–10.
10. Faraj AA, Moulton A, Sirivastava VM. Snapping iliotibial band. Report of ten cases and review of the literature. Acta Orthop Belg. 2001;67:19–23.
11. Ilizaliturri Jr VM, Martinez-Escalante FA, Chaidez PA. Endoscopic iliotibial band release for external snapping hip syndrome. Arthroscopy. 2006;22:505–10.
12. Byrd JWT. Snapping hip. Oper Tech Sports Med. 2005;13(1):46–54.
13. Byrd JWT. Hip arthroscopy for non-structural hip problems. In: Berry DJ, Lieberman JR, editors. Surgery of the hip. Elsevier, Philadelphia, PA.
14. Fery A, Sommelet J. The snapping hip. Late results of 24 surgical cases. Int Orthop. 1988;12:277–82.
15. White RA, Hughes MS, Burd T. A new operative approach in the correction of external coxa saltans: the snapping hip. Am J Sports Med. 2004;32:1504–8.
16. Ilizaliturri V. External snapping hip syndrome. In: Byrd JWT, Guanche C, editors. ANNA advanced arthroscopy: the hip. Philadelphia: Saunders; 2010. p. 138–41.

Abductor Tendinopathies and Repair

23

Patrick Jost, Christopher Walsh, Asheesh Bedi,
and Bryan T. Kelly

Introduction

Lateral hip pain is a common clinical problem. Greater trochanteric pain syndrome (GTPS) was initially defined as pain over the proximal greater trochanter that is reproducible with direct palpation or resisted abduction [1]. This term has been expanded to include patients with trochanteric bursitis, external snapping hip, and tears of the gluteus medius and minimus tendons [2]. Patients with this syndrome are often successfully treated with corticosteroid injection [1, 3, 4]. GTPS has also been described in patients treated for osteoarthritis; Howell found a 20% prevalence of abductor pathology in patients undergoing total hip arthroplasty (THA). Farmer et al. encountered a 4.6% rate of trochanteric bursitis after THA [5], of which 80% responded to corticosteroid injection. Arthroscopic bursectomy is an option in recalcitrant cases [6, 7]. However, in patients with GTPS who do not respond to conservative treatment or injection, tears of the abductor tendons should be suspected, and MRI may be

indicated [8, 9]. In patients with recalcitrant GTPS who underwent MRI, Bird et al. found that 46% of patients had a tear of the gluteus medius and another 38% had gluteus medius tendinopathy without tear [10]. These tears are commonly found at the anterior portion of the lateral facet and can be treated successfully by open [11] or arthroscopic repair [12].

Natural History

Tears of the gluteus medius and minimus tendons likely represent chronic, attritional injuries similar to rotator cuff tears of the shoulder. The gluteus medius and minimus are analogous to the supraspinatus and subscapularis, respectively, in many ways. The medius inserts on the lateral and posterosuperior facets, creating a force vector similar to the supraspinatus [13]. The minimus inserts on the anterior facet and, in most functional positions, provides internal rotation similar to the subscapularis [14]. Similar to the tendons of the rotator cuff, gluteus medius tears appear to be more common than tears of the minimus. Howell estimated that 25% of women and 10% of men will develop a tear of the gluteus medius [15]. The incidence of tears is more common in women than men by a ratio of approximately 4:1. Such a difference in demographics suggests that there may be an underlying mechanical etiology based upon the different force vectors subjected to the abductor tendons in the female pelvis compared to the male pelvis.

Insertional Anatomy

The gluteus medius inserts into both the posterosuperior and lateral facets. The lateral facet also contains a bald spot just anterosuperior to the medius tendon insertion. Immediately anterior to the bald spot lies the anterior facet, where the gluteus minimus inserts (Fig. 23.1) [13]. When repairing tears of the gluteus medius, familiarity with the normal anatomy is

P. Jost, M.D.
Milwaukee Orthopedic Group,
1218 W Kilbourn Ave, Suite 301, Milwaukee, WI 53233, USA
e-mail: pwjost@gmail.com

C. Walsh, M.D.
Department of Orthopaedic Surgery,
University of Michigan Health System,
1500 E. Medical Center Drive, 2912 Taubman Center,
Box 0328, Ann Arbor, MI 48109-5328, USA
e-mail: chris.walshmd@gmail.com

A. Bedi, M.D.
MedSport,
Ann Arbor, MI, USA

Sports Medicine and Shoulder Surgery, Department of Orthopaedic
Surgery, Hospital for Special Surgery,
24 Frank Lloyd Wright Drive, Lobby A, Ann Arbor, MI 48106, USA
e-mail: abedi@umich.edu

B.T. Kelly, M.D.(✉)
Center for Hip Preservation, Hospital for Special Surgery,
525 East 70th Street, New York, NY 10021, USA
e-mail: kellyb@hss.edu

J.W.T. Byrd (ed.), *Operative Hip Arthroscopy*,
DOI 10.1007/978-1-4419-7925-4_23, © Springer Science+Business Media New York 2013

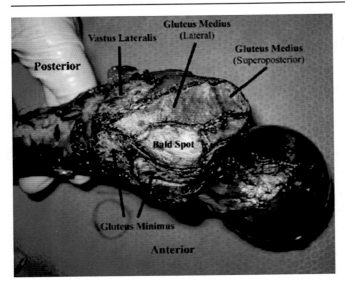

Fig. 23.1 Cadaveric dissection of greater trochanter demonstrating gluteus medius insertion footprints at the superoposterior (*SP*) and lateral facets, and their relationship to the vastus tubercle and gluteus minimus insertion. Also demonstrated is the bald spot located between the insertion of the gluteus medius on the lateral facet and the insertion of the gluteus minimus on the anterior facet (Reprinted from Robertson et al. [13]. With permission from Elsevier)

essential to recreate the true footprint of the tendon. Care must be taken to avoid placing anchors in and reattaching tissue to the bald spot of the trochanter [16].

History and Physical Examination

A detailed history is invaluable in the diagnostic workup of a patient with hip pain. Groin pain generally suggests intra-articular pathology, while lateral pain that can be reproduced with deep palpation over the trochanter generally represents GTPS. However, there is significant overlap with regard to pain location, and patients often present with more than one clinical problem. Patients with external coxa saltans (snapping hip syndrome) will complain of an audible or palpable snap as the hip moves from flexion to extension. This can usually be reproduced during clinical examination. Abductor tendon tears and trochanteric bursitis both commonly present with tenderness over the greater trochanter and pain with resisted abduction, but patients with torn abductors often have a more acute clinical course and will frequently have frank weakness of abduction or a Trendelenburg gait.

The examination begins with observation and inspection. The patient is asked to walk and should be observed for a limp, coxalgic or antalgic gait, or frank Trendelenburg gait. The patient is then asked to lie supine on the table, and the hip is taken through a full range of motion, taking note of positions that provoke pain. Isolated range of motion of other joints can also aid in reaching a diagnosis. Pain that is most pronounced at extremes of hip motion, especially flexion and internal rotation, is most likely due to impingement. Pain that changes with lumbar spine or knee range of motion suggests pathology at those sites. The patient is then asked to lie in the lateral position to allow the clinician access to the lateral hip for palpation. Lateral hip pain can arise from a variety of etiologies, including lumbar spine disease, GTPS, and intra-articular hip pathology. Direct palpation can be very helpful in the differential diagnosis and should be performed at each specific location systematically. Palpation begins at the ileal and sacral origins of the gluteus maximus. The insertion should then be palpated for tenderness at the posterolateral insertion into the linea aspera of the proximal femur as well as the iliotibial band. The gluteus medius is then palpated beginning with its origin at the anterolateral ilium, followed by its two insertions onto the lateral and superoposterior facets. The gluteus minimus origin is deep to the gluteus medius and is difficult to isolate with palpation. The distal portion, however, can be palpated as it inserts into the anterior facet of the greater trochanter. Finally, the trochanteric bursa itself can be palpated overlying the bald spot of the lateral and posterior facets [13].

Each muscle group is then carefully evaluated for strength. The hip is placed in flexion to test the tensor fascia lata, in neutral to evaluate the gluteus medius, and extension for the gluteus maximus. Tears of the gluteus medius can present with pain or weakness with resisted abduction. This is similar to the presentation of trochanteric bursitis, and differentiating between them is difficult without advanced imaging or further diagnostic testing.

Imaging

Upon initial presentation with hip pain, patients are evaluated with an AP pelvis radiograph as well as a Dunn elongated neck lateral. This view is performed with the hip in 90° of flexion and 20° of abduction and provides an orthogonal view of the femoral head and neck to the view provided by the AP pelvis.

If abductor or other soft tissue pathology is suspected, high-quality magnetic resonance imaging (MRI) can prove invaluable. The MRI sequences include a screening examination of the entire pelvis and high-resolution cartilage-sensitive sequences of the hip in three planes. Magnetic resonance arthrography can be used to evaluate for intra-articular hip pathology. Dwek classified abductor tears based on their MRI appearance and divided the greater trochanter into the superoposterior, lateral, anterior, and posterior facets (Figs. 23.2 and 23.3a–d) [8]. Figure 23.3a shows an under-surface tear of the gluteus minimus tendon off of the anterior

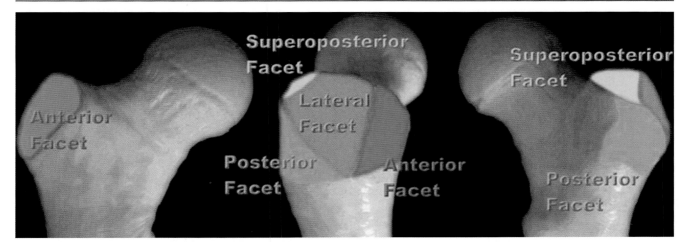

Fig. 23.2 The four facets of greater trochanter (Reprinted from Dwek et al. [8]. With permission from Elsevier)

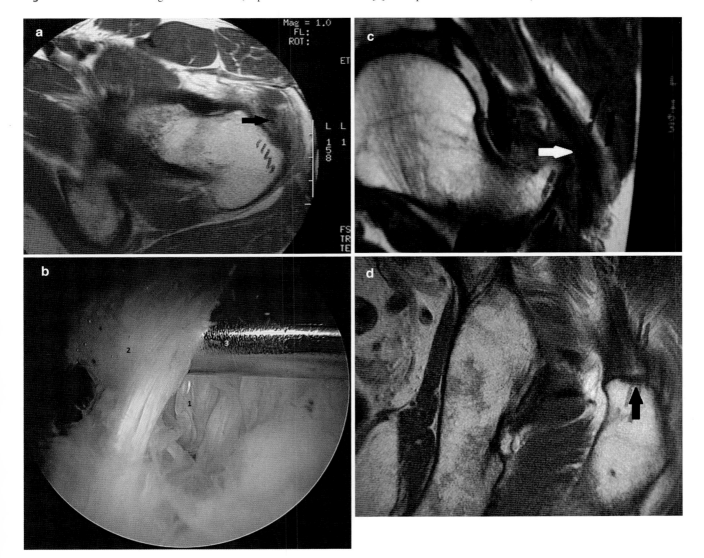

Fig. 23.3 (**a**) Axial image of a left hip demonstrating partial undersurface tears of the gluteus minimus tendon off of the anterior facet (*black arrow*). (**b**) Arthroscopic image of an undersurface tear of the gluteus minimus. The shredded fibers of the gluteus minimus are labeled (*1*), which lie beneath the intact fibers of the gluteus medius (*2*), which is being elevated off of the anterior facet using a switching stick (*3*). (**c**) Coronal image demonstrating undersurface tears of the anterior fibers of the gluteus medius tendon off of the lateral facet (*white arrow*). (**d**) Coronal image demonstrating partial tear of the posterior fibers of the gluteus medius tendon off of the superoposterior facet (*black arrow*)

facet with a representative arthroscopic view of the same tendon tear demonstrated in Fig. 23.3b. Figure 23.3c shows a coronal image demonstrating partial tearing of the anterior fibers of the gluteus medius tendon off of the lateral facet. Figure 23.3d shows a coronal image demonstrating partial tearing of the posterior fibers of the gluteus medius tendon off of the superoposterior facet. The posterior facet is the only facet that does not have any distinct tendon attachment but is the primary location of the largest bursae of the peritrochanteric space and thus is the likely source of primary pain in patients with true isolated trochanteric bursitis without associated tendon tear.

Ultrasound can be used to guide diagnostic or therapeutic injections, as well as evaluate the gluteus medius and minimus tendons. Dynamic ultrasound can be used to evaluate for external coxa saltans.

Surgical Technique

(See Video 23.1: http://goo.gl/yMGZB) Before entering the peritrochanteric space, routine diagnostic arthroscopy of the central and peripheral compartments is performed. The anterior or midanterior portal can be used for entry into the peritrochanteric space. We prefer to use a midanterior portal that is 2–3 cm distal and lateral to the standard anterior portal, directly anterior to the lateral prominence of the greater trochanter (Fig. 23.4). The midanterior portal provides safe access to the joint by reducing the risk of injury to the lateral femoral cutaneous nerve, which is in close proximity to the standard anterior portal [17]. It also allows an easier angle into the peritrochanteric space than the standard anterior portal. A well-placed midanterior portal should lie distal to the gluteus medius muscle belly and proximal to the vastus lateralis, avoiding injury to both structures and facilitating abductor repair. Fluoroscopy can aid in proper portal placement by confirming placement directly over the lateral prominence of the greater trochanter (Fig. 23.5).

Once the desired portals are established and evaluation of the central and peripheral compartments is complete, the cannula is directed from the midanterior portal posterolaterally into the peritrochanteric space. Traction should be completely released, and the leg is placed in 20–25° of abduction, 10° of flexion, and 15° of internal rotation to facilitate entry into the space [16]. Moving the hip into abduction increases the space between the iliotibial band and the greater trochanter and facilitates viewing and working in the potential space. The cannula is then swept back and forth, similar to the technique used to gain access to the subacromial space of the shoulder. The space is then distended with 50–70 mmHg of fluid pressure and a 70° scope is introduced into the potential space between the iliotibial band and the greater trochanter.

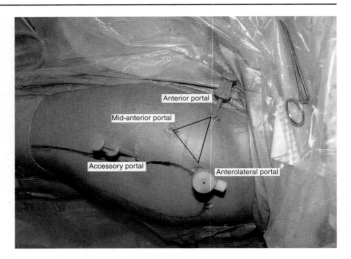

Fig. 23.4 Portal placement for entry into the peritrochanteric space typically uses the midanterior portal as the initial viewing portal. This portal can be placed directly over the lateral prominence of the trochanter to avoid inadvertent disruption of the gluteus medius muscle fibers proximal to the trochanteric tip and the vastus lateralis muscle fibers distal to the vastus ridge. The three most common working portals (anterolateral, midanterior, and anterior portals) form a triangle such that each portal should be separated from one another by a minimum of 5–6 cm to optimize the available space for instruments (Reprinted from Robertson and Kelly [17]. With permission from Elsevier)

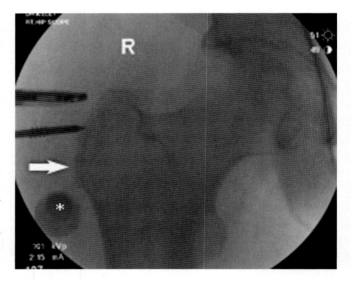

Fig. 23.5 Fluoroscopic image of a right hip. A metal cap (*asterisk*) is being used to externally palpate the general area of the lateral prominence of the greater trochanter (*arrow*). It is important to direct the initial entry point at this lateral prominence to avoid inadvertent injury to the gluteus medius fibers proximally or the vastus lateralis fibers distally. Fluoroscopy can also be used to confirm that the direction of entry of suture anchors is perpendicular to the lateral facet

Upon entry into the peritrochanteric space, the distal anterolateral accessory portal is established. The proper location for this portal is in line with the anterolateral portal, 4–5 cm directly distal to it. A motorized shaver is inserted into the

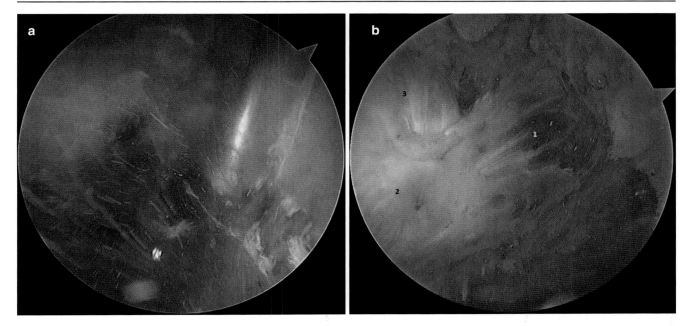

Fig. 23.6 (**a**) Initial viewing within the peritrochanteric space is made with the 70° arthroscope in the midanterior facet with the light source directed distally. Visualization is facilitated by a thorough bursectomy. (**b**) Orientation can be facilitated with the use of fluoroscopic imaging at the initial stage of the bursectomy when the view is not yet well established. Once the bursa is cleared and the space is more easily viewed, then orientation toward the gluteus medius (*1*), gluteus minimus (*2*), and lateral facet (*3*) can be made

peritrochanteric space through this portal, and the trochanteric bursa is thoroughly cleared (Fig. 23.6a, b). The bursectomy begins distally at the gluteus maximus insertion and progresses proximally in a systematic fashion. This should allow easy visualization of the iliotibial band and greater trochanter, which define the lateral and medial borders of the space. The standard anterolateral portal can then be used as a third working or viewing portal, improving proximal access or distal visualization. A thorough inspection then begins at the gluteus maximus insertion into the linea aspera and vastus lateralis, which should be the distal and posterior extent of any dissection (Fig. 23.7). The sciatic nerve lies 3–4 cm posterior to the maximus insertion. The origin of the vastus lateralis is then evaluated leading up the vastus tubercle, with the arthroscope directed just anterior to the lateral facet (Fig. 23.8). The gluteus medius muscle and insertion are then evaluated at the anterior and lateral facets. Both facets and the entire tendon should be inspected and carefully probed. Partial tears are often on the undersurface and difficult to see arthroscopically (Fig. 23.9a, b). The gluteus minimus is often covered by medius muscle and can be difficult to visualize. A switching stick can be used to gently retract medius muscle to see the tendinous insertion of the gluteus minimus onto the anterior facet. The arthroscope should then be turned laterally to evaluate the iliotibial band. If external coxa saltans is present, the insertional fibers of the gluteus medius may appear inflamed and injected (Fig. 23.10a) and the adjacent posterior third of the iliotibial band may appear thickened

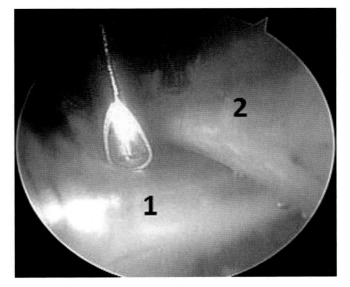

Fig. 23.7 With the 70° scope in the midanterior portal the most clearly identifiable landmark is the distal insertion of the gluteus maximus tendon into the femur (*1*). The sciatic nerve lies approximately 3–4 cm posterior to the insertion of the gluteus maximus tendon, so visualization of this tendon can help confirm that the sciatic nerve is not at risk during the procedure. The distal extent of the bursectomy can be identified by the clear insertion of the gluteus maximus tendon posterior to the longitudinal fibers of the vastus lateralis. The gluteus maximus tendon inserts just posterior to the longitudinal fibers of the vastus lateralis (*2*), which can be seen, as the scope is turn toward the femur

and irritated (Fig. 23.10b). Arthroscopic iliotibial band release can be performed at this point if necessary and is described elsewhere in this text.

If a tear in the gluteus medius is identified, it must be assessed for retraction and repairability by assessing tissue mobility and quality, similar to tears of the rotator cuff

(Fig. 23.11a, b). If the tear is repairable, the tendon edge is debrided back to healthy, robust tissue. The bony footprint of the torn tendon should also be prepared; soft tissue is cleared and the bone is decorticated to bleeding cancellous bone (Fig. 23.12a, b). Suture anchors are then placed into the footprint. A spinal needle is placed first and positioned with arthroscopic and fluoroscopic guidance to find the ideal location and trajectory. Anchors are then placed into the footprint through stab incisions, followed by confirmation of anchor position by fluoroscopy (Fig. 23.13a, b). Tears of the gluteus medius off the lateral facet are generally repaired with 2–4 anchors spaced evenly across the tendon footprint. After anchor placement, sutures are passed sequentially through the free tendon edge using a suture-passing device (Fig. 23.14a–c). The tendon edge can be captured with a needle penetrating device placed through the distal anterolateral portal. Sutures are then parked in the midanterior portal. Alternatively, sutures can be passed using a penetrating suture-passing device. All sutures should be passed through cannulas to avoid soft tissue entrapment. Knots are then tied using standard arthroscopic knot tying techniques to reduce the tendon anatomically to the footprint (Fig. 23.15). Partial-thickness undersurface tears that are seen on MRI are often difficult to see arthroscopically. The tendon should be carefully probed and inspected, and high-grade partial-thickness tears may be taken down and repaired with the standard technique. Alternatively, a transtendinous repair technique has been described [18].

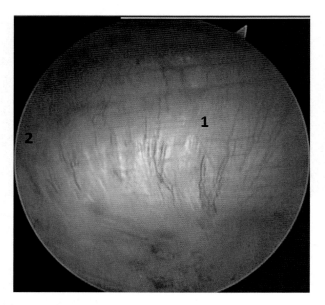

Fig. 23.8 The longitudinal fibers of the vastus lateralis (*1*) should be clearly visualized as the scope is brought proximal toward the vastus ridge (*2*)

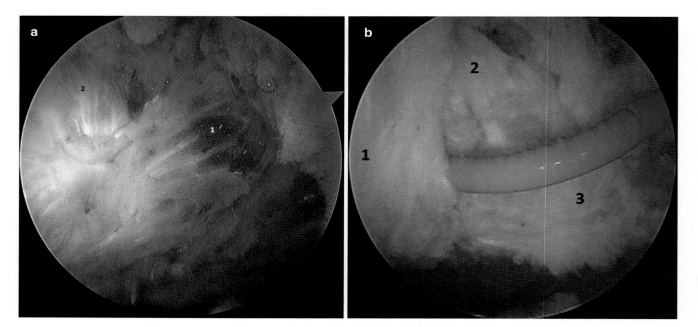

Fig. 23.9 (**a**) Inspection of the gluteus medius (*1*) and minimus (*2*) tendon insertion requires careful palpation of the suspected area of injury, and correlation with MR imaging is essential. (**b**) Oftentimes, the tendon tears are undersurface, and the scope must be moved to the anterior aspect of the medius insertion (*1*), and the tendon needs to be retracted manually with a probe to fully appreciate the area of tendon tearing (*2*). Here the vastus lateralis (*3*) is seen distal to the more proximal tendon tears involving the anterior fibers of the gluteus medius (*1*) and the undersurface fibers of the gluteus minimus (*2*)

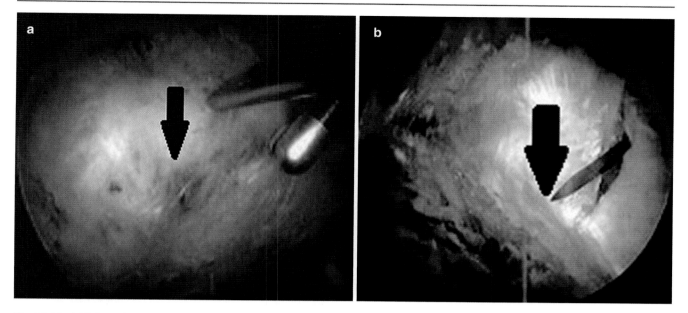

Fig. 23.10 (**a**) Inflamed and injected fibers of the gluteus medius fibers at their insertion site at the lateral facet (*black arrow*). (**b**) As the 70° scope is turned lateral, a clear view of the thickened fibers of the iliotibial band is seen and is oftentimes thickened and irritated in the setting of external coxa saltans (*black arrow*). Under direct visualization of the area of contact against the greater trochanter, the iliotibial band can be selectively released from the inside out

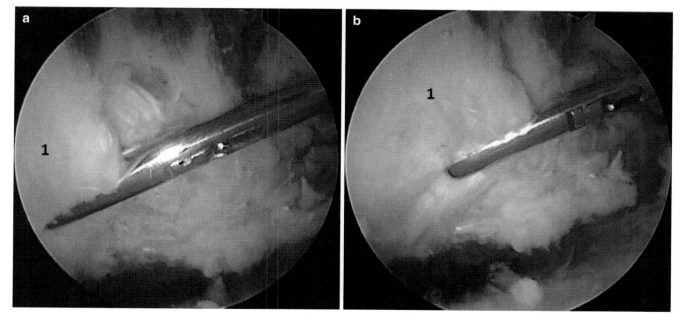

Fig. 23.11 (**a**) Once the tendon edge is clearly demarcated, the degenerated tendon is debrided and the free edge of the tendon (*1*) is assessed for mobility. (**b**) The edge of the gluteus medius (*1*) is being held by a suture grasper and pulled distally to its normal insertion site at the footprint of the lateral facet. If the tendon is retracted and cannot be mobilized, then conversion to an open procedure may be necessary, although this can usually be determined preoperatively based upon the MRI findings

In patients that preoperatively have excessively tight iliotibial band (positive Ober's test) or who have evidence of inflammation induced by direct contact of the ITB directly adjacent to the abductor repair sight, then a concomitant ITB release can be performed using a standard cruciate technique (Fig. 23.16).

Postoperative Management

Following gluteus medius repair, all patients are given crutches and a hip abduction brace set at 10° of abduction and allowed 20 lb of foot flat weight bearing for the first 6 weeks. Continuous passive motion is started immediately for 2–4 h/day, and a

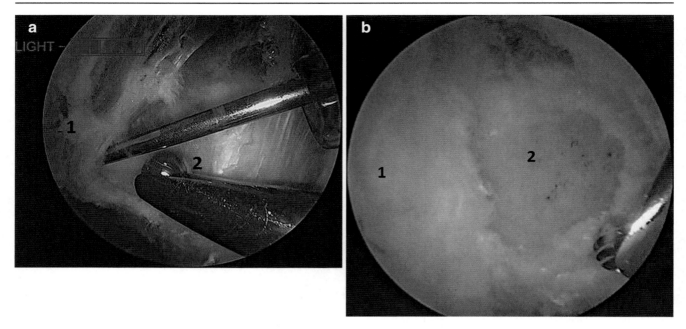

Fig. 23.12 (**a**) The torn edge of the gluteus medius tendon can be retracted to allow direct access to the bony footprint of the tendon. (**b**) Once the footprint is clearly exposed and the gluteus medius tendon (*1*) is protected, the footprint should be abraded with a motorized burr or shaver to create a bleeding bed of bone to facilitate tendon healing (*2*)

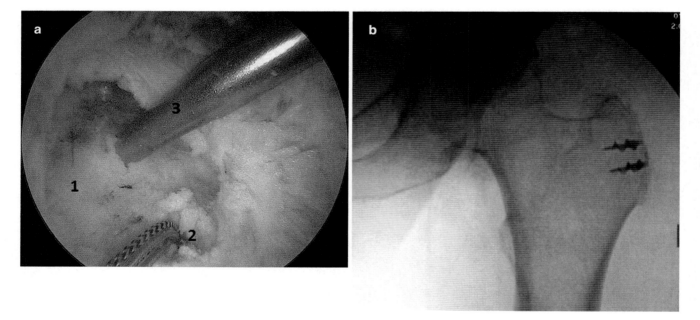

Fig. 23.13 (**a**) Placement of the anchors requires clear visualization of the footprint (*1*). In this example, the first more posterior anchor has been placed, seen with the double-loaded sutures coming out of the bone (*2*). The second anchor is being placed percutaneously (*3*). (**b**) Fluoroscopic imaging should be used during anchor placement to confirm that they are placed perpendicular to the trochanter

stationary bike is used for 20 min/day. Passive hip flexion to 90° is allowed, as is passive hip abduction. Patients are instructed to avoid active abduction and internal or external rotation or passive adduction past neutral and external rotation past 30° for a minimum of 6 weeks after the repair. Two weeks after surgery, patients begin isometric strengthening of the hip extensors, adductors, and external rotators, as well as quadriceps neuromuscular stimulation. At 4–6 weeks, patients begin hip flexor and quadriceps strengthening. Gradual progression to full weight bearing begins at 6–8 weeks. At 10 weeks, weight bearing, all lower extremity strengthening, and core strengthening are progressed as tolerated. By 3–6 months, patients should have minimal pain, achieve quadriceps and hamstring strength near to the contralateral limb,

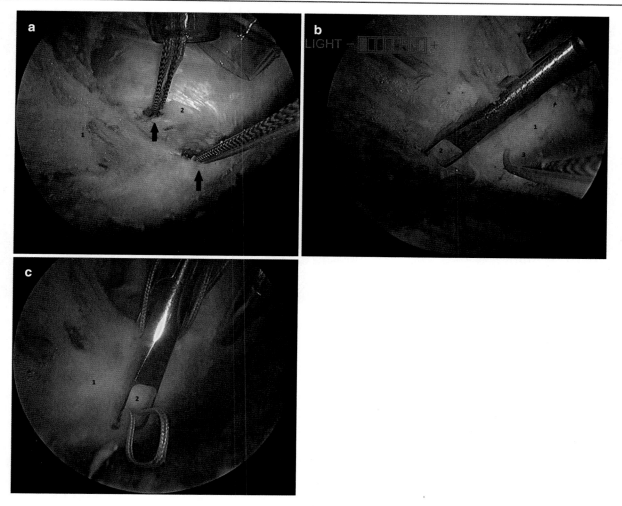

Fig. 23.14 (**a**) In this example, two anchors (*arrows*) are placed just distal to the torn edge of the gluteus medius tendon (*1*) in the anterior and posterior regions of the lateral facet (*2*). (**b**) Once the anchors are strategically placed within the prepared bony footprint, the sutures are passed through the free edge of the tendon (*1*) using a standard suture passing device (*2*). Placement of the sutures should be planned to maximize tendon apposition against bone (*3*). (**c**) Although each tear requires individualized planning, a combination of horizontal mattress and simple suture passage through the free edge of the gluteus medius (*1*) typically allows for a "double row" equivalent suture fixation (*2*), with good, strong, anatomic footprint restoration

and have a normal step down test. Running is allowed when the patient demonstrates near equal abductor strength, and the ability to support the pelvis with single-leg stance.

Outcomes

Conservative treatment of GTPS and trochanteric bursitis has led to generally good results and usually includes physical therapy and corticosteroid injections [1, 4]. Surgical treatment of recalcitrant cases by trochanteric bursectomy, with or without iliotibial band release, has also led to good results. [6, 7]

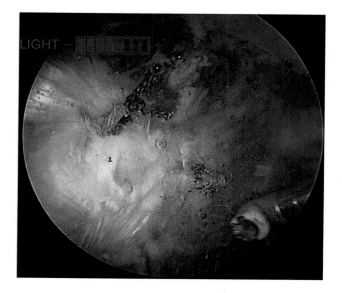

Fig. 23.15 Once the sutures are tied and tensioned, final inspection should ensure that the footprint of the tendon (*1*) lies anatomically against the involved facet

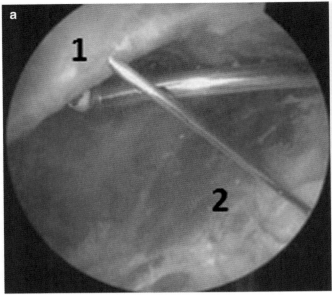
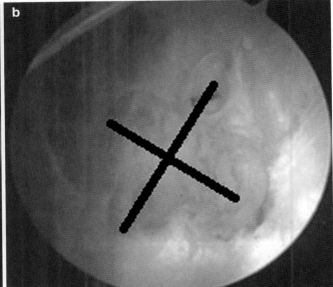

Fig. 23.16 If there appears to be excessive pressure of the iliotibial band (*1*) on the greater trochanter (*2*), then a cruciate release of the ITB can be performed under direct visualization. (**a**) Inflamed and injected fibers of the gluteus medius fibers at their insertion site at the lateral facet. (**b**) Then a cruciate release can be performed using a standard inside out technique (*lines*)

Few results of abductor tendon tears have been reported. Kagan et al. reported on seven patients who were treated with iliotibial band release for recalcitrant GTPS and were found to have full-thickness tears of the gluteus medius tendon. Suture-only open repairs were performed, and all seven patients had excellent outcomes [11]. Voos et al. reported on the arthroscopic repair technique described in this chapter. Ten patients were followed for 12–31 months. At final follow-up, all ten patients were pain-free and nine of ten regained full hip strength [12].

GTPS is a common clinical entity that usually responds well to conservative management. However, when patients do not respond to conservative management, further evaluation is necessary to rule out tears of the abductor tendons. When properly indicated, surgical repair can provide excellent outcomes and predictable return to function.

References

1. Karpinski MR, Piggott H. Greater trochanteric pain syndrome. A report of 15 cases. J Bone Joint Surg Br. 1985;67(5):762–3.
2. Strauss EJ, Nho SJ, Kelly BT. Greater trochanteric pain syndrome. Sports Med Arthrosc. 2010;18(2):113–9.
3. Schapira D, Nahir M, Scharf Y. Trochanteric bursitis: a common clinical problem. Arch Phys Med Rehabil. 1986;67(11):815–7.
4. Ege Rasmussen KJ, Fano N. Trochanteric bursitis. Treatment by corticosteroid injection. Scand J Rheumatol. 1985;14(4):417–20.
5. Farmer KW, Jones LC, Brownson KE, Khanuja HS, Hungerford MW. Trochanteric bursitis after total hip arthroplasty: incidence and evaluation of response to treatment. J Arthroplasty. 2010;25(2):208–12.
6. Baker Jr CL, Massie RV, Hurt WG, Savory CG. Arthroscopic bursectomy for recalcitrant trochanteric bursitis. Arthroscopy. 2007;23(8):827–32.
7. Farr D, Selesnick H, Janecki C, Cordas D. Arthroscopic bursectomy with concomitant iliotibial band release for the treatment of recalcitrant trochanteric bursitis. Arthroscopy. 2007;23(8):905.e1–5.
8. Dwek J, Pfirrmann C, Stanley A, Pathria M, Chung CB. MR imaging of the hip abductors: normal anatomy and commonly encountered pathology at the greater trochanter. Magn Reson Imaging Clin N Am. 2005;13(4):691–704, vii.
9. Cvitanic O, Henzie G, Skezas N, Lyons J, Minter J. MRI diagnosis of tears of the hip abductor tendons (gluteus medius and gluteus minimus). AJR Am J Roentgenol. 2004;182(1):137–43.
10. Bird PA, Oakley SP, Shnier R, Kirkham BW. Prospective evaluation of magnetic resonance imaging and physical examination findings in patients with greater trochanteric pain syndrome. Arthritis Rheum. 2001;44(9):2138–45.
11. Kagan 2nd A. Rotator cuff tears of the hip. Clin Orthop Relat Res. 1999;368:135–40.
12. Voos JE, Shindle MK, Pruett A, Asnis PD, Kelly BT. Endoscopic repair of gluteus medius tendon tears of the hip. Am J Sports Med. 2009;37(4):743–7.
13. Robertson WJ, Gardner MJ, Barker JU, Boraiah S, Lorich DG, Kelly BT. Anatomy and dimensions of the gluteus medius tendon insertion. Arthroscopy. 2008;24(2):130–6.
14. Beck M, Sledge JB, Gautier E, Dora CF, Ganz R. The anatomy and function of the gluteus minimus muscle. J Bone Joint Surg Br. 2000;82(3):358–63.
15. Howell GE, Biggs RE, Bourne RB. Prevalence of abductor mechanism tears of the hips in patients with osteoarthritis. J Arthroplasty. 2001;16(1):121–3.
16. Voos JE, Rudzki JR, Shindle MK, Martin H, Kelly BT. Arthroscopic anatomy and surgical techniques for peritrochanteric space disorders in the hip. Arthroscopy. 2007;23(11):1246.e1–5.
17. Robertson WJ, Kelly BT. The safe zone for hip arthroscopy: a cadaveric assessment of central, peripheral, and lateral compartment portal placement. Arthroscopy. 2008;24(9):1019–26.
18. Domb BG, Nasser RM, Botser IB. Partial-thickness tears of the gluteus medius: rationale and technique for trans-tendinous endoscopic repair. Arthroscopy. 2010;26(12):1697–705.

Subgluteal Space and Associated Disorders

24

Hal David Martin

Introduction

Understanding the subgluteal space of the hip is important in the evaluation of patients presenting with posterior hip pain. The source of posterior hip pain can include osseous, capsular labral, musculotendinous, and neurovascular pathologic conditions. Posterior hip pain can be confused with the lumbar spine and pelvic (genitourinary and abdominal) pathology emphasizing the importance of a comprehensive history and physical examination. The complexity of this region requires a thorough understanding of the anatomy, biomechanics, and pathokinematics. There are four sources of posterior extra-articular hip pain for which the surgeon should be aware: deep gluteal syndrome, hamstring pathology, pudendal nerve, and ischiofemoral impingement. The objective of this chapter will be to review pertinent aspects of the subgluteal space anatomy, define this region, and introduce potential sources of extra-articular hip pathology.

The subgluteal space is anterior and beneath the gluteus maximus and posterior to the posterior border of the femoral neck, the linea aspera (lateral), the sacrotuberous and falciform fascia (medial), the inferior margin of the sciatic notch (superior), and the hamstring origin (inferior) (Fig. 24.1). Within this region of great importance are the sciatic nerve, piriformis, obturator internus/externus, gemelli, quadratus femoris, hamstrings, superior and inferior gluteal nerves, lateral ascending vessels of the medial femoral circumflex artery, ischium, sacrotuberous and sacrospinous ligaments, and origin of the ischiofemoral ligament. Pathologic conditions can occur in a chronic insidious fashion and involve inflammatory, tumorous, or acute injury.

H.D. Martin, DO
The Hip Clinic, Oklahoma Sport Science and Orthopaedics,
6205 N Santa Fe, Suite 200, Oklahoma City, OK 73118, USA
e-mail: haldavidmartin@yahoo.com

A comprehensive examination of the hip is imperative in establishing diagnoses of each layer of hip pathology: osseous, capsulolabral, musculotendinous, and neurovascular.

Anatomy and Biomechanics

The anatomy of the subgluteal space is complex and must be understood in order to appreciate the clinical presentation and treatment of deep gluteal syndrome or other pathologic conditions. At the sciatic notch, between the iliotibial band and the greater trochanter deep to the gluteal muscles is the piriformis muscle, which arises from the ventrolateral surface of the sacrum. The piriformis inserts superior and posterior to the greater trochanter (Fig. 24.2a). Distal to the piriformis muscle is the cluster of short external rotators: the gemellus superior, obturator internus, and gemellus inferior. The gemelli blend with the tendon of the obturator internus and insert on the anterior part of the medial surface of the greater trochanter [3]. Often, the piriformis tendon is partially blended with the common tendon of the obturator/gemelli complex [2, 4] (Fig. 24.2b). The obturator internus arises from the inner surface of the anterolateral wall of the pelvis and exits the pelvis through the lesser sciatic foramen [2, 3]. The superior gemellus arises for the outer surface of the ischial spine and the inferior gemellus arises from the ischial tuberosity. Inferior to the obturator/gemelli complex is the quadratus femoris muscle arising from the upper part of the external border of the ischial tuberosity and inserting on the posterior surface of the femur along the intertrochanteric crest [3]. The quadratus femoris assists in external rotation, and the piriformis, obturator internus, and gemelli muscles assist external rotation and abduction of the flexed hip. At the ischium, the biceps femoris and semitendinosis have a common tendinous origin and separate an average of 9.9 cm from the proximal border of origin [5]. The inferior border of the gluteus maximus is an average of 6.3 cm from the proximal border of the semitendinosis/biceps femoris origin [5].

Fig. 24.1 Schematic of the subgluteal space. *HS* hamstring origin, *LA* linea aspera, *LT* lesser trochanter, *OI* obturator internus, *PF* piriformis, *SSL* sacrospinous ligament, *STL* sacrotuberous ligament

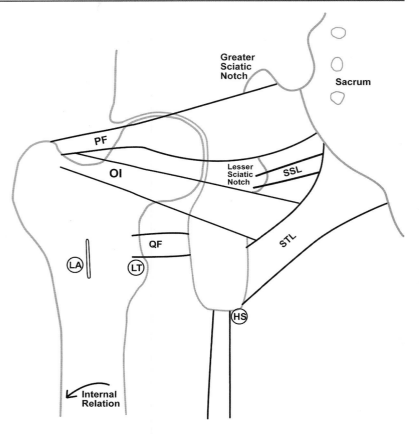

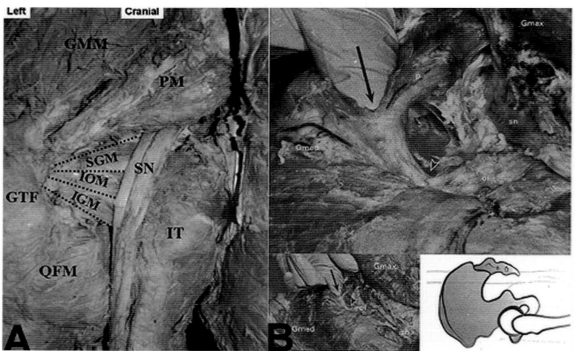

Fig. 24.2 Musculature within the subgluteal space. (**a**) Left subgluteal region. *Dashed lines* represent separation of external rotator musculature. *GMM* gluteus maximus muscle, *GTF* greater trochanter of the femur, *IGM* inferior gemellus muscle, *IOM* internal obturator muscle, *IT* ischial tuberosity, *PM* piriformis muscle, *SN* sciatic nerve, *QF* quadratus femoris muscle (Reprinted from Guvencer et al. [1]. With permission from Springer Science+Business Media). (**b**) Lateral photograph and diagram of a left hemipelvis. The superior gemellus at times is fused with the obturator internus (*OI*) and combines with piriformis (*P*) to make conjoint tendon. The gluteus medius (*Gmed*), P, and OI are shown approaching the greater trochanter. The dissector's index finger elevates and exposes the large connection between Gmed and P (*black arrow*) before P joins OI to form the conjoint tendon (*black arrowhead*). *SN* sciatic nerve (Reprinted from Solomon et al. [2]. With permission from The British Editorial Society of Bone & Joint Surgery)

Fig. 24.3 Nerve anatomy of the posterior pelvis. Schematic illustrating nerve anatomy of the posterior pelvis (Reprinted from Filler and Kline [6]. With permission from Elsevier)

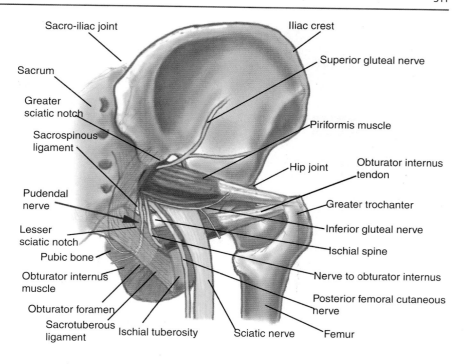

Six neural structures exit the pelvis through the greater sciatic notch: the sciatic nerve, the pudendal nerve, the posterior femoral cutaneous nerve, the superior gluteal nerve, the inferior gluteal nerve, and the nerve to the obturator internus (Fig. 24.3). The superior and inferior gluteal arteries also exit through the greater sciatic notch. The sciatic nerve, formed by L4–S3 sacral roots, courses distally through the subgluteal space anterior to the piriformis muscle and posterior to the obturator/gemelli complex and quadratus femoris. The superior and inferior gluteal arteries branch off of the internal iliac artery within the pelvis (lumbosacral region) The superior gluteal artery descends out of the pelvis through the upper greater sciatic notch, and the inferior gluteal artery descends out of the pelvis through the lower greater sciatic notch [3]. The superior gluteal artery and nerve divides 1–2 cm above the superior border of the piriformis and fans out in a course anterior and distal to the greater sciatic foramen between the gluteus minimus and gluteus medius supplying the gluteus medius, gluteus minimus, and tensor fascia lata [7] (Fig. 24.4). The inferior gluteal nerve and artery enters the pelvis at the greater sciatic notch medial to the sciatic nerve passing between the piriformis muscle and coccygeus muscles [3]. It descends along with the sciatic nerve and posterior femoral cutaneous nerve between the greater trochanter and ischial tuberosity. The inferior gluteal artery gives rise to two branches underlying the external rotators contributing to the perfusion of the acetabulum and capsule [8]. A superficial arterial branch of the inferior gluteal artery crosses the sciatic nerve laterally between the piriformis and superior gemellus muscles (Fig. 24.5) [8].

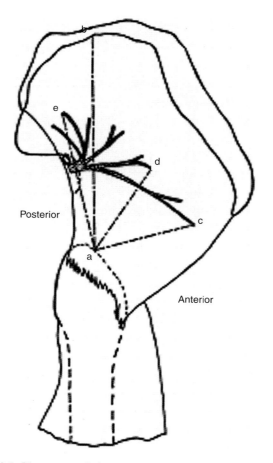

Fig. 24.4 The course of the superior gluteal nerve. Course of the superior gluteal nerve as it exits through the greater sciatic notch superior to the piriformis muscle (Reprinted from Jacobs and Buxton [7]. With permission from JBJS) (*a*) superior border of the greater trochanter; (*b*), iliac crest; line (*a–b*), mid-lateral line; (*c, d, e*) terminal distributions of the superior gluteal artery

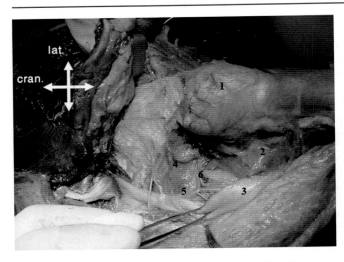

Fig. 24.5 Distal branch of the inferior gluteal artery. Posterior aspect of the right hip, demonstrating the distal branch of the inferior gluteal artery. (*1*) Greater trochanter, (*2*) quadratus femoris muscle, (*3*) sciatic nerve, (*4*) inferior gemellus muscle, (*5*) inferior gluteal artery, and (*6*) branch of the inferior gluteal artery to the hip capsule and acetabulum. Cran, cranial; lat, lateral (Reprinted from Kalhor et al. [8]. With permission from JBJS)

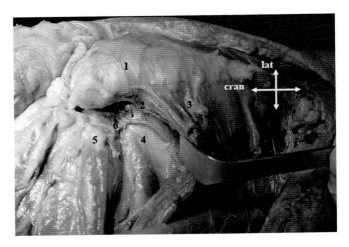

Fig. 24.6 Deep branch of the medial femoral circumflex artery. Posterior aspect of the right hip, demonstrating the anatomic position of the deep branch of the medial femoral circumflex artery. (*1*) Greater trochanter, (*2*) trochanteric branch of the medial femoral circumflex artery, (*3*) quadratus femoris muscle, (*4*) obturator externus muscle, (*5*) obturator internus and gemellus muscles, and (*6*) anastomotic branch to the inferior gluteal artery. Cran, cranial; Lat, lateral (Reprinted from Kalhor et al. [8]. With permission from JBJS)

The anatomic position of the medial circumflex artery is relevant within the subgluteal space as it follows the inferior border of the obturator externus and crosses over its tendon and under the external rotators and piriformis muscle (Fig. 24.6) [8].

Distal to the piriformis are the nerve to the gemellus superior/obturator internus (arising from L5, and S1, 2) and the nerve to the gemellus inferior/quadratus femoris (arising

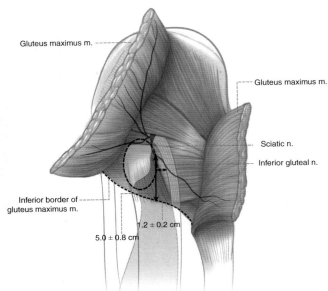

Fig. 24.7 Anatomic relationship of hamstrings origin with the sciatic nerve. At the lateral border of the ischium, the inferior gluteal nerve is an average 5.0±0.8 cm from the distal border of the gluteal maximus. The sciatic nerve lies an average of 1.2±0.2 cm from the most lateral aspect of the ischial tuberosity (Reprinted from Miller et al. [9]. With permission from JBJS)

from L4,5, and S1) [3]. The course of the obturator nerve is through the obturator foramen then divides into anterior and posterior branches innervating the adductor muscles. In a cadaveric study by Miller et al., the sciatic nerve was located at an average of 1.2±0.2 cm from the most lateral aspect of the ischial tuberosity, and the inferior gluteal nerve and artery was 5 cm to the inferior border of the gluteus maximus [9] (Fig. 24.7). The proximal origin of the hamstrings was found to have an intimate relationship with the inferior gluteal nerve and artery and sciatic nerve [9].

The pudendal nerve arises from S2 to S4 and exits the pelvis with the internal pudendal vessels through the greater sciatic foramen. The pudendal nerve then enters the Alcock (pudendal) canal formed by the obturator fascia and sacrotuberous ligament (STL) [10, 11] (Fig. 24.8). The STL is a strong support ligament controlling movement of the lower portion of the sacrum and is an important consideration for the pudendal nerve [12] (Fig. 24.9). Anterior and superior to the STL is the sacrospinous ligament (Fig. 24.10) attached to the lateral margins of the sacrum and coccyx and extending laterally to the ischial spine [3].

Under normal conditions, the sciatic nerve is able to stretch and glide in order to accommodate moderate strain or compression associated with joint movement. During a straight leg raise with knee extension, the sciatic nerve experiences a proximal excursion of 28.0 mm [13] medial, toward the hip joint. Strain of the sciatic nerve increases

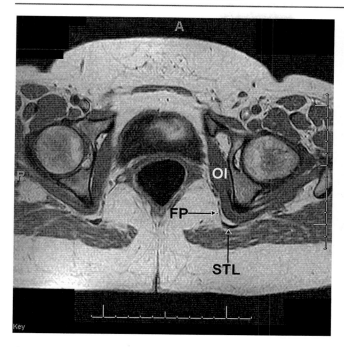

Fig. 24.8 MRI of the sacrotuberous ligament and falciform process. The falciform process (*FP*) extends off the sacrotuberous ligament (*STL*) and fuses with the fascia of the obturator internus (*OI*)

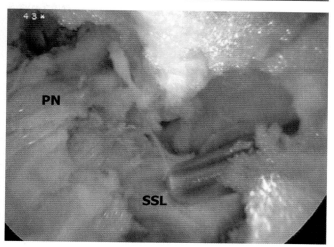

Fig. 24.10 Sacrospinous ligament. Endoscopic view of a cadaveric sacrospinous ligament (*SSL*) and its relationship to the pudendal nerve (*PN*)

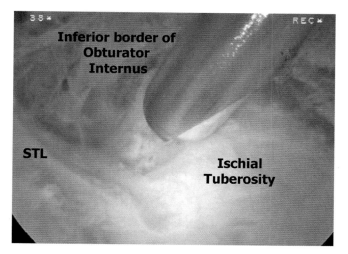

Fig. 24.9 Sacrotuberous ligament. Endoscopic view of the sacrotuberous ligament (*STL*) as it attaches to the ischial tuberosity

6.6% relative to the extended hip [3, 13]. The bony morphometry alterations during hip flexion, adduction, and internal rotation may influence sciatic nerve kinematics [14]. Hip flexion, adduction, and internal rotation increase the distance between the greater trochanter and posterior superior iliac spine and the distance between the greater trochanter and ischial tuberosity. This hip position stretches the piriformis muscle and causes a narrowing of the space between the inferior border of the piriformis, the superior gemellus, and sacrotuberous ligament [1].

Sciatic Nerve Entrapment/Deep Gluteal Syndrome

Entrapment of the sciatic nerve is characterized by nondiscogenic, extrapelvic nerve compression presenting with symptoms of pain and dysesthesias in the buttock area, hip, or posterior thigh and/or as radicular pain [15]. It was first theorized that the piriformis muscle was the source of entrapment by Yeoman in 1928 [16], who described the possibility of sciatic nerve entrapment by the piriformis [17]. In 1934, Freiberg and Vinke described the clinical finding of the Lasègue sign and tenderness at the sciatic notch attributed to sciatica caused by the piriformis muscle [18]. The nomenclature "piriformis muscle syndrome" was introduced in 1947 by Robinson, who described a tender sausage-shaped mass over the piriformis area [16]. While the diagnosis of piriformis syndrome in the early years was largely based on clinical findings, diagnostic techniques have improved somewhat. It is now known that a number of structures within the subgluteal space can entrap the sciatic nerve. Etiologies of sciatic nerve entrapment include the piriformis muscle [14, 16–25], fibrous bands containing blood vessels [14, 17, 25], gluteal muscles [26], hamstring muscles [27, 28], the gemelli-obturator internus complex [29, 30], ischial tuberosity [31–33], and acetabular reconstruction surgery [34]. Additionally, vascular abnormalities [15, 22, 35], prolonged surgery in the seated position [36], after total hip replacement [37], and secondary to space-occupying lesions [18, 19] have been reported to cause sciatic nerve compression. Due to the variation of anatomical entrapment, the term "deep gluteal syndrome" [26] may be a more accurate description of this nondiscogenic sciatica.

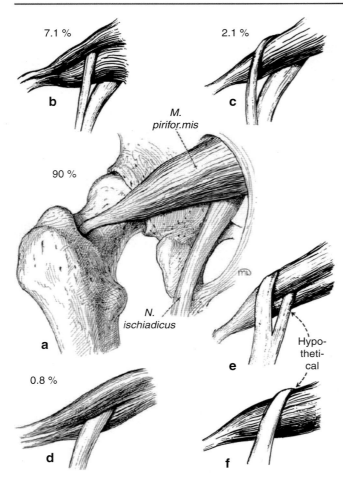

Fig. 24.11 Schematic of piriformis/sciatic nerve variants. Six types of arrangement of the sciatic nerve, or of its subdivisions in relation to the piriformis muscle, arranged in the order of frequency. Gluteal (external) view. The percentage incidence in 240 examples is indicated. (**e, f**) Hypothetical in 1938. (**a**) Nerve undivided passes out of greater sciatic foramen, below piriformis muscle; (**b**) divisions of nerve pass through and below heads of muscle; (**c**) divisions above and below undivided muscle; (**d**) nerve undivided between the heads of muscle; (**e**) divisions of nerve between and above heads; and (**f**) undivided nerve above undivided muscle (Reprinted from Beaton and Anson [38]. With permission from JBJS)

The piriformis muscle is the most common source of sciatic nerve entrapment. Variations exist concerning the relationship between the piriformis muscle and sciatic nerve. The fact that these piriformis-sciatic nerve anomalies exist is important for the surgeon to recognize; however, the anomaly itself may not be the etiology of DGS symptoms. Six categories of piriformis-sciatic nerve variations have been classified (Fig. 24.11) [38], and the prevalence of anomalies was 16.9% in a meta-analysis of cadaveric studies (Table 24.1) and 16.2% in published surgical case series [42].

There are a number of structures at the level of the piriformis. Hughs and Goldstein [22] report on 5 cases of extrapelvic compression of the sciatic nerve. Three cases involved the piriformis muscle, two category B and one category A with a thick tendon below the belly of the PM. Two involved persistent sciatic artery and venae comitantes. We reported on 35 patients endoscopically treated for deep gluteal syndrome and 18 involved the piriformis muscle (Video 24.1: http://goo.gl/sZHXk). The piriformis muscle was characterized as split, bulging split with the sciatic nerve passing through the body, split tendon with an anterior and posterior component, and split in two distinct components with one dorsally and one inferiorly going between a bifurcated sciatic nerve [14]. In many cases, a thick tendon can hide under the belly of the piriformis overlying the nerve [14, 22] (Fig. 24.12) (Video 24.2: http://goo.gl/p8Tn7 and Video 24.3: http://goo.gl/SzSW0) (see also Video 22.1: http://goo.gl/APn1g).

Hypertrophy of the piriformis muscle has also been attributed to sciatic nerve entrapment [19, 21, 22, 43]. However, of 14 patients with posttraumatic piriformis syndrome, Benson and Schutzer found that only 2 had larger piriformis muscles on the symptomatic side and 7 appeared smaller than the unaffected side [16].

Atypical fibrovascular scar bands and greater trochanteric bursae hypertrophy were present in many cases of sciatic nerve entrapment [14, 25] (Fig. 24.13) (Video 24.1: http://goo.gl/sZHXk). In 27 of the 35 patients previous described by Martin et al., the greater trochanteric bursa was found to be excessively thickened, and large fibrovascular scar bands were present in many patients [14]. The fibrovascular bands extended from the posterior border of the greater trochanter to the gluteus maximus on to the sciatic nerve and extended up to the greater sciatic notch [14] (Video 24.1 http://goo.gl/sZHXk). The hamstring tendon insertion can be thickened over the ischium and onto the sciatic nerve due to trauma or avulsion of the hamstring [5, 14]. The obturator internus/gemelli complex is commonly overlooked in association with sciatica-like pain [4, 14, 29, 30]. As the sciatic nerve passes under the belly of the piriformis and over the superior gemelli/obturator internus, a scissor effect between the two muscles can be the source of entrapment [4, 14, 30]. In one case, we found the obturator internus penetrating the sciatic nerve (Fig. 24.14) (see Video 24.2: http://goo.gl/p8Tn7 and Video 24.3: http://goo.gl/SzSW0).

Ischial Tunnel syndrome is described as pain in the lower buttock region that radiates down the posterior thigh to the popliteal fossa and is commonly associated with hamstring weakness. Puranen and Orava first reported on the surgical release of the sciatic nerve from adhesions in the proximal hamstring area [27]. At the lateral insertion of the hamstring tendons to the ischial tuberosity, these tight tendinous structures and adhesions were thought to be the result of scarring or a fibrotic band between the tendons and sciatic nerve [26, 27]. Patients experience pain with sitting and stretching and with exercise, primarily running (sprinting and acceleration) [27, 44]. Palpable tenderness is located around the

Table 24.1 Characteristics of cadaveric studies: piriformis and sciatic nerve variants

Investigator	Number of cadavers (number of sides included)		Percentage of female cadavers	Laterality of the anomalies		Notes
				Unilateral (%)	Bilateral (%)[a]	
Parsons and Keith [75]	69	(138)	"Mostly men"	–	–	
Bardeen [82]	123	(246)[b]	30	–	–	
Trotter [86]	232	(464)	21	24	48 (63.6)	
Beaton and Anson [83][c]	60[b]	(120)	–	5	14 (73.6)	
Beaton and Anson [38][e]	60	(120)	–	3	2 (40.0)	Results presented in this study included data from a previous study
Ming-Tzu [84]	70	(140)	"Mostly men"	22	24 (52.2)	
Mirsa [85]	150	(300)	–	–	–	
Anson and McVay [81][d]	1,004[b]	(2,000)	–	–	–	This data set incorporated data from Beaton and Anson's two previous studies
Nizankowski et al. [74]	100	(200)	45	–	–	
Lee and Tsai [73]	84	(168)	13	–	–	
Pecina [76]	65	(130)	–	–	–	
Chiba [69]	257	(511)	46	–	–	Three lower limbs of males excluded
Chiba et al. [70]	221	(442)	–	–	–	
Pokorny et al. [78]	51	(102)	–	–	–	
Fishman et al. [71]	38	(76)	–	1	10 (91.0)	This data was found in a study presenting data on the usage of H-reflex latencies for diagnosing piriformis syndrome
Benzon et al. [68]	36	(66)	–	1	0	In six cadavers, only one side was studied
Agur and Dalley [80]	320[b]	(640)	–	–	–	
Ugrenovic et al. [79]	100	(200)	–	–	–	This study was carried out on human fetuses
Pokorny et al. [77]	91	(182)[b]	–	–	–	
Guvencer et al. [72]	25	(50)	0	–	–	
Total	See Table 3			56	98 (63.6)[e]	

This table is a reprint from [42], with permission

[a]Total number of cadavers used as a denominator

[b]Information derived from data presented in the text

[c]This study had inconsistencies in its reporting of statistics

[d]Omitted from total as these results have been included in Anson and McVay [81]

[e]95% confidence interval = 55.5–71.2%

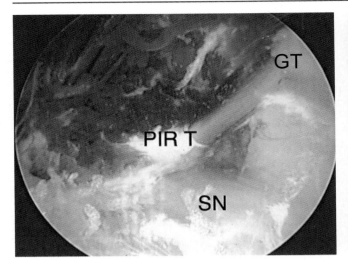

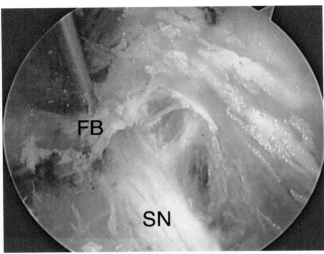

Fig. 24.12 Entrapment of the sciatic nerve by the piriformis muscle tendon. Endoscopic view of a right hip with sciatic nerve (*SN*) entrapment by the piriformis tendon (*PIR T*) medial to its insertion on the greater trochanter (*GT*) (Reprinted Martin et al. [14]. With permission from Elsevier)

Fig. 24.13 Sciatic nerve entrapment by fibrous bands. Endoscopic view of a right hip with sciatic nerve (*SN*) entrapment by fibrous scar bands (*FB*) near the piriformis muscle (*PM*) (Reprinted Martin et al. [14]. With permission from Elsevier)

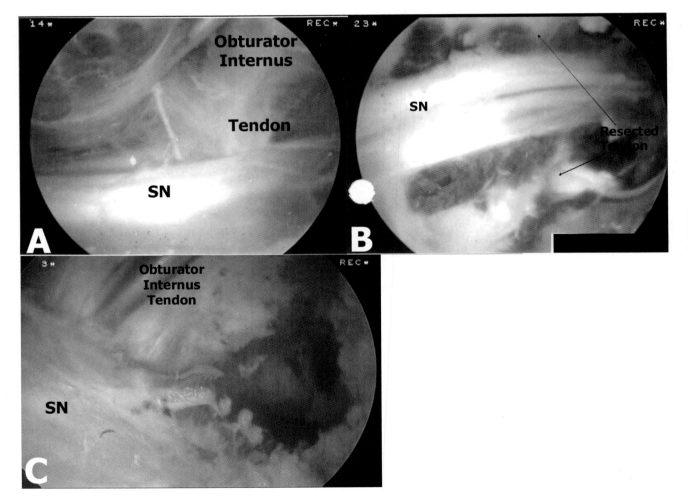

Fig. 24.14 Entrapment of the sciatic nerve by the obturator internus. Following release of the piriformis (proximal to the obturator internus), the SN did not achieve adequate mobility with internal/external rotation or by probing. (**a**) A branch of the obturator internus tendon piercing the sciatic nerve (*SN*). (**b**) Post-release of obturator internus tendon with the sciatic nerve together. (**c**) Endoscopic view of a large obturator internus tendon piercing the SN

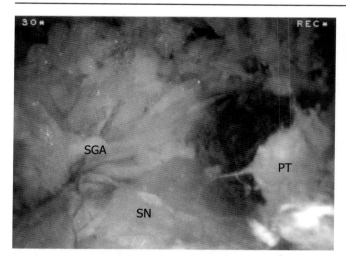

Fig. 24.15 Entrapment of the sciatic nerve by superior gluteal artery. A branch of the superior gluteal artery (*SGA*) is in diastole crossing the sciatic nerve (*SN*) distal to the sciatic notch. The piriformis tendon (*PT*) is seen released to the right

ischial tuberosity in the proximal hamstring region. Hamstring tears alone differ where the pain is located more distal in the muscle belly commonly with a palpable defect from the tear [28]. Clinically, Young et al., reported that the straight leg raise test (Lasègue test) is variable, no neurological deficit, and marked weakness of the hamstring muscle at 30° knee flexion yet normal strength at 90° knee flexion, could assist in diagnosis [28]. Hamstring avulsions can lead to hamstring syndrome involving the sciatic nerve by scarring around the sciatic nerve or the formation of tight fibrotic bands in the area of the ischial tuberosity [14, 45, 46].

Other sources of sciatic nerve entrapment include malunion of the ischium or healed avulsions, lesser trochanter (Video 24.4: http://goo.gl/R4Pe3), greater trochanter (Video 24.7: http://goo.gl/2keh8), tumor, vascular abnormalities (Video 24.3: http://goo.gl/SzSW0) (Fig. 24.15) [15, 22, 32], gluteus maximus (from a prior iliotibial band release), or as a result of acetabular fracture or post-hip reconstruction [34, 37].

Clinical Presentation

Physical Examination and Ancillary Testing

A comprehensive physical examination, a detailed history, and standardized radiographic interpretation are paramount in evaluating hip pain [14, 47, 48]. When assessing posterior hip pain, the physical examination will allow for an assessment of osseous, capsular labral, musculotendinous, and neurovascular sources and etiologies. Additionally, it is important to recognize the coexistence of many of these pathologies. The lumbar spine, abdominal, genitourinary

problems are ruled out by history, physical examination, and ancillary testing. Symptoms of deep gluteal syndrome and sciatica can be variable. In all cases of suspected nerve entrapment, the spine must first be ruled out by MRI and history/physical examination. Patients presenting with sciatic nerve entrapment often have a history of trauma and symptoms of sit pain (inability to sit for more than 30 min), radicular pain of the lower back or hip, and paresthesias of the affected leg [14, 16]. Some symptoms may mimic a hamstring tear or inter-articular hip pathology such as aching, burning sensation, or cramping in the buttock or posterior thigh. These symptoms should be sorted by the physical examination. The pudendal nerve should also be evaluated in patients with sit pain, which is distinguished by pain more medial to the ischium and is discussed later in the chapter. Upon palpation of the piriformis, Robinson described a tender sausage-shaped mass as a key feature of what he termed "piriformis muscle syndrome" [49]. Physical examination tests that have been used for the clinical diagnosis of sciatic nerve entrapment include passive stretching tests and active contraction tests. The space narrows with flexion, adduction, and internal rotation [1]. Lasègue sign is pain with straight leg raise testing (to 90° hip flexion) [50, 51]. Pace's sign is pain and weakness with resisted abduction and external rotation of the hip [52]. Freiberg's sign is pain with internal rotation of the extended hip [50, 51]. A variant of the Freiberg test involves flexion, adduction, and internal rotation of the hip with the knee flexed (relaxing the sciatic nerve), sometimes referred to as the FAIR test [15, 16]. We have found these tests to be quite variable and have found them to be more reproducible with the knee in extension.

The seated piriformis stretch test (Fig. 24.16a) is a flexion and adduction with internal rotation test performed with the patient in the seated position [53]. The examiner extends the knee (engaging the sciatic nerve) and passively moves the flexed hip into adduction with internal rotation while palpating 1 cm lateral to the ischium (middle finger) and proximally at the sciatic notch (index finger). A positive test is the recreation of the posterior pain at the level of the piriformis or external rotators. An active piriformis test is performed by the patient pushing the heel down into the table, abducting and externally rotating the leg against resistance, while the examiner monitors the piriformis (Fig. 24.16b). The active piriformis test is similar to Pace's sign, which is pain and weakness on resisted abduction and external rotation of the thigh in the seated position [53].

A useful palpation test for sit pain is shown in Fig. 24.17. The physician palpates in three positions of the gluteal area: the piriformis (lateral/superior), at the level of the external rotators, and lateral to the ischium. If pain is localized at the ischium, rule out the hamstring bursa or hamstring tears, and if the pain is more medial, one should evaluate the

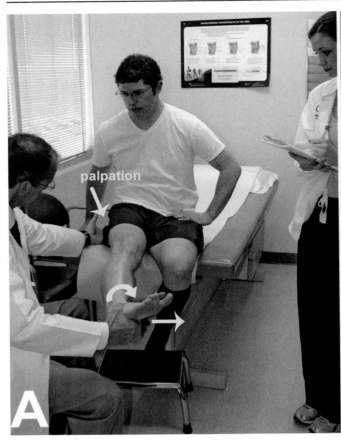

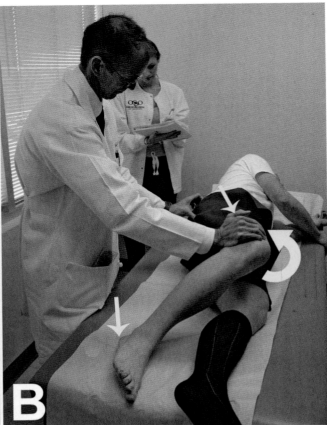

Fig. 24.16 Seated piriformis stretch test and active piriformis test. (**a**) The patient is in the seated position with knee extension. The examiner passively moves the flexed hip into adduction with internal rotation while palpating 1 cm lateral to the ischium (*middle finger*) and proximally at the sciatic notch (*index finger*). (**b**) With the patient in the lateral position, the examiner palpates the piriformis. The patient drives the heel into the examining table thus initiating external hip rotation while actively abducting and externally rotating against resistance (Reprinted from Martin [53]. With permission from Elsevier)

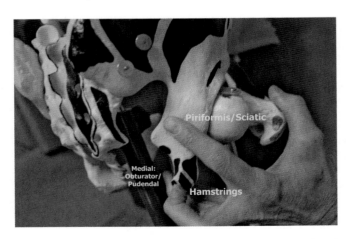

Fig. 24.17 Seated palpation test. The physician palpates the gluteal area: lateral/superior at the piriformis muscle/sciatic nerve (*index finger*), ischium at the hamstring/hamstring tendinosis or avulsion (*middle finger*), medial at the obturator internus/pudendal nerve (*ring finger*). Pain lateral to the ischium, particularly with hip extension, may be ischiofemoral/sciatic nerve

pudendal nerve more carefully. Some patients may present with neurological symptoms of abnormal reflexes or motor weakness [15]. Symptoms related to nerves other than the sciatic nerve may be observed such as weakness of the gluteus medius and minimus muscles (superior gluteal nerve), weakness of the gluteus maximus (inferior gluteal nerve), perineal sensory loss (pudendal nerve), or loss of posterior cutaneous sensation (posterior femoral cutaneous nerve) (Fig. 24.18) [55].

Injection tests have been advocated for supporting the diagnosis of DGS when the piriformis is involved. Pace and Nagle used a double injection technique of an anesthetic and corticosteroids toward the piriformis muscle which relieved the pain in 41 of 45 patients [52]. Guided injections utilizing CT, fluoroscopy, ultrasound, or open MRI to the piriformis muscle have been used to avoid injection to an incorrect site [21]. Pain relief following one or two injections was obtained in 37 of 162 patients with piriformis syndrome [21].

Fig. 24.18 Innervation of the perineum. Sensory zones of the perineum (Reprinted from Labat et al. [54]. With permission from John Wiley & Sons, Inc.)

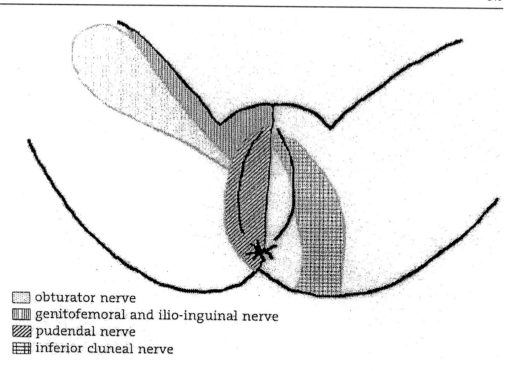

obturator nerve
genitofemoral and ilio-inguinal nerve
pudendal nerve
inferior cluneal nerve

EMG and nerve conduction studies are beneficial to the diagnosis of deep gluteal syndrome. Patients presenting with symptoms of sciatic nerve entrapment may fail to exhibit paraspinal denervation even when radiculopathy coexists [56]. Electrophysiological considerations include positive sharp waves in the peroneus longus, brevis, tertius, and the anterior tibialis, but absent in the gastrocnemius, posterior tibialis, or plantar intrinsics. Reduction of the sural sensory nerve action potential on the affected side is suggestive of injury distal to the ganglia [56]. Piriformis entrapment of the sciatic nerve is often indicated by H-reflex disturbances of the tibial and/or perineal nerves [40, 56]. Special attention should be given to patient positioning. With the knee in extension, the H-reflex will result as normal; however, with the hip in flexion, adduction, and internal rotation (patient in the lateral position) and the knee in flexion, the H-reflex will be delayed. This position will tighten the piriformis muscle compressing the sciatic nerve sufficiently to disturb nerve conduction distally. When positioning the leg in FADDIR, it is important to maintain a neutral pelvis, as anterior pelvic tilt will reduce the degree of adduction. We have found it also to be helpful to extend the knee and compare side to side.

When no other etiological finding is identified, piriformis syndrome could be established by physical examination and injection test and distinguish intra-articular source of pain by intra-articular injection and physical examination [14]. At least one author has proposed the value of MR neurography, which may be helpful in selected patients with sciatica as an aid to diagnosis [21].

Nonoperative Treatment for Sciatic Nerve Entrapment/Deep Gluteal Syndrome

Nonoperative treatment for deep gluteal syndrome begins with a conservative approach addressing the suspected site of impingement. Impingement from a hypertrophied, contracted, or inflamed muscle (piriformis, quadratus femoris, obturator internus, superior/inferior gemellus) begins with rest anti-inflammatories, muscle relaxants, and physical therapy. The physical therapy program should include stretching maneuvers aimed at the external rotators. The piriformis stretch, or FAIR, involves placing the leg in flexion, adduction, and internal rotation (Fig. 24.19). Patients with CAM impingement, anterior pincer impingement, or acetabular retroversion may not be able to stretch adequately into this position and should be evaluated and treated primarily as most will resolve with appropriate surgical intervention. In a seated position, the patient brings the knee into the chest and across midline and pulls the knee to the opposite shoulder. Gradually progress the stretching by increasing duration and intensity until a maximal stretch is obtained. Additional physical therapy techniques that may be helpful include ultrasound and electrical stimulation.

Injections of a muscle anesthetic or corticosteroid can provide pain relief in patients not responding to physical therapy. It is important to administer the injection to the correct site and technique options include fluoroscopic guidance (with or without a radiographic dye), CT, ultrasound, electromyographic guidance, and MRI guidance. A trial of three

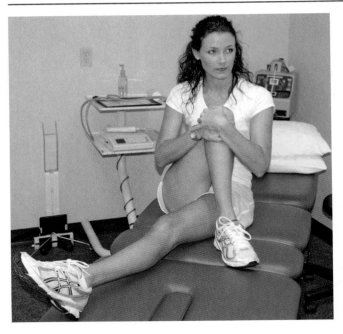

Fig. 24.19 Piriformis stretch. In a seated position, the patient brings the knee into the chest and across midline and pulls the knee to the opposite shoulder

injections has been recommended before opting for more aggressive therapy, taken on a case by case basis [15, 21, 57]. Most cases of deep gluteal syndrome/sciatic nerve entrapment will respond to conservative nonoperative measures.

Operative Treatment

Operative treatment options include open and arthroscopic techniques. The open transgluteal approach has been described to effectively perform piriformis muscle resection and neuroplasty of the sciatic and posterior femoral cutane-

ous nerves [21, 25]. Open operative treatment has been successful in a number of case studies, and the largest case series have reported good to excellent outcomes in 75–100% of the procedures [16, 21, 28]. Additionally, release of the hamstrings and neurolysis of the sciatic nerve at the hamstring origin has been performed. Young et al. performed 47 open surgical proximal hamstring releases, and 86% achieved satisfactory results with significant pain relief and increased hamstring strength [28]. Contrasting release is surgical repair. Hamstring avulsions can lead to sciatica by scarring around the sciatic nerve or the formation of tight fibrotic bands in the area of the ischial tuberosity [14, 45, 46]. Surgical repair is recommended early to avoid involvement of the sciatic nerve [45, 46]. The principal indications for primary repair of proximal hamstring injuries include a complete avulsion of the semitendinosis, semimembranosis, and biceps femoris [5]. Retraction seen on MRI of ≥2 cm of two tendons associated with an injury of the third tendon in young (<50 years old) active individuals is a relative indication for surgical repair [5]. Injury to a single tendon or multiple tendons with <2 cm retraction and elderly or sedentary patients are contraindications for surgery [5]. The surgical technique has been outlined by Miller et al. [5]. The concepts of treatment in this area continue to evolve. Table 24.2 is a summary of open technique results for treatment of sciatic nerve entrapment.

Endoscopic Release

Endoscopy is an effective and minimally invasive approach to the treatment of sciatic nerve entrapment. In 2003, Dezawa et al., reported on six cases of endoscopic piriformis muscle release [20]. We reported on a case series of 35 patients presenting with deep gluteal syndrome [14]. Average duration of symptoms was 3.7 years with an average preoperative verbal analog score of 7, which decreased to 2.4 postoperatively.

Table 24.2 Surgical treatment: open results summary

Author	Number of procedures	Results
Miller et al. [31]	1	Immediate pain relief; 2.5 years post-op, no pain yet decreased sensation over the posterolateral aspect of thigh
Vandertop and Bosma [25]	1	4 years post-op, doing well
Chen [19]	1	Pain resolved in 1 week; motor weakness of the ankle extensors and toes for 3 months; 4 years post-op, asymptomatic
Hughes et al. [22]	5	At 1 year, (1) no pain, slight residual tenderness in buttock; (2) asymptomatic; (3) no pain, slight residual tenderness in buttock; (4) no pain; and (5) excellent
Sayson et al. [24]	1	6 months post-op: no pain
Benson and Schutzer [16]	15	2 years post-op: 11 excellent, 4 good
Meknas et al. [30]	12	No pain decrease at 6 months; 8 years post-op, significant decrease in pain
Filler et al. [21]	64	2 years post-op: excellent, 59%; good, 23%; no benefit, 17%; worse, 2%
Lewis et al. [39]	4	2 months post-op: 3 excellent, 1 still experiencing pain
Issack et al. [34]	10	1 year post-op: partial to complete relief of radicular pain, of diminished sensation, and of paresthesias
Young et al. [28]	44 Hamstring	53 months post-op: 33 satisfied, 5 somewhat satisfied, 6 not satisfied
Beauchesne and Schutzer [18]	1	Immediate pain relief, residual numbness and limp resolved in 4 weeks
Jones et al. [41]	1	Immediate pain relief, 6 weeks post-op: complete resolution of symptoms

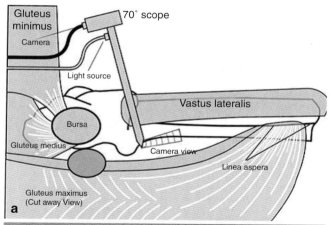

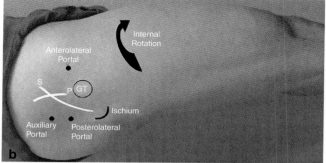

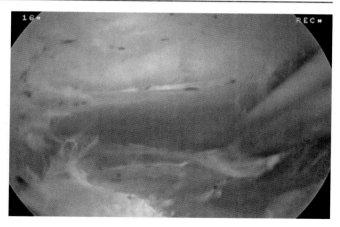

Fig. 24.21 Sciatic nerve decompression/inspection: bursectomy. The greater trochanteric bursa can be excessively thickened with fibrous scar bands extending to near the sciatic nerve up to the sciatic notch

Fig. 24.20 Peritrochanteric space and portal placement. (**a**) Peritrochanteric space and anatomical landmarks with orientation of the arthroscope and light source. The scope is introduced into the PTS and turned around to introduce the Auxiliary portal (Reprinted from Martin [60]. With permission from Slack, Inc.). (**b**) The anterolateral portal placement is 1 cm anterior and 1 cm superior to the greater trochanter (*GT*). The posterolateral portal placement is 3 cm posterior to the greater trochanter and in line with the anterolateral portal. The auxiliary portal is positioned 3 cm posterior and 3 cm superior to the greater trochanter. The course of the sciatic nerve (*S*) and piriformis (*P*) is depicted in relation to the greater trochanter and ischium (Reprinted Martin et al. [14]. With permission from Elsevier)

Preoperative modified Harris Hip Score was 54.4 and increased to 78 postoperatively. Twenty-one patients reported preoperative use of narcotics for pain; two remained on narcotics postoperatively (unrelated to initial complaint). Eighty-three percent of patients had no postoperative sciatic sit pain (inability to sit for >30 min) [14].

The supine technique developed by Byrd [58] is utilized and modified by positioning the table in maximal contralateral patient tilt. Nerve conduction and EMG is monitored intraoperatively. Inspection of the subgluteal space is best performed using a 70° long arthroscope and adjustable/lengthening cannulas. The peritrochanteric space is entered through the anterolateral and posterolateral portals, and systematic inspection of the peritrochanteric space is performed [59]. Shown in Fig. 24.20a is the starting position, and once orientation has been established, turn the arthroscope proximal, initiate bursectomy, and establish the auxiliary posterolateral portal. The auxiliary posterolateral portal is

made 3 cm posterior and 3 cm superior to GT (Fig. 24.20b), which allows for better visualization of the sciatic nerve up to the sciatic notch. Initiate bursectomy noting the extent of the fibrous bands (Video 24.1: http://goo.gl/sZHXk) (Fig. 24.21). The kinematic excursion of the sciatic nerve is then assessed with the leg in flexion with internal/external rotation and full extension with internal/external rotation [13, 14]. Identify the sciatic nerve at the level of the quadratus femoris releasing any fibrous bands (Video 24.1: http://goo.gl/sZHXk) (Fig. 24.22). Inspect the sciatic nerve distal to the quadratus femoris and beneath the proximal end of the linea aspera insertion of the gluteus maximus and release any fibrous congestion around the nerve. Inspect adjacent to the ischium and check the ischial tunnel (Video 24.1: http://goo.gl/sZHXk and Video 24.4: http://goo.gl/R4Pe3): (Fig. 24.23). Looking back proximal, in the region of the obturator internus, identify a branch of the inferior gluteal artery which must be cauterized or ligated (if large) (Video 24.3: http://goo.gl/SzSW0) and released prior to inspection of the piriformis (Video 24.1: http://goo.gl/sZHXk and 24.3: http://goo.gl/SzSW0) (Fig. 24.24). Release any fibrovascular congestion in the obturator internus region. Identify the piriformis muscle and tendon (Video 24.1: http://goo.gl/sZHXk, Video 24.2: http://goo.gl/p8Tn7 and Video 24.3: http://goo.gl/SzSW0) (Fig. 24.25a). The piriformis tendon is often hidden under the belly of the muscle. Release the tendon with arthroscopic scissors (Video 24.1: http://goo.gl/sZHXk, Video 24.2: http://goo.gl/p8Tn7 and Video 24.3: http://goo.gl/SzSW0) (Fig. 24.25b). Perform a dynamic assessment of the sciatic nerve with flexion, internal, and external rotation (Video 24.1: http://goo.gl/sZHXk and Video 24.6: http://goo.gl/MgIkA) (Fig. 24.26). Probe the sciatic nerve up to the sciatic notch. Proceed with caution at the sciatic notch as the superior gluteal neurovascular structures are within this area (Video 24.1: http://goo.gl/sZHXk) (Fig. 24.27). Thoroughly probe around and under the sciatic nerve to identify and

Fig. 24.22 Sciatic nerve decompression/inspection: at the quadratus femoris. Identify the sciatic nerve at the level of the quadratus femoris. Gross appearance of the sciatic nerve before decompression can be hypovascular or significantly entrapped by scar tissue and fibrous bands

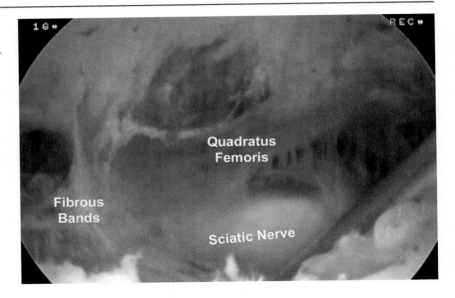

Fig. 24.23 Sciatic nerve decompression/inspection: distal to the quadratus femoris. Endoscopic view of the left hip through the posterolateral portal looking distal to the quadratus femoris. With internal and external rotation of the hip, inspect and release fibrous bands adjacent to the ischium and check the ischial tunnel

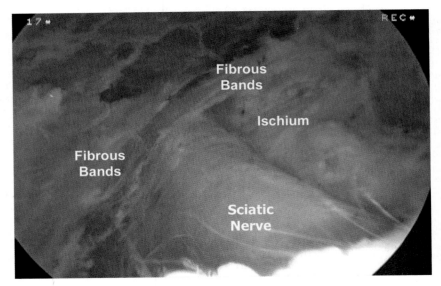

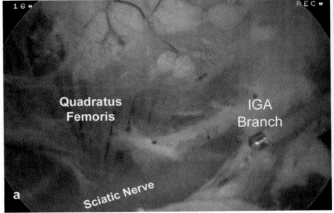
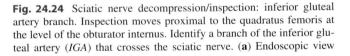
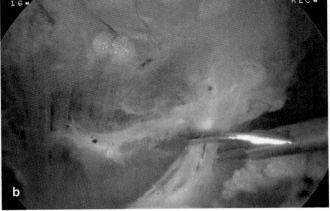

Fig. 24.24 Sciatic nerve decompression/inspection: inferior gluteal artery branch. Inspection moves proximal to the quadratus femoris at the level of the obturator internus. Identify a branch of the inferior gluteal artery (*IGA*) that crosses the sciatic nerve. (**a**) Endoscopic view through the anterolateral portal with a 70° scope; cauterize (ligate if very large) the IGA branch and (**b**) dissect carefully before inspection of the piriformis muscle

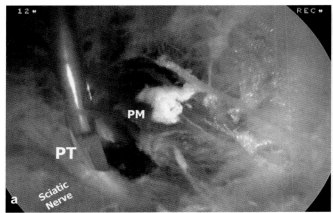

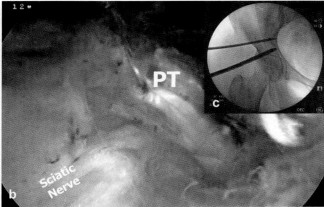

Fig. 24.25 Sciatic nerve decompression/inspection: piriformis muscle. (**a**) Endoscopic view of a right hip with the scope in the posterolateral portal and arthroscopic scissors through the auxiliary portal. The piriformis muscle (*PM*) must be probed, and often, the tendon (*PT*) lies under the muscle belly. (**b**) The PT is lifted up off the sciatic nerve for resection using arthroscopic scissors (the arthroscope is in the same position for **a** and **b**). (**c**) Fluoroscopic view showing location at the sciatic notch

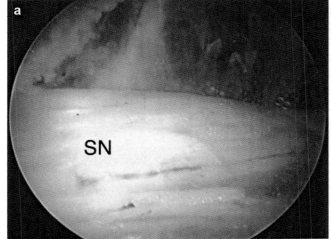

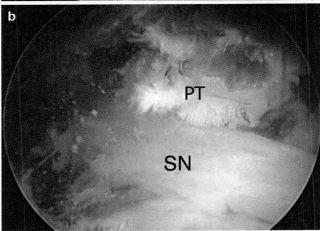

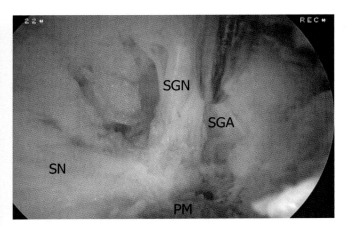

Fig. 24.27 Sciatic nerve decompression/inspection: superior gluteal nerve and artery area of caution. Endoscopic view as the sciatic nerve (*SN*) exits the greater sciatic notch proximal to the piriformis (*PM*) encountering the superior gluteal nerve (*SGN*) and superior gluteal artery (*SGA*)

release any ancillary musculotendinous branches that may be binding the nerve. Consideration may be given for resection of the obturator internus tendon if necessary (Video 24.1: http://goo.gl/sZHXk) (Fig. 24.14).

The sciatic nerve is vulnerable to entrapment by various structures within the subgluteal space. The sciatic nerve can also be entrapped in the intrapelvic region. Familiarity with the anatomy, clinical presentation (history/physical examination), and ancillary testing of deep gluteal syndrome is key for diagnosis. The majority of literature regarding sciatic nerve entrapment has been published in neurological journals; however, interest in orthopedic journals is increasing. The hip surgeon should be aware of continuum of data and evolution of sciatic nerve entrapment studies. Table 24.3 provides a summary of works involving sciatic nerve entrapment.

Fig. 24.26 Sciatic nerve decompression/inspection: dynamic inspection. Endoscopic view of the sciatic nerve (*SN*) post-decompression. The kinematic excursion of SN was checked with internal (**a**) and external rotation (**b**) of the hip to ensure adequate glide of the nerve. Resect 1–2 cm of the piriformis tendon (*PT*) (Reprinted Martin et al. [14]. With permission from Elsevier)

Table 24.3 Summary of sciatic nerve entrapment studies

Author	Entrapment source	Clinical	Diagnostic
Miller et al. [31]	Ischial tuberosity avulsion fracture, fragment within the substance of the biceps femoris tendon impinging and piercing the SN	Tender sciatic notch, decreased sensation posterior thigh, radicular pain, SLR	AP radiograph/CT osseous fragment, myelogram, and EMG; needle EMG mild abnormality
Vandertop [25]	Case report: fibrovascular band, piriformis, and inferior gluteal vessels	Paresthesia; radiating pain to toes; sensory and DTR deficits; tenderness from piriformis down to midthigh; positive Pace, Freiberg, and FAIR tests	Injection, temporary relief; CT, small L5–S1 disc herniation; EMG nonspecific
Chen et al. [19]	Piriformis pyomyositis	Tender gluteal area, radicular pain, SLR, Freiberg, Pace	CT, swelling piriformis / intramuscular abscess
Hughes et al. [22]	5 cases: (1) Bifid PM, split SN at the notch. (2) Bifid PM, hourglass-shaped constriction of peroneal division between the two heads of muscle. (3) PM appeared normal, thick tendinous band on the undersurface of PM found to indent the SN. (4) Pulsatile vascular mass. (5) Persistent sciatic vessels	N/A	N/A
Sayson et al. [24]	Case report: inflamed PM and thick fibrous band crossing the sciatic nerve	Radiating pain, paresthesia, pain walking, sitting, bending at the waist, tender to palpation	N/A
Benson and Shutzer [16]	14 cases: piriformis syndrome	Trauma, buttock paint, sit pain, tenderness at the greater sciatic notch, FAIR, and radicular pain	Hip and lumbar spine radiographs, MRI, CT, and 6 of 8 with abnormal EMG
Meknas et al. [4]	Internal obturator muscle	Buttock pain, tender sciatic notch, sit pain, Pace, Freiberg	N/A
Dezawa et al. [20]	Piriformis muscle	Buttock pain, pain with palpation of the piriformis	N/A
Filler et al. [21]	Piriformis muscle, distal foraminal entrapment, ischial tunnel, discogenic pain with referred leg pain, pudendal nerve/ sacrospinous ligament, distal sciatic entrapment	Buttock and leg pain; back pain; resisted ABD or ADD of flexed IR; sciatic notch tender or pain at the GT; pain sitting	MRI, MR neurography, open MRI-guided injections
Cox and Bakkum [29]	Possible source: gemelli-obturator internus complex	Cadaver study	N/A
Lewis et al. [39]	12 of 14 showed increased fluid-attenuated inversion recovery signal, at sciatic notch or just inferior to the level of PM	N/A	MR neurography
Mayrand et al. [23]	Case report: piriformis syndrome, secondary to avulsion of the ischial tuberosity	Shooting pain from buttock to lateral foot, posterior thigh and calf, paresthesia, restricted hip range of motion	X-ray of bony overgrowth of ischial tuberosity
Issack et al. [34]	Acetabular fracture, SN released from scar and heterotopic bone	Radicular pain, decreased sensation, paresthesia, motor loss, foot drop	N/A
Young et al. [28]	Hamstring tendons	Tender proximal hamstring/ischial tuberosity, weakness	Ultrasound, MRI, nerve conduction
Torriani et al. [33]	Ischiofemoral impingement, narrowing of ischiofemoral space, and abnormal quadratus femoris	Radiating pain, back pain, snapping hip	MRI
Meknas et al. [30]	Internal obturator tendon	8-year follow-up: decrease in pain	N/A
Jawish et al. [40]	Piriformis syndrome. 1 case: SN was bifid under the hypertrophied PM. 1 case: bifid PM and bifid SN with one through PM and one proximal. 1 case: PM and sacrosciatic ligament. 2 cases: PM hypertrophied with SN directly below. 1 case: a transverse fibrous band compressing SN	Constancy of signs: (1) no spinal path on MRI, (2) tender sciatic spine and none lower back or SIJ, (3) sit pain, (4) sit pain with leg crossed, (5) IR and Max ADD, (6) H-reflex of CPN gone with IR ADD	MRI, EMG dynamic
Beauchesne and Schutzer [18]	Piriformis muscle, myositis ossificans	Trauma, radicular pain, neuropathy	CT, MRI
Jones et al. [41]	Posterior paralabral cyst	Trauma, radicular pain, deep gluteal pain, SLR	MRI

SN sciatic nerve, SLR straight leg raise, AP anterior posterior, CT computed tomography, EMG electromyogram, DTR deep tendon reflexes, FAIR flexion/adduction/internal rotation, PM piriformis muscle, N/A not available, ABD abduction, ADD adduction, IR internal rotation, GT greater trochanter, MRI magnetic resonance imaging, MR magnetic resonance, SIJ sacroiliac joint

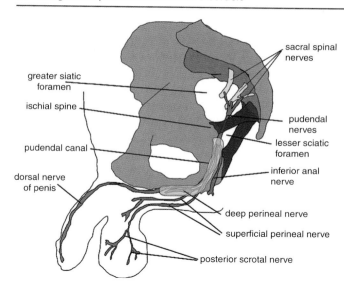

Fig. 24.28 The course of the pudendal nerve. The pudendal nerve exits the pelvis through the greater sciatic notch passing over the sacrospinous ligament and reenters the pelvis through the lesser sciatic notch then enters the Alcock (*yellow*) canal formed by the obturator fascia and sacrotuberous ligament (Reprinted from Moore and Dalley [61]. With permission from Lippincott Williams & Wilkins)

Pudendal Nerve

The goal in developing this section is to raise awareness of a very disabling form of posterior hip pain: neuropathic pain in the distribution of the pudendal nerve (Fig. 24.28) with sensations of burning, tearing, stabbing lightning-like, electrical, sharp shooting, and/or foreign body sensation [62]. Pain is made worse with sitting, reduced with standing, and absence upon awakening and progressing through the day. The common historical etiologies that include childbirth, prolonged sitting, trauma, and cycling exercises have been thought as causative. The etiology of pudendal nerve entrapment requires further definition. However, suspicion of this pathology can be validated through thorough history, physical examination, and appropriate ancillary tests especially including injections.

Anatomy

The pudendal nerve can become entrapped in several locations from the greater sciatic notch to the lesser sciatic notch and even distally to the obturator internus/levator ani fascia. The anatomy of the pudendal nerve can have significant individual variation. In 87 of 100 cadaveric hips, the sacrotuberous ligament (STL) has been found to be composed of the two parts: a ligamentous band and a membranous falciform process [11]. The attachment of the falciform process to the ischial ramus showed two variations. Most commonly, the falciform process continued toward and along the ischial

ramus to the obturator fascia. The second type coursed along the ischial ramus, fused with the obturator fascia, and continued to the ischioanal fossa. The medial border of the falciform process descended to fuse with the lateral anococcygeal ligament. Superior to the STL is the sacrospinous ligament. A very rare anomaly of the pudendal nerve was discovered in a cadaver involving the pudendal nerve and vessels coursing posterior to the STL [11].

Pudendal nerve relationship with the sacrospinous ligament is varied and could be prone to entrapment [63]. Four main types of pudendal nerve entrapment are based upon the location of entrapment, which is very important for injections [12]: Type I, at the exit of the greater sciatic notch accompanied by piriformis muscle spasm; Type II, at the ischial spine, sacrotuberous ligament, and lesser sciatic notch entrance; Type III, at the entrance of the Alcock canal associated with the obturator internus muscle spasm; and Type IV, distal entrapment of terminal branches [12].

Diagnostic Criteria

The diagnosis of pudendal neuralgia has been primarily clinical and empirical [54]; however, progress in clinical nerve imaging and injection techniques is aiding in the differential diagnosis of pudendal nerve entrapment [12]. In 2008, Labat et al. validated the Nantes criteria with five essential diagnostic criteria: (1) pain in the anatomical territory of the pudendal nerve (Fig. 24.18), (2) worsened by sitting (although no pain when sitting on a toilet seat), (3) the pain does not wake the patient at night, (4) pain with no objective sensory impairment, and (5) pain is relieved by diagnostic pudendal nerve block [54]. Also defined in the report are complementary diagnostic criteria, exclusion criteria, and associated signs not excluding the diagnosis [54]. Neurophysiologic testing techniques have been used to aid in diagnosis [62]. The physical examination is useful for preliminarily sorting patients into four categories: Type I, sciatic notch tenderness only; Type II, midischial tenderness; Type IIIa, obturator internus muscle tenderness only; Type IIIb, obturator and piriformis muscle tenderness; and Type IV, no palpable tenderness. MR neurography or MRI can then be helpful to identify abnormalities in nerve or adjacent muscles/vessels [12]. Positive MRI findings will lead to injection sites according to category: for Type I, piriformis injection; Type II, block the pudendal nerve at the ischial spine; Type IIIa, obturator internus injection; Type IIIb, piriformis and obturator internus injection; and Type IV, block the pudendal nerve in the area of the Alcock canal [12]. If no relief and no specific aggravation, evaluate immune/rheumatological issues and end-organ causes, which if negative, consider a ganglion block. A repeat injection may be required if necessary for diagnosis and treatment.

Treatment

Surgical treatment involves open minimal access approaches usually on an outpatient or overnight-stay basis. Electromyography of the pudendal nerve, sciatic nerve, nerve to the obturator internus, and the inferior and superior gluteal nerves is recommended intraoperatively for identification and protection. Surgical procedures include a superior transgluteal approach, a medial transgluteal approach, an inferior transgluteal approach, or a transischial approach [12, 62]. Recommended surgical treatments are for Type I, piriformis resection and neuroplasty of the pudendal nerve inside the sciatic notch and as it exits the sciatic notch; Type II, neuroplasty of the pudendal nerve inside at the ischial spine with sectioning of the sacrotuberous or sacrospinous ligaments, if needed; Type IIIa, neuroplasty of the nerve to the obturator internus and the pudendal nerve in the inferior retrosciatic space, through the lesser sciatic notch, and the proximal Alcock canal; Type IIIb, perform operation Type I and Type IIIa; and Type IV, neuroplasty of the distal pudendal nerve [12].

Outcomes

Antolak reviewed the responses to perineural injections of patients originally evaluated in 2005, 56% had continued pain free status at 24 months [67]. Filler reported on 200 patients with pudendal nerve entrapment and 12% achieved long-standing relief (over 1 year) with injection alone [12]. One hundred and eighty-five operations were performed (some patients bilateral). The surgical procedures achieved good to excellent outcome in 87% of the patients. In most cases, improvement was reported within 4 weeks, whereas some continued to improve for up to 12 months [12]. Popeney et al. reported on 58 patients with pudendal nerve entrapment, and 60% were classified as responders [62].

Ischiofemoral Impingement

Ischiofemoral impingement as an etiology of posterior hip pain has recently been reported [32, 33, 64]; however, the surgical technique for treatment has yet to be published. Ischiofemoral impingement syndrome is described as a narrowing of the ischiofemoral space and an abnormal quadratus femoris muscle MR signal intensity [32, 33] (Video 24.4: http://goo.gl/R4Pe3 and Video 24.5: http://goo.gl/0KchA) (Fig. 24.29). The ischiofemoral space is defined as the smallest distance between the lateral cortex of the ischial tuberosity and medial cortex of the lesser trochanter. The quadratus femoris space is defined as the smallest space for passage of the quadratus femoris muscle delimited by the superolateral surface of the hamstring tendons and the posteromedial surface of the iliopsoas tendon or lesser trochanter. The ischiofemoral (Video 24.4: http://goo.gl/R4Pe3 and Video 24.5: http://goo.gl/0KchA) (Fig. 24.30) and quadratus femoris spaces have been found to be significantly narrower in affected subjects compared with normal [33]. Suggested cut-off values are ≤17 mm for the ischiofemoral space and ≤8 mm for the quadratus femoris space [33]. Abnormalities

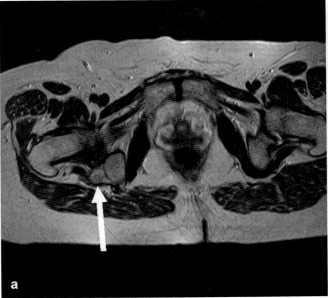
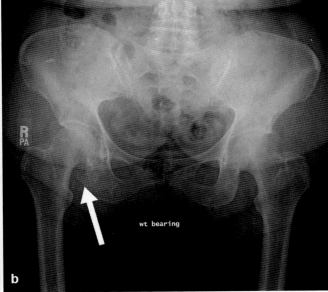

Fig. 24.29 Imaging of ischiofemoral impingement. (**a**) MRI showing a large bony outgrowth (*arrow*) on the right ischium. (**b**) Standing AP radiograph of the same patient showing a large bony outgrowth (*arrow*) on the right ischium

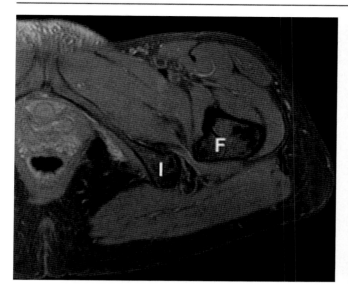

Fig. 24.30 MRI of ischiofemoral impingement. Left side MRI of a narrowed ischiofemoral tunnel. The distance between the lateral cortex of the ischial tuberosity (*I*) and medial cortex of the lesser trochanter of the femur (*F*) is 10.9 mm

of the quadratus femoris muscle included edema (100%), partial tear (33%), and fatty infiltration (8%). The hamstring tendons of affected subjects showed evidence of edema (50%) and partial tears (25%) [33]. Of 239 patients with non-discogenic sciatica, 4.7% were diagnosed with ischial tunnel syndrome [12]. These patients experience tenderness to palpation at the lateral surface of the ischial tuberosity, which is distinguished from pain at the medial surface of the ischial tuberosity often associated with obturator internus pain and pudendal nerve entrapment [12]. This can be differentiated by pain at terminal hip extension while walking and MRI hyperintensity. Currently, there are no published data; there have been good short-term outcomes with quadratus femoris resection or bony resection [65, 66] (Video 24.4: http://goo.gl/R4Pe3 and Video 24.5: http://goo.gl/0KchA) (Fig. 24.31).

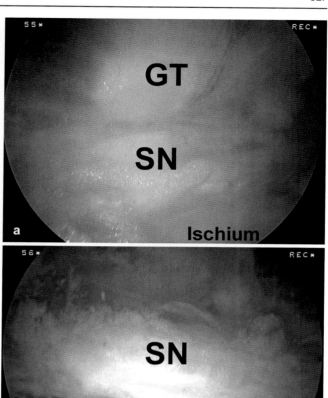

Fig. 24.31 Endoscopic decompression of ischial impingement of the sciatic nerve. (**a**) Endoscopic view of the sciatic nerve (*SN*) trapped between the greater trochanter (*GT*) and ischium. With hip flexion and external rotation, the sciatic nerve was not able to move due to the ischial outgrowth of bone. (**b**) Endoscopic view following bone resection of the ischium

Acknowledgements I would like to thank Ian J. Palmer [PhD] and Munif Hatem [MD] for their assistance in preparing this chapter.

Summary

This chapter has reviewed the anatomy, defined the region, and focused on the potential sources of extra-articular hip pathology within the subgluteal space. The subgluteal space and associated disorders are complex and can be difficult to diagnose and treat. Posterior hip pain can result from osseous, capsular labral, musculotendinous, and neurovascular etiologies; therefore each layer must be assessed. A detailed understanding of anatomy, biomechanics, and pathokinematics is required to appreciate disorders of the subgluteal space. Through a comprehensive history and physical examination, a differential diagnosis can be made to direct ancillary testing and appropriate treatment considerations.

References

1. Guvencer M, Akyer P, Iyem C, Tetik S, Naderi S. Anatomic considerations and the relationship between the piriformis muscle and the sciatic nerve. Surg Radiol Anat. 2008;30:467–74.
2. Solomon LB, Lee YC, Callary SA, Beck M, Howie DW. Anatomy of piriformis, obturator internus and obturator externus: implications for the posterior surgical approach to the hip. J Bone Joint Surg Br. 2010;92:1317–24.
3. Clemente C. Gray's Anatomy: anatomy of the human body. 13th ed. Baltimore: Williams and Wilkins; 1985.
4. Meknas K, Christensen A, Johansen O. The internal obturator muscle may cause sciatic pain. Pain. 2003;104:375–80.
5. Miller SL, Webb GR. The proximal origin of the hamstrings and surrounding anatomy encountered during repair. Surgical technique. J Bone Joint Surg Am. 2008;90(Suppl 2 Pt 1):108–16.

6. Filler AG, Kline DG. General principles in evaluating and treating peripheral nerve pathology, injuries, and entrapments and their historical context. In: Winn HR, editor. Youmans neurological surgery. Philadelphia: Saunders; 2009.

7. Jacobs LG, Buxton RA. The course of the superior gluteal nerve in the lateral approach to the hip. J Bone Joint Surg. 1989;71:1239–43.

8. Kalhor M, Beck M, Huff TW, Ganz R. Capsular and pericapsular contributions to acetabular and femoral head perfusion. J Bone Joint Surg. 2009;91:409–18.

9. Miller SL, Gill J, Webb GR. The proximal origin of the hamstrings and surrounding anatomy encountered during repair. A cadaveric study. J Bone Joint Surg. 2007;89:44–8.

10. Kirici Y, Yazar F, Ozan H. The neurovascular and muscular anomalies of the gluteal region: an atypical pudendal nerve. Surg Radiol Anat. 1999;21:393–6.

11. Loukas M, Louis Jr RG, Hallner B, Gupta AA, White D. Anatomical and surgical considerations of the sacrotuberous ligament and its relevance in pudendal nerve entrapment syndrome. Surg Radiol Anat. 2006;28:163–9.

12. Filler AG. Diagnosis and treatment of pudendal nerve entrapment syndrome subtypes: imaging, injections, and minimal access surgery. Neurosurg Focus. 2009;26:E9.

13. Coppieters MW, Alshami AM, Babri AS, Souvlis T, Kippers V, Hodges PW. Strain and excursion of the sciatic, tibial, and plantar nerves during a modified straight leg raising test. J Orthop Res. 2006;24:1883–9.

14. Martin HD, Shears SA, Johnson JC, Smathers AM, Palmer IJ. The endoscopic treatment of sciatic nerve entrapment/deep gluteal syndrome. Arthroscopy. 2011;27:172–81.

15. Papadopoulos EC, Khan SN. Piriformis syndrome and low back pain: a new classification and review of the literature. Orthop Clin North Am. 2004;35:65–71.

16. Benson ER, Schutzer SF. Posttraumatic piriformis syndrome: diagnosis and results of operative treatment. J Bone Joint Surg. 1999;81:941–9.

17. Adams JA. The piriformis syndrome – report of four cases and review of the literature. S Afr J Surg. 1980;18:13–8.

18. Beauchesne RP, Schutzer SF. Myositis ossificans of the piriformis muscle: an unusual cause of piriformis syndrome. A case report. J Bone Joint Surg. 1997;79:906–10.

19. Chen WS. Sciatica due to piriformis pyomyositis. Report of a case. J Bone Joint Surg. 1992;74:1546–8.

20. Dezawa A, Kusano S, Miki H. Arthroscopic release of the piriformis muscle under local anesthesia for piriformis syndrome. Arthroscopy. 2003;19:554–7.

21. Filler AG, Haynes J, Jordan SE, Prager J, Villablanca JP, Farahani K, et al. Sciatica of nondisc origin and piriformis syndrome: diagnosis by magnetic resonance neurography and interventional magnetic resonance imaging with outcome study of resulting treatment. J Neurosurg. 2005;2:99–115.

22. Hughes SS, Goldstein MN, Hicks DG, Pellegrini Jr VD. Extrapelvic compression of the sciatic nerve. An unusual cause of pain about the hip: report of five cases. J Bone Joint Surg. 1992;74:1553–9.

23. Mayrand N, Fortin J, Descarreaux M, Normand MC. Diagnosis and management of posttraumatic piriformis syndrome: a case study. J Manipulative Physiol Ther. 2006;29:486–91.

24. Sayson SC, Ducey JP, Maybrey JB, Wesley RL, Vermilion D. Sciatic entrapment neuropathy associated with an anomalous piriformis muscle. Pain. 1994;59:149–52.

25. Vandertop WP, Bosma NJ. The piriformis syndrome. A case report. J Bone Joint Surg. 1991;73:1095–7.

26. McCrory P, Bell S. Nerve entrapment syndromes as a cause of pain in the hip, groin and buttock. Sports Med (Auckland, NZ). 1999;27:261–74.

27. Puranen J, Orava S. The hamstring syndrome. A new diagnosis of gluteal sciatic pain. Am J Sports Med. 1988;16:517–21.

28. Young IJ, van Riet RP, Bell SN. Surgical release for proximal hamstring syndrome. Am J Sports Med. 2008;36:2372–8.

29. Cox JM, Bakkum BW. Possible generators of retrotrochanteric gluteal and thigh pain: the gemelli-obturator internus complex. J Manipulative Physiol Ther. 2005;28:534–8.

30. Meknas K, Kartus J, Letto JI, Christensen A, Johansen O. Surgical release of the internal obturator tendon for the treatment of retrotrochanteric pain syndrome: a prospective randomized study, with long-term follow-up. Knee Surg Sports Traumatol Arthrosc. 2009;17:1249–56.

31. Miller A, Stedman GH, Beisaw NE, Gross PT. Sciatica caused by an avulsion fracture of the ischial tuberosity. A case report. J Bone Joint Surg. 1987;69:143–5.

32. Patti JW, Ouellette H, Bredella MA, Torriani M. Impingement of lesser trochanter on ischium as a potential cause for hip pain. Skeletal Radiol. 2008;37:939–41.

33. Torriani M, Souto SC, Thomas BJ, Ouellette H, Bredella MA. Ischiofemoral impingement syndrome: an entity with hip pain and abnormalities of the quadratus femoris muscle. Am J Roentgenol. 2009;193:186–90.

34. Issack PS, Kreshak J, Klinger CE, Toro JB, Buly RL, Helfet DL. Sciatic nerve release following fracture or reconstructive surgery of the acetabulum. Surgical technique. J Bone Joint Surg. 2008;90(Suppl 2 Pt 2):227–37.

35. Papadopoulos SM, McGillicuddy JE, Albers JW. Unusual cause of 'piriformis muscle syndrome'. Arch Neurol. 1990;47:1144–6.

36. Brown JA, Braun MA, Namey TC. Piriformis syndrome in a 10-year-old boy as a complication of operation with the patient in the sitting position. Neurosurgery. 1988;23:117–9.

37. Uchio Y, Nishikawa U, Ochi M, Shu N, Takata K. Bilateral piriformis syndrome after total hip arthroplasty. Arch Orthop Trauma Surg. 1998;117:177–9.

38. Beaton L, Anson B. The sciatic nerve and the piriformis muscle: their interrelation and possible cause of coccygodynia. J Bone Joint Surg Am. 1938;20:686–8.

39. Lewis AM, Layzer R, Engstrom JW, Barbaro NM, Chin CT. Magnetic resonance neurography in extraspinal sciatica. Arch Neurol. 2006;63:1469–72.

40. Jawish RM, Assoum HA, Khamis CF. Anatomical, clinical and electrical observations in piriformis syndrome. J Orthop Surg Res. 2010;5:3.

41. Jones HG, Sarasin SM, Jones SA, Mullaney P. Acetabular paralabral cyst as a rare cause of sciatica. A case report. J Bone Joint Surg. 2009;91:2696–9.

42. Smoll NR. Variations of the piriformis and sciatic nerve with clinical consequence: a review. Clin Anat. 2010;23:8–17.

43. Filler AG. Piriformis and related entrapment syndromes: diagnosis & management. Neurosurg Clin N Am. 2008;19:609–22, vii.

44. Migliorini S, Merlo M. The hamstring syndrome in endurance athletes. Br J Sports Med. 2011;45:363.

45. Chakravarthy J, Ramisetty N, Pimpalnerkar A, Mohtadi N. Surgical repair of complete proximal hamstring tendon ruptures in water skiers and bull riders: a report of four cases and review of the literature. Br J Sports Med. 2005;39:569–72.

46. Wood DG, Packham I, Trikha SP, Linklater J. Avulsion of the proximal hamstring origin. J Bone Joint Surg. 2008;90:2365–74.

47. Martin HD. Clinical examination of the hip. Oper Tech Orthop. 2005;15:177–81.

48. Martin HD, Kelly BT, Leunig M, Philippon MJ, Clohisy JC, Martin RL, et al. The pattern and technique in the clinical evaluation of the adult hip: the common physical examination tests of hip specialists. Arthroscopy. 2010;26:161–72.

49. Freiberg AH, Vinke TH. Sciatica and the sacroiliac joint. J Bone Joint Surg Am. 1934;16:126–36.

50. Robinson DR. Piriformis syndrome in relation to sciatic pain. Am J Surg. 1947;73:355–8.

51. Freiberg AH. Sciatic pain and its relief by operations on muscle and fascia. Arch Surg. 1937;34:337–50.

52. Pace JB, Nagle D. Piriform syndrome. West J Med. 1976;124:435–9.

53. Martin H. Clinical examination and imaging of the hip. In: Byrd J, Guanche C, editors. AANA advanced arthroscopy: the hip. Philadelphia: Saunders; 2010.

54. Labat JJ, Riant T, Robert R, Amarenco G, Lefaucheur JP, Rigaud J. Diagnostic criteria for pudendal neuralgia by pudendal nerve entrapment (Nantes criteria). Neurourol Urodyn. 2008;27:306–10.

55. McCrory P. The "piriformis syndrome" – myth or reality? Br J Sports Med. 2001;35:209–10.

56. Fishman LM, Wilkins AN. Piriformis syndrome: electrophysiology vs. anatomical assumption. In: Fishman LM, Wilkins AN, editors. Functional electromyography. New York: Springer; 2011.

57. Barton PM. Piriformis syndrome: a rational approach to management. Pain. 1991;47:345–52.

58. Byrd JW. Hip arthroscopy utilizing the supine position. Arthroscopy. 1994;10:275–80.

59. Voos JE, Rudzki JR, Shindle MK, Martin H, Kelly BT. Arthroscopic anatomy and surgical techniques for peritrochanteric space disorders in the hip. Arthroscopy. 2007;23:1246 e1–5.

60. Martin H. Diagnostic arthroscopy. In: Kelly BT, Philippon MJ, editors. Arthroscopic techniques of the hip: a visual guide. Thorofare: Slack Inc; 2009.

61. Moore K, Dalley A. Essential clinical anatomy. 4th ed. Philadelphia: Lippincott Williams & Wilkins; 1999.

62. Popeney C, Ansell V, Renney K. Pudendal entrapment as an etiology of chronic perineal pain: diagnosis and treatment. Neurourol Urodyn. 2007;26:820–7.

63. Mahakkanukrauh P, Surin P, Vaidhayakarn P. Anatomical study of the pudendal nerve adjacent to the sacrospinous ligament. Clin Anat. 2005;18:200–5.

64. Johnson KA. Impingement of the lesser trochanter on the ischial ramus after total hip arthroplasty. Report of three cases. J Bone Joint Surg. 1977;59:268–9.

65. Byrd JW. Arthroscopy association of North America annual meeting. Hollywood, FL; 2010.

66. Martin H. American academy of orthopaedic surgeons annual meeting. San Diego, CA; 2011.

67. Antolak SJ. Surgical care in pudendal neuralgia. In workshop Pudendal Neuralgia: Diagnosis and Management. Chair: Gordon A. Pain Res Manag (Abstract 26C) 2010;15:87.

68. Benzon HT, Katz JA, Benzon HA, Iqbal MS. Piriformis syndrome: anatomic considerations, a new injection technique, and a review of the literature. Anesthesiology 2003;98:1442–8.

69. Chiba S. [Multiple positional relationships of nerves arising from the sacral plexus to the piriformis muscle in humans]. Kaibogaku zasshi 1992;67:691–724.

70. Chiba S, Ishibashi Y, Kasai T. [Perforation of dorsal branches of the sacral nerve plexus through the piriformis muscle and its relation to changes of segmental arrangements of the vertebral column and others]. Kaibogaku zasshi 1994;69:281–305.

71. Fishman LM, Dombi GW, Michaelsen C, Ringel S, Rozbruch J, Rosner B, et al. Piriformis syndrome: diagnosis, treatment, and outcome--a 10-year study. Archives of physical medicine and rehabilitation 2002;83:295–301.

72. Guvencer M, Iyem C, Akyer P, Tetik S, Naderi S. Variations in the high division of the sciatic nerve and relationship between the sciatic nerve and the piriformis. Turkish neurosurgery 2009;19:139–44.

73. Lee CS, Tsai TL. [The relation of the sciatic nerve to the piriformis muscle]. Taiwan yi xue hui za zhi 1974;73:75–80.

74. Nizankowski C, Slociak J, Szybejko J. [Variations in the anatomy of the sciatic nerve in man]. Folia morphologica 1972;31:507–13.

75. Parsons FG, Keith A. Sixth Annual Report of the Committee of Collective Investigation of the Anatomical Society of Great Britain and Ireland, 1895–96. Journal of anatomy and physiology 1896;31:31–44.

76. Pecina M. Contribution to the etiological explanation of the piriformis syndrome. Acta anatomica 1979;105:181–7.

77. Pokorny D, Jahoda D, Veigl D, Pinskerova V, Sosna A. Topographic variations of the relationship of the sciatic nerve and the piriformis muscle and its relevance to palsy after total hip arthroplasty. Surg Radiol Anat 2006;28:88–91.

78. Pokorny D, Sosna A, Veigl P, Jahoda D. [Anatomic variability of the relation of pelvitrochanteric muscles and sciatic nerve.]. Acta chirurgiae orthopaedicae et traumatologiae Cechoslovaca 1998;65:336–9.

79. Ugrenovic S, Jovanovic I, Krstic V, Stojanovic V, Vasovic L, Antic S, et al. [The level of the sciatic nerve division and its relations to the piriform muscle]. Vojnosanitetski pregled 2005;62:45–9.

80. Agur A, Dalley A. Grant's Atlas of Anatomy. Baltimore: Lippincott Williams and Wilkins; 2005.

81. Anson B, McVay C. Surgical anatomy. Philidelphia: W.B. Saunders Company; 1971.

82. Bardeen K. A statistical study of the variations in the formation and position of the lumbosacral plexus in man. Anat Anz 1901;9:209–38.

83. Beaton L, Anson B. The relation of the sciatic nerve and of its subdivisions to the piriformis muscle. Anat Rec 1937;70:1–5.

84. Ming-Tzu P. The relation of the sciatic nerve to the piriformis muscle in the Chinese. Am J Phys Anthropol 1941;28:375.

85. Misra B. The relations of the sciatic nerve to the piriformis in Indian cadavers. J Anat Soc India 1954;3:28–33.

86. Trotter M. The relation of the sciatic nerve to the piriformis muscle in American Whites and Negroes. Anat Rec 1932;52:321–3.

Endoscopic Hamstring Repair and Ischial Bursectomy

Carlos A. Guanche

Introduction

Hamstring injuries are common in athletic populations and can affect all levels of athletes [1–4]. There is a continuum of injuries that can range from musculotendinous strains to avulsions, and most are strains that occur at the musculotendinous junction [1, 2]. By definition, a strain is a partial or complete disruption of the musculotendinous unit [1, 4, 5]. Hamstring strains can result in significant pain and time lost to sport [1, 2]. Most do not require surgical intervention and resolve with a variety of modalities and rest.

Avulsions of the proximal hamstring tendons, however, can cause more significant disabilities. These typically avulse from the ischium and are much less common [6–8]. The diagnosis of a complete avulsion can be difficult to make without the appropriate imaging, and delay in diagnosis can complicate the management, especially when patients present chronically [2, 8–10]. While treatment of the common hamstring strain is uncomplicated, treatment of proximal hamstring avulsions is controversial in the literature [2, 7, 9, 11].

Another aspect that has been poorly documented in the literature is refractory ischial bursitis secondary to partial ruptures of the hamstring origin. Whether the pain is due to the partial rupture or simply due to a painful tendinopathy that may masquerade as ischial bursitis has not really been determined. These injuries can be debilitating and often lead to significant limitations of activities in the population most affected by the problem, namely, runners. There is limited data concerning the treatment of partial avulsions [12, 13]. Cohen et al. recommends consideration of nonoperative treatment for acute partial avulsions [12]. Lempainen et al. reported good results with repair of partial avulsion that had failed initial nonoperative treatment [13].

With the recent expansion of hip arthroscopy, the natural progression has been to explore other areas that may perhaps be amenable to endoscopic or arthroscopic visualization and perhaps treatment. With that in mind, this chapter will discuss the clinical presentation, evaluation, management, and endoscopic treatment of hamstring proximal avulsion injuries and chronic partial tearing with ischial bursitis.

Anatomy

With the exception of the short head of the biceps femoris, the hamstring complex originates from the ischial tuberosity and inserts distally below the knee on the proximal tibia. The tibial branch of the sciatic nerve innervates the semitendinosus, semimembranosus, and the long head of biceps femoris, while the short head of the biceps femoris is innervated by the peroneal branch of the sciatic nerve [3].

The proximal hamstring complex has a strong bony attachment on the ischial tuberosity (Fig. 25.1). Their footprint on the ischium is comprised of the semitendinosus and the long head of biceps femoris beginning as a common proximal tendon and footprint, while there is a distinct semimembranosus footprint [14]. The semimembranosus footprint is lateral (and anterior) to the crescent-shaped footprint of the common insertion of the semitendinosus and long head of the biceps femoris (Fig. 25.1).

The sciatic nerve is the most important neurovascular structure of the posterior thigh. It typically lies immediately lateral to the proximal hamstring tendon complex at an average of 1.2 cm from the ischial tuberosity (Fig. 25.2) [15]. Certainly, this structure needs to be carefully identified during any surgical repair. Additionally, sciatic nerve neurolysis is sometimes indicated during surgical treatment of chronic proximal avulsions. The posterior femoral cutaneous nerve, which supplies sensation to the posterior thigh, is located in the subcutaneous tissue. It begins above the ischial tuberosity and travels lateral to the ischium and into the subcutaneous tissues at the level of the buttock crease (Fig. 25.3). Deep

C.A. Guanche, M.D.
Southern California Orthopedic Institute,
6815 Noble Avenue, Van Nuys, Los Angeles, CA 91405, USA
e-mail: cguanche@scoi.com

J.W.T. Byrd (ed.), *Operative Hip Arthroscopy*,
DOI 10.1007/978-1-4419-7925-4_25, © Springer Science+Business Media New York 2013

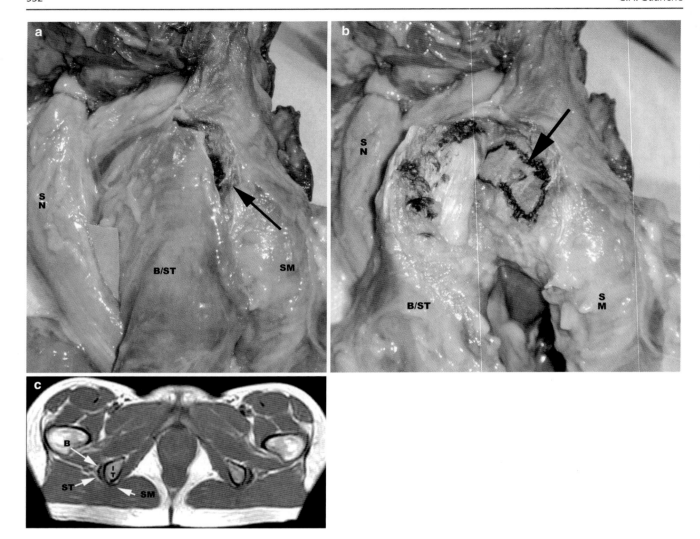

Fig. 25.1 Anatomical dissection of the left hamstring origin, viewed from posteriorly. (**a**) The hamstring origin begins at the lateral aspect of the ischium with a common biceps and semitendinosus (*B/ST*) origin as well as a separate semimembranosus (*SM*) footprint. The sciatic nerve (*SN*) is lateral to the ischium. In this image, the two origins have been split along the *arrow*. (**b**) In this figure, the B/ST portion has been everted to show its origin and footprint on the ischium (*arrow*) (*SN* sciatic nerve). (**c**) Axial T2 image of hamstring origin at the level of the ischium. The image is pointing to the right hip (*B* biceps femoris, *SM* semimembranosus, *ST* semitendinosus, *IT* ischial tuberosity)

to the gluteus maximus muscle is the inferior gluteal nerve and artery; it is found at the proximal one-third of the structure and is approximately 5 cm, on average, above the distal tip of the ischial tuberosity [14]. Immediately medial is the pelvic floor and the rectum. Superiorly, and slightly medial is the insertion of the sacrotuberous ligament.

Mechanism of Injury

The typical mechanism of an acute injury is a forced hip flexion with the knee in extension, as is classically observed in waterskiing [2, 16–18]. However, the injury can result from a wide variety of sporting activities that require rapid acceleration and deceleration [2, 8].

Proximal hamstring avulsion injuries can be classified as acute or chronic depending on the time from injury. Injuries can be categorized as complete tendinous avulsions, partial tendinous avulsions, apophyseal avulsions, and degenerative (tendinosis) avulsions [8]. Degenerative tears of the hamstring origin are more insidious in onset and are commonly seen as an overuse injury in middle- and long-distance runners. The mechanism of injury in these patients is presumably repetitive irritation of the medial aspect of the hamstring tendon (typically along the lateral aspect of the tuberosity, where the bursa resides) ultimately causing an attritional tear of the tendon.

Symptoms of ischial bursitis include buttock pain or hip pain, and localized tenderness overlying the ischial tuberosity. Additional symptoms of chronic ischial bursitis may

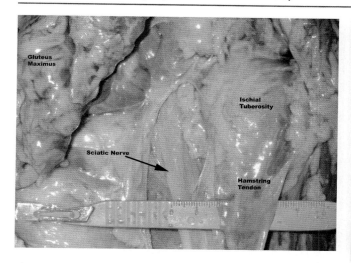

Fig. 25.2 The relationship between the sciatic nerve and the ischial tuberosity. The nerve lies at an average of 1.2 cm lateral to the tuberosity. The posterior femoral cutaneous nerve is typically lateral and posterior to the main nerve and inserts into the subcutaneous tissue below the level of the tuberosity. View is of a left hip, posterior aspect (*SN* sciatic nerve, *H* common hamstring tendon)

include tingling into the buttock that spreads down the leg. This is presumably from local inflammation and swelling in the area of the sciatic nerve. The symptoms usually worsen while sitting. Clinically, those most affected tend to sit with the painful buttock elevated off their seat.

Clinical Examination and Imaging

Physical examination is typically performed with the patient in the prone position. Examination with the knee slightly flexed will limit muscle spasms and make examination more comfortable in acute ruptures. Inspection and palpation of the posterior thigh may reveal muscle spasm. Ecchymoses may only be observed if the fascial covering is also disrupted. Palpation of the entire posterior thigh is very important to localize the injury. In the acute injuries, there is typically focal tenderness and swelling. However, with delayed presentation, there is more likely to be diffuse swelling and tenderness. Low-grade strains typically have limited swelling and tenderness, while in the more severe strains, a palpable defect may be appreciated.

Although, the diagnosis of a common strain is usually made by history and physical examination, plain radiographs are indicated to assure there is not a bony component to the injury. This is especially true in the skeletally immature where an ischial apophyseal avulsion is more likely (Fig. 25.4). Typical radiographic views would be an anteroposterior view of the pelvis, as well as anteroposterior and lateral views of the femur. An MRI examination is indicated to assess the degree of damage and the location of the injury [6, 11, 19, 20]. A hamstring strain is diagnosed via increased

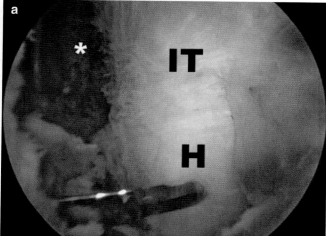

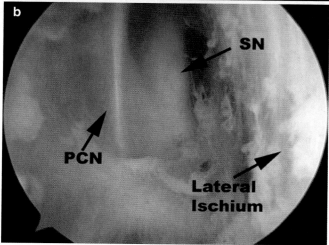

Fig. 25.3 Endoscopic view of the sciatic nerve and posterior femoral cutaneous branch (PCN) in a left hip (*IT* ischial tuberosity, *H* hamstring tendon). (**a**) View at the site of the hamstring origin with the distal tuberosity/hamstring origin exposed and the sciatic nerve (*) in the background. (**b**) View further anterior with the more lateral aspect of the tuberosity visualized and the sciatic nerve (*SN*) as well as the posterior femoral cutaneous nerve (*PCN*) visualized

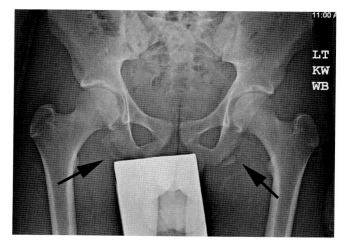

Fig. 25.4 AP radiograph of bilateral ischial tuberosity avulsion injuries (*arrows*) in a 14-year-old track athlete

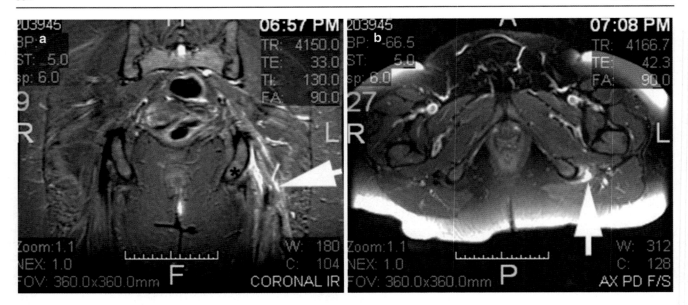

Fig. 25.5 Complete hamstring avulsion after a slip and fall in a 55-year-old patient. (**a**) Coronal T2-weighted image depicting a complete avulsion of the common hamstring origin (*arrow*) (* ischial tuberosity).

(**b**) Axial T2-weighted image depicting the degree of retraction of the common biceps and semitendinosus origin (*arrow*)

signal intensity on T2-weighted sequences, which represents edema and hemorrhage. Frank tears in the musculotendinous unit can also be seen. With full thickness tears, the diagnosis is obvious with retraction of the tendon from its attachment at the ischium. Sagittal and coronal T2-weighted sequences best delineate the injury and can estimate the retraction of the hamstring tendon (Fig. 25.5). In situations where there is chronic ischial bursitis and only partial tearing, a more careful analysis of the imaging studies must be undertaken. Typically, the MRI often reveals tendon degeneration, associated thickening, and surrounding soft tissue edema as well as ischial bursitis (Fig. 25.6). Ultrasound examination may be alternative imaging modality for patients unable to undergo MRI, especially if there is access to an experienced technologist familiar with musculoskeletal techniques [3, 4, 19, 21].

Treatment

There is increasing literature demonstrating good to excellent outcomes with open surgical management of acute complete avulsions [8, 16, 22, 23]. Blasier and Morawa were one of the first to report surgical management of a complete tendinous avulsion in a water skier [16]. Orava and Kujala reported good outcomes in their series, which included four repairs, done within 2 months of injury [17]. Klingele and Sallay reported good to excellent outcomes in their series of 11 complete proximal tendinous avulsions (7 acute, 4 chronic) [8]. Ten of the 11 were satisfied with the outcome, and 7 of the 9 athletically active patients were able to return to sport at average of

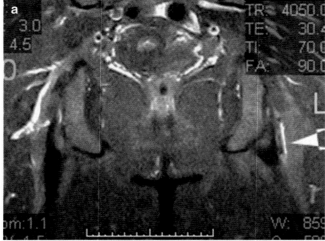

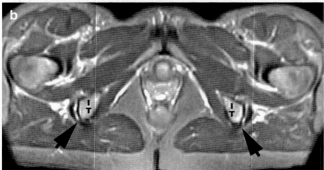

Fig. 25.6 MRI imaging of partial tearing of the hamstring origin in a 50-year-old marathon runner. (**a**) Coronal T2-weighted image depicting the fluid within the bursa left ischial bursa (*arrowhead*) as well as the partial tearing of the hamstring origin. (**b**) Axial T2-weighted image with a view of both ischial tuberosities and the fluid in the ischial bursae (*arrows*) (*IT* ischial tuberosity)

6 months. Isokinetic testing revealed an average of 91% return of hamstring function. Folsom and Larson reported on 20 acute primary repairs in their series [22]. At final follow-up, 75% were able to return to sport and 95% said they would have surgery again.

There is limited data, however, concerning the treatment of partial avulsions [12, 13]. Cohen et al. recommend consideration of nonoperative treatment for acute partial avulsions (one tendon ruptures) [12]. Lempainen et al. reported on a series of 48 partial avulsion repairs, all of which failed initial nonoperative treatment [13]. The conjoint tendon of the biceps femoris and semitendinosus was involved in all cases. They reported good and excellent results in 88% of the cases, and 41 were able to return to their previous level of sports at an average of 5 months. They suggested that excellent outcomes are possible, even in delayed repair of partial avulsions. They further noted that the surgical procedure was technically less demanding in the acute phase as there was less need for sciatic nerve neurolysis. They recommended that surgical repair be considered even in partial avulsions.

To date, there has been no report of endoscopic management of these injuries. After developing experience in the open management of these injuries, the author has subsequently developed an endoscopic technique that allows a safe approach to the area of damage in most of these tears. It is expected that the benefits of a more direct approach, without elevating the gluteus maximus and with the use of endoscopic magnification to protect the sciatic nerve, will improve the management of these injuries and reduce the morbidities associated with the open approach.

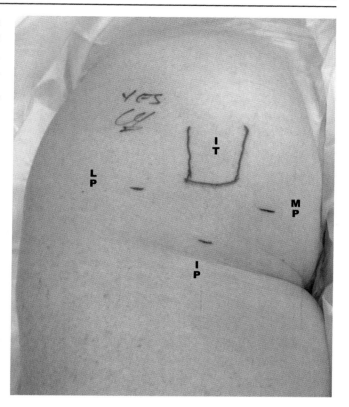

Fig. 25.7 Prone positioning of the patient with the leg and thigh draped free. The left ischium and the appropriate portal position have been marked (*IT* ischial tuberosity, *LP* lateral portal, *MP* medial portal, *IP* inferior portal)

Endoscopic Technique

(See Video 25.1: http://goo.gl/xAPst) Following the induction of anesthesia, the patient is placed in the prone position, with all prominences and neurovascular structures protected. The posterior aspect of the hip is then sterilized assuring that the leg and thigh are also so that the leg and hip can be repositioned intraoperatively (Fig. 25.7).

Two portals are then created, 2 cm medial and 2 cm lateral to the palpable ischial tuberosity (Fig. 25.8). The lateral portal is established first. This is done using blunt dissection with a switching stick, as the gluteus maximus muscle is penetrated and the submuscular plane is created. The switching stick serves to palpate the prominence of the tuberosity and identify the medial and lateral borders of the ischium. The medial portal is then established, taking care to palpate the medial aspect of the ischium. A 30° arthroscope is then inserted in the lateral portal, and an electrocautery device is placed in the medial portal. Any remaining fibrous attachments between the ischium and the gluteus muscle are then released, taking care to stay along the central and medial

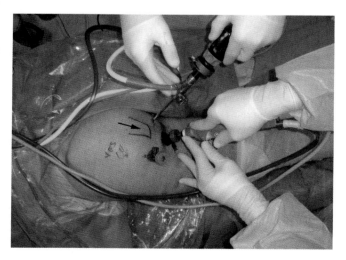

Fig. 25.8 Portals for endoscopic hamstring repair. The arthroscope is in the medial portal, while a shaver is inserted in the inferior portal. The lateral portal has a cannula in place (*arrow* ischial tuberosity)

portions of the ischium to avoid injury to the sciatic nerve. The tip of the ischium and the medial aspect are delineated; the lateral aspect is then exposed with the use of a switching stick as a soft tissue dissector. With the lateral aspect identified, the dissection continues anteriorly and laterally

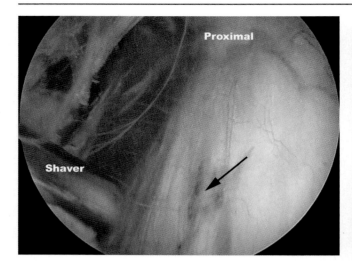

Fig. 25.9 A partial hamstring origin detachment in a marathon runner. A split in the tendon origin is noted (*arrow*). The view is of a left hip

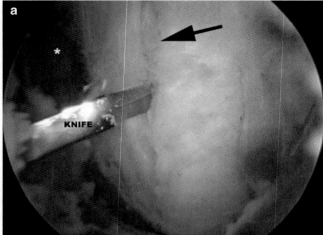

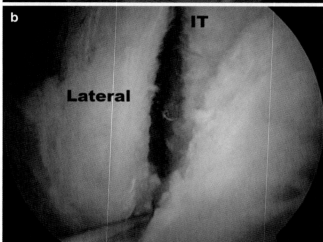

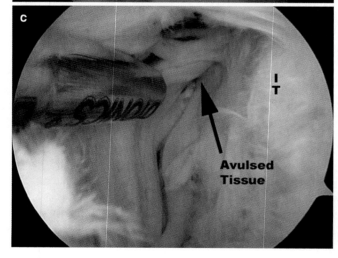

toward the known area of the sciatic nerve (Fig. 25.3). Very careful and methodical release of any soft tissue bands is then undertaken in a proximal to distal direction in order to mobilize the nerve and protect it throughout the exposure and ultimate repair of the hamstring tendon.

With the nerve identified and protected, attention is then directed once again to the area of the tendinous avulsion. The tip of the ischium is identified through palpation with the instruments. The tendinous origin is then inspected to identify any obvious tearing (Fig. 25.9). In acute tears, the area is obvious and the tendon is often retracted distally. In these cases, there is occasionally a large hematoma that needs to be evacuated. It is especially important to protect the sciatic nerve during this portion of the procedure, as it is sometimes obscured by the hematoma.

Once the area of pathology is identified (in incomplete tears), an endoscopic knife can be employed to longitudinally split the tendon along its fibers (Fig. 25.10). Often, this can be identified through palpation, as there is typically softening over the area of the detachment, making the tissue ballottable against the ischium. The hamstring is then undermined and the partial tearing debrided with an oscillating shaver, as well the lateral wall of the ischium is cleared of devitalized tissue. The lateral ischium is debrided of devitalized tissue, and a bleeding corticocancellous bed is prepared in preparation for the tendon repair (Fig. 25.11).

An inferior portal is then created approximately 4 cm distal to the tip of the ischium and equidistant from the medial and lateral portals (Fig. 25.8). This portal is employed for insertion of suture anchors, as well as suture management. A variety of suture passing devices can then be used for the repair. The principles are essentially the same as those

Fig. 25.10 Completion of a partial tear with the use of an endoscopic knife. The views are of a left hip. (**a**) An endoscopic knife is being employed for longitudinally splitting the hamstring tendon (*arrow*) at its origin, visualized from the medial portal, with the knife in the lateral portal. The sciatic nerve (*) can be seen in the background (*IT* ischial tuberosity). (**b**) The completed split with the lateral ischium, now clearly visualized (*IT* ischial tuberosity). (**c**) Elevating the lateral tissue clearly shows the chronically avulsed tissue of the hamstring origin (*IT* ischial tuberosity)

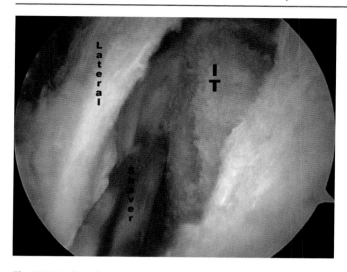

Fig. 25.11 Completed preparation of the lateral wall of the ischium in anticipation of hamstring repair in a left hip (*IT* ischial tuberosity)

employed in arthroscopic rotator cuff repair. Once all of the sutures are passed through the tissue of the avulsed hamstring, the sutures are tied and a solid repair of the tendon is completed. In general, one suture anchor is used per centimeter of detachment (Fig. 25.12).

Postoperatively, the patient is fitted with a hinged knee brace that is fixed at 90° of flexion for 4 weeks in order to not only limit weight bearing but also to restrict excursion of the hamstring tendons and protect the repair. At 4 weeks, the knee is gradually extended by about 30° per week in order to allow full weight bearing by 6–8 weeks, while maintaining the use of crutches. Physical therapy is instituted at this point, with the initial phase focused on hip and knee range of motion. Hamstring strengthening is begun at 10–12 weeks, predicated on full range of motion and a painless gait pattern. Full, unrestricted activity is allowed at approximately 4 months.

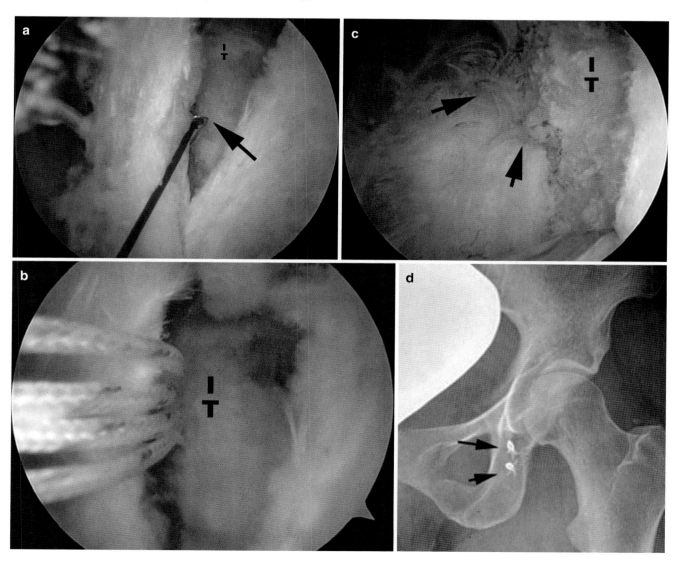

Fig. 25.12 Hamstring tendon repair with ischial bursectomy in a patient with chronic pain and inability to run as a result of chronic ischial pain. Views are of left hip (*IT* ischial tuberosity). (**a**) Suture passer in position (*arrow*). (**b**) Two mattress sutures in place. (**c**) Final hamstring repair with sutures approximated (*arrows*). (**d**) AP pelvic radiograph showing the position of the suture anchors (*arrows*)

Summary

The evolution of hip arthroscopy has helped generate much interest in the diagnosis and treatment of hip and pelvic injuries. As a result of the focus on intra-articular hip pathology, many additional anatomic and clinical studies have been undertaken that have advanced the treatment of previously ignored or undertreated areas. The current technique described in this chapter is one such offshoot of the improvement in the treatment of athletic hip and pelvic injuries. Expansion of endoscopic methods such as this provides a much less invasive approach for a problem that can be challenging for the physician and disabling for the patient. As a novel technique, the results and potential complications remain to be elucidated.

References

1. Brown TD. Thigh. In: DeLee JC DD, Miller MD, editors. Orthopaedic sports medicine. Principles and practice, vol. 2. Philadelphia: Saunders; 2003. p. 1481–523.
2. Clanton TO, Coupe KJ. Hamstring strains in athletes: diagnosis and treatment. J Am Acad Orthop Surg. 1998;6:237–48.
3. Garrett Jr WE. Muscle strain injuries. Am J Sports Med. 1996;24(6 Suppl):S2–8.
4. Garrett Jr WE, Rich FR, Nikolaou PK, Vogler 3rd JB. Computed tomography of hamstring muscle strains. Med Sci Sports Exerc. 1989;21:506–14.
5. Burkett LN. Causative factors in hamstring strains. Med Sci Sports. 1970;2:39–42.
6. Brandser EA, el-Khoury GY, Kathol MH, et al. Hamstring injuries: radiographic, conventional tomographic, CT, and MR imaging characteristics. Radiology. 1995;197:257–62.
7. Heiser TM, Weber J, Sullivan G, et al. Prophylaxis and management of hamstring muscle injuries in intercollegiate football players. Am J Sports Med. 1984;12:368–70.
8. Klingele KE, Sallay PI. Surgical repair of complete proximal hamstring tendon rupture. Am J Sports Med. 2002;30:742–7.
9. Cross MJ, Vandersluis R, Wood D, Banff M. Surgical repair of chronic complete hamstring tendon rupture in the adult patient. Am J Sports Med. 1998;26:785–8.
10. Kujala UM, Orava S, Jarvinen M. Hamstring injuries. Current trends in treatment and prevention. Sports Med. 1997;23:397–404.
11. Pomeranz SJ, Heidt Jr RS. MR imaging in the prognostication of hamstring injury. Work in progress. Radiology. 1993;189:897–900.
12. Cohen S, Bradley J. Acute proximal hamstring rupture. J Am Acad Orthop Surg. 2007;15:350–5.
13. Lempainen L, Sarimo J, Heikkila J, et al. Surgical treatment of partial tears of the proximal origin of the hamstring muscles. Br J Sports Med. 2006;40:688–91.
14. Miller SL, Gill J, Webb GR. The proximal origin of the hamstrings and surrounding anatomy encountered during repair. A cadaveric study. J Bone Joint Surg Am. 2007;89:44–8.
15. Miller A, Stedman GH, Beisaw NE, Gross PT. Sciatica caused by an avulsion fracture of the ischial tuberosity. A case report. J Bone Joint Surg Am. 1987;69:143–5.
16. Blasier RB, Morawa LG. Complete rupture of the hamstring origin from a water skiing injury. Am J Sports Med. 1990;18:435–7.
17. Orava S, Kujala UM. Rupture of the ischial origin of the hamstring muscles. Am J Sports Med. 1995;23:702–5.
18. Sallay PI, Friedman RL, Coogan PG, Garrett WE. Hamstring muscle injuries among water skiers. Functional outcome and prevention. Am J Sports Med. 1996;24:130–6.
19. Koulouris G, Connell D. Evaluation of the hamstring muscle complex following acute injury. Skeletal Radiol. 2003;32:582–9.
20. Slavotinek JP, Verrall GM, Fon GT. Hamstring injury in athletes: using MR imaging measurements to compare extent of muscle injury with amount of time lost from competition. AJR Am J Roentgenol. 2002;179:1621–8.
21. Garrett Jr WE, Califf JC, Bassett 3rd FH. Histochemical correlates of hamstring injuries. Am J Sports Med. 1984;12:98–103.
22. Folsom GJ, Larson CM. Surgical treatment of acute versus chronic complete proximal hamstring ruptures: results of a new allograft technique for chronic reconstructions. Am J Sports Med. 2008;36:104–9.
23. Ishikawa K, Kai K, Mizuta H. Avulsion of the hamstring muscles from the ischial tuberosity. A report of two cases. Clin Orthop Relat Res. 1988;232:153–5.

Hip Instability

Carlos A. Guanche

26

Introduction

Although the hip depends primarily on its osseous anatomy for stability, its unique soft tissue envelope also plays a role in its stability, particularly when there are variants from normal [1]. It is therefore critical to assess both the osseous and soft tissue components of the hip in cases of suspected instability. In addition, a history of any trauma, no matter how remote, and an assessment of chronic/congenital abnormalities must be entertained when assessing a patient.

The first and most critical assessment is in making the decision of whether the problem is traumatic or not. The spectrum of symptoms can range from frank dislocation to a subluxation. Atraumatic hip instability can result from repetitive rotational stresses, and the mechanism of injury in these patients is a subclinical capsular laxity that has a mild hip dysplasia [2]. Generalized laxity may also cause atraumatic instability.

The treatment algorithm of hip instability is based on the underlying cause, and as such, diagnosing the etiology of hip instability begins with a proper history and physical examination, followed by plain radiographs. Further imaging and specialized radiographs may then be indicated. Treatment may consist of conservative care, and in refractory cases, surgical repair may be necessary. In those with severe dysplasia or with progression to arthritis, periacetabular osteotomy or total joint arthroplasty may be considered.

Anatomy

Although this chapter will not be a thorough discussion of the anatomy, certain salient points need to be delineated. Once fused, the acetabular surface is oriented approximately 45° caudally and 15–20° anteriorly. Significant alterations in acetabular version or inclination, as well as its orientation relative to the femoral head/neck, can affect the joint capsule and ligaments. In addition, the suction effect that relies on joint congruency for its function may be compromised [1]. These factors may become etiologic in the development of hip instability.

Hip stability is complemented by the acetabular labrum and capsuloligamentous complex. In the neutral anatomic position, the anterior part of the femoral head is not engaged in the acetabulum. The acetabular labrum compensates for this by covering this portion of the femoral head. The labrum is attached to the transverse acetabular ligament anteriorly and posteriorly at the base of the fovea and proceeds to run around the circumference of the acetabular rim [1]. The labrum adds 22% to the depth of the socket and aids in developing the suction effect that provides additional hip stability [3]. Absence of the labrum can lead to a loss of this suction effect, as well as increased cartilage consolidation and increasing contact pressures of the femoral head on the acetabulum [4–7]. Proprioceptors and nociceptors have been identified within the labrum and capsule that may explain the decreased proprioception and increased pain with a torn labrum [8]. In addition, a complex neuromuscular loop exists that maintains the appropriate position between the femoral head and acetabulum with balanced muscular regulation that is assessed by proprioceptive feedback provided both from the position of the body and receptors in the capsule and labrum. Any divergence from this mechanism as a result of injury may lead to instability [9]. Much like the meniscus in the knee, the labrum is largely avascular except for the most peripheral portion near the capsule, diminishing its ability to heal [4].

The labrum is not, however, a stand-alone structure. It functions in conjunction with the capsuloligamentous complex. Anteriorly, this complex primarily consists of the iliofemoral ligament (ligament of Bigelow) [1]. This ligament, which is 12–14 mm thick and shaped like an inverted Y, provides resistance to hip extension beyond neutral and resists external rotation [1]. The pubofemoral ligament (from the pubic portion of

C.A. Guanche, M.D.
Southern California Orthopedic Institute,
6815 Noble Avenue, Van Nuys, Los Angeles,
CA 91405, USA
e-mail: cguanche@scoi.com

J.W.T. Byrd (ed.), *Operative Hip Arthroscopy*,
DOI 10.1007/978-1-4419-7925-4_26, © Springer Science+Business Media New York 2013

339

the acetabular rim to blend with the most inferior fibers of the iliofemoral ligament) reinforces the inferior and anterior capsule, resisting extension and abduction [1]. A third structure, the ischiofemoral ligament, reinforces the posterior surface of the capsule and has a spiraling pattern [1]. Finally, the zona orbicularis is a deep layer of fibers within the capsule that forms a circular pattern around the femoral neck, constricting the capsule and restricting distraction [1].

The position of maximum hip joint stability is in full extension because this is where the twisted orientation of the capsular ligaments causes a screw home effect [1]. However, the articular surfaces of the hip joint are not in optimal contact in this position (the "close-packed" position). Optimal contact occurs in the loose-packed position of flexion and external rotation as the ligaments uncoil [1]. The greatest risk of traumatic dislocation, then, is when the joint is in neither the close-packed or the maximally congruent position. This occurs in the flexed and adducted position [1].

The ligamentum teres and psoas tendon are two other structures about the hip that deserve additional discussion [1]. The ligamentum has no real stabilizing effect on the hip joint while the psoas protects the anterior intermediate capsule, which is devoid of ligamentous protection [1].

Clinical Evaluation

Hip instability can manifest as overtly as frank traumatic dislocation or can be as obscure as occult groin pain or clicking. The picture can be further complicated by referred pain from the lumbosacral region as well as the genitourinary tract and abdominal wall [10]. Age also plays a significant role in determining a differential diagnosis for hip pain [11]. In children, hip dislocation, bony avulsions, apophyseal injuries, fractures, SCFE, Perthes, DDH, and toxic and septic arthritis are all potential causes [11, 12]. In the adult, the spectrum of potential injuries is at least as great as in the child [10, 11].

The history should include a qualitative assessment of the main complaint to determine if it is primarily pain, clicking, catching, or instability. Precipitating factors, as well as potential referred or systemic causes, must be assessed. Specific examination maneuvers should be considered in cases of possible instability [13]. Antalgic gait patterns where there is shortening of the stance phase and of step length on the affected side can result from instability. A Trendelenburg gait may indicate an attempt to bring the center of gravity over the affected side to decrease the moment arm across that hip joint [12]. The patient with atraumatic instability may be able to demonstrate subluxation or dislocation of the involved hip, although this is rare. A positive axial distraction test can be confirmed with a positive vacuum sign on dynamic fluoroscopy [1] (Fig. 26.1). Anterior apprehension may also be elicited with the patient in the lateral decubitus position, while suspending the affected leg in slight abduction (Fig. 26.2).

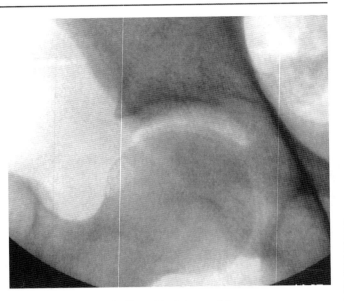

Fig. 26.1 Suction seal effect of the joint – axial x-ray

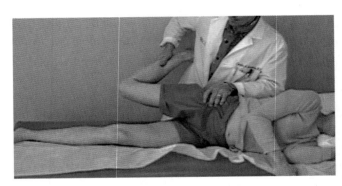

Fig. 26.2 Anterior apprehension examination. The patient is placed in the lateral decubitus position. The affected extremity is then extended and internally and externally rotated in an attempt to reproduce the sensation of instability or giving way of the hip

Finally, hip instability can manifest with pain on prone extension/external rotation of the involved hip, and this is specific for residual anterior instability.

Imaging should always begin with plain radiographs. The standard views are an AP pelvis, as well as an AP and lateral of the affected hip [14]. Apart from being able to detect the common radiographic features of trauma, plain radiographs can also help detect evidence of femoroacetabular impingement.

Several radiographic indices have been described to differentiate normal from abnormal osseous anatomy based on the AP pelvis radiograph. The Tonnis angle is used to assess lateral subluxation of the femoral head and subsequent increased forces across the weight-bearing acetabulum (Fig. 26.3). A measurement of <10° is considered normal [15, 16].

Another measurement is the center-edge angle of Wiberg, which assesses acetabular inclination (Fig. 26.4). This angle

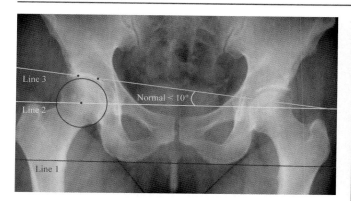

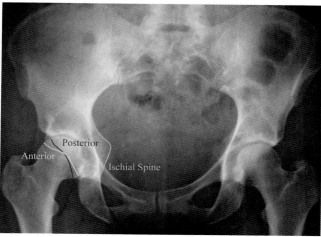

Fig. 26.3 An AP radiograph showing the technique of measuring the Tönnis angle. The Tönnis angle is normally < 10°. The *red line* (line 1) connecting the ischial tuberosities is the reference line. The *yellow line* (line 2) is drawn parallel to line 1 through the center of the femoral head. The angle that is formed between line 2 and line 3 connecting two points demarcating the "sourcil" or weight-bearing surface of the acetabulum is the Tönnis angle

Fig. 26.5 An AP radiograph demonstrating the crossover sign indicating acetabular retroversion. The *yellow line* (representing the anterior wall of the acetabulum) crosses the *red line* (representing the posterior wall of the acetabulum). Also of note is the visualization of the ischial spine (*blue line*), which is normally superimposed by the acetabulum, but easily visible with retroversion

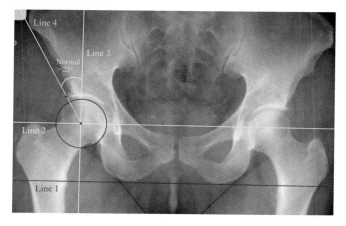

Fig. 26.4 An AP radiograph showing the center-edge angle of Wiberg. The *red line* (line 1) represents the initial reference line through the tuberosities that provides the parallel line for line 2 through the femoral head. Line 3 is a line directly perpendicular to line 2, and the angle between this line and line 4 (a line from the center of the femoral head to the lateral edge of the acetabulum). This angle should be greater than 25°, with 20–25° being considered borderline

When evaluating a patient with potential dysplasia, the faux profile view is often used to evaluate anterior and lateral coverage of the femoral head by the acetabulum. While plain radiographs are sufficient for making the diagnosis in most cases, there are pathologic entities that require further investigation. Among the choices for more advanced imaging are bone scan; ultrasound; computed tomography (CT), including CT arthrography and 3D reconstructions; magnetic resonance imaging (MRI); and MRI arthrography [10, 14, 20].

Imaging of bony lesions about the hip is best accomplished using computed tomography as it provides the greatest spatial resolution of bony structures. Cases of questionable hip dysplasia should employ CT in preoperative planning. The use of intra-articular contrast in CT arthrography can increase the contrast between cartilage and labral tissue [10, 14, 21].

Magnetic resonance imaging has become the most reliable means of diagnosing unresolved hip pathology outside of direct visualization and is often useful in cases of instability. MRI has been shown to effectively demonstrate inflammatory arthropathies and joint effusions [14, 22] but has been less accurate in assessing articular cartilage lesions [23–26]. Contrast MRI studies in patients with a torn labrum or torn iliofemoral ligament can result in a larger volume of intra-articular contrast and thus indirectly confirm the diagnosis of instability (Fig. 26.6) [1].

Atraumatic Instability

As is the case in the shoulder, where numerous types of instability have been described, the separation between traumatic and atraumatic instability in the hip is often difficult.

should measure at least 20–25° to be considered normal inclination [17, 18].

One can estimate acetabular version using the AP pelvis by looking for a "crossover sign" (Fig. 26.5). The two lines involved estimate the posterior and anterior rims of the acetabulum. The posterior rim is traced from the ischial tuberosity superolaterally to the roof of the acetabulum. The anterior rim is traced from the teardrop in a superior and lateral direction along the rim to the roof. If these lines cross, it is estimated that the acetabulum is retroverted [15, 17, 19]; if not, it is assumed that the acetabular version is within the normal 10–15° of anterior version.

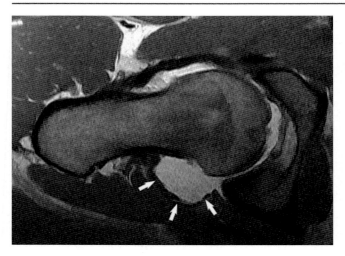

Fig. 26.6 Capsular redundancy after trauma. Axial, T2-weighted, MRI arthrogram of a patient with a posterior subluxation. Note the excess posterior capsular volume (*arrows*)

For the purpose of this chapter, we will consider only those instability syndromes that are the direct result of a distinct, traumatic event that caused a discrete subluxation or frank dislocation as truly traumatic instability. All other congenital dysplasias and connective tissue disorders, as well as repetitive use injuries and idiopathic syndromes, will be considered atraumatic.

Congenital connective tissue disorders can predispose a patient to atraumatic hip instability. There have been very few reports in the literature of habitual hip dislocation that have not been accompanied by Ehlers-Danlos syndrome, arthrochalasis multiplex congenita, Marfan's syndrome, Down's syndrome, or congenital or acquired hip dysplasia [1]. As opposed to frank episodes of subluxation or dislocation that may be seen in atraumatic shoulder instability, idiopathic hip instability often presents more subtly.

In a review of five cases of presumed coxa saltans, or snapping hip syndrome, Bellabarba et al. described a syndrome of "idiopathic hip instability [2]." In this series, all patients presented with a long history of snapping in the groin, gait disturbances, and pain in the provocative position of hip flexion, adduction, and internal rotation that had escaped diagnosis. It seemed as if the patients should fit into one of the previously described categories of snapping hip: internal, external, and intra-articular [27–41]. These patients, by contrast, had physical examinations consistent with generalized ligamentous laxity and AP pelvis radiographs suggestive of mild dysplasia, as evidenced by a slightly lower center-edge angle [2]. They complained of symptoms of popping and snapping when rising from a chair or in other instances when the hip was subjected to flexion adduction and internal rotation. Both the exacerbating and alleviating maneuvers were analogous to the Barlow and Ortolani signs used in infants for diagnosing developmental hip dysplasia, which suggests a posterior direction to the instability. Furthermore, when the unanesthetized, non-sedated patient had the affected hip subjected to gentle

manual traction without counter traction, 4–10 mm of inferior subluxation was seen. The force used to "subluxate" the hip in this instance was much less than the 400 N of axial force described by Arvidsson as necessary to create the radiographic vacuum sign that suggests subluxation [42]. All of the above evidence led the authors to postulate that subclinical hip dysplasia, combined with capsuloligamentous laxity, caused a break in the suction mechanism of the hip during gait, causing a popping sensation [2]. Presuming that the instability was largely posteriorly directed and that preoperative arthrography showed posterior capsular redundancy, one patient of the five underwent open posterior capsular plication.

Atraumatic instability has also been attributed to a deficient labrum associated with redundant capsular/ligament tissue [1]. This deficient complex can create an abnormal load distribution due to a transiently incongruent joint from subtle subluxation. The previously mentioned screw home mechanism caused by the dynamic nature of the hip capsule and its associated ligaments may help explain why pelvic rotation and external rotation of the hip commonly elicit the symptoms of hip instability previously described. In a computational model developed to analyze the effect of bony deficiency on stress distributions (and indirectly the likelihood of instability), it was found that the less the bony coverage (depicted by lower center-edge angles), the higher the acetabular rim stresses noted [42].

Professional and high-level athletes that participate in sports that require repeated hip rotation (football, golf, gymnastics, soccer, ballet, and baseball) are susceptible to overuse injuries to the labrum and capsuloligamentous complex [1, 43, 44]. Tears of the labrum or iliofemoral ligament can result in insufficiency of the buffer mechanism and result in increased tension on the joint capsule that can be further exacerbated by slight superior and lateral inclination of the acetabulum [1]. Labral degeneration combined with subtle rotational hip instability secondary to redundant capsular tissue as a common injury pattern has been seen in elite athletes [1]. In ten patients treated with arthroscopic labral debridement and thermal capsulorrhaphy, all patients had improvement in their Harris hip scores as compared to preoperatively with 83% having significant improvement in their symptoms at 12–24 months' follow-up [1]. In contrast, Villar reported only 67.5% success in 58 cases at a mean 3.5-year follow-up with labral debridement without capsular treatment [45]. Alternatively, plication can also be performed by passing nonabsorbable, braided suture through the capsule, thus imbricating the capsular tissue [46] (Fig. 26.7) (Video 26.1: http://goo.gl/NI0Km).

Although the preliminary results of thermal capsulorrhaphy in the hip have been promising, more long-term follow-up is needed as is suggested by the shoulder literature. These studies show that thermal energy delivered to tissue via laser or radiofrequency resulted in shrinkage of the tissue by disrupting intramolecular cross-links in collagen [47, 48]. The amount of tissue shrinkage is directly related to the temperature applied, and the optimal temperature appears to be between 65°C and

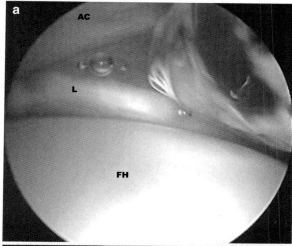

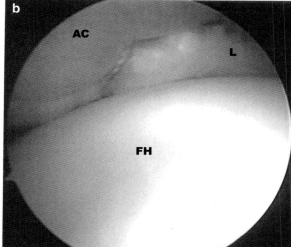

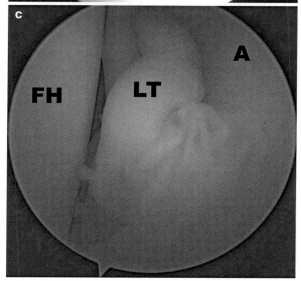

Fig. 26.7 Patient with anterior capsular laxity. *AC* anterior capsule, *L* labrum, *FH* femoral head. (**a**) Initial view with large sublabral recess. (Image is of a left hip viewed from the anterior portal.) (**b**) View from same vantage point, showing obliteration of recess. Note suture in labrum in the middle of the field of view. (Image is of a left hip viewed from the anterior portal.) (**c**) View of an attritional ligamentum teres tear in the same patient, with no history of a frank dislocation event. (Image is of a left hip viewed from the anterolateral portal)

75°C [49–52]. Thermal treatment causes immediate collagen and cell damage, resulting in decreased mechanical stiffness that lasts at least 2 weeks. After this, the tissue undergoes active repair and by 12 weeks has similar mechanical properties and cellular components to the native capsule [53, 54]. Several studies in the shoulder have shown good results when anterior instability is treated by thermal capsulorrhaphy combined with anterior Bankart repair [55–58]. These studies are hard to interpret, however, as they combine two procedures.

Miniaci and McBirnie used only thermal capsulorrhaphy in the treatment of MDI and had 47% recurrent instability [59]. In addition to recurrent instability, complications such as capsule destruction, nerve injuries, and cartilage damage that can lead to massive chondrolysis and premature osteoarthritis can occur [60–64]. Heat capsulorrhaphy in the hip, therefore, should be used with caution at this time.

While subtle hip dysplasia combined with capsular laxity and labral pathology can lead to symptomatic hip instability amenable to arthroscopic treatment, care must be taken to recognize more significant dysplasia. Overtly dysplastic hips typically share common abnormalities that occur to a greater or lesser extent depending on the severity [65]. The true acetabulum is usually shallow, lateralized, anteverted, and deficient anteriorly and superiorly. There may be underdevelopment of the entire pelvis. On the femoral side, the femoral head is usually small and the neck is usually excessively anteverted and short with an increased neck-shaft angle. The greater trochanter may be displaced posteriorly, and the femoral canal may be narrow [66]. The presence of significant hip dysplasia in the adult can be ascertained with plain radiography. AP pelvis and false profile lateral films of the affected hip allow for measurement of the anterior center-edge angle of Lequesne and de Seze [65], the lateral center-edge angle of Wiberg [66], the horizontal position of the hip joint center [67], acetabular roof obliquity [67, 68], and the integrity of Shenton's line.

A patient that presents with radiographic evidence of dysplasia but little or no symptoms should be treated nonsurgically with strengthening and proprioceptive training of the hip and trunk musculature [69]. NSAIDS can be used and combined with cessation of high impact activities. The potential natural history of increasing instability and the development of degenerative arthritis should be discussed. Reexamination and repeat radiographs should be documented at 1- to 2-year intervals [13, 69]. Surgical intervention should be reserved for those patients that fail conservative management and have persistent symptoms. Arthroscopic treatment for mildly dysplastic hips may be appropriate but is not indicated in the patient with significant dysplasia. Significant labral hypertrophy occurs in these patients. The role of this excess labral tissue has not been completely elucidated, but it may be significant in its effect on joint stability. Aggressive resection of this tissue can accelerate degenerative changes and possibly lead to early arthritis. Pelvic and femoral osteotomies, arthrodesis, resection arthroplasty, and replacements have all been described as potential options [69]. Osteotomies that may be expected to slow the progression of degenerative changes by better distributing weight-bearing forces across the hip joint have been described. These procedures may also provide better preservation of bone stock for potential subsequent arthroplasty [69].

Pelvic reconstructive osteotomies are indicated for patients in whom articular congruity is achievable and are intended to restore more normal hip anatomy and biomechanics with the goal of improving symptoms and preventing degenerative changes [69]. Patients for which a pelvic osteotomy may be indicated include young patients with symptomatic dysplasia without excessive proximal migration of the center of rotation, reasonably well-maintained range of motion, and no more than mild degenerative changes as classified by Tönnis [68, 69].

A commonly performed procedure is the Bernese periacetabular osteotomy (PAO), which is indicated in patients with symptoms of hip mechanical overload, impingement, or instability resulting from insufficient acetabular coverage [70]. Siebenrock et al. showed that at an average follow-up of 11.3 years, excellent correction can be maintained and the hip joint preserved in 82% of patients, while 73% reported good to excellent results [71]. Similar results have been obtained by several other authors [72–75]. Due to the complex nature of the operation, complications have been reported that include nerve injury (particularly to the lateral femoral cutaneous and peroneal branch of the sciatic nerve), inadvertent intra-articular extension of the osteotomy, heterotopic ossification, and excessive anteriorization [76–79].

Other reconstructive osteotomies have been described, including the Salter innominate [80]. Most of the procedures, however, have largely been replaced by the Bernese [81–89]. Salvage osteotomies, such as the Chiari and Shelf osteotomies, are indicated in severely dysplastic hips with issues beyond the scope of this chapter [69].

Femoral osteotomies are indicated in the rare instance where the femur is the primary location of deformity or when pelvic osteotomy does not provide adequate coverage [69]. Combined femoral and acetabular osteotomies have been reported in up to 27% of cases [69–75].

Traumatic Instability

The spectrum of hip instability ranges from subtle changes such as snapping and pain to acute subluxations and frank traumatic dislocations. The most common mechanism for hip dislocation is a dashboard motor vehicle injury with a posteriorly directed force against a flexed knee and hip. During athletics, dislocations may occur via a forward fall onto a flexed knee with the hip flexed or a blow from behind while down on all four limbs [90]. Sports such as American football, skiing, jogging, gymnastics, basketball, biking, and soccer have all

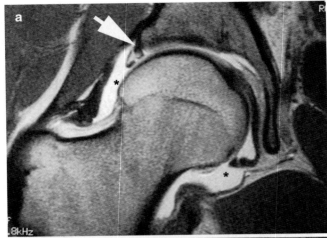

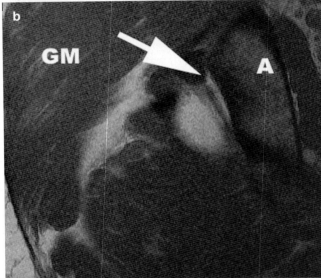

Fig. 26.8 Capsular disruption and labral tear after dislocation of the hip. (**a**) Coronal, T1-weighted image showing a labral tear (*arrow*) as well as generalized capsular distension (*asterisks*). (**b**) Coronal image, further posterior showing the posterior capsular disruption (*arrow*). *A* acetabulum, *GM* gluteus maximus

had reports of traumatic dislocations [91–94]. Excessive capsular laxity has been associated with these types of dislocations [30, 40, 95–100]. Irrespective of the degree of initial trauma, if normal capsular healing fails to occur, persistent laxity may occur and predispose the patient to instability (Fig. 26.8). Two cases of posterior dislocation following minor trauma while playing soccer have been reported. The patients developed recurrent posterior dislocation with trivial incidents secondary to large posterior capsular redundancy [101]. Similarly, recurrent anterior dislocations have occurred as a result of excessive anterior capsular redundancy [102]. These patients have been treated nonoperatively with brief immobilization, physical therapy, and activity modification. Open capsular shift/repair has been particularly successful in preventing further dislocation [103].

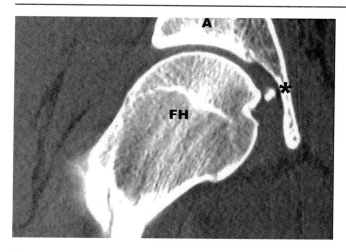

Fig. 26.9 CT scan image of a patient with a history of a transient dislocation event. Note the loose body (*asterisk*) in the fossa. *A* acetabulum, *FH* femoral head

Hip arthroscopy has been shown to be an important part of the armamentarium in the effort to at least delay the onset of posttraumatic degenerative joint disease (DJD) following traumatic dislocation [104–107]. Residual intra-articular bony or osteochondral fragments may be responsible for the development of DJD in complex dislocations [102, 108–111] (Fig. 26.9). The incidence of osteoarthritis secondary to traumatic hip dislocation has been reported between 24% and 57%, depending on the severity of the trauma [112–116]. Simple dislocations, or those without radiographic evidence of fracture, have been shown to have the lowest incidence of subsequent DJD. However, the incidence of posttraumatic DJD in these injuries is still 24% [116].

Nonconcentric reduction after a traumatic dislocation is considered an absolute indication for operative intervention. The presence of loose bodies, however, has been considered a relative indication, particularly if the reduction is concentric and the loose bodies are located below the fovea [117–119]. An in vivo rabbit model has shown that free cartilaginous loose particles inside the joint increase chondrolytic enzyme activity and induce secondary arthrosis [107, 117]. In the 1990s, hip arthroscopy was begun to be used to remove loose bodies seen on plain radiography or CT, largely due the concern that these fragments could eventually lead to posttraumatic arthritis [102, 108–110]. While performing these arthroscopies, previously unrecognized cartilaginous loose bodies were frequently found [105, 107]. Since 24% of "simple" dislocations have been shown to develop subsequent DJD, the literature would support that these loose bodies that had been previously undetected could actually contribute significantly to the development of posttraumatic DJD and that they should be addressed prophylactically with arthroscopic removal [105, 116].

Mullis and Dahners reported on a series of 36 patients treated with hip arthroscopy following dislocation [105].

Excluding procedures in which a repeat arthroscopy was performed for retained loose bodies, the average time to arthroscopy was 15 days. Twenty-five of 36 (69%) patients had radiographic evidence of loose bodies (nonconcentric reduction and/or radiographically visible loose bodies). In nine patients, there was a concentric reduction without radiographic evidence of loose bodies. Intraoperatively, 33 of 36 (92%) patients were found to have loose bodies. Seven of the nine (78%) patients with no preoperative radiographic evidence of loose bodies had loose bodies found at arthroscopy.

Yamamoto et al. documented a 15-year experience with hip arthroscopy after traumatic dislocation [104]. Ten joints in nine patients were treated 1–7 days post-dislocation. Seven hips were classified as Thompson-Epstein (TE) I injuries, two type II, one type IV, and one central fracture dislocation. All dislocations had arthroscopic lavage and debridement. One TE I fracture underwent arthroscopic osteosynthesis of the femoral head fracture, and one TE II had extraction of the fragment. The other TE II injury and two of the TE I injuries as well as the TE IV injury had subsequent ORIF of the fragment. At arthroscopy, seven of ten (70%) joints revealed loose osteochondral fragments that were not recognized preoperatively with radiographs or CT scan. At a minimum of 5 years' follow-up, eight of ten joints were asymptomatic. One joint (Pipkin type 3 femoral head fracture) went on to develop femoral head AVN that was not symptomatic. The one TE IV injury developed hip joint DJD at 1 year. These results prompted the authors to recommend arthroscopic debridement for all TE type I and type II dislocations, but not types III and IV.

Most recently, Philippon et al. have documented the findings in 14 professional athletes sustaining a dislocation of the hip [107]. In these athletes, all patients had chondral defects and six had chondral injuries on both surfaces. All of the patients had labral tears. Eleven patients had partial or complete tears of the ligamentum teres, and two patients had a capsular tear.

Interestingly, there were nine patients in this study with evidence of femoroacetabular impingement. It appears that perhaps these patients are more likely to experience traumatic dislocations with a relatively small amount of trauma as a result of their underlying bony morphology. Presumably, this anatomical variant would relatively increase the risk of subluxation or dislocation of the hip joint as a result of the levering effect of the head and neck junction on the acetabular rim.

There has been some concern regarding the timing of arthroscopy after traumatic dislocation in terms of the risk of AVN [46], prompting those concerned to recommend a 6 week waiting period post-dislocation before performing arthroscopy. In the two previously discussed, however, arthroscopic surgery was performed in the first 7 days by Yamamota and in the first 2 weeks by Dahners [104, 105]. The only complications observed in the Dahners study were three repeat procedures for retained loose bodies and some fluid extravasation into the gluteal compartment that resolved without incident [105]. Yamamoto et al. had one case of AVN that developed in a patient with a Pipkin type 3 injury [104].

Conclusion

The spectrum of hip instability is wide and includes symptoms that range from that which is similar to a simple snapping hip to a complete dislocation that results in persistent repeated dislocations. A thorough history and physical examination combined with the appropriate imaging studies are essential in determining where on this spectrum the patient's complaints fit. It is critical to recognize the patients that have obvious bony findings leading to the instability in order to appropriately manage them without simply resorting to arthroscopic repair of what is typically the most obvious problem, i.e., a labral tear.

The treatment of these disorders also covers a wide range. Conservative care that includes temporary immobilization, followed by activity modification, physical therapy, and the eventual return to activity, can be effective for those with mild capsular or musculotendinous injuries. More involved instability that includes labral injury, capsular laxity, and possibly mild acetabular dysplasia can be treated effectively with open capsular plication or, more recently, arthroscopic capsular plication, thermal capsulorrhaphy, and labral debridement (or repair). Hip dysplasia that involves bony abnormalities that cannot be addressed by arthroscopic or open capsular means can be treated using periacetabular osteotomy, while dysplasia that involves significant DJD is better treated with total hip arthroplasty. Finally, traumatic dislocations with retained loose bodies and/or femoral head fractures can be treated with open or arthroscopic loose body removal, as well as arthroscopic or open femoral head/acetabular fixation.

References

1. Philippon MJ. The role of arthroscopic thermal capsulorrhaphy in the hip. Clin Sports Med. 2001;20:817–29.
2. Bellabarba C, Sheinkop M, Kuo K. Idiopathic hip instability. Clin Orthop. 1998;355:261–71.
3. Takechi H, Nagashima H, Ito S. Intra-articular pressure of the hip joint outside and inside the limbus. J Jpn Orthop Assoc. 1982;56:529–36.
4. Kelly BT, Williams RJ, Philippon MJ. Hip arthroscopy: current indications, treatment options, and management issues. Am J Sports Med. 2003;316:1020–37.
5. Ferguson SJ, Bryant JT, Ganz R, et al. An in vitro investigation of the acetabular labral seal in hip joint mechanics. J Biomech. 2003;36:171–8.
6. Ferguson SJ, Bryant JT, Ganz R, et al. The acetabular labrum seal: a pro-elastic finite element model. Clin Biomech. 2000;15:463–8.
7. Ferguson SJ, Bryant JT, Ganz R, et al. The influence of the acetabular labrum on hip joint cartilage consolidation: a pro-elastic finite element model. J Biomech. 2000;33:953–60.
8. Kim YT, Azuma H. The nerve endings of the acetabular labrum. Clin Orthop. 1995;320:176–81.
9. Torry MR, Schenker ML, Martin HD, et al. Neuromuscular hip biomechanics and pathology in the athlete. Clin Sports Med. 2006;25:179–97, vii.
10. Kallas KM, Guanche CA. Physical examination and imaging of hip injuries. Oper Tech Sports Med. 2002;10:176–83.
11. Scopp JM, Moorman III CT. The assessment of athletic hip injury. Clin Sports Med. 2001;20:647–59.
12. Paletta Jr GA, Andrish JT. Injuries about the hip and pelvis in the young athlete. Clin Sports Med. 1995;14:591–628.
13. Hoppenfeld S. Physical examination of the hip and pelvis. In: Hoppenfeld S, editor. Physical exam of the spine and extremities. Norwalk: Appleton and Lange; 1976. p. 143.
14. Erb RE. Current concepts in imaging the adult hip. Clin Sports Med. 2001;20:661–96.
15. Tonnis D, Heinecke A. Acetabular and femoral anteversion: relationship with osteoarthritis of the hip. J Bone Joint Surg Am. 1999;81(12):1747–70.
16. Tonnis D, Legal H, Graf R, editors. Congenital dysplasia and dislocation of the hip in children and adults. Berlin: Springer; 1987.
17. Delaunay S, Dussault RG, Kaplan PA, et al. Radiographic measurements of dysplastic adult hips. Skeletal Radiol. 1997;26(2):75–81.
18. Wenger DR, Bomar JD. Human hip dysplasia: evolution of current treatment concepts. J Orthop Sci. 2003;8(2):264–71.
19. Reynolds D, Lucas J, Klaue K. Retroversion of the acetabulum. A cause of hip pain. J Bone Joint Surg Br. 1999;81(2):281–8.
20. DePaulis F, Cacchio A, Michelini O, et al. Sports injuries in the pelvis and hip: diagnostic imaging. Eur J Radiol. 1998;27 Suppl 1:S49–59.
21. Kneeland JB. MR imaging of sports injuries of the hip. Magn Reson Imaging Clin N Am. 1999;7:105–15.
22. Beltran J, Caudill JL, Herman LA, et al. Rheumatoid arthritis: MR imaging manifestations. Radiology. 1987;165:153–7.
23. Edwards DJ, Lomas D, Villar RN. Diagnosis of the painful hip by magnetic resonance imaging and arthroscopy. J Bone Joint Surg Br. 1995;77B:374–6.
24. Hodler J, Trudell D, Pathria MN, et al. Width of the articular cartilage of the hip: quantification by using fat suppression spin echo MRI in cadavers. AJR Am J Roentgenol. 1992;192:351–5.
25. Potter HG, Montgomery KD, Heise CW, et al. MRI of acetabular fractures: value in detecting femoral head injury, intraarticular fragments, and sciatic nerve injury. AJR Am J Roentgenol. 1994;163:881–6.
26. Czerny C, Kramer J, Neuhold A, et al. MRI and magnetic resonance arthrography of the acetabular labrum: comparison with surgical findings [in German]. Roto Fortschr Ged Rontgenstr Neuen Bildgeb Verfahr. 2001;173:702–7.
27. Allen WC, Cope R. Coxa saltans: the snapping hip revisited. J Am Acad Orthop Surg. 1995;3:303–8.
28. Tietz CC, Garrett WE, Miniaci A, et al. Tendon problems in athletic individuals. J Bone Joint Surg. 1997;79A:138–52.
29. Jacobsen T, Allen WC. Surgical correction of the snapping iliopsoas tendon. Am J Sports Med. 1990;18:470–4.
30. Lieberman J, Altchek D, Salvati E. Recurrent dislocation of a hip with a labral lesion. Treatment with a modified bankart repair. J Bone Joint Surg. 1993;75A:1524–7.
31. Nunziata A, Blumenfeld I. Cadera a resort: a proposito de una variedad. Prensa Med Argent. 1951;38:1997–2001.
32. Schaberg JE, Harper MC, Allen WC. The snapping hip syndrome. Am J Sports Med. 1984;12:361–5.
33. Staple TW, Jung D, Mork A. Snapping tendon syndrome: hip tenography with fluoroscopic monitoring. Radiology. 1988;166:873–4.

34. Binnie JF. The snapping hip. Ann Surg. 1913;58:59–66.

35. Mayer L. Snapping hip. Surg Gynecol Obstet. 1919;29:425–8.

36. Zoltan DJ, Clancy Jr WG, Keene JS. A new operative approach to snapping hip and refractory trochanteric bursitis in athletes. Am J Sports Med. 1986;14:201–4.

37. Altenberg AR. Acetabular labrum tears: a cause of hip pain and degenerative arthritis. South Med J. 1977;70:174–5.

38. Dorrell JH, Catterall A. The torn acetabular labrum. J Bone Joint Surg. 1986;68B:400–3.

39. Ikeda T, Awaya G, Suzuki S. Torn acetabular labrum in young patients: arthroscopic diagnosis and management. J Bone Joint Surg. 1988;70B:13–6.

40. Sullivan CR, Bickel WH, Lipscomb PR. Recurrent dislocation of the hip. J Bone Joint Surg. 1955;37A:1256–70.

41. Suzuki S, Awaya G, Okada Y. Arthroscopic diagnosis of ruptured acetabular labrum. Acta Orthop Scand. 1986;57:513–5.

42. Chegini S, Beck M, Ferguson SJ. The effects of impingement and dysplasia on stress distributions in the hip joint during sitting and walking: a finite element analysis. J Orthop Res. 2009;27:195–201.

43. Arvidsson I. The hip joint: forces needed for distraction and appearance of the vacuum phenomenon. Scand J Rehabil Med. 1990;22:157–61.

44. Bombelli R, editor. Structure and function in normal and abnormal hips. 3rd ed. New York: Springer; 1993.

45. Santori N, Villar R. Acetabular labral tears: result of arthroscopic partial limbectomy. Arthroscopy. 2000;16(1):11–5.

46. Shindle MK, Ranawat AS, Kelly BT. Diagnosis and management of traumatic and atraumatic hip instability in the athletic patient. Clin Sports Med. 2006;25:309–26.

47. Flory PJ, Garrett RR. Phase transition in collagen and gelatin systems. J Am Chem Soc. 1958;80:4836–45.

48. Flory PJ, Weaver ES. Helix coil transition in dilute aqueous collagen solutions. J Am Chem Soc. 1959;82:4518–25.

49. Hayashi K, Hecht P, Thabit III G, et al. The biologic response to laser thermal modification in an in vivo sheep model. Clin Orthop Relat Res. 2000;373:265–76.

50. Hecht P, Hayashi K, Cooley AJ, et al. The thermal effect of monopolar radiofrequency energy on the properties of joint capsule: an in vivo histologic study using a sheep model. Am J Sports Med. 1998;26:808–14.

51. Liao WL, Hedman TP, Vangsness Jr CT. Thermal profile of radiofrequency energy in the inferior glenohumeral ligament. Arthroscopy. 2004;20:603–8.

52. Medvecky MJ, Ong BC, Rokito AS, Sherman OH. Thermal capsular shrinkage: basic science and clinical applications [review]. Arthroscopy. 2001;17:624–35.

53. Hecht P, Hayashi K, Lu Y, et al. Monopolar radiofrequency energy effects on joint capsular tissue: potential treatment for joint instability. An in vivo mechanical and biomechanical, morphological and biochemical study using an ovine model. Am J Sports Med. 1999;27:761–71.

54. Miniaci A, Codsi MJ. Thermal capsulorrhaphy for the treatment of shoulder instability. Am J Sports Med. 2006;34(8):1356–63.

55. Gartsman GM, Roddey TS, Hammerman SM. Arthroscopic treatment of bidirectional glenohumeral instability: 2–5 year follow-up. J Shoulder Elbow Surg. 2001;10:28–36.

56. Mishra DK, Fanton GS. Two-year outcome of arthroscopic bankart repair and electrothermal-assisted capsulorrhaphy for recurrent anterior shoulder instability. Arthroscopy. 2001;17:844–9.

57. Noonan TJ, Tokish JM, Briggs KK, Hawkins RJ. Laser assisted thermal capsulorrhaphy [review]. Arthroscopy. 2003;19:815–9.

58. D'Alessandro DF, Bradley JP, Fleischli JE, Connor PM. Prospective evaluation of thermal capsulorraphy for shoulder instability: indications and results, 2–5 year follow-up. Am J Sports Med. 2004;32:21–33.

59. Miniaci A, McBirnie J. Thermal capsular shrinkage for treatment of multidirectional instability of the shoulder. J Bone Joint Surg Am. 2003;85:2283–7.

60. Levine WN, Clark Jr AM, D'Alessandro DF, Yamaguchi K. Chondrolysis following arthroscopic thermal capsulorrhaphy to treat shoulder instability: a report of 2 cases. J Bone Joint Surg Am. 2005;87:616–21.

61. Petty DH, Jazraxi LM, Estrada LS, Andrews JR. Glenohumeral chondrolysis after shoulder arthroscopy: case reports and review of the literature. Am J Sports Med. 2004;32:509–15.

62. Rath E, Richmond JC. Capsular disruption as a complication of thermal alteration of the glenohumeral capsule. Arthroscopy. 2001;17:E10.

63. Wong KL, Williams GR. Complications of thermal capsulorrhaphy of the shoulder. J Bone Joint Surg Am. 2001;83(Suppl 2 Pt 2): 151–5.

64. Good C, Shindle MK, Kelly BT, Wanich T, Warren RF. Glenohumeral chondrolysis after shoulder arthroscopy with thermal capsulorrhaphy. Arthroscopy. 2007;23(7):797.e1–e5.

65. Lequesne M, de Seze. False profile of the pelvis. A new radiographic incidence for the study of the hip. Its use in dysplasias and different coxopathies. Rev Rhum Mal Osteoartic. 1961;28:643–52. French.

66. Wiberg G. Studies on dysplastic acetabular and congenital subluxation of the hip joint. With special reference to the complication of osteoarthritis. Parts HV. Acta Chir Scand Suppl. 1939;58:7–38.

67. Matsui M, Masuhara K, Nakata K, Nishii T, Sugano N, Ochi T. Early deterioration after modified rotational acetabular osteotomy for the dysplastic hip. J Bone Joint Surg Br. 1997;79:220–4.

68. Massie WK, Howorth MB. Congenital dislocation of the hip. Part 1. Methods of grading results. J Bone Joint Surg Am. 1950;32: 519–31.

69. Sanchez-Sotelo J, Trousdale RT, Berry DJ, Cabanela ME. Surgical treatment of developmental dysplasia of the hip in adults: 1. Non-arthroplasty options. J Am Acad Orthop Surg. 2002;10:321–33.

70. Ganz R, Klaue K, Vinh TH, Mast JW. A new periacetabular osteotomy for the treatment of hip dysplasias: technique and preliminary results. Clin Orthop. 1988;232:26–36.

71. Siebenrock KA, Scholl E, Lottenbach M, Ganz R. Bernese periacetabular osteotomy. Clin Orthop. 1999;363:9–20.

72. Crockarell Jr J, Trousdale RT, Cabanela ME, Berry DJ. Early experience and results with the periacetabular osteotomy: the mayo clinic experience. Clin Orthop. 1999;363:64–72.

73. Trousdale RT, Ekkernkamp A, Ganz R, Wallrichs SL. Periacetabular and intertrochanteric osteotomy for the treatment of osteoarthrosis in dysplastic hips. J Bone Joint Surg Am. 1995;77:73–85.

74. Matta JM, Stover MD, Siebenrock K. Periacetabular osteotomy through the Smith-Petersen approach. Clin Orthop. 1999;363: 21–32.

75. Trumble SJ, Mayo KA, Mast JW. The periacetabular osteotomy: minimum 2 year follow-up in more than 100 hips. Clin Orthop. 1999;363:54–63.

76. Hussel JG, Mast JW, Mayo KA, Howie DW, Ganz R. A comparison of different surgical approaches for the peri-acetabular osteotomy. Clin Orthop. 1999;363:64–72.

77. Hussel JG, Rodriguez JA, Ganz R. Technical complications of the Bernese periacetabular osteotomy. Clin Orthop. 1999;363:81–92.

78. Ping ME, Trousdale RT, Cabanela ME, Harper CM. Intraoperative electromyographic monitoring during periacetabular osteotomy. Clin Orthop. 2002;400:158–64.

79. Myers SR, Eijer H, Ganz R. Anterior femoroacetabular impingement after periacetabular osteotomy. Clin Orthop. 1999;363: 93–9.

80. Wong-Chung J, Ryan M, O'Brien TM. Movement of the femoral head after Salter osteotomy for acetabular dysplasia. J Bone Joint Surg Br. 1990;72:563–7.

81. Sutherland DH, Greenfield R. Double innominate osteotomy. J Bone Joint Surg Am. 1977;59:1082–91.

82. Le Coeur P. Corrections des defauts d'orientation de l'articulation coxofemorale par oteotomie de l'os iliaque. Rev de Chir Orthop. 1965;51:211–2.

83. Hopf A. Hip acetabular displacement by double pelvic osteotomy in the treatment of hip joint dysplasia and subluxation in young people and adults [German]. Z Orthop Ihre Grenzgeb. 1966;101:559–86.

84. Steel HH. Triple osteotomy of the innominate bone. J Bone Joint Surg Am. 1973;55:343–50.

85. Carlioz H, Khouri N, Hulin P. Osteotomie pelvienne triple juxtacotyloidienne. Rev de Chir Orthop. 1982;68:497–501.

86. Tonnis D, Behrens K, Tsharani F. A modified technique of triple pelvic osteotomy. J Pediatr Orthop. 1981;1:241–9.

87. Eppright RH. Abstract: dial osteotomy of the acetabulum in the treatment of dysplasia of the hip. J Bone Joint Surg Am. 1975;57:1172.

88. Wagner H, editor. Experiences with spherical acetabular osteotomy for the correction of the dysplastic acetabulum. Acetabular dysplasia: skeletal dysplasias in childhood. Berlin: Springer; 1978. p. 131–45.

89. Sanchez-Sotelo J, Berry DJ, Trousdale RT, Cabanela ME. Surgical treatment of developmental dysplasia of the hip in adults: II. Arthroplasty options. J Am Acad Orthop Surg. 2002;10:334–44.

90. Chudik S, Lopez V. Hip dislocations in athletes. Sports Med Arthrosc. 2002;10:123–33.

91. Giza E, Mithofer K, Matthews H, et al. Hip fracture-dislocation in football: a report of two cases and review of the literature. Br J Sports Med. 2004;38:E17.

92. Lamke LO. Traumatic dislocations of the hip. Follow-up on cases from the Stockholm area. Acta Orthop Scand. 1970;41:188–98.

93. Mitchell JC, Giannoudis PV, Millner PA, et al. A rare fracture-dislocation of the hip in a gymnast and review of the literature. Br J Sports Med. 1999;33:283–4.

94. Stiris MG. Magnetic resonance arthrography of the hip joint in patients with suspected rupture of the labrum acetabulare. Tidsskr Nor Laegeforen. 2001;121:698–700.

95. Dameron Jr T. Bucket-handle tear of the acetabular labrum accompanying posterior dislocation of the hip. J Bone Joint Surg Am. 1959;41:131–4.

96. Nelson C. Traumatic recurrent dislocation of the hip. Report of a case. J Bone Joint Surg Am. 1970;52:128–30.

97. Rasleigh-Belcher H, Cannon S. Recurrent dislocation of the hip with a bankart-type lesion. J Bone Joint Surg Br. 1966;68:398–9.

98. Simmons R, Elder J. Recurrent post-traumatic dislocations of the hip in children. South Med J. 1972;65:1463–6.

99. Slavic M, Dungl P, Spindrick J, et al. Recurrent traumatic dislocation of the hip in a child. Significance of early arthrography. Arch Orthop Trauma Surg. 1986;104:385–8.

100. Hunter GA. Posterior dislocation and fracture-dislocation of the hip: a review of fifty-seven patients. J Bone Joint Surg Br. 1969;51:38–44.

101. Liebenberg F, Dommisse G. Recurrent posttraumatic dislocation of the hip. J Bone Joint Surg Br. 1969;51:632–7.

102. Dall D, MacNab I, Gross A. Recurrent anterior dislocation of the hip. J Bone Joint Surg Am. 1970;52:574–6.

103. Heinzelmann P, Nelson C. Recurrent traumatic dislocation of the hip. Report of a case. J Bone Joint Surg Am. 1976;58:895–6.

104. Yamamoto Y, Takatoshi I, Ono T, Hamada Y. Usefulness of arthroscopic surgery in hip trauma cases. Arthroscopy. 2003;19:269–73.

105. Mullis BH, Dahners LE. Hip Arthroscopy to remove loose bodies after traumatic dislocation. J Orthop Trauma. 2006;20:22–6.

106. Svoboda S, Williams DM, Murphy KP. Hip arthroscopy for osteochondral loose body removal after a posterior hip dislocation. Arthroscopy. 2003;19:777–81.

107. Philippon MJ, Kuppersmith DA, Wolf AB, et al. Arthroscopic findings following traumatic hip dislocation in 14 professional athletes. Arthroscopy. 2009;25:169–74.

108. DeLee JC. Fractures and dislocations of the hip. In: Rockwood CA, Green DP, editors. Fractures in adults. 2nd ed. Philadelphia: J. B. Lippincott; 1984. p. 1211–356.

109. Letournel E. Acetabular fractures. Clin Orthop. 1980;151:81–106.

110. Matta JM, Anderson LM, Epstein HC. Fracture of the acetabulum. Clin Orthop. 1986;205:230–50.

111. Rowe CR, Lowell JD. Prognosis of fractures of the acetabulum. J Bone Joint Surg Am. 1961;43:30–59.

112. Thompson VP, Epstein HC. Traumatic dislocation of the hip. J Bone Joint Surg Am. 1951;33:746–78.

113. Armstrong JR. Traumatic dislocation of the hip: review of 101 dislocations. J Bone Joint Surg Br. 1948;30:430–45.

114. Stewart MJ, McCarroll HR, Mulhollan JS. Fracture dislocation of the hip. Acta Orthop Scand. 1975;46:507–25.

115. Brav CEA. Traumatic dislocation of the hip. J Bone Joint Surg Am. 1962;44:1115–34.

116. Upadhyay SS, Moulton A, Srikrishnamurthy K. An Analysis of the late effects of traumatic posterior dislocation of the hip without fracture. J Bone Joint Surg Br. 1983;65:150–2.

117. Epstein HC. Posterior fracture-dislocations of the hip: long term follow-up. J Bone Joint Surg Am. 1974;56:1103–27.

118. Epstein HC. Traumatic dislocations of the hip. Clin Orthop. 1973;92:116–42.

119. Evans CH, Mazzocchi RA, Nelson DD, et al. Experimental arthritis induced by intra-articular injection of allogenic cartilaginous particles into rabbit knees. Arthritis Rheum. 1984;27:200–7.

Adhesive Capsulitis and Arthrofibrosis

J.W. Thomas Byrd

Introduction

In 2006, we published the first and, to date, only case series reporting on arthroscopic management of adhesive capsulitis of the hip [1]. Any hope for a correct diagnosis and something more than serendipitous treatment begins with an awareness of the disorders. As has been stated, "The eyes cannot see what the mind does not know." Or as was more eloquently stated by Dr. Jack Hughston: "You may not have seen it, but it's seen you." Adhesive capsulitis of the hip is not common, but it is also not exceedingly rare. Any clinician involved in the treatment of hip disorders will be faced with patients presenting with adhesive capsulitis as either a primary or contributing diagnosis.

Our known experience in the treatment of adhesive capsulitis began in 2000. A 41-year-old female with recalcitrant hip pain and MRA evidence of a labral tear was undergoing arthroscopic surgery (Figs. 27.1 and 27.2). Examining her hip under anesthesia revealed limited range of motion. A modestly vigorous effort to see if the hip was really that stiff resulted in a series of audible cracks and immediately greater rotational motion. X-ray revealed no evidence of a femoral neck fracture, so we proceeded with arthroscopy which revealed a miniscule labral tear, but extensive hemorrhagic fibrinous debris which was removed mostly for the purposes of visualization (Fig. 27.3). Postoperatively, the patient had immediate resolution of symptoms that has endured to this day.

Retrospectively, we probably unknowingly encountered this a couple of years prior. A middle-aged female with long-standing fairly incapacitating hip pain underwent arthroscopy. With her small frame and normal radiographs, we anticipated an easy procedure. However, the hip was stiff and the procedure difficult. No major structural damage was encountered and very little was done. Postoperatively, the patient remained

incapacitated by her unexplained pain. We suspect that had we been aware of the diagnosis, performed a manipulation, and followed this with a properly directed structured rehab program, then this case might also have been a home run instead of a source of extreme disappointment.

Presentation

Adhesive capsulitis of the hip shares the same clinical demographics as adhesive capsulitis in the shoulder [2]. There is a particular predilection for middle-aged females, especially in the fourth and fifth decades. However, men and younger or older women are not immune. There does appear to be an association with diabetes mellitus, especially Type II, and in these patients, the treatment can be even more challenging, both for conservative and surgical measures.

When patients present, the nature of the onset of their symptoms is variable and of no specific diagnostic value. In some patients, the problem may have been precipitated by an injury, or they may recount some sort of acute episode, or it may simply have become more noticeable over time.

Patients may describe specific symptoms with turning, twisting maneuvers, catching when rising from a seated position, or discomfort with prolonged sitting. However, often they may describe simply pain that is constant or independent of any particular activities.

Physical Exam

Like adhesive capsulitis in the shoulder, the principal examination finding is just that the hip hurts with range of motion in virtually any direction. The level of discomfort may cause the patient to guard, and the examiner may question whether the patient is overreacting or demonstrating symptom magnification.

The most important single differentiating physical examination feature of adhesive capsulitis is that the greatest pain and restriction is in external rotation. Flexion with internal

J.W.T. Byrd, M.D.
Nashville Sports Medicine Foundation,
2011 Church Street, Suite 100, Nashville, TN 37203, USA
e-mail: byrd@nsmfoundation.org

J.W.T. Byrd (ed.), *Operative Hip Arthroscopy*,
DOI 10.1007/978-1-4419-7925-4_27, © Springer Science+Business Media New York 2013

Fig. 27.1 A 41-year-old female with recalcitrant left hip pain and unremarkable AP (**a**) and lateral (**b**) radiographic images. (All rights are retained by Dr. Byrd)

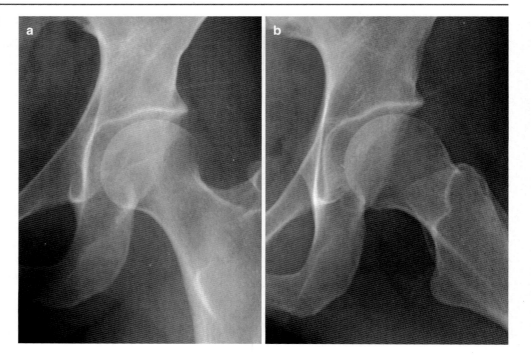

Fig. 27.2 Sagittal MRI (**a**) and MRA (**b**) images both reveal evidence of an anterior labral tear (*arrows*). (All rights are retained by Dr. Byrd)

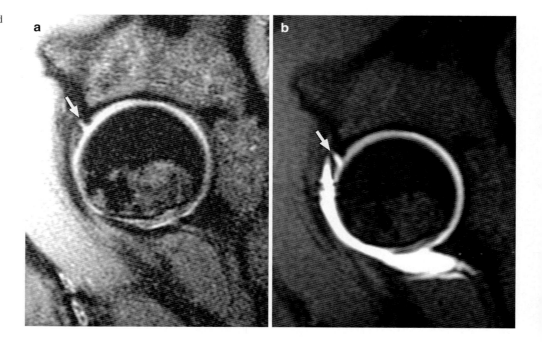

rotation may be uncomfortable as is commonly seen with most irritable hips, but it is external rotation that is more painful and restricted in comparison to the contralateral side. The patient will also describe that this is especially notice-able when trying to sit cross-legged.

Posterior impingement is relatively uncommon but can also result in selectively worse pain with hip external rota-tion [3]. However, this is usually easily distinguished from adhesive capsulitis because of the more global nature of the pain pattern with a frozen hip.

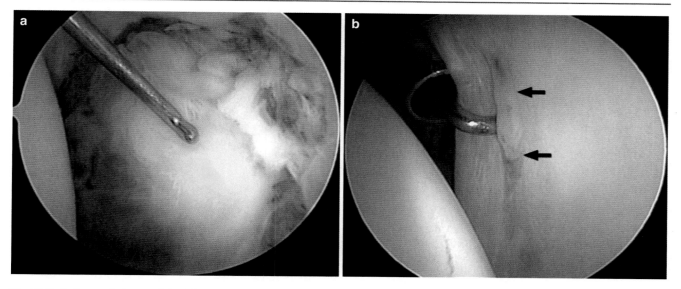

Fig. 27.3 Arthroscopic image of the left hip from the anterolateral portal. (**a**) Viewing medially reveals hemorrhagic fibrinous debris contained within the acetabular fossa. (**b**) Viewing anterior, the small anterior labral tear is identified (*arrows*). (All rights are retained by Dr. Byrd)

Recording rotational motion, the examiner will find significant limitation of the involved compared to the uninvolved side. There may be some loss of internal rotation, but the greatest restriction is in external rotation.

Imaging

Our experience has been that there is nothing specific about any imaging method that is enlightening about the diagnosis of adhesive capsulitis. Imaging studies are important to rule out other causes of a stiff painful hip. Also, while one-third of patients may present with primary adhesive capsulitis, in two-thirds of the cases, there is some underlying intra-articular pathology that may secondarily trigger the adhesive capsulitis. Thus, a proper investigation is important to look for potential concomitant underling pathology.

Routine radiographs are obtained as they would be in the initial evaluation of any hip disorder. There are no radiographic features to tip the diagnosis of adhesive capsulitis. However, there is ample evidence that various radiographic abnormalities such as FAI may exist among asymptomatic individuals; so the clinician must be careful in assessing the clinical relevance of study findings [4]. Radiographs are still helpful to rule out advanced degenerative disease, severe impingement, or other disorders that could provide an explanation for a stiff hip.

Conventional magnetic resonance imaging (MRI) is unrevealing as far as findings of adhesive capsulitis. It is logical that adhesive capsulitis results in substantially reduced fluid volume of the joint. Early reports suggested that arthrography could help in the diagnosis; however, our experience with gadolinium arthrography with MRI (MRA) has not revealed any telltale signs of adhesive capsulitis [1, 5, 6]. In fact, when imaging reports describe difficulty accessing the joint for an intra-articular injection, it is hard to surmise whether this was due to a tight hip or simply whether the person performing the injection was having a difficult time. These studies are still important to rule out other disorders such as sepsis, transient regional osteoporosis, avascular necrosis, or other conditions that could potentially mimic adhesive capsulitis.

Radionuclide scans are infrequently obtained in the evaluation of hip disorders and are usually not necessary in the assessment of adhesive capsulitis. However, it is worthwhile to remember that a bone scan may help to assess the osseous homeostasis around the joint and serve as a useful screening tool to look at surrounding areas. In complex cases, it may have some value.

Conservative Treatment

If a preliminary working diagnosis of adhesive capsulitis has been reached, a trial of conservative treatment is appropriate. The first step is pain control. This includes an effort to identify and modulate provoking activities and usually a trial of non-narcotic medication. Supervised physical therapy is usually recommended, but it must be with a knowledgeable therapist who can understand the idiosyncrasies of adhesive capsulitis. Sometimes, this may begin just with modalities to diminish discomfort. Ultimately, the solution to adhesive

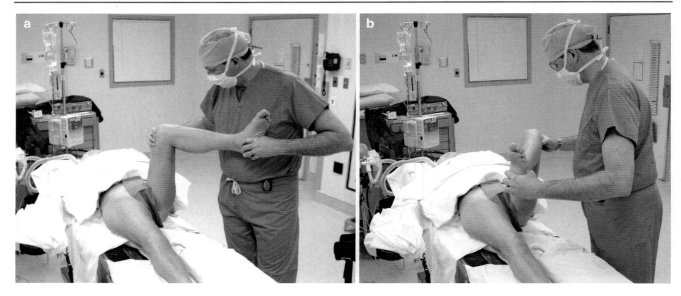

Fig. 27.4 Examination under anesthesia assess for rotational motion with the hip in a 90° flexed position, checking both internal (**a**) and external (**b**) rotations. (All rights are retained by Dr. Byrd)

capsulitis focuses on regaining range of motion. Just like in the shoulder, patients must be warned that the efforts to regain motion may result in a transient phase of increased soreness, and only once full mobility has been accomplished, then will the results of diminished pain start to be truly perceived. Like in the shoulder, this can be a challenge and again necessitates a therapist knowledgeable and skilled in the treatment which includes a heavy emphasis on manual therapy.

One concern that will often be raised by the patient is whether efforts to improve range of motion can cause more damage in the joint. This is highly unlikely, and the consequence of not trying conservative treatment is of potentially greater consequence. If patients can respond to conservative treatment and avoid surgery, that is always a plus. Also, anything that can be gained preoperatively will also place the patient in a better position for the postoperative recovery. Therapy can also serve as a useful gauge for the clinician to interpret the patient's motivation and willingness to participate in their own recovery.

For recalcitrant cases, a trial of an intra-articular injection of cortisone is appropriate. Concomitant injection of long-acting anesthetic is traditionally used for its diagnostic value to substantiate that the hip is the principal source of symptoms. However, like in the shoulder, the response to an injection in the hip for a patient with adhesive capsulitis is variable. Some patients do not experience a noticeable response to the anesthetic and the therapeutic response to the cortisone can be disappointing. This is explained by the fact that this is more of an intrinsic capsular disease rather than an intra-articular problem.

Arthroscopic Treatment

(See Video 27.1: http://goo.gl/PdUU2) There are many circumstances under which arthroscopy may be appropriate. For patients with clinical evidence of intra-articular pathology, this may be the reason for surgery. However, the component of adhesive capsulitis must be recognized and incorporated as part of the strategy in the surgical management as well as the postoperative rehabilitation.

In the presence of recalcitrant adhesive capsulitis, it must be kept in mind that the majority of patients will have some underlying intra-articular damage. Arthroscopy is rarely necessary as part of the specific treatment for adhesive capsulitis. Arthroscopy is more to precisely assess and address any underlying intra-articular damage. In addition to labral tears, FAI, and other common intra-articular problems, several reports have reflected on adhesive capsulitis associated with synovial chondromatosis [5, 6]. This has been our observation as well, and sometimes the diagnosis of synovial chondromatosis may not be obvious on the preoperative studies.

Any arthroscopic procedure begins with an examination under anesthesia (Fig. 27.4). At this time, the true nature of the restricted rotational motion will be evident and documented. In fact, there is one paradox regarding examination

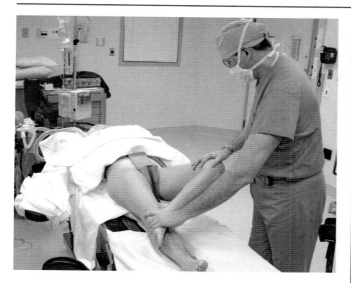

Fig. 27.5 With the affected hip in a figure-of-four position, downward manual pressure is applied to the medial side of the ipsilateral knee. With gentle constant pressure, crepitus can be felt and heard, characteristic of the disrupting adhesions. The knee will lower closer to the table, equal to the unaffected side. Once the characteristic capsular pattern of constriction has been released, it is then easier to further stretch the hip in internal and external rotation, achieving full passive range of motion (Reprinted from Byrd [1]. With permission from Elsevier). (All rights are retained by Dr. Byrd)

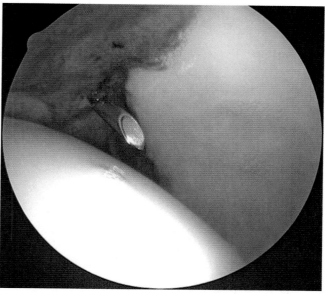

Fig. 27.6 Viewing from the anterolateral portal in this left hip, the fluid has been evacuated and a spinal needle positioned for the anterior portal. (All rights are retained by Dr. Byrd)

under anesthesia of the hip compared to other joints. For most joints, when the patient is relaxed, the documented range of motion may be greater than recorded during an earlier examination. However, in the hip, patients become adept at compensating for restricted hip motion with increased pelvic motion. This is a subconscious adaptation and can be difficult to account for during a normal exam. Thus, when the patient is asleep, they may be found to actually have less rotational motion than might have been documented on a previous awake examination. This is not unique to adhesive capsulitis but is simply a generalization of observations on hip range of motion. As previously mentioned with adhesive capsulitis, the greatest restriction is in external rotation.

Manipulation under anesthesia is essential to being able to effectively and safely perform the arthroscopic procedure (Fig. 27.5). The manipulation is carried out by placing the leg in a figure-of-four position with the ankle across the front of the contralateral knee. One hand then stabilizes the contralateral iliac crest while gentle pressure is applied to the medial aspect of the ipsilateral distal thigh. Typically, with gently-applied pressure, the adhesions can be felt to break loose. Steady constant application is performed without forceful maneuvers. Once this has been performed, usually essentially full rotational motion in both directions will be achieved.

Arthroscopy is then carried out in a standard fashion. However, following the manipulation, a significant hemarthrosis will be encountered when the arthroscope is initially introduced. This must be cleared before the subsequent portals can be safely placed with arthroscopic visualization. Attempting to flush fluid through the scope cannula will not clear the blood. Fluid egress is achieved by placing a 17-gauge spinal needle anteriorly. This requires triangulation skills to place the needle in front of the arthroscope and comes with experience. Precise needle positioning is not critical; it is simply a matter of having the needle in the joint, establishing fluid egress, which will usually clear the field of view.

An alternative method is to evacuate all fluid from the joint after the arthroscope has been placed. With a dry field, positioning of the anterior portal can be performed with reasonably good visualization (Fig. 27.6).

Once all portals have been placed, systematic inspection is performed, and the characteristic hemorrhagic fibrinous debris is removed from the central space and capsulolabral reflection (Fig. 27.7). Within the fossa, the pulvinar will typically have been transformed to dense hemorrhagic fibrous material that is also debrided. The principal purpose of clearing the joint is to thoroughly assess for intra-articular damage that may have precipitated the adhesive capsulitis. This accompanying damage is then addressed as indicated. Interestingly, the peripheral compartment is often spared of many signs of synovitis other than amorphous fibrotic changes of the undersurface of the capsule (Fig. 27.8).

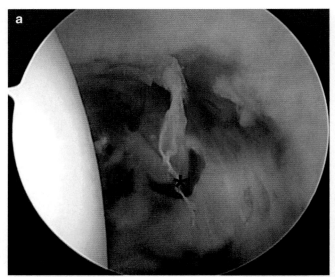

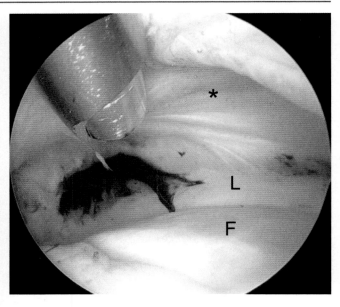

Fig. 27.8 Viewing the peripheral compartment of this left hip, the capsular side of the labrum (*L*) and femoral head (*F*) are evident. A little clot is present but the peripheral space has been relatively spared of hemorrhagic changes other than mild amorphous fibrosis of the undersurface of the capsule (*asterisk*). (All rights are retained by Dr. Byrd)

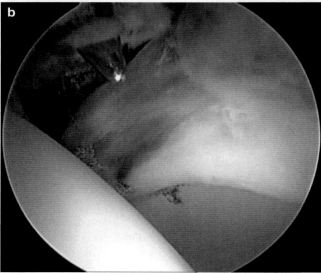

Fig. 27.7 Viewing from the anterolateral portal of this left hip, (**a**) characteristic hemorrhagic fibrinous material is identified in the central space (*asterisk*). (**b**) Hemorrhagic changes are identified at the capsulolabral reflection which is being probed by the obturator. (All rights are retained by Dr. Byrd)

Postoperative Rehabilitation

For adhesive capsulitis, the main focus of the early postoperative rehab is to maximize range of motion; although this may need to be modulated depending on what other intra-articular pathology was addressed. A regional anesthetic block may be helpful to control pain and facilitate early postoperative rehabilitation. Therapy may be implemented on a daily basis for the first few weeks depending on the severity of the tightness and how the patient tolerates the recovery strategy.

Arthrofibrosis

(Video 27.2: http://goo.gl/Z3Bl6) Arthrofibrosis and adhesive capsulitis are two distinctly different entities. The treatment strategies can be quite different and thus the two should not be confused with one another. Adhesive capsulitis is a primary intrinsic capsular disorder that can respond readily to manipulation. Arthrofibrosis is a much more global problem of the capsule and surrounding soft tissues. This is often the result of previous trauma or surgery. Some cases of FAI with severely restricted motion also behave like arthrofibrosis and may share a similar treatment strategy.

Select cases of arthrofibrosis may be appropriately managed with arthroscopy, especially when no other more appealing alternatives are available. In these cases where dense adhesions and scar are the problem, open surgery may simply begot more scar. Also, for some of these cases where the symptoms are severe, considering an arthroplasty might prove to be an unwise choice. If the problem is soft tissue scarring and not advanced arthritis, a replacement does not solve the problem and may result in an equal amount of pain with the arthroplasty.

With arthrofibrosis, manipulation under anesthesia usually has little effect on increasing range of motion and also does little to improve distractibility of the joint. Thus, repeated forceful attempts at manipulation should be avoided.

Accessing a stiff hip, whether from arthrofibrosis or severe FAI, introduces particular challenges (Fig. 27.9). Because of limited joint space separation and sometimes abnormal bony morphology, extra steps may be necessary to avoid creating excessive iatrogenic damage to the joint. The sequence of steps for portal placements is as has been previously described in the joint access chapter with the following modifications.

Traction is applied, assessing the amount of joint space separation. Venting the joint with a spinal needle and then distending the joint with fluid through the needle may variously provide a little more space. Distending the joint also separates the capsule from the labrum so that the needle can then be repositioned, decreasing the likelihood penetrating the labrum.

The arthroscope cannula is then advanced over the guide wire. For a tight hip, forcing the cannula into the joint can cause unnecessary damage. In these circumstances, the cannula is advanced only to the level of the capsule and the arthroscope is introduced with the inflow attached. "Peeking" through the capsule, the labrum is viewed from the outside. The anterior portal is then established for introduction of another cannula. The needle must be positioned through the capsule, directly in front of the arthroscope, peripheral to the labrum (Fig. 27.10a, b). This challenges the surgeon's triangulation skills because of the small area in which to place the needle. This becomes easier with experience and reflects why these types of cases are not for beginners.

Once the needle has been positioned, a cannula can be advanced to the level of the capsule. A capsulectomy is then begun connecting the anterior and anterolateral por-

tals (Fig. 27.11). At this point, no attempt has yet been made to enter the joint. For most stiff hips, an extensive capsulectomy is performed, extending anteromedially and lateral. As the posterolateral labrum is visualized, a posterolateral portal can be established (Fig. 27.12). Sometimes, this may just be a small inflow cannula, allowing for a separate inflow. With the pump removed from the arthroscope cannula, a smaller diameter cannula can be used, which can be very advantageous within the tight quarters of a stiff hip.

Occasionally, with the arthroscope "peeking" through the capsule, it may be easier to view posterior than anterior. Either way, the purpose is to position a needle through the capsule where it can be visualized safely away from the labrum and femoral articular surface. Then the capsulectomy is begun with known reference to the location of the joint structures. The capsulectomy can then be extended in any direction to accomplish the necessary complete exposure.

The aggressive capsulectomy is therapeutic in helping to achieve more freedom of movement of the joint. It also then allows the joint to be entered with clear arthroscopic visualization of the important intra-articular structures. Hopefully, excising the capsule may also aid in achieving better joint space separation, but this is not always the case.

Dienst has described an alternative method of first accessing the hip via the peripheral compartment without traction [7]. Once the instrumentation has been positioned in the periphery, traction can then be applied and the central compartment entered. With his technique, as well as the one described by us, it is important to see the hip joint structures before passing the instruments into the joint. For both techniques, the biggest challenge may remain simply accomplishing adequate joint space separation. Again, we have observed that sometimes even extensive capsular excision does little to alter the force necessary to distract the hip. We prefer our technique of accessing the joint with traction applied because the preoperative patient positioning for traction is very important to make sure that a safe traction process has been used. Altering the position of the hip and applying traction after the patient has been draped requires extra attention to make sure that the counterforce perineal post remains in the proper position relative to the genitalia.

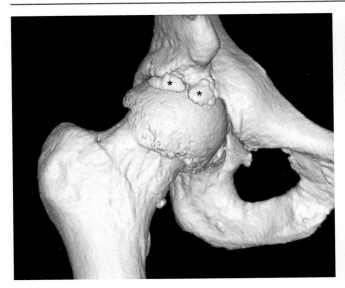

Fig. 27.9 A 3D CT reconstruction of a right hip illustrates severe impingement with bone fragments (*asterisks*) creating a structural barrier to the joint. (All rights are retained by Dr. Byrd)

Summary

Adhesive capsulitis will be encountered by most surgeons treating hip disorders. It may occur as a primary entity or in conjunction with other hip pathology. A sense of awareness is important for correctly making the diagnosis. With recognition of the entity, an appropriate treatment strategy can be integrated into the patient's care.

Arthrofibrosis is a bigger challenge and one for which the surgeon must have a well-planned treatment strategy. While there is no published data on arthroscopy specifically for arthrofibrosis, our experience suggests that this is a preferable approach for most cases that require surgical intervention. Also, as we are tackling more severe forms of FAI with stiffer hips, many of these border on requiring the strategy first developed for arthrofibrosis. These are challenging problems that may necessitate an aggressive approach. However, the methodology must be deliberate and well planned in order to modulate the greater risk of iatrogenic problems that goes along with these challenging cases.

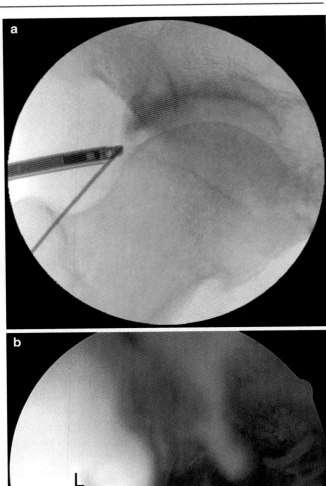

Fig. 27.10 (**a**) Intraoperative fluoroscopic image illustrates the scope perched at the edge of the lateral capsule and a needle being positioned for the anterior portal. (**b**) The needle is viewed directly above the femoral head (*F*) peripheral to the ossified portion of the labrum (*L*). (All rights are retained by Dr. Byrd)

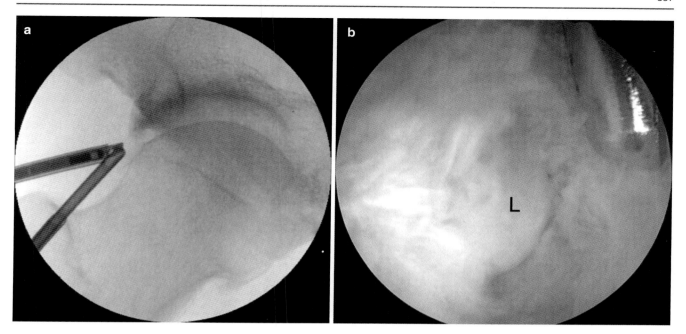

Fig. 27.11 (**a**) Fluoroscopic image now shows the shaver placed from the anterior portal. (**b**) A capsulotomy is begun, starting to better reveal the ossified fragment of labrum (*L*). (All rights are retained by Dr. Byrd)

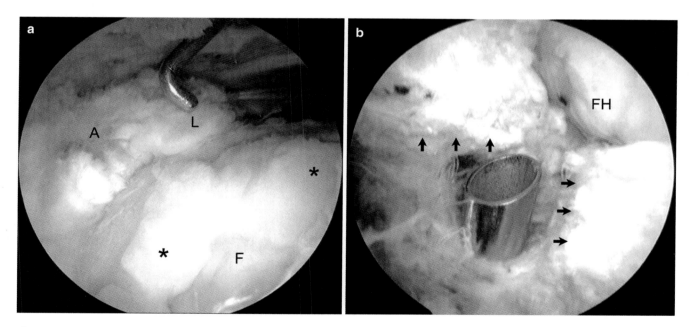

Fig. 27.12 (**a**) More extensive capsulectomy has been performed, better demonstrating the ossified labrum (*L*), acetabulum (*A*), and spurring (*asterisk*) of the femoral head (*F*). (**b**) Viewing posteriorly, a posterolateral portal has been positioned within the wedge-shaped area of the capsulotomy (*arrows*), adjacent to the femoral head (*FH*). (All rights are retained by Dr. Byrd)

References

1. Byrd JWT. Adhesive capsulitis of the hip. Arthroscopy. 2006;22(1): 89–94.

2. Hannafin JA, Chiaia TA. Adhesive capsulitis. A treatment approach. Clin Orthop. 2000;372:95–109.

3. Parvizi J, Leunig M, Ganz R. Femoroacetabular impingement. J Am Acad Orthop Surg. 2007;15(9):561–70.

4. Laborie LB, Lehmann TG, Engesaeter IO, et al. Prevalence of radiographic findings thought to be associated with femoroacetabular impingement in a population-based cohort of 2081 healthy young adults. Radiology. 2011;260(2):494–502. Epub 2011 May 25.

5. Murphy WA, Siegel MJ, Gilula LA. Arthrography in the diagnosis of unexplained chronic hip pain with regional osteopenia. AJR Am J Roentgenol. 1977;129:283–7.

6. Lequesne M, Becker J, Bard M, Witvoet J, Postel M. Capsular constriction of the hip: arthrographic and clinical considerations. Skeletal Radiol. 1981;6:1–10.

7. Dienst M, Seil R, Kohn DM. Safe arthroscopic access to the central compartment of the hip. Arthroscopy. 2005;21(12):1510–4.

Total Hip Arthroplasty

28

J.W. Thomas Byrd

Introduction

Arthroscopy can be performed in the presence of a total hip arthroplasty. There are only a few scientific articles on this subject, reflecting that it is not commonly indicated. The clinical workup of a painful total hip replacement is extensive and beyond the scope of this text [1]. The largest two published series were by McCarthy ($n = 14$), looking at conventional arthroplasties, and Pattyn ($n = 15$), in a series of resurfacing arthroplasties [2, 3].

There are many causes of a symptomatic total hip replacement but only a few that are amenable to arthroscopic intervention. Removal of fragments such as methyl methacrylate, broken wires, metallic beads, or loose screws has been described [4–6]. There are several reports on the role of arthroscopy in the treatment of a septic arthroplasty. Most commonly, this has been purported for patients who are medically compromised and would have a difficult time withstanding the systemic stresses of an open procedure [7]. However, it is likely that arthroscopic debridement and lavage would be an appropriate first surgical choice for any septic joint.

For properly selected cases, arthroscopy may have diagnostic value in assessing problems associated with a painful arthroplasty. It is not a substitute for a comprehensive diagnostic workup, but soft tissue disease and loosening can be evaluated and biopsies obtained [8]. In fact, McCarthy and Pattyn have both described diagnosing occult infection by arthroscopy with tissue cultures in patients with previous culture-negative aspirates [2, 3].

The most common reason for arthroscopy in the presence of an arthroplasty is management of a painful iliopsoas tendon. Iliopsoas tendinitis or iliopsoas impingement by the component is being more commonly encountered. There are two reasons for this. Larger heads are being used for greater stability with a tendency toward larger acetabular components which can be proud anteriorly, creating friction against the iliopsoas. Secondly, resurfacing procedures are popular for younger adult males in whom the osteoarthritis is commonly caused by FAI. Residual deformity of the preserved portion of the joint can similarly result in friction against the iliopsoas. For these circumstances, endoscopic release of the iliopsoas can be performed with minimal morbidity and, for properly selected cases, is a preferable first line of surgical treatment compared to revising the components. Pattyn has also described femoroplasty to correct residual impingement caused by reduced anterior femoral offset as being successful at relieving symptoms among a small subset of resurfacing arthroplasties [3].

Two Techniques for Arthroscopy of a Conventional Total Hip Arthroplasty

There are two methods for accessing the central compartment of a hip arthroplasty. The choice is determined by whether or not the components can be adequately distracted. With either technique, the paramount issue is to minimize contact between the arthroscopic instruments and the bearing surfaces of the prosthesis. Regardless of whether the surface is metallic, ceramic, or polyethylene, any contact can alter the surface characteristics and negatively influence its low coefficient of friction and long-term wear.

Positioning is performed as would be done with any routine arthroscopic procedure [9]. Traction is applied. If there is good separation of the components, adequate to assure easy clearance of the instruments within the joint, then arthroscopy is performed essentially as would be normally carried out for a native hip (Fig. 28.1). Particular care is taken with initial placement of the arthroscope cannula to minimize any contact with the bearing surfaces. Once the

J.W.T. Byrd, M.D.
Nashville Sports Medicine Foundation,
2011 Church Street, Suite 100, Nashville,
TN 37203, USA
e-mail: byrd@nsmfoundation.org

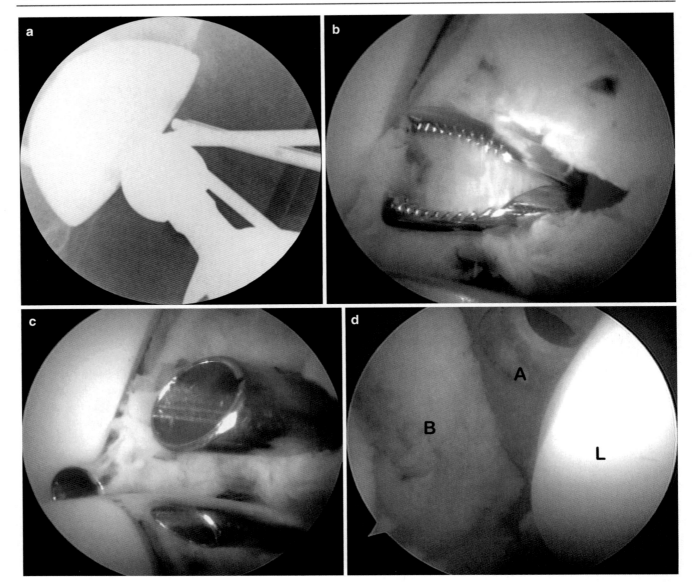

Fig. 28.1 A 59-year-old man with a painful left total hip arthroplasty. (**a**) AP fluoroscopic view demonstrates distraction of the joint allowing placement of the three standard arthroscopic portals. (**b**) Fibrinous tissue is present and being biopsied. (**c**) Viewing from the anterior portal, the relationship of the lateral two portals is demonstrated within the joint, also illustrating the intact articulating surfaces of the prosthesis. (**d**) The interface of the bone (*B*) and acetabular shell (*A*) is visualized behind the acetabular liner (*L*). (All rights are retained by Dr. Byrd)

arthroscope has been introduced, other portals can then be placed under direct arthroscopic visualization, watching exactly how the instruments enter the joint. Even for patients who have undergone a previous complete capsulectomy, a generous pseudo-capsule usually reforms and is entered much like a native joint. The consistency of the tissues may be different, and the amount of resistance encountered as cannulas are placed may have a different feel. This can change the sense of control as the cannula is advanced, and the surgeon should just be careful not to inadvertently plunge the instruments into the joint.

Sometimes, dense tissue constrains the hip and does not allow for effective distraction. Arthroscopy can still be performed with an alternative technique. The arthroscope cannula is first placed directly on the neck of the femoral component (Fig. 28.2). There will be at least a small space present where a subsequent working portal can be established, also along the neck. This requires some experience with triangulation technique in order to position a spinal needle directly in front of the arthroscope lens. Once the working portal has been established, soft tissue debridement can then proceed to develop a larger space and subsequently

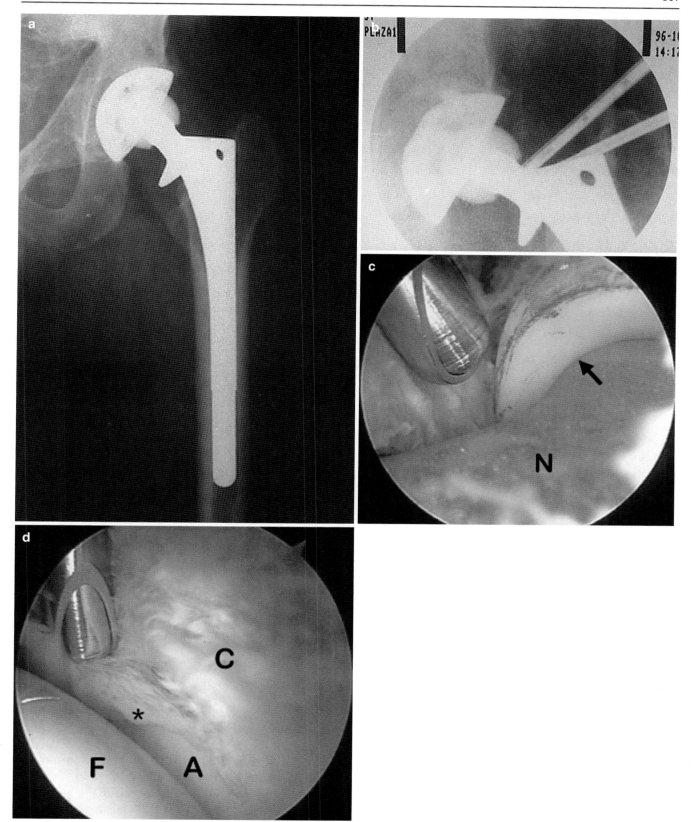

Fig. 28.2 A 38-year-old male with unexplained left hip pain 21 months following a total hip replacement. (**a**) AP radiograph reveals a well-positioned press-fit prosthesis with no evidence of loosening. (**b**) Fluoroscopic view demonstrates the position of the arthroscope and shaver along the base of the neck, thus avoiding the articular surface of the prosthesis. (**c**) Debridement of the fibrous tissue exposes the neck of the prosthesis (*N*) and its junction with the ceramic head (*arrow*). (**d**) A dense portion of fibrous tissue (*asterisk*) was entrapped between the polyethylene liner of the acetabulum (*A*) and the femoral head component (*F*). Peripheral to this is the reformed capsule (*C*). (All rights are retained by Dr. Byrd)

bring into view the rest of the joint and the components. Entering on the neck of the prosthesis will avoid inadvertently contacting the bearing surfaces. Subsequent dissection and exposure then must proceed in a methodical controlled fashion, assuring good visualization at every step, in order to avoid any potential harm to the prosthesis. Other portals can be introduced as needed.

Arthroscopy in the Presence of a Resurfacing Arthroplasty

Arthroscopy in the presence of a resurfacing arthroplasty comes closer to the technique of arthroscopy for a natural hip joint. Standard portals can be used with strict precautions to avoid contacting the bearing surfaces [9]. Much of the work may be performed in the periphery, and various supplementary portals can be used. Work in the periphery may include assessing for signs of residual bony impingement, synovial disease, or iliopsoas impingement/friction against the prosthesis [3, 10].

Painful Iliopsoas Tendon

Diagnosing the iliopsoas tendon as a source of pain in the presence of an arthroplasty is sometimes straightforward and sometimes elusive. This is a distinctly different entity than a troublesome snapping iliopsoas tendon occasionally encountered in a native hip [11]. The snapping hip is usually more distinct in both the diagnosis and in gauging the response to treatment. An arthroplasty always requires a thorough workup to rule out causes other than a painful iliopsoas [1]. Assuming those other etiologies have been ruled out as thoroughly as possible, there are features that will tip one to the diagnosis of an iliopsoas problem.

Weight-bearing pain is usually absent, which would be more indicative of component loosening as a problem. Ambulating on a level surface may be difficult because of firing of the iliopsoas, but ascending and descending inclines and steps are usually even more problematic. Rising from a seated position can be painful or any activity that results in concentric or eccentric firing of the iliopsoas moving across the anterior surfaces of the prosthesis.

On examination, passive flexion and rotational motion should typically not cause much discomfort because the psoas is not firing. Active flexion and often just lowering the leg against gravity can be quite painful. Stretching the hip in maximal extension has also been reported to elicit iliopsoas pain [12]. Sometimes these clinical findings are clear, and sometimes the observations are mixed as far as indicating the etiology of symptoms. Rarely is snapping present as would be observed with coxa saltans of the native hip.

Plain radiographs are necessary in all cases. These are important to assess the positioning and alignment of the components as well as looking for any signs of loosening or other bony abnormality. Particular attention is given looking for anterior prominences, from either the components or residual bone that would suggest a mechanical reason for friction with the iliopsoas (Fig. 28.3). An MRI may be appropriate. The artifact is typically severe due to the prosthetic components, but newer techniques are getting better at diminishing the amount of scatter. Even with the artifact, it may be helpful to look at the iliopsoas and its surrounding bursa. Often, there may be no findings at all, but edema within the iliopsoas or surrounding bursitis may be evident (Fig. 28.4). Occasionally, even hemorrhagic iliopsoas bursitis may occur when friction against the edge of the component results in fraying of the tendon (Fig. 28.5). Beyond these findings, the workup usually centers more on loosening or other causes for a painful arthroplasty.

Injection around the iliopsoas tendon can be a useful diagnostic test, but the results are not always conclusive. Blind injection is of limited usefulness because of the lack of certainty on knowing the location of instillate. In the office setting, ultrasound guidance is a preferred method for precise injection [13]. If fluid is present within the bursa, aspiration can also be performed for cytology and culture. Alternatively, an injection can be performed under fluoroscopy with a few cc's of contrast to substantiate positioning within the bursa [14].

Injecting long-acting anesthetic and cortisone is performed for diagnostic and potentially therapeutic purposes. However, the response to injection is not always conclusive. The space around the iliopsoas and the bursa is not especially well contained, and there may be ample communication with the joint. Even in a native hip, there is a significant incidence of communication between the joint and the iliopsoas bursa [15]. Thus, the response to injection can be useful but not necessarily definitive for a problem of the iliopsoas.

Release of the iliopsoas tendon can be effectively performed by endoscopic methods, and for this purpose, there appears to be no advantage of an open procedure. Release of the iliopsoas tendon can be performed either at the joint itself or distally from the lesser trochanter. The appeal of releasing the tendon from within the joint or pseudo capsule is the potential to view if the damaged tendon is rubbing against an exposed anterior rim of the acetabulum or other aspect of the component. However, this technique necessitates the care that must be taken to avoid harming the bearing surfaces. Alternatively, the tendon can be released from the lesser trochanter within the iliopsoas bursa (Fig. 28.6) [9]. The advantage of this method is that it avoids the prosthesis altogether. As the tendinous insertion is released, some of the iliopsoas may still be adherent to the anterior pseudo capsule. This can be observed and dissected free from within the iliopsoas

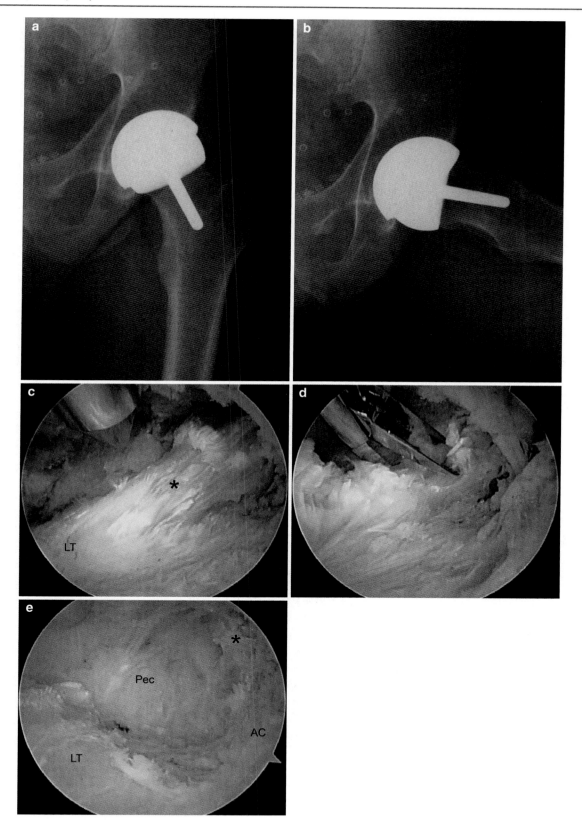

Fig. 28.3 A 50-year-old male with a 10-month history of recalcitrant left hip flexor pain following resurfacing. Two previous iliopsoas injections had provided temporary relief. (**a** and **b**) AP and lateral radiographs reveal the prosthesis to be well seated, but some prominence of the acetabular cup. (**c**) The iliopsoas tendon (*asterisk*) is identified at its insertion to the lesser trochanter (*LT*). (**d**) The tendon is being divided with a basket. (**e**) Division is complete between the lesser trochanter (*LT*) and proximal stump (*asterisk*). A fibrous layer covers the area of the pectineus muscle medially (*Pec*) and anterior capsule (*AC*). (All rights are retained by Dr. Byrd)

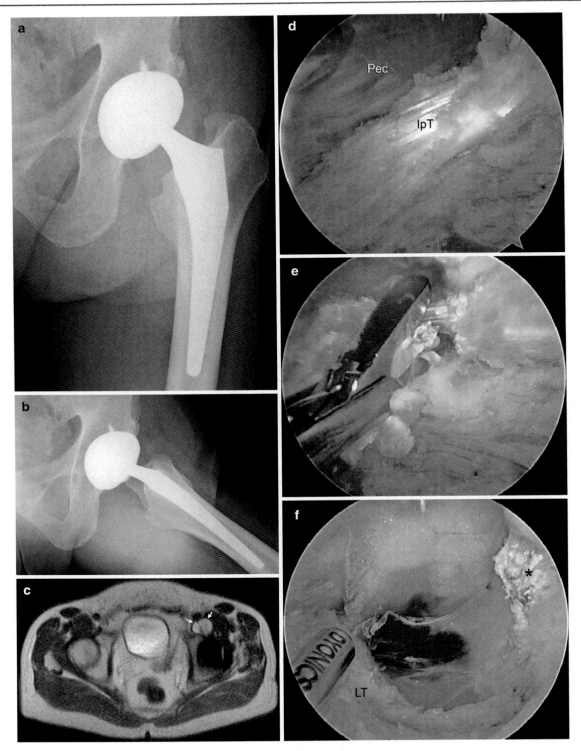

Fig. 28.4 A 59-year-old male orthopedic surgeon developed recurrent painful bursal swelling 3 years following a left total hip arthroplasty. Two previous aspirations provided temporary alleviation and were culture negative. (**a** and **b**) AP and lateral radiograph of the left hip reveal the prosthesis to be properly seated. (**c**) Axial pelvis MRI reveals significant bursal fluid accumulation (*arrows*) evident despite artifact from hip arthroplasty. (**d**) The iliopsoas tendon (*IpT*) is silhouetted by the pectineus (*Pec*). (**e**) The tendon is being released with a basket. (**f**) Division is complete with the tendon stump (*asterisk*) separated from the lesser trochanter (*LT*). (All rights are retained by Dr. Byrd)

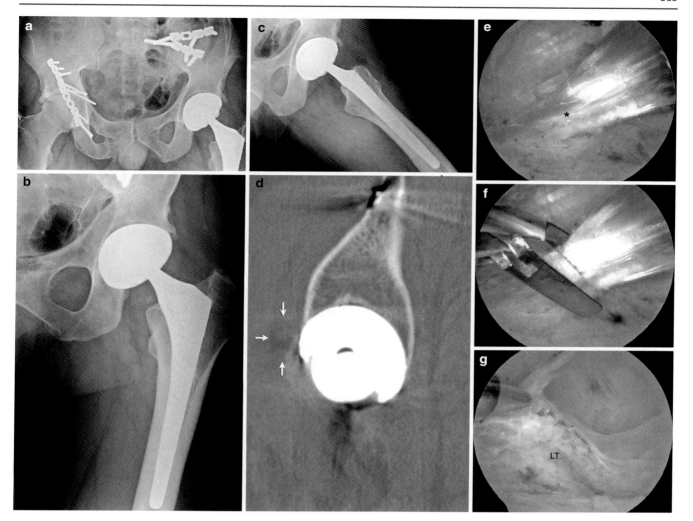

Fig. 28.5 A 31-year-old male developed recurrent painful bursal hematomas 3 years following a left total hip arthroplasty performed for polytrauma. (**a**) AP pelvis demonstrates sequela of the previous injury. (**b** and **c**) AP and lateral radiograph of the left prosthesis reveal it to be properly seated. (**d**) A sagittal CT reconstruction reveals prominence of the anterior acetabular rim and adjacent fluid within the iliopsoas bursa (*arrows*). (**e**) The enthesis of the iliopsoas (*asterisk*) is exposed. (**f**) Division is being performed with a basket. (**g**) Release is complete, exposing the bony surface of the lesser trochanter (*LT*). (All rights are retained by Dr. Byrd)

bursa. This is our preferred method unless there is a compelling reason to need to inspect the prosthetic components centrally.

Regardless of the method selected for releasing the iliopsoas tendon, any surgery of this structure is known to carry a significant incidence of postsurgical heterotopic ossification [16]. Thus, we recommend a one-time low-dose radiation treatment with standard recognized protocol as prophylaxis against the development of heterotopic ossification [17]. Remember that this procedure is most commonly performed for subjective reasons of pain, which is not always precisely localized. If the patient were to develop heterotopic ossification, that could just add further complexities to deciphering a patient's pain.

Fig. 28.6 The schematic illustrates release of the iliopsoas tendon from the lesser trochanter. The hip is flexed approximately 20° and externally rotated. Two laterally based portals are centered within the iliopsoas bursa at the lesser trochanter. (All rights are retained by Dr. Byrd)

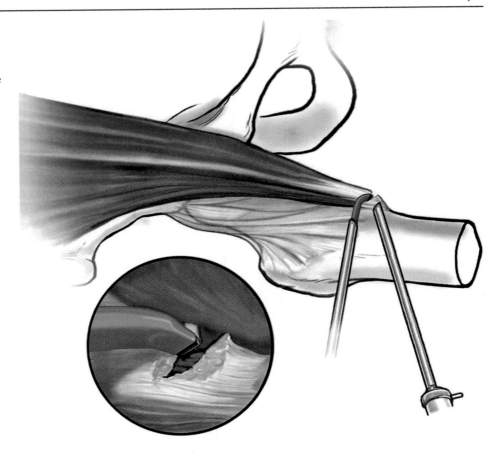

Summary

Arthroscopy can be performed in the presence of a total hip arthroplasty. It is not a substitute for a proper and thorough workup including history, examination, and imaging studies. However, for properly selected cases, it may have both diagnostic and therapeutic value.

References

1. Bozic KJ, Rubash HE. The painful total hip replacement. Clin Orthop Relat Res. 2004;420:18–25.
2. McCarthy JC, Jibodh SR, Lee JA. The role of arthroscopy in evaluation of painful hip arthroplasty. Clin Orthop Relat Res. 2009;467:174–80.
3. Pattyn C, Verdonk R, Audenaert E. Hip arthroscopy in patients with painful hip following resurfacing arthroplasty. Knee Surg Sports Traumatol Arthrosc. 2011;19:1514–20. doi:10.1007/S00167–011–1467–7.
4. Shifrin L, Reis N. Arthroscopy of a dislocated hip replacement: a case report. Clin Orthop. 1980;146:213–4.
5. Vakili F, Salvati EA, Warren RF. Entrapped foreign body within the acetabular cup in total hip replacement. Clin Orthop. 1980;150:159–62.
6. Nordt W, Giangarra CE, Levy IM, et al. Arthroscopic removal of entrapped debris following dislocation of a total hip arthroplasty. Arthroscopy. 1987;3(3):196–8.
7. Hyman JL, Salvati EA, Laurencin CT, et al. The arthroscopic drainage, irrigation and debridement of late, acute total hip arthroplasty infections: average 6-year follow-up. J Arthroplasty. 1999;14(8):903–10.
8. Fontana A, Zecca M, Sala C. Arthroscopic assessment of total hip replacement and polyethylene wear: a case report. Knee Surg Sports Traumatol Arthrosc. 2000;8(4):244–5.
9. Byrd JWT. Routine arthroscopy & access: central & peripheral compartments, iliopsoas bursa, peritrochanteric and subgluteal spaces. In: Byrd JWT, editor. Operative hip arthroscopy, 3rd ed. New York: Springer. 2012;11:131–160.
10. Khanduja V, Villar RN. The role of arthroscopy in resurfacing arthroplasty of the hip. Arthroscopy. 2008;24(1):122.e1–3.
11. Byrd JWT. Evaluation and management of the snapping iliopsoas tendon. Instr Course Lect. 2006;55:347–55.
12. Lachiewicz PF, Kauk JR. Anterior iliopsoas impingement and tendinitis after total hip arthroplasty. J Am Acad Orthop Surg. 2009;17(6):337–44.
13. Sofka CM, Saboeiro G, Adler RS. Ultrasound-guided adult hip injections. J Vasc Interv Radiol. 2005;16(8):1121–3.
14. Erb R. Adult hip imaging. In: Byrd JWT, editor. Operative hip arthroscopy. 2nd ed. New York: Springer; 2005. p. 51–69.
15. Chandler S. Iliopsoas bursa in man. Anat Rec. 1934;58(3):235–40.
16. Velasco AD, Allan DB, Wroblewski BM. Psoas tenotomy and heterotopic ossification after Charnley low-friction arthroplasty. Clin Orthop Relat Res. 1993;291:193–5.
17. Balboni TA, Gobezie R, Mamon HJ. Heterotopic ossification: pathophysiology, clinical features and the role of radiotherapy for prophylaxis. Int J Radiat Oncol Biol Phys. 2006;65(5):1289–99.

Hip Arthroscopy in Adolescence and Childhood

29

Yi-Meng Yen and Mininder S. Kocher

Introduction

Hip pain in the young active patient has multiple etiologies and can range from developmental to traumatic to infectious. Some of these diagnoses occur during certain stages of childhood. Developmental dysplasia of the hip occurs usually in infants, Legg-Calve-Perthes disease generally occurs in children aged 4–10, slipped capital femoral epiphysis (SCFE) occurs in children before skeletal maturity, and labral pathology occurs in older pediatric and adolescent patients [1]. Osteomyelitis or septic arthritis, transient synovitis, and trauma can occur at any stage.

The application of hip arthroscopy to the pediatric and adolescent patient requires a thorough understanding of all these hip disorders. There are a number of intra- and extra-articular etiologies for pain that have been described. This is due to the close proximity of structures around the hip joint. These disorders include apophyseal injuries, tendon injuries, hip dislocation, as well as femoroacetabular impingement (FAI) which can account for early development of osteoarthritis in the young adult. The majority of soft tissue injuries around the hip heal with nonoperative treatment. However, with the advent of less invasive methods and the development of more advanced imaging of the hip through magnetic resonance imaging (MRI), internal

derangements of the hip such as labral tears, loose bodies, and chondral injuries due to conditions such as SCFE, Perthes, and FAI are being diagnosed and treated with increased frequency.

The traditional approach to managing intra-articular problems in pediatrics and adolescent patients has been to use open methods, including the surgical dislocation approach popularized by Ganz [2]. Hip arthroscopy has obvious advantages compared to arthrotomy and surgical dislocation in the pediatric population. It is significantly less invasive than arthrotomy and allows for quicker recovery and return to activities. Most of the experience in hip arthroscopy has been with treating hip disorders in adults with the role of hip arthroscopy, and results in children and adolescents have been less well characterized. This may in part be due to the periarticular and physeal related issues that are unique to the skeletally immature patient.

The first reported experience of arthroscopy in the pediatric age group was described in 1977 by Gross [3], who found that the procedure did not aid in diagnosis or therapeutic intervention, thus perhaps diminishing early efforts of hip arthroscopy in younger patients. However, two series in 1981 and 1986 reported more favorable results with the use of arthroscopy in the pediatric hip for juvenile chronic arthritis for accurately diagnosing the cartilage damage and severity of the synovitis [4, 5]. In 1992, Futami et al. reviewed their experience with arthroscopy for slipped capital femoral epiphysis by performing a diagnostic arthroscopy prior to in situ pinning [6]. He concluded from the erosion of cartilage and labral pathology that the pathomechanics of SCFE are traumatic in nature and that the arthroscopy was useful for diagnosis and decompression of the hematoma from the SCFE.

Historically, the most common indication for hip arthroscopy in the pediatric and adolescent population has been in the case of Legg-Calve-Perthes disease, both for the diagnosis of the severity of the disease and the therapeutic removal of loose bodies [7]. Suzuki reported on a series of 19 children undergoing arthroscopy for LCP. They visualized significant synovial proliferation in the acetabular fossa and

Y.-M. Yen, M.D., Ph.D.
Division of Sports Medicine, Department of Orthopaedic Surgery, Children's Hospital Boston, Harvard Medical School, 300 Longwood Avenue, Boston, MA 02115, USA
e-mail: yi-meng.yen@childrens.harvard.edu

M.S. Kocher, M.D., MPH (✉)
Division of Sports Medicine, Department of Orthopaedic Surgery, Children's Hospital Boston, Harvard Medical School, 300 Longwood Avenue, Boston, MA 02115, USA

Department of Orthopaedic Surgery, Harvard Medical School, 300 Longwood Avenue, Boston, MA, USA
e-mail: mininder.kocher@childrens.harvard.edu

J.W.T. Byrd (ed.), *Operative Hip Arthroscopy*,
DOI 10.1007/978-1-4419-7925-4_29, © Springer Science+Business Media New York 2013

also hypervascularity of the labrum and capsule and thereby postulated that the mass effect and hypervascularity added to the instability and femoral head coverage [8]. Bowen et al. described arthroscopic chondroplasty of the femoral head after skeletal maturity in patients with Legg-Calve Perthes disease as children [9].

In a later study, Schindler and colleagues reviewed 24 arthroscopies for varied diagnoses and conclude that hip arthroscopy was effective for synovial biopsy and loose body removal; however, as a purely diagnostic procedure, arthroscopy only supported the diagnosis in 54% of patients [10]. This has been supported in a larger series on adults in which diagnostic hip arthroscopy was useful in only specific cases, and the authors noted that the improvements in imaging modalities may significantly decrease the indications for purely diagnostic arthroscopy [11].

As the understanding of hip disease and our arthroscopic experience continues to evolve, the use of hip arthroscopy will undoubtedly become more widespread. The surgeon must be precise in the role of hip arthroscopy for diagnosis and treatment in the pediatric and adolescent population.

Anatomy

The acetabulum is the convergence point of three ossification centers: the ischium, pubis, and ilium. The triradiate cartilage assumes a Y-shape with the anterior slanted portion of the "Y" dividing the ilium and pubis, the posterior slanted portion separating the ilium and ischium, and the inferior limb separating the ischium and pubis. The physis of the triradiate cartilage is bipolar, with the germinal zone running in the center of each arm of the "Y" [12]. The major role of the triradiate cartilage is to facilitate a progressive radial increase in size of the acetabulum while maintaining spherical congruency in response to growth of the proximal femur [13]. As adolescence is reached, secondary ossification centers (os acetabulum) develop in the periphery of the acetabulum [14]. The os acetabulum is the epiphysis of the pubis and forms the anterior wall of the acetabulum while the epiphysis of the ilium forms the majority of the superior edge of the acetabulum [12]. The triradiate closes at approximately age 12 in girls and age 14 in boys, with the secondary ossification centers fully fusing around skeletal maturity.

The three main growth centers of the proximal femur are the physis of the proximal femur, which is usually contained within the sphericity of the femoral head, the growth plate of the greater trochanter developing directly above the lateral metaphysis, and the femoral neck isthmus. Around age 8, an indentation in the ossification center where the ligamentum attaches forms, and the final anteversion of the proximal femur is determined. Of the active growth regions around the proximal femur, the capital femoral physis is the first to close, beginning centrally. The proximal femoral physeal

plate contributes approximately 30% to the overall growth of the length of the femur and about 10% of the growth of the entire limb. Damage to the growth plate usually results in a varus deformity because of the continued growth of the femoral neck and greater trochanter [15, 16]. Closure of the proximal femoral physis occurs approximately between ages 16 and 18.

Physical Exam

The goal of the history and physical examination of the hip is to differentiate between intra-articular and extra-articular etiologies of hip pain. The clinician needs to be able to determine the onset, frequency, severity, location, chronicity, inciting factors, radiation of pain, and mechanical symptoms (i.e., catching, popping, snapping, locking, or giving way). Mechanical symptoms such as clicking and locking can be seen with labral tears, whereas audible or visible snapping may be associated with coxa saltans interna or externa. Intra-articular hip pain usually presents as groin pain, and patients often demonstrate the "C-sign" placing their hands cupped over their greater trochanter [17, 18]. However, in the pediatric and adolescent patients, hip pain may not be the presenting symptom. Due to the referral pattern of pain, hip pathology should be strongly suspected in a patient with knee pain, especially with a normal examination of the knee. Another frequent pediatric presentation is the limping child with no known injury. A history of preceding illness should direct the physician to consider the diagnosis of transient synovitis; however, septic arthritis needs to be worked up [19].

The physical examination should be thorough. The patient's gait should be noted, and any leg-length discrepancies assessed. Examination of the lumbar spine including motor function, sensation, range of motion, reflexes, and straight-leg raises must be performed to rule out lumbar spine pathology as the cause of symptoms. The hip examination begins with palpation of bony prominences about the hip and a thorough assessment of the range of motion, particularly the rotational profile. Pain with passive flexion and internal rotation of the hip has been identified as predictors of intra-articular pathology, which has been corroborated in young patients [20, 21]. The impingement test (flexion to 90° and maximal internal rotation and adduction) should be performed in the supine position. A Trendelenburg test and thorough neurological assessment should be conducted. Comparison to the contralateral hip must be a part of each examination.

Imaging

Plain radiographs are perhaps the most useful imaging tool for the initial evaluation of hip complaints when performed correctly. Radiographic evaluation begins with an anteroposterior radiograph of the pelvis with the beam centered at the mid-point of the pelvis with the coccyx 1–3 cm above the pubis symphysis. The radiograph is used to assess degenerative changes, bony lesions, dysplasia, the presence of osteochondral loose bodies, as well as factors that predispose to FAI. Additionally, morphologic changes of the acetabulum such as retroversion, coxa profunda, and protrusio can be identified, though excessive lordosis and rotation will make assessment of the acetabular version inaccurate [22]. Although there has been shown to be no difference in the height of the weight-bearing surface of an AP pelvis taken supine versus standing [23], a standing AP pelvis can emphasize evidence of mild dysplasia by showing lateralization of the femoral head. The faux profile view is a true lateral of the acetabulum performed with the patient standing and the pelvis turned approximately 25° toward the beam and the ipsilateral foot and knee and the film perpendicular to the beam [24]. This demonstrates the degree of anterior acetabular coverage. Finally, a lateral view of the proximal femur is obtained, either a cross table, frog leg, or Dunn lateral of the hip. We prefer the Dunn lateral of the hip to best see the offset of the anterolateral head-neck junction of the proximal femur (Fig. 29.1a, b). Additionally, computed tomography (CT) can be performed to aid in diagnosis but is not widely used in pediatric patients due to the radiation dosage.

Magnetic resonance imaging (MRI) is generally obtained to further assess or confirm hip pathology. While an MRI allows improved visualization of the soft tissues, early degenerative changes, stress reactions, and osteonecrosis [25], it has been shown that plain MRI may not accurately identify labral defects and other intra-articular structures compared to MR arthrogram [26]. There are, however, newer imaging protocols that may be more capable of visualizing these defects without the arthrogram [27, 28]. MRI is also useful for the evaluation of the morphology of the femoral head-neck junction, although conventional axial, sagittal, and coronal cuts may underestimate the magnitude of a cam lesion. We routinely obtain radial sequence images around the femoral head to better define cam lesions due to FAI (Fig. 29.2a, b) [29].

Although MRI arthrogram offers improved evaluation of the chondral surface, this technique has been shown to have a high false-negative rate, thus limiting its usefulness in identifying true articular surface damage [25, 26]. Gadolinium-based biochemical MRI in the form of dGEMRIC (delayed gadolinium-enhanced MRI of cartilage) has now been established as an important modality in articular cartilage imaging. Negatively charged gadolinium contrast is administered intravenously, and there is uptake in hyaline cartilage at an inverse proportion to the GAG content. Degenerated cartilage contains less GAG, and the concentration of infiltrated gadolinium will be high compared to the relatively low amount that accumulates in healthy cartilage. Thus, T1 MRI measurements

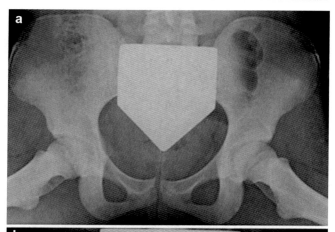

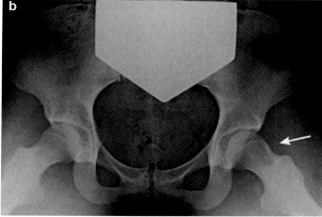

Fig. 29.1 (a) Frog leg lateral radiograph of the pelvis. Due to the version of the femur, it is difficult to visualize the femoral head-neck junction. (b) Dunn lateral of the same patient. The decreased offset of the right head-neck junction is more evident on this lateral view (shown by *arrow*)

can give an indirect reflection of the underlying tissue charge and GAG content of cartilage which reflects chondral injury [30, 31].

Hip Arthroscopy

Hip arthroscopy is performed either in the supine or lateral decubitus position [32, 33]. We prefer the supine position because it allows easier use of the image intensifier and more straightforward instrument handling. A standard fracture table or a specialized hip arthroscopy extension on a regular OR table can be utilized. Traction is placed on the lower extremities with both feet in stirrups or boots. A large padded perineal post is used to protect the pudendal nerve. Adequate traction typically requires 50–75 lb of force in order to distract approximately 1 cm. C-arm is used to confirm the amount of traction and for facilitation of portal placement. Portal placement includes anterior, mid-anterior, anterolateral, posterolateral, and peripheral portals; we typically only use 2–3 portals.

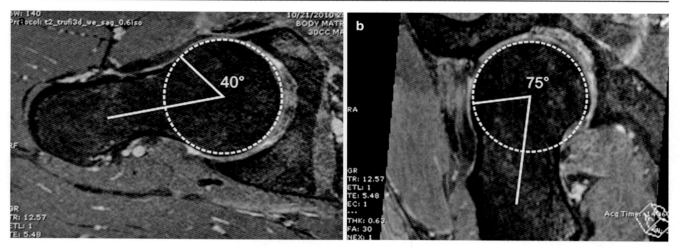

Fig. 29.2 (a) Axial oblique T2-weighted sequence MRI of the right hip. Alpha angle of the femoral head-neck junction is normal in these views. (b) Radial T2-weighted sequences of the same hip. Asphericity of the anterolateral femoral head-neck junction is demonstrated with an abnormal alpha angle

Once the arthroscope is inserted, a complete diagnostic examination of the hip joint should be performed. Synovitis is debrided and chondral injuries are addressed in the same manner as adults. Chondral flaps should be debrided carefully with a full radius shaver with or without arthroscopic biters. The chondroplasty should be performed to give a stable edge of cartilage. Thermal chondroplasty has been described, but due to the potential of damage to the chondrocytes, we do not routinely use radio frequency ablation [34, 35].

Adolescent or pediatric patients with grade IV chondromalacia of the cartilage are troubling due to this chondral damage at an early age. These chondral lesions are rarely degenerative in this population and are usually the result of trauma or CAM impingement, particularly from SCFE. Microfracture can be performed on areas of exposed bone in either cam or pincer impingement [36]. However, microfracture is more commonly performed in the focal lesions due to cam impingement, while the rim chondrosis in pincer impingement can be removed during acetabular rim trimming. To perform the microfracture procedure, first, the unstable cartilage is debrided, and exposed bone is prepared by removing the calcified cartilage layer while preserving the subchondral plate [37, 38]. Arthroscopic awls with an angle that allows the tip of the awl to be perpendicular to the subchondral bone surface are used to make multiple holes ("microfractures") in the exposed subchondral bone plate. As many holes as possible are created, leaving about 3–4 mm between each with a depth of approximately 2–4 mm to access the marrow elements. When the irrigation pressure is decreased, the release of fat droplets and blood from the holes can be observed indicating successful microfracture (Fig. 29.3a, b).

The labrum is examined, and irreparable tears are debrided. Labral repair is performed in the same manner as in adults, with preparation of the acetabular rim and placement of suture anchors to secure the labrum to bone. If the triradiate cartilage is still open, care should be taken to avoid placing an anchor into the cartilaginous portion between the ilium and pubis. Additionally, we attempt to minimize the number of suture anchors in order to avoid iatrogenic damage to the secondary ossification centers around the acetabulum. We prefer to repair the labrum in all possible cases.

Acetabular retroversion is corrected with labral separation (if necessary) and the use of a motorized burr. The amount of resection is determined by the lateral and anterior center edge angle. In patients that are just prepubertal, the perichondral ring of the acetabulum can be disrupted, but we have not seen any adverse sequelae from careful rim trimming. Coxa profunda can also be addressed with rim trimming or alternatively with a triradiate epiphyseodesis.

Once the central compartment work has been performed, the peripheral compartment is entered by releasing traction and flexing the hip. Resection of the CAM lesion is performed in this compartment using a motorized burr. The CAM lesion is often visible as a discoloration or fibrillation of the chondral surface with a visible protrusion. The CAM lesion is often sclerotic and the resection should proceed just proximal or to the level of the physis. Depending upon the physiologic age of the child, if there is significant growth remaining, the resection is done just to the level of the physis, checking with liberal use of fluoroscopy, although we have not seen any adverse reactions to some resection proximal to the physis in patients older than 10–11. Usually, we routinely resect just proximal to the physis, visualizing the physis arthroscopically (Fig. 29.4).

Once the arthroscopy is concluded, if the patient has mild dysplasia or is significantly ligamentously lax, we close the capsule with number 1 Vicryl; otherwise, the capsule is left

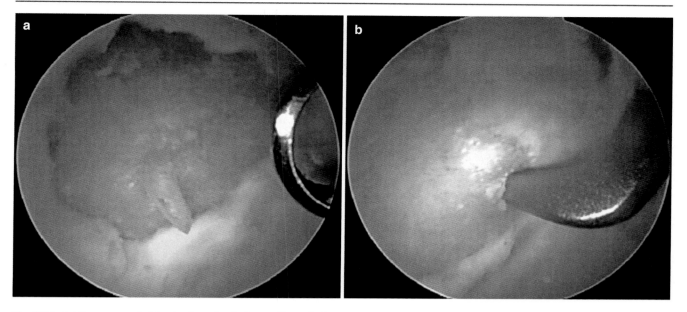

Fig. 29.3 (**a**) Large area of delamination of articular cartilage. A ring curette was used to debride the loose cartilage and remove the calcified layer. (**b**) An arthroscopic awl is used to create multiple microfracture holes in the exposed bone

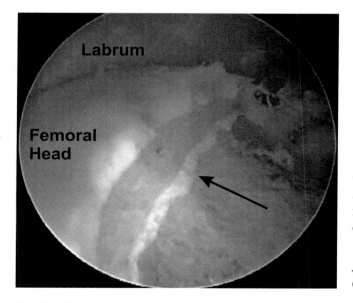

Fig. 29.4 Resection of cam lesion of a right hip with exposed physis just distal to level of resection. Viewing portal is anterolateral, the *arrow* denotes the physis

open. The portals or incisions are closed in standard fashion, and sterile dressings placed over the wounds, along with a cryotherapy device.

Postoperative Management

The patients are either discharged as a day surgery or kept for brief overnight stay for optimal pain control. A continuous passive motion (CPM) machine is used for 3–4 weeks and in the case of microfracture for an 8-week period. Crutch-assisted touchdown weight bearing is maintained for 2–3 weeks, but for 6–8 weeks with microfracture. Patients are encouraged to start physical therapy utilizing modifications of the techniques described by Stalzer et al. [39]. Initial physical therapy consists of passive motion progressing to active-assisted motion and eventually active motion with particular emphasis on regaining hip internal rotation. The early phase of physical therapy should focus primarily on achieving range of motion. Stationary bicycle exercises without resistance are begun in the immediate postoperative period. This phase is followed by an emphasis on muscular endurance. The last phase of therapy focuses on the return of power and strength. Impact sports are delayed until at least 4–6 months postoperatively.

Complications

Complications associated with arthroscopy of the hip include all of those for adults, such as nerve palsies and recurrent injury or under-resection, as well as potential complications that are unique to the pediatric population including proximal femoral physeal separation and growth disturbances. In a review of 218 pediatric hip arthroscopies, Nwachukwu et al. [40, 41] reported an overall complication rate of 1.8% which included transient pudendal nerve palsy, instrument breakage, and suture abscess, but no cases of osteonecrosis or growth disturbance of the acetabulum or proximal femur. Additionally, both Kocher et al. [41] and Schindler et al. [10] showed complete pudendal nerve functional return and relatively low complication rate for most pediatric hip arthroscopies.

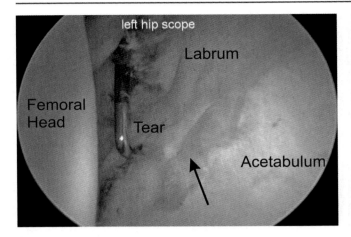

Fig. 29.5 Fraying and tearing of the acetabular labrum of the left hip shown by the probe with chondral flaps evident adjacent to the tear is denoted with the *arrow*. The probe is in the anterior portal, and the viewing portal is anterolateral

Results from Literature

There have been relatively few results published on the use of hip arthroscopy in pediatric hip disease. In the largest consecutive case series of 54 hip arthroscopies for a variety of pediatric conditions, including isolated labral tear, LCP, labral tear after prior periacetabular osteotomy, spondyloepiphyseal dysplasia, SCFE, avascular necrosis, and osteochondral fracture, outcomes were good at 1 year [41]. Overall, there was significant improvement of the modified Harris hip score from 53 to 83 with 83% of patients improved after 1 year. The remaining is a summary of studies conducted in the pediatric population.

Hip Dysplasia

Hip dysplasia can lead to the development of osteoarthritis if left completely untreated. Frequently, hip dysplasia leads to pain from intra-articular pathology including torn hypertrophic labrums and chondral abnormalities (Fig. 29.5) [42, 43]. If left untreated, these intra-articular abnormalities can affect later acetabular realignment procedures [44, 45]. While there have been older reports on the efficacy of labral debridement improving 85% of dysplasia patients [46], recent data cautions against the role of labral debridement in the dysplastic hip as the sole surgery [47]. We and others have used arthroscopy as a useful adjunct to open surgery in order to evaluate the hip joint prior to an acetabular osteotomy [43]. The improved visibility of the cartilage and labrum allows for prognostic evaluation of the joint, and the choice of reconstructive or salvage procedure may be influenced by the diagnostic arthroscopy. Labral pathology, if present can

be addressed with a repair or debridement prior to osteotomy. Moreover, hip arthroscopy for labral debridement *after* hip dysplasia has been corrected by a periacetabular osteotomy has been shown to be useful [41].

Arthroscopy of the hip has also been reported in the management of dysplasia in children less than 2 years of age [48, 49]. The indication is an adjunct to closed reduction of the dysplastic hip. Arthroscopic debridement of the pulvinar and ligamentum teres allows for closed reduction of the dislocated hip without performing an open reduction. Additionally, the iliopsoas and transverse acetabular ligament can be released for further stabilization of the hip. We have no experience with these methods, but this appears to be a useful method in allowing a more minimally invasive surgery than a traditional open reduction.

Legg-Calve-Perthes Disease

Historically, the most common indication for hip arthroscopy in the pediatric and adolescent population has been in the case of Legg-Calve-Perthes disease, both for diagnosis of the severity of the disease and the removal of loose bodies [7, 50]. Gross reported on areas of flattening of the femoral head, fibrillation of the cartilage, and dilation of the vascular ring of the perichondrium in patients with LCP [3]. Suzuki et al. reported on a series of 19 children undergoing arthroscopy for LCP and showed pronounced synovial proliferation in the acetabular fossa and hypervascularity of the labrum and corresponding capsule. They postulated that the mass effect and hypervascularity add to the instability and femoral head coverage [8]. Bowen et al. described arthroscopic chondroplasty of the femoral head after skeletal maturity in patients with Legg-Calve-Perthes disease as children [9]. At this time, during active LCP disease, there is little indication for hip arthroscopy; however, adolescents and young adults can present with the long-term sequelae of LCP including labral and ligamentum teres tears, chondral damage, loose bodies, osteochondritis dissecans, and defects of the femoral head [7–9, 51]. Arthroscopy can address the chondral and labral issues, and osteoplasty of the femoral head-neck junction can be performed, but due to the magna and breva deformities of the proximal femur, it can be technically quite challenging.

Avascular Necrosis

Hip arthroscopy has also been used in avascular necrosis of the older patient for diagnostic staging and treatment of labral pathology and chondral damage. Hip arthroscopy has been particularly useful for the staging of the disease process and has been shown to be more accurate than MRI or plain radiographs [52, 53]. Kloen et al. noted anterosuperior

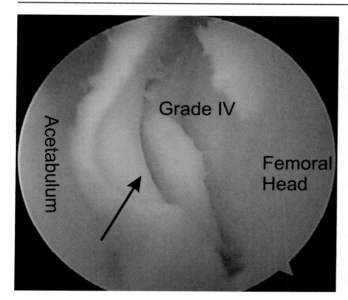

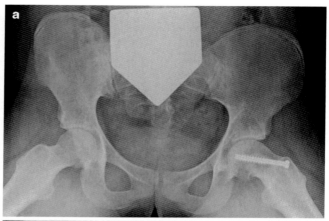

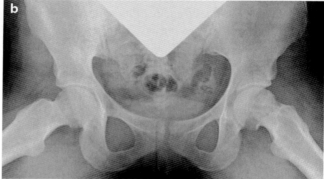

Fig. 29.6 Patient with spondyloepiphyseal dysplasia with multiple layers of delamination (onion-skinning) of the cartilage of the femoral head of a right hip. The camera is in the anterolateral portal. The chondral flaps are denoted with an *arrow*

flattening of the femoral heads in AVN resulting in cam impingement with lesions of the labrum and acetabular cartilage correlating to the cam lesion [54].

Epiphyseal Dysplasia

Multiple epiphyseal dysplasia and spondyloepiphyseal dysplasia can produce loose bodies and/or chondral flaps [43]. Arthroscopy can be useful to remove the loose bodies and debride the chondral flaps [41, 43] (Fig. 29.6). Additionally, avascular necrosis of the femoral head has been shown to occur in a large proportion of patients with epiphyseal dysplasia [55], which could lead to the same sequelae as LCP. McCarthy et al. also advocated the use of hip arthroscopy to treat the mechanical symptoms of early avascular necrosis including loose bodies, synovitis, chondral flaps, and labral tears [56].

Slipped Capital Femoral Epiphysis

In 1992, Futami et al. reviewed their experience with arthroscopy prior to in situ pinning for slipped capital femoral epiphysis. Due to the anterosuperior cartilage erosion and posterolateral labrum injury, Futami concluded that the pathomechanics of SCFE are traumatic in nature and that the arthroscopy was useful for diagnosis and decompression of the hematoma from the SCFE [6]. Using a three-dimensional computer model, Rab showed that the metaphyseal impingement of SCFE could erode the anterosuperior acetabular

Fig. 29.7 (**a**) Left hip SCFE that underwent in situ pinning with resultant cam lesion. (**b**) Removal of in situ screw and resection of cam lesion

cartilage and damage the posterolateral labrum [57]. In a study of surgical dislocation for the management of SCFE, Leunig et al. found a constant area of damage in the superomedial acetabulum with tears of the labrum and partial to full-thickness cartilage loss [58]. Oftentimes, the anterior femoral metaphysis is level or extends past the epiphysis which needs to be resected during the osteoplasty of the femoral head-neck junction. Our findings demonstrate similar changes at the time of arthroscopy as Leunig's findings. Arthroscopic cam decompression and the treatment of intra-articular lesions can be performed in mild to moderate slips (Fig. 29.7a, b). In severe deformity, a realignment osteotomy may be necessary with arthroscopy performed as an adjunct to the procedure [59].

Femoroacetabular Impingement (FAI)

FAI has become a common indication for hip arthroscopy in the adult population. Two distinct types of FAI, pincer and cam types, have been identified, with a mixed type occurring as well [60]. Philippon et al. have reported on the treatment of FAI in the athletic adolescent patient. 16 patients with a mean age of 15 were treated for idiopathic FAI. All had labral pathology and underwent arthroscopic rim trimming and limited femoral head-neck osteoplasty. The modified Harris hip scores increased from 55 to 90, while hip outcome score for activities of daily living and sports increased from 58 to 94 and 33 to 89, respectively. Mean patient satisfaction was 9 out of 10 at 1 year. While the standard for FAI has been open surgical dislocation, arthroscopic treatment has been increasing [61]. Both types of FAI are increasingly being recognized in the adolescent population, and we are routinely performing arthroscopic decompression with good success.

Septic Arthritis and Trauma

Arthroscopic lavage has been used for the treatment of septic arthritis, particularly in the pediatric age group. Two groups have reported good success with arthroscopic irrigation and debridement followed by medical therapy for treating hip infection [62, 63]. A recent comparative study of 20 hips treated with either open arthrotomy or arthroscopy followed by antibiotics showed no difference in outcome. Hospital stay was significantly shorter for the group that underwent arthroscopic management [64].

Loose bodies following hip dislocations have been described in adults [65–67], and hip arthroscopy has been used for removal of loose bodies in adults but has not been widely used in the pediatric population. Torn ligamentum teres, osteochondral fragments, and acetabular epiphysis-labrum entrapment have been reported as impediments to relocation [68–70]. Kashiwagi described a case of arthroscopic resection of the ligamentum teres following a traumatic hip dislocation in a 10-year-old [71]. In the pediatric age group, open arthrotomy has been recommended for incongruous reductions. Immediate use of hip arthroscopy may lead to excessive extravasation of fluid into the soft tissue or abdominal cavity because of the immense disruption of the hip capsule and surrounding tissues. The procedure for removal of loose bodies following dislocation is generally performed several weeks after the injury.

Conclusion

As the experience with hip arthroscopy expands, so, too, will the ability to recognize the various injury patterns to the chondral surfaces of the hip. Hip arthroscopy offers potential advantages over traditional open arthrotomy and surgical dislocation in terms of limited invasiveness and diminished morbidity. Most of the experience in hip arthroscopy has been with hip disorders in adults, the indications and results of hip arthroscopy in children and adolescents have been less well characterized. The pediatric hip has unique conditions, including Legg-Calve-Perthes disease, slipped capital femoral epiphysis, developmental dysplasia of the hip, septic arthritis, coxa vara, juvenile rheumatoid arthritis, and chondrolysis. Further development of hip arthroscopy in children and adolescents is necessary to refine indications, evaluate longer-term results, and develop pediatric-specific instrumentation.

References

1. Skinner HB, Scherger JE. Identifying structural hip and knee problems. Patient age, history, and limited examination may be all that's needed. Postgrad Med. 1999;106(7):51–2, 5–6, 61–4 passim.
2. Ganz R, Gill TJ, Gautier E, Ganz K, Krugel N, Berlemann U. Surgical dislocation of the adult hip a technique with full access to the femoral head and acetabulum without the risk of avascular necrosis. J Bone Joint Surg Br. 2001;83(8):1119–24.
3. Gross RH. Hip arthroscopy in the pediatric population. Orthop Rev. 1977;6:43–9.
4. Holgersson S, Brattstrom H, Mogensen B, Lidgren L. Arthroscopy of the hip in juvenile chronic arthritis. J Pediatr Orthop. 1981;1(3):273–8.
5. Rydholm U, Wingstrand H, Egund N, Elborg R, Forsberg L, Lidgren L. Sonography, arthroscopy, and intracapsular pressure in juvenile chronic arthritis of the hip. Acta Orthop Scand. 1986;57(4):295–8.
6. Futami T, Kasahara Y, Suzuki S, Seto Y, Ushikubo S. Arthroscopy for slipped capital femoral epiphysis. J Pediatr Orthop. 1992;12(5):592–7.
7. Kuklo TR, Mackenzie WG, Keeler KA. Hip arthroscopy in Legg-Calve-Perthes disease. Arthroscopy. 1999;15(1):88–92.
8. Suzuki S, Kasahara Y, Seto Y, Futami T, Furukawa K, Nishino Y. Arthroscopy in 19 children with Perthes' disease. Pathologic changes of the synovium and the joint surface. Acta Orthop Scand. 1994;65(6):581–4.
9. Bowen JR, Kumar VP, Joyce 3rd JJ, Bowen JC. Osteochondritis dissecans following Perthes' disease. Arthroscopic-operative treatment. Clin Orthop Relat Res. 1986;209:49–56.
10. Schindler A, Lechevallier JJ, Rao NS, Bowen JR. Diagnostic and therapeutic arthroscopy of the hip in children and adolescents: evaluation of results. J Pediatr Orthop. 1995;15(3):317–21.
11. Dorfmann H, Boyer T. Arthroscopy of the hip: 12 years of experience. Arthroscopy. 1999;15(1):67–72.
12. Ponseti IV. Growth and development of the acetabulum in the normal child. Anatomical, histological, and roentgenographic studies. J Bone Joint Surg Am. 1978;60(5):575–85.
13. Portinaro NM, Murray DW, Benson MK. Microanatomy of the acetabular cavity and its relation to growth. J Bone Joint Surg Br. 2001;83(3):377–83.
14. Zander G. "Os acetabuli" and other bone nuclei, periarticular calcifications at the hip joint. Acta Radiol. 1943;24:317–27.
15. Iwersen LJ, Kalen V, Eberle C. Relative trochanteric overgrowth after ischemic necrosis in congenital dislocation of the hip. J Pediatr Orthop. 1989;9(4):381–5.
16. Siffert RS. Patterns of deformity of the developing hip. Clin Orthop Relat Res. 1981;160:14–29.
17. Byrd JW. Hip arthroscopy: patient assessment and indications. Instr Course Lect. 2003;52:711–9.
18. Domb BG, Brooks AG, Byrd JW. Clinical examination of the hip joint in athletes. J Sport Rehabil. 2009;18(1):3–23.
19. Kocher MS, Zurakowski D, Kasser JR. Differentiating between septic arthritis and transient synovitis of the hip in children: an evidence-based clinical prediction algorithm. J Bone Joint Surg Am. 1999;81(12):1662–70.
20. DeAngelis NA, Busconi BD. Assessment and differential diagnosis of the painful hip. Clin Orthop Relat Res. 2003;406:11–8.

21. McCarthy JC. The diagnosis and treatment of labral and chondral injuries. Instr Course Lect. 2004;53:573–7.

22. Clohisy JC, Carlisle JC, Beaule PE, et al. A systematic approach to the plain radiographic evaluation of the young adult hip. J Bone Joint Surg Am. 2008;90 Suppl 4:47–66.

23. Pessis E, Chevrot A, Drape JL, et al. Study of the joint space of the hip on supine and weight-bearing digital radiographs. Clin Radiol. 1999;54(8):528–32.

24. Lequesne MG, Laredo JD. The faux profile (oblique view) of the hip in the standing position. Contribution to the evaluation of osteoarthritis of the adult hip. Ann Rheum Dis. 1998;57(11):676–81.

25. Newberg AH, Newman JS. Imaging the painful hip. Clin Orthop Relat Res. 2003;406:19–28.

26. Keeney JA, Peelle MW, Jackson J, Rubin D, Maloney WJ, Clohisy JC. Magnetic resonance arthrography versus arthroscopy in the evaluation of articular hip pathology. Clin Orthop Relat Res. 2004;429:163–9.

27. Czerny C, Hofmann S, Neuhold A, et al. Lesions of the acetabular labrum: accuracy of MR imaging and MR arthrography in detection and staging. Radiology. 1996;200(1):225–30.

28. Mintz DN, Hooper T, Connell D, Buly R, Padgett DE, Potter HG. Magnetic resonance imaging of the hip: detection of labral and chondral abnormalities using noncontrast imaging. Arthroscopy. 2005;21(4):385–93.

29. Domayer SE, Mamisch TC, Kress I, Chan J, Kim YJ. Radial dGEMRIC in developmental dysplasia of the hip and in femoroacetabular impingement: preliminary results. Osteoarthritis Cartilage. 2010;18(11):1421–8.

30. Bittersohl B, Hosalkar HS, Haamberg T, et al. Reproducibility of dGEMRIC in assessment of hip joint cartilage: a prospective study. J Magn Reson Imaging. 2009;30(1):224–8.

31. Bittersohl B, Hosalkar HS, Kim YJ, Werlen S, Siebenrock KA, Mamisch TC. Delayed gadolinium-enhanced magnetic resonance imaging (dGEMRIC) of hip joint cartilage in femoroacetabular impingement (FAI): are pre- and postcontrast imaging both necessary? Magn Reson Med. 2009;62(6):1362–7.

32. Byrd JW. Hip arthroscopy utilizing the supine position. Arthroscopy. 1994;10(3):275–80.

33. Glick JM, Sampson TG, Gordon RB, Behr JT, Schmidt E. Hip arthroscopy by the lateral approach. Arthroscopy. 1987;3(1):4–12.

34. Kaplan LD, Ernsthausen JM, Bradley JP, Fu FH, Farkas DL. The thermal field of radiofrequency probes at chondroplasty settings. Arthroscopy. 2003;19(6):632–40.

35. Lu Y, Edwards 3rd RB, Cole BJ, Markel MD. Thermal chondroplasty with radiofrequency energy. An in vitro comparison of bipolar and monopolar radiofrequency devices. Am J Sports Med. 2001;29(1):42–9.

36. Crawford K, Philippon MJ, Sekiya JK, Rodkey WG, Steadman JR. Microfracture of the hip in athletes. Clin Sports Med. 2006;25(2):327–35, x.

37. Steadman JR, Miller BS, Karas SG, Schlegel TF, Briggs KK, Hawkins RJ. The microfracture technique in the treatment of full-thickness chondral lesions of the knee in national football league players. J Knee Surg. 2003;16(2):83–6.

38. Steadman JR, Rodkey WG, Rodrigo JJ. Microfracture: surgical technique and rehabilitation to treat chondral defects. Clin Orthop Relat Res. 2001 Oct; (391 Suppl):S362–9.

39. Stalzer S, Wahoff M, Scanlan M. Rehabilitation following hip arthroscopy. Clin Sports Med. 2006;25(2):337–57.

40. Nwachukwu BU, McFeely ED, Nasreddine AY, Krcik JA, Frank J, Kocher MS. Complications of hip arthroscopy in children and adolescents. J Pediatr Orthop. 2011;31(3):227–31.

41. Kocher MS, Kim YJ, Millis MB, et al. Hip arthroscopy in children and adolescents. J Pediatr Orthop. 2005;25(5):680–6.

42. Fujii M, Nakashima Y, Jingushi S, et al. Intraarticular findings in symptomatic developmental dysplasia of the hip. J Pediatr Orthop. 2009;29(1):9–13.

43. Roy DR. Arthroscopy of the hip in children and adolescents. J Child Orthop. 2009;3(2):89–100.

44. Byrd JW, Jones KS. Hip arthroscopy in the presence of dysplasia. Arthroscopy. 2003;19(10):1055–60.

45. Ilizaliturri Jr VM, Chaidez PA, Valero FS, Aguilera JM. Hip arthroscopy after previous acetabular osteotomy for developmental dysplasia of the hip. Arthroscopy. 2005;21(2):176–81.

46. McCarthy JC, Mason JB, Wardell SR. Hip arthroscopy for acetabular dysplasia: a pipe dream? Orthopedics. 1998;21(9):977–9.

47. Parvizi J, Bican O, Bender B, et al. Arthroscopy for labral tears in patients with developmental dysplasia of the hip: a cautionary note. J Arthroplasty. 2009;24(6 Suppl):110–3.

48. Bulut O, Ozturk H, Tezeren G, Bulut S. Arthroscopic-assisted surgical treatment for developmental dislocation of the hip. Arthroscopy. 2005;21(5):574–9.

49. McCarthy JJ, MacEwen GD. Hip arthroscopy for the treatment of children with hip dysplasia: a preliminary report. Orthopedics. 2007;30(4):262–4.

50. McCarthy RE. Avascular necrosis of the femoral head in children. Instr Course Lect. 1988;37:59–65.

51. Roy DR. Arthroscopic findings of the hip in new onset hip pain in adolescents with previous Legg-Calve-Perthes disease. J Pediatr Orthop B. 2005;14(3):151–5.

52. Ruch DS, Sekiya J, Dickson Schaefer W, Koman LA, Pope TL, Poehling GG. The role of hip arthroscopy in the evaluation of avascular necrosis. Orthopedics. 2001;24(4):339–43.

53. Sekiya JK, Ruch DS, Hunter DM, et al. Hip arthroscopy in staging avascular necrosis of the femoral head. J South Orthop Assoc. 2000;9(4):254–61.

54. Kloen P, Leunig M, Ganz R. Early lesions of the labrum and acetabular cartilage in osteonecrosis of the femoral head. J Bone Joint Surg Br. 2002;84(1):66–9.

55. Mackenzie WG, Bassett GS, Mandell GA, Scott Jr CI. Avascular necrosis of the hip in multiple epiphyseal dysplasia. J Pediatr Orthop. 1989;9(6):666–71.

56. McCarthy J, Puri L, Barsoum W, Lee JA, Laker M, Cooke P. Articular cartilage changes in avascular necrosis: an arthroscopic evaluation. Clin Orthop Relat Res. 2003;406:64–70.

57. Rab GT. The geometry of slipped capital femoral epiphysis: implications for movement, impingement, and corrective osteotomy. J Pediatr Orthop. 1999;19(4):419–24.

58. Leunig M, Casillas MM, Hamlet M, et al. Slipped capital femoral epiphysis: early mechanical damage to the acetabular cartilage by a prominent femoral metaphysis. Acta Orthop Scand. 2000;71(4):370–5.

59. Akkari M, Santili C, Braga SR, Polesello GC. Trapezoidal bony correction of the femoral neck in the treatment of severe acute-on-chronic slipped capital femoral epiphysis. Arthroscopy. 2010;26(11):1489–95.

60. Ganz R, Parvizi J, Beck M, Leunig M, Notzli H, Siebenrock KA. Femoroacetabular impingement: a cause for osteoarthritis of the hip. Clin Orthop Relat Res. 2003;417:112–20.

61. Peters CL, Erickson JA. Treatment of femoro-acetabular impingement with surgical dislocation and debridement in young adults. J Bone Joint Surg Am. 2006;88(8):1735–41.

62. Chung WK, Slater GL, Bates EH. Treatment of septic arthritis of the hip by arthroscopic lavage. J Pediatr Orthop. 1993;13(4):444–6.

63. Kim SJ, Choi NH, Ko SH, Linton JA, Park HW. Arthroscopic treatment of septic arthritis of the hip. Clin Orthop Relat Res. 2003;407:211–4.

64. El-Sayed AM. Treatment of early septic arthritis of the hip in children: comparison of results of open arthrotomy versus arthroscopic drainage. J Child Orthop. 2008;2(3):229–37.

65. Mullis BH, Dahners LE. Hip arthroscopy to remove loose bodies after traumatic dislocation. J Orthop Trauma. 2006;20(1):22–6.

66. Owens BD, Busconi BD. Arthroscopy for hip dislocation and fracture-dislocation. Am J Orthop. 2006;35(12):584–7.

67. Svoboda SJ, Williams DM, Murphy KP. Hip arthroscopy for osteochondral loose body removal after a posterior hip dislocation. Arthroscopy. 2003;19(7):777–81.

68. Barrett IR, Goldberg JA. Avulsion fracture of the ligamentum teres in a child. A case report. J Bone Joint Surg Am. 1989;71(3):438–9.

69. Olsson O, Landin LA, Johansson A. Traumatic hip dislocation with spontaneous reduction and capsular interposition. A report of 2 children. Acta Orthop Scand. 1994;65(4):476–9.

70. Shea KP, Kalamchi A, Thompson GH. Acetabular epiphysis-labrum entrapment following traumatic anterior dislocation of the hip in children. J Pediatr Orthop. 1986;6(2):215–9.

71. Kashiwagi N, Suzuki S, Seto Y. Arthroscopic treatment for traumatic hip dislocation with avulsion fracture of the ligamentum teres. Arthroscopy. 2001;17(1):67–9.

Complex Hip Reconstruction

30

Trevor R. Gaskill and Marc J. Philippon

Introduction

Arthroscopic management of hip disorders continues to be a rapidly progressing subspecialty within orthopedic sports medicine. Over the past decade, the most common indication for arthroscopic hip surgery has been for diagnostic or debridement procedures. More recently, it has been recognized that hip disorders are a significant cause of disability in active, young adult patients [1–6].

Currently, it is common practice at many centers to repair labral tissue, address cartilage injuries, and perform bony osteoplasties. The structural significance of the ligamentum teres and hip capsule to femoroacetabular stability [7–10] is also gaining recognition. Early clinical evidence suggests these techniques may result in improved outcomes, as compared to simple debridement procedures [11–16].

As knowledge regarding structural deficiencies of the hip increases, innovative reconstructive techniques are beginning to emerge [11, 12, 17, 18]. These surgical procedures allow difficult hip pathologies to be treated, which may have otherwise gone untreated due to limited surgical alternatives. These techniques include reconstruction of deficient labral tissue, femoroacetabular microfracture, osteochondral transplantation, and capsular or ligamentum teres reconstruction. The early results of these complex reconstructive techniques are encouraging in the properly indicated patient. This chapter provides an overview of the rationale, indications, and surgical technique for these reconstructive procedures of the hip.

Iliotibial Band Labral Reconstruction

The function of the acetabular labrum remains to be fully understood; however, it appears to play a critical role in hip biomechanics and stability [19–22]. Several studies suggest that the labrum is capable of forming a seal with the femoral head [20–22]. Moreover, the loss of this seal results in a greater efflux of fluid into the peripheral space resulting in a significant increase in the rate of cartilage compression [20]. This increases contact stress seen by the cartilage by as much as 92% in cadaveric models [20]. It is thought that this may lead to an increased coefficient of friction in the hip and could contribute to premature cartilage degeneration [2, 20]. The loss of the normal suction seal may additionally lead to femoroacetabular microinstability, thereby compounding the biomechanical implications of labral damage [19]. For these reasons, greater attention is being placed on repair of labral tears.

Though prospective randomized studies do not exist, early clinical data is beginning to suggest that patients experience superior outcomes with labral preservation as opposed to debridement [5, 23, 24]. In some circumstances, however, the presence of a severely degenerative labrum, complex tear pattern, or segmental deficiency precludes standard labral repair. Moreover, some patients continue to experience pain after subtotal or total labrectomy. For these reasons, we typically recommend labral reconstruction to help restore this important labral anatomy [11, 12].

Technique

(See Video 30.1: http://goo.gl/0X5K1) A standard preparation and draping is performed with the patient in a modified supine position. Two standard arthroscopic portals are utilized

Research performed at the Steadman Philippon Research Institute, Vail, CO, USA.

T.R. Gaskill, M.D.
Bone & Joint Sports Medicine Institute, Naval Medical Center Portsmouth, 620 John Paul Jones Circle, Portsmouth, VA 23708, USA

Steadman Philippon Research Institute, The Steadman Clinic, Vail, CO, USA
e-mail: gaski011@gmail.com

M.J. Philippon, M.D. (✉)
Department of Hip Arthroscopy, Steadman Philippon Research Institute and Steadman Clinic, 181 West Meadow Dr. Suite 1000, Vail, CO 81657, USA
e-mail: mjp@sprivail.org, drphilippon@sprivail.org

J.W.T. Byrd (ed.), *Operative Hip Arthroscopy*,
DOI 10.1007/978-1-4419-7925-4_30, © Springer Science+Business Media New York 2013

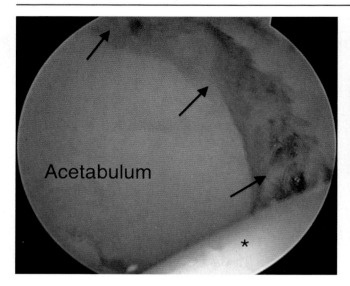

Fig. 30.1 Arthroscopic image of right hip viewing from the anterolateral peritrochanteric portal in the supine position. Note absence of labrum from the 12 o'clock to 3 o'clock positions (*arrows*). Acetabulum and femoral head (*) can also be visualized

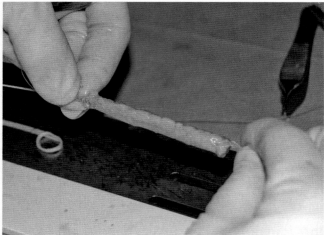

Fig. 30.2 Intraoperative photograph of prepared iliotibial band graft after tubularization with heavy absorbable suture

including the anterolateral peritrochanteric portal and the mid-anterior portal. A complete diagnostic arthroscopy is performed, and all concomitant pathology is treated. If the labrum is deemed irreparable, its remnant is resected to robust, stable borders. The magnitude of labral deficiency is then assessed, and the acetabular rim is prepared using a mechanical burr (see Fig. 30.1). It is typical for 1–3 cm of labral tissue to be deficient in these cases.

The arthroscope is removed from the hip and traction is released. Through an additional skin incision just distal to the anterolateral portal, a segment of iliotibial band (15 mm wide) is removed from the junction of the central and posterior thirds of the tendon. The length of the graft should be 30% longer than the measured labral defect. A trochanteric bursectomy is performed, and the iliotibial band is closed using absorbable sutures. Internal and external rotation of the hip is done to confirm snapping does not occur secondary to the graft harvest.

The graft is then tubularized with heavy absorbable sutures to encourage host tissue incorporation into the graft after it has been cleared of any muscular or fatty tissue (see Fig. 30.2). If a 15-mm graft width is used, tubularization typically results in a 7–8-mm-diameter graft. A suture loop is placed on one end of the graft to facilitate intra-articular orientation and fixation. The hip is placed back into traction, and a suture anchor is placed at the anterior and posterior extents of the labral deficiency. A suture from the anterior anchor is delivered through an arthroscopic cannula placed through the mid-anterior portal. This suture is passed through the anterior portion of the graft using a free needle ex vivo. An arthroscopic knot pusher is then utilized to advance the graft into the hip, orient it along the deficient acetabular

segment, and secure it into place anteromedially. Similarly, a suture from the posterior anchor is passed through the suture loop using a grasping device and subsequently secured. Additional anchors are placed at 1 cm intervals to secure the central portion of the graft. To achieve a congruent fit with the femoral head and neck, sutures are placed through or around the graft to appropriately evert it.

As with any labral repair, traction is released, and dynamic examination of hip motion is done. If the labral graft is not well approximated to the femoral head or is lifted by femoral neck bony dysmorphology, anchor fixation or the femoral neck osteoplasty is revisited. It is our goal for the reconstructed labrum and femoral head-neck junction to represent a smooth, congruent relationship throughout all ranges of motion (see Fig. 30.3). A routine capsular closure or plication is then performed based on clinical evaluation of capsular laxity.

Clinical Results

To date, we have performed more than 200 labral reconstructions for deficient or irreparable labral injuries (see Fig. 30.4). In an early series of 47 patients, Philippon et al. reported a significant improvement in Modified Harris Hip Scores at 1-year follow-up [11]. Mean patient satisfaction was an eight, on a scale of 1–10, with ten being very satisfied. Increased age and joint space less than 2 mm were found to be independent risk factors for less optimal outcomes. Sierra et al. have also reported labral reconstruction during surgical hip dislocation using ligamentum teres capitis in a series of five patients [13]. No complications were reported, and clinical function was improved after a minimum of 5 months' follow-up. These data indicate labral reconstruction may be a viable alternative to labral debridement in appropriately selected patients; however, long-term follow-up and further biomechanical research is still necessary.

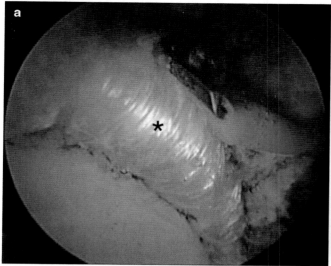

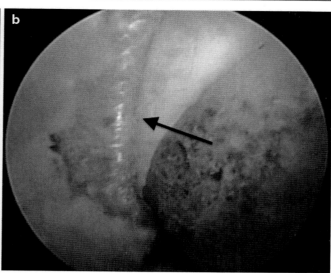

Fig. 30.3 Arthroscopic image of a right hip viewing from the antero-lateral peritrochanteric portal in the supine position. Completed iliotibial band labral reconstruction (*) is shown after it has been secured to the acetabulum (**a**) and demonstrating satisfactory conformity (*arrow*) to the femoral head (**b**)

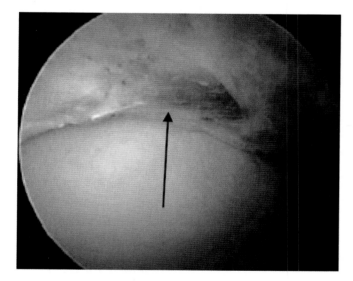

Fig. 30.4 Arthroscopic image of a right hip viewing from the antero-lateral peritrochanteric portal in the supine position. The reconstructed labrum is visualized 1 year from index procedure (*arrow*)

Ligamentum Teres Reconstruction

The role of the ligamentum teres remains controversial. It is recognized as an important vascular supply to the femoral head in the skeletally immature patients [25]. However, it is traditionally viewed as a vestigial remnant with no biomechanical or vascular role in the adult hip and is routinely sacrificed during open surgical dislocations [7, 10, 26].

More recent evidence, however, suggests that the ligamentum teres is a potential source of hip pain and may provide some degree of mechanical stability to the hip [10]. Recently, a porcine model found the ligamentum teres to have a tensile strength similar to that of the anterior cruciate ligament [27]. Therefore, it may be an important femoroacetabular stabilizer in flexion, adduction, and internal rotation [7]. Histologically, the ligamentum teres also appears to undergo degenerative changes similar to those seen in other tendons, which may indicate similar loading patterns [28]. It has been transferred clinically as an adjunct to open relocation of the dislocated pediatric hip with promising early results [29]. Each of these findings suggests that the ligamentum teres may represent more than a vestigial remnant.

The diagnosis of a ligamentum teres tear remains a difficult clinical diagnosis since distinction from other sources of intra-articular hip pain is complicated. Though the mechanism of injury is unclear, the ligamentum teres is reported to be abnormal in approximately 4–15% of sports-related hip arthroscopic procedures [7, 9, 30]. Ligamentum teres injuries are also an elusive radiologic diagnosis. In a series of 23 hips with arthroscopically proven ligamentum teres ruptures, only 39% (9/23) were prospectively identified [30]. For this reason, an injury to the ligamentum teres is currently best diagnosed arthroscopically.

Partial tearing of the ligamentum teres is managed with selective radio-frequency ablation or debridement [30]. We believe the ligamentum teres to be an important stabilizer of the femoroacetabular joint in patients capable of extreme motion arcs such as ballet dancers. To this end, it is intuitive that acetabular containment must be decreased compared to normal hips for these extremes of motion to be possible. Therefore, the hip may become more dependent on soft tissue structures for stability, which is in some ways analogous to the glenohumeral joint. If this patient population exhibits the acute onset of symptoms, femoroacetabular instability on

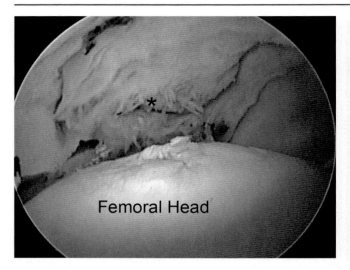

Fig. 30.5 Intraoperative image of a right hip viewing from the antero-lateral peritrochanteric portal of a right hip in the supine position. Note the absence of the ligamentum teres in cotyloid fossa (*)

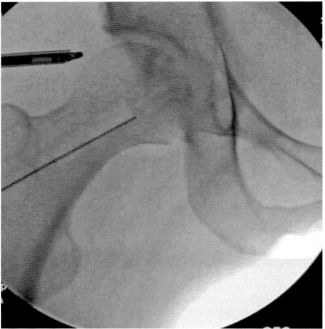

Fig. 30.6 Intraoperative fluoroscopic image of a right hip demonstrating guide pin placement for ligamentum teres reconstruction. The guide pin should exit within the femoral fovea as confirmed arthroscopically

clinical examination, a ruptured ligamentum teres, and fails nonsurgical measures, a ligamentum teres reconstruction may be required. If femoroacetabular impingement or labral damage is present concomitantly, it is our practice to treat this pathology first. Reconstruction of the ligamentum teres should be undertaken if symptoms persist after labral repair.

Technique

A standard preparation and draping is performed with the patient in a modified beach chair position. Typical anterolateral peritrochanteric and mid-anterior portals are established and diagnostic arthroscopy performed. After confirmation of ligamentum teres rupture, the remnant ligament is resected (see Fig. 30.5). Similar to arthroscopic labral reconstruction, an iliotibial band graft is harvested from the junction of its middle and posterior thirds. A typical graft measures 15 mm in width by 50 mm in length and is tubularized using heavy absorbable suture. If adequate iliotibial band is not available we have utilized tibialis anterior allograft.

Under fluoroscopic visualization a 2-mm guide wire is placed through the femoral neck in a retrograde fashion to exit at the center of the fovea capitis as confirmed arthroscopically (see Fig. 30.6). An 8-mm femoral tunnel is then reamed. Through this tunnel, a double-loaded 2.9-mm anchor is placed in the ligamentum teres footprint, and sutures are retrieved through an arthroscopic cannula in the mid-anterior portal. These sutures are passed through one end of the prepared graft, and it is shuttled into the joint and secured to the cotyloid fossa (see Fig. 30.7). The distal end of the graft is then passed into the femoral tunnel using shuttling sutures.

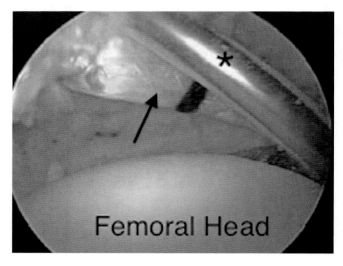

Fig. 30.7 Arthroscopic image of a right hip viewing from the antero-lateral peritrochanteric portal in the supine position. The iliotibial band ligamentum teres graft (*arrow*) is sutured to the cotyloid fossa using an arthroscopic knot pusher (*)

Graft tensioning occurs in the position of hip external rotation and extension, leaving approximately 2.5 cm within the joint. The femoral portion of the graft is secured within the tunnel using a 9-mm by 30-mm interference screw (see Fig. 30.8).

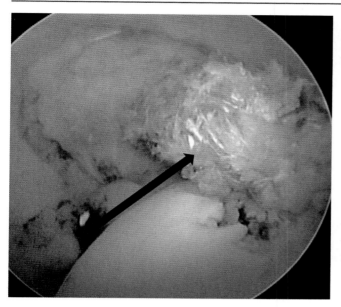

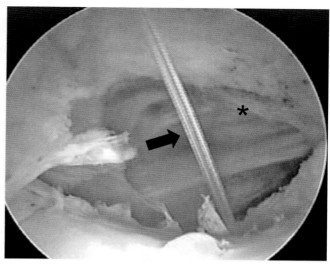

Fig. 30.8 Arthroscopic image of a right hip viewing from the antero-lateral peritrochanteric portal in the supine position. The completed ligamentum teres reconstruction (*arrow*) is visualized

Fig. 30.9 Arthroscopic image of a right hip viewing from the antero-lateral peritrochanteric portal in the supine position. A large anterior capsular deficiency (*) is noted in a patient with hip instability. The initial suture anchor (*arrow*) along the anterior acetabular rim has been placed (*arrow*)

Clinical Results

Only one published case, to our knowledge, exists describing the clinical outcome of a ligamentum teres reconstruction [17]. In this case, an artificial graft was utilized to reconstruct the ligamentum teres in a 20-year-old dancer with symptomatic hip instability. This was anchored within the acetabulum using a button-type device and a femoral interference screw. This successfully eliminated preoperative symptoms, however, resulted in a decrease in external rotation to 50% of the contralateral hip. At 8 months' follow-up, the patient's non-arthritic hip score improved from 42 to 89 points. We have performed a similar reconstruction in four patients and have anecdotally seen satisfactory results with respect to symptomatic resolution and patient satisfaction scores. Though indications continue to be defined, these techniques may improve stability in appropriately selected patients. The potential loss of motion, however, should be discussed with the patient preoperatively.

Capsular Reconstruction

The hip capsule is an underappreciated yet critical structure to the innate stability of the hip. Specific focal thickenings of the hip capsule have been identified and help provide stability at the end ranges of motion [31–33]. These ligaments include the iliofemoral, pubofemoral, and ischiofemoral ligaments which restrict extension, abduction, and internal rotation, respectively [33]. The iliofemoral ligament is noted

to have a greater cross-sectional area and maximal failure load as compared to the ischiofemoral ligament [33]. Capsulotomies are capable of disrupting the iliofemoral ligament and may contribute to hip instability if not appropriately closed.

Symptomatic hip instability may also occur secondary to collagen disorders or traumatic events that damage these soft tissue restraints [34]. These patients typically experience apprehension in a flexed, abducted, and internally rotated position and often have a positive external rotation dial or axial traction apprehension test [35]. Under anesthesia with muscle relaxation, the hip is typically able to be distracted with manual axial traction. This creates a "vacuum sign" when viewed radiographically. When symptomatic, an arthroscopic or open capsular plication may be required to reduce redundant capsule. However, in cases where the capsular tissue is absent or would not support plication, a capsular reconstruction may be necessary.

Technique

A standard preparation and draping in the modified supine position is completed and standard anterolateral and mid-anterior portals are established. A diagnostic arthroscopy is performed noting any capsular deficiencies (see Fig. 30.9). The size of identified defects is noted, and iliotibial band is harvested from the junction of its posterior and middle thirds though a separate incision distal to the anterolateral portal.

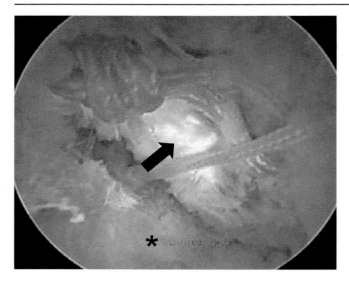

Fig. 30.10 Arthroscopic image of a right hip viewing form the antero-lateral peritrochanteric portal in the supine position. The completed capsular augmentation is visualized with graft in place (*arrow*). The acetabular rim is also visualized (*)

The graft is then cleaned of any muscular or fatty tissue and is passed through the mid-anterior portal into the hip joint. With the hip in traction, suture anchors are used to fix the iliotibial graft medially to the anterior acetabulum. The remainder of the graft is then sewn to the lateral remnant capsule using an interrupted suture technique, thereby augmenting the capsular defect (see Fig. 30.10). Anterior capsular reconstructions are tensioned in extension to prevent motion limitations.

Rehabilitation

Our standard hip rehabilitation protocol is utilized after each of these reconstructive procedures with few modifications. As with all arthroscopic hip procedures, immediate range of motion is initiated to prevent adhesion formation. Patients are allowed 20-lb flat-foot weight bearing and are instructed to use a continuous passive motion machine over the first two postoperative weeks. If microfracture is performed, the weight-bearing restrictions and continuous passive motion machine use is extended to 6–8 weeks, as dictated by the lesion size. This restriction is designed to minimize compression of the femoral head into the lesion while the marrow clot matures.

Anti-rotational bands are routinely utilized for the first 14–21 days to protect our capsular closure or plication. If a ligamentum teres reconstruction is completed, external rotation is limited for a minimum of 21 days using a Bledsoe hip brace and de-rotational bands. Patients also are prescribed 2 weeks of indomethacin to prevent heterotopic bone formation. Similarly, hip extension and external rotation past neutral are not allowed for 6–12 weeks after a capsular reconstruction is performed.

Passive hip circumduction remains a critical portion of all postoperative rehabilitation programs and has resulted in a considerable decrease in adhesion formation. After passive motion is maximized, active motion and strength conditioning begin. Rehabilitation is continued until good pelvic stability and normalized gait are achieved.

Acknowledgements No financial support in the form of grants, equipment, or other items was received in relation to the completion of this work.

Vail Valley Medical Center IRB approval (PRO# 2002–03) was received for completion of this manuscript.

References

1. Clohisy JC, Knaus ER, Hunt DM, et al. Clinical presentation of patients with symptomatic anterior hip impingement. Clin Orthop Relat Res. 2009;467:638–44.
2. Ganz R, Parvizi J, Beck M, et al. Femoroacetabular impingement: a cause for osteoarthritis of the hip. Clin Orthop Relat Res. 2003;417:112–20.
3. Larson CM, Giveans MR. Arthroscopic management of femoroacetabular impingement: early outcomes measures. Arthroscopy. 2008;24:540–6.
4. Parvizi J, Leunig M, Ganz R. Femoroacetabular impingement. J Am Acad Orthop Surg. 2007;15:561–70.
5. Philippon MJ, Briggs KK, Yen YM, et al. Outcomes following hip arthroscopy for femoroacetabular impingement with associated chondrolabral dysfunction: minimum two-year follow-up. J Bone Joint Surg Br. 2009;91:16–23.
6. Philippon MJ, Maxwell RB, Johnston TL, et al. Clinical presentation of femoroacetabular impingement. Knee Surg Sports Traumatol Arthrosc. 2007;15:1041–7.
7. Cerezal L, Kassarjian A, Canga A, et al. Anatomy, biomechanics, imaging, and management of ligamentum teres injuries. Radiographics. 2010;30:1637–51.
8. Kashiwagi N, Suzuki S, Seto Y. Arthroscopic treatment for traumatic hip dislocation with avulsion fracture of the ligamentum teres. Arthroscopy. 2001;17:67–9.
9. Rao J, Zhou YX, Villar RN. Injury to the ligamentum teres. Mechanism, findings, and results of treatment. Clin Sports Med. 2001;20:791–9, vii.
10. Bardakos NV, Villar RN. The ligamentum teres of the adult hip. J Bone Joint Surg Br. 2009;91:8–15.
11. Philippon MJ, Briggs KK, Hay CJ, et al. Arthroscopic labral reconstruction in the hip using iliotibial band autograft: technique and early outcomes. Arthroscopy. 2010;26:750–6.
12. Philippon MJ, Schroder e Souza BG, Briggs KK. Labrum: resection, repair and reconstruction sports medicine and arthroscopy review. Sports Med Arthrosc. 2010;18:76–82.
13. Sierra RJ, Trousdale RT. Labral reconstruction using the ligamentum teres capitis: report of a new technique. Clin Orthop Relat Res. 2009;467:753–9.
14. Philippon MJ, Schenker ML, Briggs KK, et al. Can microfracture produce repair tissue in acetabular chondral defects? Arthroscopy. 2008;24:46–50.
15. Meyers MH. Resurfacing of the femoral head with fresh osteochondral allografts. Long-term results. Clin Orthop Relat Res. 1985;197:111–4.
16. Evans KN, Providence BC. Case report: fresh-stored osteochondral allograft for treatment of osteochondritis dissecans the femoral head. Clin Orthop Relat Res. 2010;468:613–8.

17. Simpson JM, Field RE, Villar RN. Arthroscopic reconstruction of the ligamentum teres. Arthroscopy. 2011;27:436–41.

18. Crawford K, Philippon MJ, Sekiya JK, et al. Microfracture of the hip in athletes. Clin Sports Med. 2006;25:327–35.

19. Crawford MJ, Dy CJ, Alexander JW, et al. The 2007 Frank Stinchfield Award. The biomechanics of the hip labrum and the stability of the hip. Clin Orthop Relat Res. 2007;465:16–22.

20. Ferguson SJ, Bryant JT, Ganz R, et al. An in vitro investigation of the acetabular labral seal in hip joint mechanics. J Biomech. 2003;36:171–8.

21. Ferguson SJ, Bryant JT, Ganz R, et al. The influence of the acetabular labrum on hip joint cartilage consolidation: a poroelastic finite element model. J Biomech. 2000;33:953–60.

22. Ferguson SJ, Bryant JT, Ganz R, et al. The acetabular labrum seal: a poroelastic finite element model. Clin Biomech (Bristol, Avon). 2000;15:463–8.

23. Espinosa N, Beck M, Rothenfluh DA, et al. Treatment of femoroacetabular impingement: preliminary results of labral refixation. Surgical technique. J Bone Joint Surg Am. 2007;89(Suppl 2 Pt.1): 36–53.

24. Byrd JW, Jones KS. Hip arthroscopy for labral pathology: prospective analysis with 10-year follow-up. Arthroscopy. 2009;25:365–8.

25. Trueta J. The normal vascular anatomy of the human femoral head during growth. J Bone Joint Surg Br. 1957;39:358–94.

26. Kapandji IA. The physiology of the ligamentum teres. In: Kapandji IA, editor. The physiology of the joints, vol. 2. 2nd ed. New York: Churchill Livingstone; 1978.

27. Wenger D, Miyanji F, Mahar A, et al. The mechanical properties of the ligamentum teres: a pilot study to assess its potential for improving stability in children's hip surgery. J Pediatr Orthop. 2007;27:408–10.

28. Sampatchalit S, Barbosa D, Gentili A, et al. Degenerative changes in the ligamentum teres of the hip: cadaveric study with magnetic resonance arthrography, anatomical inspection, and histologic examination. J Comput Assist Tomogr. 2009;33:927–33.

29. Wenger DR, Mubarak SJ, Henderson PC, et al. Ligamentum teres maintenance and transfer as a stabilizer in open reduction for pediatric hip dislocation: surgical technique and early clinical results. J Child Orthop. 2008;2:177–85.

30. Byrd JW, Jones KS. Traumatic rupture of the ligamentum teres as a source of hip pain. Arthroscopy. 2004;20:385–91.

31. Hewitt J, Guilak F, Glisson R, et al. Regional material properties of the human hip joint capsule ligaments. J Orthop Res. 2001;19: 359–64.

32. Hewitt JD, Glisson RR, Guilak F, et al. The mechanical properties of the human hip capsule ligaments. J Arthroplasty. 2002;17: 82–9.

33. Philippon MJ. The role of arthroscopic thermal capsulorrhaphy in the hip. Clin Sports Med. 2001;20:817–29.

34. Bellabarba C, Sheinkop MB, Kuo KN. Idiopathic hip instability. An unrecognized cause of coxa saltans in the adult. Clin Orthop Relat Res. 1998;355:261–71.

35. Philippon MJ, Zehms CT, Briggs KK, et al. Hip instability in the athlete. Oper Tech Sports Med. 2007;15:189–94.

Compensatory Disorders Around the Hip

31

Sommer Hammoud, Erin Magennis, James E. Voos, Asheesh Bedi, and Bryan T. Kelly

Introduction

Evaluating the painful hip in the absence of osteoarthritis requires a comprehensive and detailed understanding of the potential underlying abnormal joint mechanics that predispose the hip joint and the associated hemipelvis to asymmetric loads. These asymmetric loads and abnormal joint kinematics secondary to underlying abnormal bony morphology can result in labral and cartilage injury, musculotendinous injury, as well as resultant injury to the neural structures about the hemipelvis. Without having a clear understanding of how mechanical factors can result in such a wide range of compensatory injury patterns about the hip, appropriate diagnosis and treatment recommendations cannot be made.

In order to help evaluate the painful hip in a comprehensive and systematic way, the senior author (BTK) has developed an algorithm to approach and understand these often complex compensatory problems. We describe it here as the "layered approach" to understanding the underlying etiologic factors contributing to pain around the hip joint and associated hemipelvis (Table 31.1). It begins with layer 1, which is the osteochondral layer. The structures within this layer are the femur, pelvis, and acetabulum. In the normal hip, these structures provide joint congruence and normal joint kinematics. Abnormalities within this layer can be subdivided into three distinct categories: (1) static overload, (2) dynamic impingement, and (3) dynamic instability. Structural variations resulting in static overload include lateral or anterior acetabular undercoverage/dysplasia, femoral anteversion, and femoral valgus. These structural mechanics lead to abnormal stress and asymmetric loads between the femoral head and acetabular socket in the axially loaded position (i.e., standing). Dynamic factors may contribute to hip pain as abnormal stress and contact between the femoral head and acetabular rim occur with hip motion. Different morphologies within layer 1 that may contribute to such dynamic impingement include FAI (cam and rim impingement), femoral retroversion, and femoral varus. When the functional range of motion required to compete in sports is greater than the amount of physiologic motion allowed by the hip, a compensatory increase in motion may be provided through layer 1. This involves increased motion and resultant stresses through the sacroiliac (SI) joint, pubic symphysis, and lumbar spine. When functional range of motion requirements are greater than physiological motion limits, forceful anterior contact occurring at the end range of internal rotation may lead to dynamic instability in the form of subtle posterior hip subluxation which occurs as the femoral head levers out of the hip socket [1].

These mechanical stresses lead to reactive hip pain related to insufficient congruency or impingement between the head and socket, leading to asymmetric wear of the chondral surfaces of the acetabulum and femoral head with or without associated instability of the hip. Thus, layer 1 has a direct effect on the inert layer of the hip or layer 2. Structures within the inert layer include the labrum, joint capsule, ligamentous complex, and ligamentum teres. These structures contribute

S. Hammoud, M.D.
Department of Sports Medicine, Massachusetts General Hospital, 175 Cambridge Street, Floor 4, 02114 Boston, MA, USA
e-mail: sommer.hammoud@gmail.com

E. Magennis, B.A. • B.T. Kelly, M.D. (✉)
Center for Hip Preservation, Hospital for Special Surgery, 525 East 70th Street, 10021 New York, NY, USA
e-mail: magennise@hss.edu; kellyb@hss.edu

J.E. Voos, M.D.
Department of Orthopaedic Surgery,
Orthopaedic and Sports Medicine Clinic of Kansas City,
3651 College Blvd., 66211 Leawood, KS, USA
e-mail: jvoos@osmckc.com

A. Bedi, M.D.
Sports Medicine and Shoulder Surgery,
Department of Orthopaedic Surgery, Hospital for Special Surgery,
24 Frank Lloyd Wright Drive, Lobby A,
48106 Ann Arbor, MI, USA

MedSport, Ann Arbor, MI, USA
e-mail: abedi@umich.edu

J.W.T. Byrd (ed.), *Operative Hip Arthroscopy*,
DOI 10.1007/978-1-4419-7925-4_31, © Springer Science+Business Media New York 2013

Table 31.1 Layered approach to clinical evaluation of the hip

Layers	Name	Structures	Purpose	Pathologies

Layer I	*Osteochondral layer*	Femur
		Pelvis
		Acetabulum
			Joint congruence and normal osteo/arthro kinematics	Dynamic Impingement
				    Cam, Rim, Femoral retroversion, Varus
				Static Overload
				    Acetabular undercoverage, femoral anteversion, femoral valgus
				Dynamic instability

Layer 2	*Inert layer*	Labrum Joint capsule Ligamentous complex Ligamentum teres	Static stability of the joint	Labral injury Ligamentum teres tear Capsular instability Adhesive capsulitis Ligament tears

Layer 3	*Contractile layer*	Peri-articular musculature
		Anterior structures
		Medial structures
		Posterior structures
		Lateral structures
		Lumbosacral and pelvic floor
			Dynamic stability of the hip, pelvis and trunk	Anterior
				    Rectus tendonopathy, Psoas, Sub-spine
				Medial
				    Adductor strain, Rectus strain, osteitis pubis
				Posterior
				    Proximal hamstring, Deep gluteal syndrome
				Lateral
				    Abductor tears; ITB syndrome; bursitis

Layer 4	*Neuromechanical layer*	Femoral nerve Lateral femoral cutaneous nerve Sciatic nerve Ilioinguinal nerve Genitofemoral nerve Pudendal Iliohypogastric nerve	Properly sequenced kinetic linking and appropriately balance neuromuscular control presence or absence of neuromechanical shortcomings	Pain syndromes Neuromuscular dysfunction Spinal referral patterns Nerve entrapments

to static stability of the hip joint. When abnormal mechanical stresses are applied to the hip joint secondary to underlying abnormalities within layer 1, pathologies such as labral injury, ligamentum teres tear, capsular instability, and various ligament tears can result. Direct injury to layer 2 structures can be predicted based upon the underlying structural mechanics of layer 1, combined with the forces that are generated through the joint and range of motion requirements of the joint that are specific to the activities that the athlete is engaged in.

Layer 3 is the contractile layer of the hip and hemipelvis. It comprises all musculature around the hemipelvis including the lumbosacral musculature and pelvic floor. This layer is responsible for the dynamic stability and muscular balance of the hip, pelvis, and trunk. Abnormal mechanics within layer 1 can lead to increased stresses of the SI joint, pubic symphysis, and ischium, and secondary increases in the strains imparted to the muscles that attach to these pelvic structures. Enthesopathies and/or tendinopathies can occur in a variety of periarticular muscular structures and can be subcategorized based upon their position relative to the hip joint (anterior, medial, posterior, and lateral). Anterior enthesopathy describes hip flexor strains, psoas impingement, and subspine impingement. Medial enthesopathy encompasses adductor and rectus tendinopathies which have traditionally been described within the realm of "sports hernia" or athletic pubalgia. Posterior

enthesopathies include mainly proximal hamstring strains but can also include injuries to the short external rotators including the piriformis and may involve a constellation of pain patterns described as "deep gluteal syndrome," which involves posterior soft tissue injury and irritation or compression of the sciatic nerve. Lateral enthesopathies involve the peritrochanteric space and injuries to the gluteus medius and minimus tendons. Specific patterns of pathology exist with certain layer 1 morphologic abnormalities associated with specific compensatory injury patterns within layer 3. One example is the classic male FAI pattern with large cam lesion and decreased internal rotation. The constellation of symptoms seen in patients with this common FAI pattern include decreased functional range of motion of the hip in flexion and internal rotation (layer 1), direct injury to the labrum and transition zone cartilage within the acetabulum (layer 2 injuries), and adductor enthesopathy and athletic pubalgia (medial enthesopathy, layer 3) (Fig. 31.1).

Layer 4 is the neurokinetic layer, including the thoracolumbosacral (TLS) plexus, lumbopelvic tissue, and lower extremity structures. This layer serves as the neuromuscular link and thus functional control of the entire segment as it functions within its environment. Compensatory injuries within this layer include nerve compression and pain syndromes, neuromuscular dysfunction, and spine referral patterns. Commonly

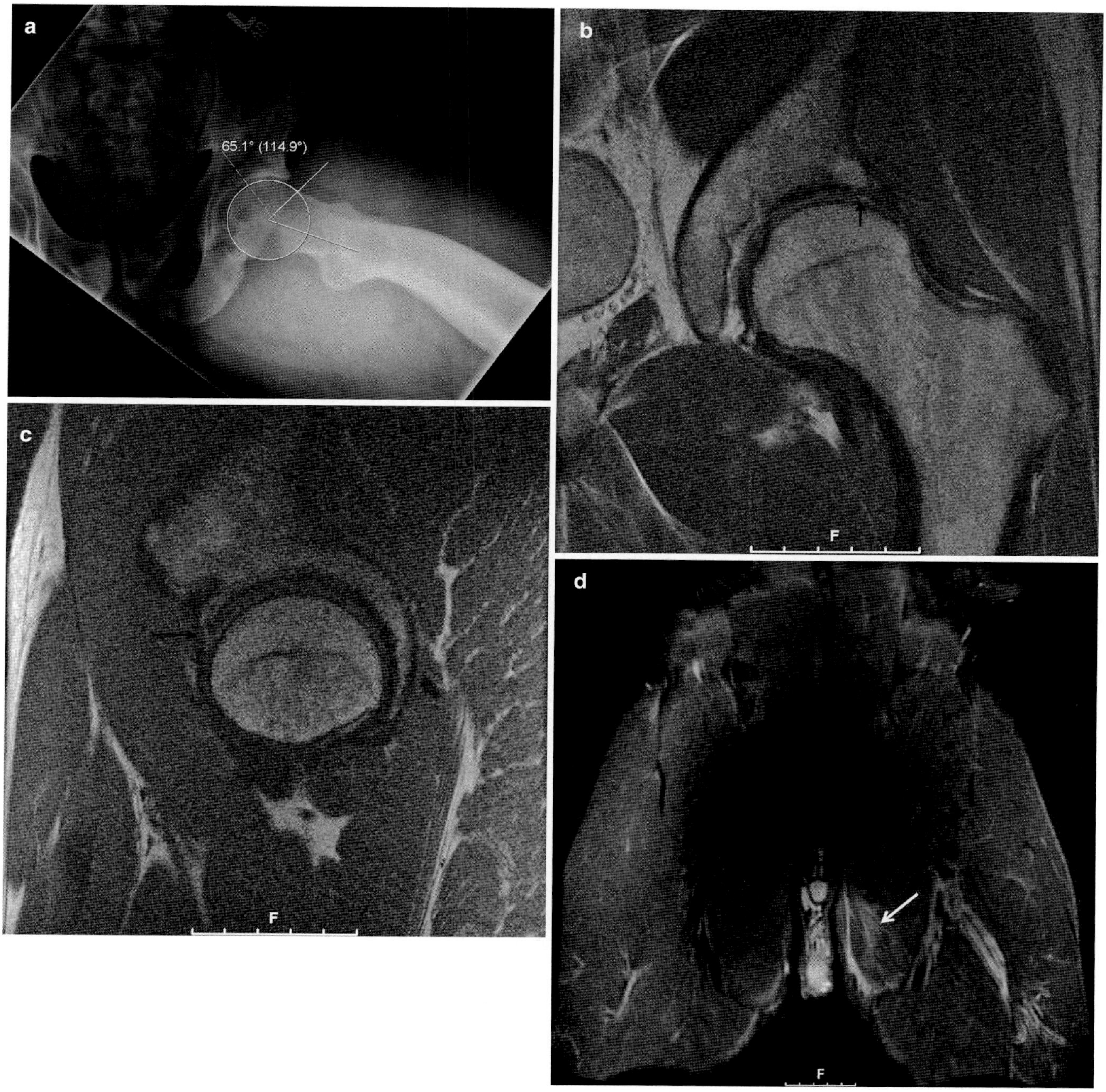

Fig. 31.1 (a) Elongated lateral plain radiograph (Dunn view) demonstrating elevated alpha angle of 65.1°. (b) Coronal MRI demonstrating cartilage thinning in the anterosuperior weight-bearing zone of the acetabulum consistent with cam-induced transition zone delamination (*arrow*). (c) Sagittal MRI demonstrating tear of the anterosuperior labrum secondary to the underlying femoroacetabular impingement-induced conflict between the femoral head and acetabulum, resulting in direct injury to the labral-chondral junction (*arrow*). (d) Coronal view of the pelvis of the same patient demonstrating secondary injury to the adductor complex due to compensatory overload of layer 3 structures (*arrow*)

involved nerves include the ilioinguinal, iliohypogastric, genitofemoral, and pudendal nerves [2–8].

In this chapter, we focus on a discussion of the compensatory soft tissue response and injury patterns to mechanical malalignment and expand the definition of compensatory injury patterns within layer 3.

Anterior Enthesopathy

Anterior enthesopathies constitutes several distinct entities that result in pain from anterior extra-articular structures that may contribute to or cause intra-articular hip injury. The three main etiologies of compensatory anterior muscular dysfunction are hip flexor strains, psoas impingement, and AIIS subspine impingement.

Hip Flexor Strain

The origin of the rectus femoris has two heads: the direct head arising from the AIIS and the reflective head from the superior acetabulum. The most common site of injury is at the musculotendinous junction [9, 10]. In addition, muscles that cross two joints from origin to insertion are more susceptible to strains [10, 11]. Imaging studies utilizing MRI have reported the indirect head as the most commonly injured site of the muscle origin [11, 12].

Avulsions of the rectus femoris are common in the adolescent, skeletally immature population [13–17]. These injuries have been reported in football, soccer, lacrosse, gymnastics, hockey, dance, and track and field [13, 14]. Proximal avulsions of the rectus in the adult, skeletally mature population are a less common entity. Several studies have reported the occurrence of proximal rectus avulsions in both professional football and soccer athletes [18–20]. Brophy et al. reported muscle-tendon lower extremity injuries to be the most common injury pattern in NFL kickers [18]. Gamradt et al. reported at total of 11 cases of proximal rectus femoris avulsions in a study of the NFL Injury Surveillance System [11]. Frequently, rectus femoris avulsions in adults or apophyseal avulsions in the skeletally immature patients are associated with clinical findings suspicious for underlying femoroacetabular impingement (FAI).

Hip flexor strains commonly occur as a noncontact injury during either eccentric contraction of the muscle or during high-velocity hip flexion such as what occurs during the kicking motion [9, 10]. Athletes often report an acute "pop" and immediate pain in the anterior hip. Ecchymosis and swelling often result. Clinical suspicion is confirmed by tenderness to palpation over the hip flexor origin, occasional step-off, and weakness and/or pain with resisted hip flexion. Assessment of hip rotation and impingement maneuvers provides clues to the involvement of associated FAI. The association with FAI is based upon a protective eccentric contraction of the hip flexor group occurring as the functional hip range of motion exceeds physiologic capacity based upon the underlying mechanical structure.

Treatment of proximal rectus avulsions is almost uniformly conservative, consisting of rest, ice, protective weight bearing for pain control, stretching, physical therapy, and gradual return to sport as symptoms allow. In the setting of American professional football, Gamradt et al. stated proximal avulsions of the rectus femoris can be treated nonoperatively with a high degree of predictability for return to full, unrestricted participation [11]. Surgical treatment is rarely indicated. In the adolescent population where a bony apophyseal avulsion has occurred, occasionally surgical intervention is warranted when the patient experiences prolonged disability despite rehabilitation or when there is significant displacement of the bony fragment [13–17, 20]. In the adult population, surgery has been described in the chronic setting where a symptomatic bony exostosis has formed and excision is necessary. The authors note several cases where a bony avulsion of the AIIS has occurred in the adult setting resulting in displacement over the rim of the acetabulum, causing secondary impingement with the femoral head-neck junction that was treated arthroscopically with fragment excision (Fig. 31.2).

Iliopsoas Impingement

The iliopsoas muscle acts as one of the main flexors of the hip joint [21]. In addition, the muscle prevents hyperextension of the hip during standing. The iliopsoas originates on the anterior border of the lumbar spine (psoas) and on the internal brim of the pelvis (iliacus). The iliopsoas inserts onto the lesser trochanter as a uniform tendon. Recent studies have addressed the theory describing the iliopsoas functioning as a hip rotator [22]. Using a computer model, Delp et al. described the iliopsoas as a small contributor to internal rotation at 0° and switched to a small external rotator at 90° of hip flexion [22]. The study concluded that although the iliopsoas does not have a significant direct influence on rotation, a short iliopsoas may indirectly contribute to internal rotation by causing hip flexion and shifting the balance of the hip rotators toward internal rotation.

When the hip is in full flexion, the iliopsoas tendon shifts laterally in relation to the center of the femoral head as it crossed the iliopectineal eminence [21]. Subsequently, with extension of the hip, the iliopsoas tendon moves medially over the femoral head. This shift of the iliopsoas over the iliopectineal eminence or at the base of the anterior inferior iliac spine (AIIS) and femoral head has been described as the source of internal coxa saltans in many patients [21].

Recently, Domb et al. described a distinct clinical entity as an etiology for anterior hip pain termed "iliopsoas impingement" (IPI) [23, 24]. IPI is based on the close proximity of the iliopsoas tendon to the capsule and anterior labrum just distal to the iliopectineal eminence. IPI has been previously described in the setting of THA where either anterior extrusion of cement or anterior overhang of the acetabular component results in irritation of the iliopsoas tendon [25].

In the native hip with IPI, the labral tear occurs at the 3 o'clock position of the right hip on the acetabulum rather than the typical 12 or 1 o'clock position seen in classic FAI [23, 24]. The inflamed capsule and iliopsoas tendon can be visualized during arthroscopy directly overlying the injured labrum. This also coincides with descriptions by several authors that during arthroscopic release of the iliopsoas for painful internal coxa saltans, a large number of cases had associated intra-articular pathology such as labral tears [25, 26].

The clinical presentation of IPI is more insidious in onset than that of a rectus femoris injury. Patients often complain of discomfort with repetitive twisting or hip flexion activities.

On occasion, the report of a sudden pop in the anterior hip via a noncontact mechanism may occur. Mechanical symptoms may be present as the iliopsoas snaps over the labrum or the torn labrum incarcerates in the joint.

On physical examination, nearly all patients have a positive flexion-adduction-internal rotation (FADIR) impingement test

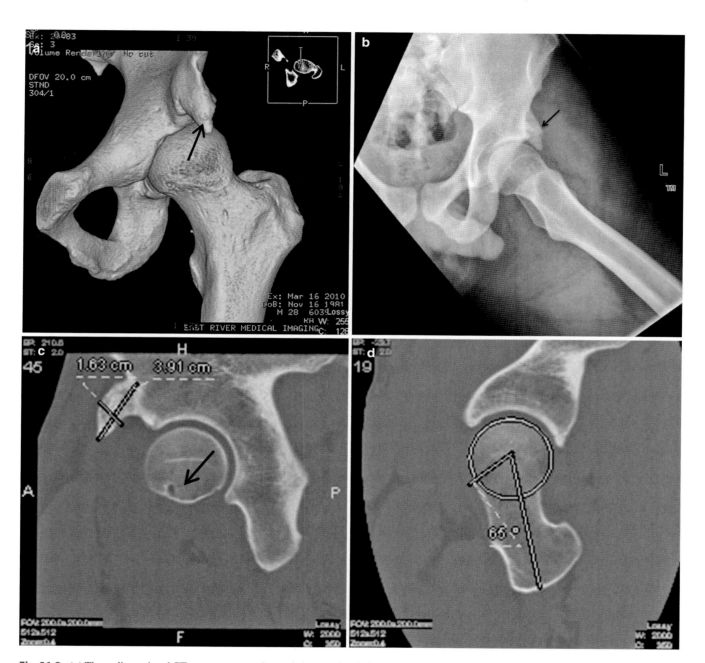

Fig. 31.2 (**a**) Three-dimensional CT scan reconstruction and elongated neck lateral (Dunn) plain radiograph (**b**) demonstrating the sequelae of a complete avulsion of the direct head of the rectus femoris in an adult athlete. Heterotopic bone formation developed along the tract of the avulsion (*arrows*), resulting in extra-articular impingement superimposed upon underlying FAI. (**c**) Sagittal reconstruction of the same patient demonstrating elongation of the anterior inferior iliac spine below the level of the acetabulum with a synovial herniation pit on the femoral head (*arrow*). (**d**) Oblique axial view of the same patient demonstrates elevated alpha angle of 65°. (**e**) Intraoperative fluoroscopy image demonstrating the severe impingement conflict between the AIIS avulsion and the cam lesion (*arrow*). (**f**) Intraoperative fluoroscopy image demonstrating arthroscopic decompression of the AIIS avulsion (*arrow*) and restoration of a normal alpha angle

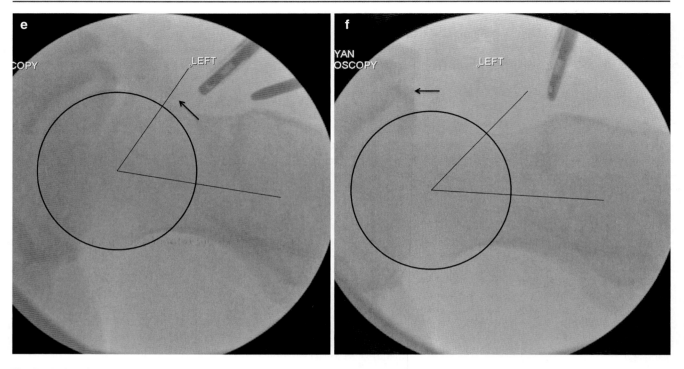

Fig. 31.2 (continued)

[23]. In addition, most patients have focal tenderness over the iliopsoas at the level of the anterior joint line. However, Domb et al. note that focal tenderness is a nonspecific finding and should not be independently used as a diagnostic criterion for IPI [23].

AP pelvis and elongated neck lateral radiographs are recommended in all patients in addition to an MRI. In 36 patients in the study by Domb et al., there was no evidence of dysplasia (center edge of Wiberg >25°), acetabular retroversion (negative crossover sign), or cam lesions (alpha angle <50°) [23]. On MRI, there were no injuries to the articular cartilage, no history of trauma or instability, and no injury in any part of the labrum other than the direct anterior 3 o'clock position.

Treatment begins uniformly with conservative options. Physical therapy is utilized for at least 3–6 months to focus on hip range of motion, strength, and iliopsoas stretching. Selective use of intra-articular and iliopsoas bursa injections provides variable relief. Hip arthroscopy is considered when conservative measures have failed [27]. A more favorable result is considered when the patient responded well to an iliopsoas injection, has a documented labral tear on MRI, and there is evidence of anterior capsule thickening where the psoas tendon crosses the acetabulum. In the study by Domb et al., all patients were treated with supine hip arthroscopy through an anterolateral and additional accessory portals as needed [23, 24]. In most cases, the distal lateral accessory portal (DLAP) is used as the primary working portal.

In cases with a tear of the labrum at the 3 o'clock position, most are debrided with a shaver. Occasionally, reattachment is required using suture anchors. To address the iliopsoas, an anterior capsulotomy approximately 1 cm in length is made directly anterior to the labral injury using the beaver blade or radiofrequency ablation device. Through this capsular window, the tendinous portion of the iliopsoas can be visualized and then tenotomized [23, 26, 28].

Domb et al. reported on 25 patients with complete follow-up (greater than 1 year) that underwent isolated, primary, unilateral iliopsoas release and either labral debridement or repair [23]. Mean postoperative outcome scores were 87, 92, and 78 for the modified Harris Hip Score, activities of daily living Hip Outcome Score, and sports-related score, respectively. In patients with increased femoral anteversion, the psoas may have an increased propensity to compress the anterior labrum as it is functioning as a dynamic stabilizer of the hip joint in external rotation. One should exercise caution in performing fractional lengthening of the iliopsoas in patients with increased femoral anteversion, as this may further destabilize the hip joint.

AIIS Subspine Impingement

Prominence of the anterior inferior iliac spine (AIIS) at the level of the acetabular rim is presented as another etiology of anterior hip impingement [29]. The senior author (BTK) has termed this AIIS subspine impingement. The rationale for this injury mechanism is that the morphology of the AIIS may result in decreased space available for soft tissue at the level of the acetabular rim during hip flexion. The result is impingement of anterior tissue (anterior capsule or iliocapsularis muscle origin) against the femoral head-neck junction (Fig. 31.3).

Pan et al. first described the treatment of AIIS impingement in a case report of a 30-year-old male who presented with anterior hip pain and limitations of hip motion that did not respond to conservative treatment [16]. Radiographs and CT scan revealed impingement between the femoral head-neck junction and a very prominent AIIS. Surgical resection of the hypertrophic AIIS was performed, resulting in resolution of pain and hip function.

Clinical findings of AIIS subspine impingement may mimic a hip flexor strain. Pain is often insidious in onset and exacerbated by deep hip flexion activities or maneuvers. If there is significant bony impingement from a low-lying AIIS, limitation in hip flexion may be noted.

Recently, a classification system for AIIS subspine impingement was submitted by the senior author (BTK) based on the clinical findings of 58 patients (33 males and 25 females) [29]. Using CT scans with 3-D reconstructions, the morphology of the AIIS and its location relevant to the superior acetabular rim is determined. When the ischium is viewed from directly posterior termed "ischium view," a horizontal line is drawn crossing at the most caudad level of the junction of the AIIS with the ilium wall. The AIIS is then classified based on the position relative to this horizontal line (Fig. 31.3). The classification system is made up of three types (I, II, and III) and two subtypes (A and B) (Table 31.2).

There may be some overlap of types II and III AIIS impingement with a history of rectus avulsion either as an adult or adolescent. Displacement of a bony fragment of the AIIS from a traumatic hip flexor avulsion may displace to the level of the acetabulum or below and ossify in continuity to the pelvis over time, resulting in anterior hip pain and restriction of motion.

Surgical decompression of the AIIS area in patients with signs of FAI and AIIS types II and III and subtype B may result in improvement of anterior impingement symptoms although no clinical series have reported this. While data is not yet available, the authors submit that adding arthroscopic decompression of the subspine area in these cases is technically feasible (Fig. 31.2). An advantage of this procedure is that subspine decompression does not remove bone from the acetabular rim itself and therefore does not jeopardize femoral head coverage. The tendon of the direct head of the rectus femoris is not compromised, as it attaches to the upper half of the AIIS.

Medial Enthesopathy

Adequate femoral head-neck offset prevents contact between the femoral neck and acetabular rim within a normal range of motion (ROM). However, with increased bone volume at the femoral head-neck junction or acetabular over coverage as seen with focal or global acetabular retroversion, insufficient clearance mechanically limits terminal range of motion in multiple planes [30, 31]. While the specific deficiencies in motion are correlated with the location of deformity, FAI has been shown to decrease maximal hip flexion, internal rotation, and abduction [31]. Moreover, internal rotation decreases with increasing flexion and adduction [31, 32].

When functional range of motion required to compete in sports is greater than the amount of physiologic motion allowed by the hip, a compensatory increase in motion and resultant stress through the SI joint, pubic symphysis, and lumbar spine may occur. Medial enthesopathies associated with this compensatory motion through the hemipelvis involve soft tissue injury to the adductor longus (adductor tendinopathy or tear), the rectus abdominis (proximal to the pubis), or the pubic symphysis itself (traditionally called "osteitis pubis"). This constellation of injuries can occur in a variety of different patterns and combinations, but constitute the fundamental basis for what has traditionally been coined "athletic pubalgia."

Osteitis Pubis

Osteitis pubis has been defined as diffuse pain, instability, inflammation, and bony changes in the pubic symphysis [33]. In athletes, it has been described as an overuse injury to the anterior pelvis [34]. It occurs most commonly in athletes participating in twisting, kicking, and turning sports such as soccer, Australian rules football, rugby, ice hockey, and American football [33–36]. The adductor muscles insert at the pubic tubercle and have been implicated in the etiology of the injury [33–36]. Moreover, limited range of motion of the hip joint has been detected in athletes diagnosed with osteitis pubis as well as in athletes with pubic bone stress injury [37, 38].

Patients most commonly complain of an insidious onset of unilateral or bilateral pain in the pubic symphysis that may radiate to the groin, lower abdomen, or perineum. Pain can be reproduced with palpation of the pubic symphysis and resisted hip adduction [33–35]. Radiographs are often normal in the acute setting. Chronic cases may display sclerosis or cystic changes [34]. Bone marrow edema at the symphysis can be seen on MRI, although its utility in diagnosis has been questioned [33–35]. In a study of the MRI findings associated with osteitis pubis, Paajanen et al. documented the presence of bone marrow edema in 100% of patients surgically treated, in 88% of those treated nonoperatively, and in 65% of asymptomatic athletes [33].

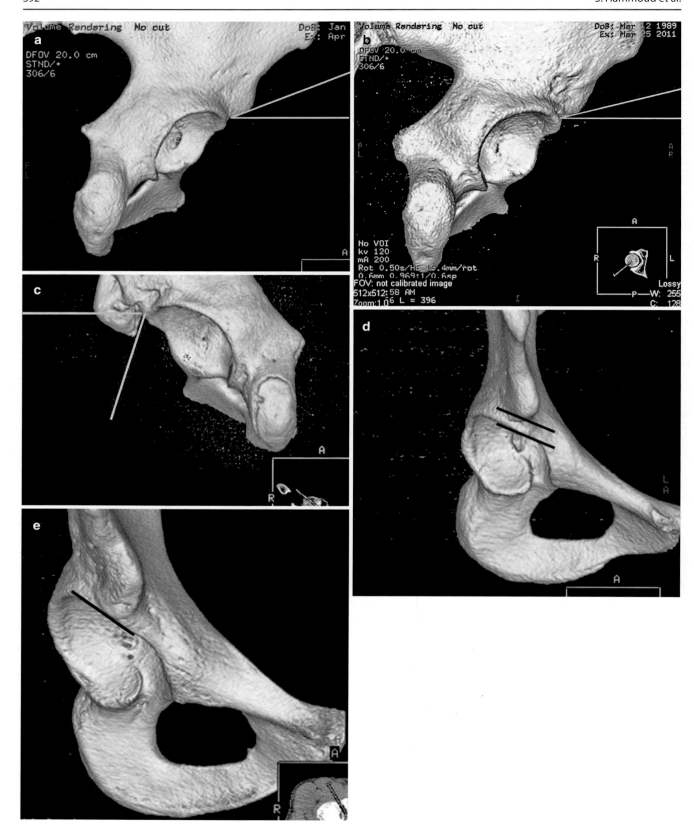

Table 31.2 AIIS morphology

Type and subtype	Description	CT definition	Suggested clinical applications
I	Upsloping	Upsloping on "ischium" view	AIIS does not contribute to impingement
II	Downsloping	Downsloping on "ischium" view, but does not cross caudad to rim in any of the views	AIIS may contribute to impingement
III	Hooked	Downsloping on "ischium" view and crosses caudad to rim in any of the views	AIIS may contribute to impingement
A	Clear subspine space	No extension of AIIS on ilium wall to rim level	Does not contribute to impingement
B	Subspine bone prominence or rim level-based AIIS	Caudad extension of AIIS on ilium wall to acetabular rim level	May contribute to impingement

Nonoperative treatment has been most commonly used with nonsteroidal anti-inflammatory drugs, core strengthening, hip range of motion therapy, and activity modifications. Local steroid injections may be used as a diagnostic and therapeutic tool [33–35]. When conservative measures have failed, surgical treatment options have been reported with success [34]. Paajanen et al. performed placement of entirely extraperitoneal endoscopic mesh behind the symphysis in 8 athletes, with 7 (88%) returning to sport at 2 months [33]. Radic et al. retrospectively evaluated 23 athletes who underwent open curettage of the pubic symphysis [34]. Twenty-one patients returned to pain-free running by 3 months, and 78% of participants felt their symptoms were better than preoperatively.

"Athletic Pubalgia"

Athletic pubalgia (AP) is one of the more difficult diagnoses to make when evaluating groin pain. Pain can be debilitating and frustrating for both the athlete and treating physician [39]. The exact etiology of the condition is difficult to ascertain and is most often attributed to overuse. AP is a weakness or tear of the posterior inguinal wall without a clinically recognizable hernia [40]. Other descriptions of pathology include attenuation of the conjoined tendon, injury at the insertion of the rectus abdominis muscle, avulsion of part of the internal oblique muscle fibers at the pubic tubercle,

tearing within the internal oblique muscle fibers at the pubic tubercle, tearing within the internal oblique musculature, or an abnormality in the external oblique aponeurosis [40, 41]. Another distinct entity known as Gilmore's groin exists in which a tear occurs in the external oblique aponeurosis, conjoined tendon, and a dehiscence between the conjoined tendon and the inguinal ligament [40, 42].

Patients with FAI may adopt an alternative motion strategy, recruiting different muscles, with an alteration in hip and pelvic biomechanics occurring even during gait [43]. During level gait, cam FAI causes a decrease in peak hip abduction and total frontal ROM, slight reduction in sagittal hip ROM, and attenuated pelvic mobility in the frontal plane [43]. It seems unlikely that these altered motions result from mechanical limitations or bony contact as would occur at the extremes of motion. This is suggestive of a soft tissue component to FAI that is adaptive in nature in order to reduce hip pain during ambulation [43]. Limited sagittal pelvic ROM has also been demonstrated in patients with FAI as compared to controls; moreover, patients with FAI could not squat as low as the control group [16]. Together these findings indicate compensatory or adaptive changes in pelvic motion and periarticular musculature secondary to FAI that may precipitate athletic pubalgia symptoms (compensatory relationship of layers 1 and 3).

In the high-performance athlete, restriction of terminal flexion and internal rotation at the hip joint (as in FAI)

Fig. 31.3 (a) Example of a Type I AIIS characterized by an "up-sloping" morphology as demonstrated by the "Ischium" view on a three-dimensional CT scan reconstruction. (b) Example of a Type II AIIS characterized by a "flat" or "down-sloping" morphology as demonstrated by the "Ischium" view on a three-dimensional CT scan reconstruction. (c) Example of a Type III AIIS characterized by a "hooked" morphology as demonstrated by the "Ischium" view on a three-dimensional CT scan reconstruction. In the Type III variant, part of the AIIS crosses caudad to the *horizontal line* on the Ischium view (c) and also obscures part of the continuity of the acetabular rim on the "Head-on" view. (d) AIIS morphologies are characterized as sub-type "A" when there is a clear smooth space without any bony prominences between the caudad level of the AIIS on the ilium wall and the acetabular rim. (e) AIIS morphologies with sub-type "B" are characterized by bony prominences between the most caudad level of the AIIS on the ilium wall (the true base) and the acetabular rim, best visualized on the "Head-on" view

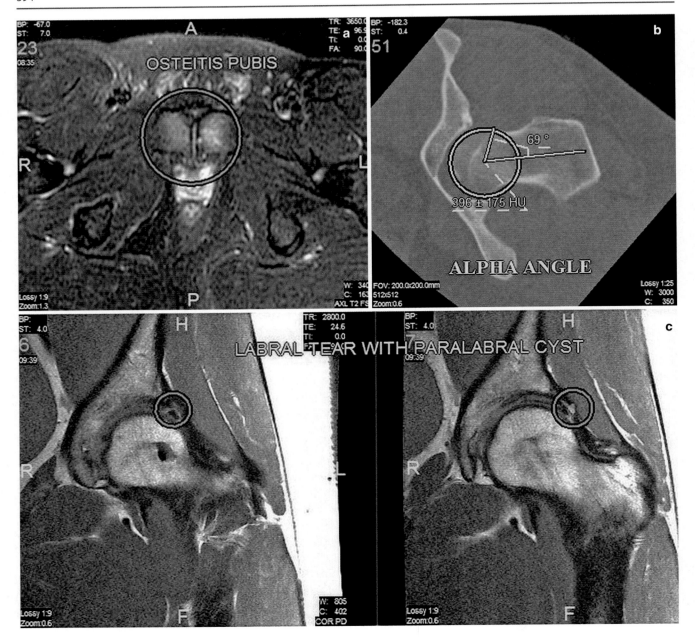

Fig. 31.4 (**a**) Axial MRI view of the pelvis demonstrated increased signal intensity in the pubic symphysis consistent with osteitis pubis. (**b**) Although radiographs may be unremarkable in the acute setting, close evaluation of the underlying bony morphology oftentimes demonstrates measurements consistent with decreased offset and increased alpha angles (69°) with associated intra-articular chondral and labral pathology seen on the coronal MRI section (**c**)

results in secondary abnormal motion of the hemipelvis. This motion may be responsible for secondary strain/injury to the central pubic musculature, defined here as medial pubalgia or medial enthesopathy (Fig. 31.4) [44]. Verrall et al. performed a prospective cohort study in order to determine whether restricted hip joint range of motion is associated with subsequent onset of athletic chronic groin injury [36]. They determined the end range of hip joint motion in 29 Australian rules football players without previous history of groin injury and then followed these players for two playing seasons for the development of chronic groin injury. Four athletes developed chronic groin injury (defined by at least 6 weeks of groin pain and missing match playing time). In these four athletes, reduced total hip joint range of motion ($P = 0.03$) was found to be associated, suggesting that limitations in hip motion is associated with later development of chronic groin injury and may be a risk factor.

In a recent study of hip injuries in the National Football League, Feeley et al. cited the most common type of hip injury was a muscle strain, followed by a contusion, intra-articular injury, and a sprain [45]. Although these injuries may occur in isolation, a "sports hip triad" has been described by the senior author (BTK) consisting of a labral tear, adductor strain, and a rectus strain [45]. Therefore, intra-articular pathology, such as FAI, may be implicated in exacerbating muscle injuries around the pelvis in athletes. Proximal hamstring tendonitis, rectus femoris avulsions, and psoas tendonitis are other causes of groin pain that may have a similar association with FAI [28, 45–47]. As with all muscle injuries, prevention is the key consisting of preseason stretching, balance, and ROM exercises. Treatment of muscle injuries consists of rest, ice, physical therapy, and range of motion exercises. Injections into the adductor enthesis have been described by Schilders et al. with success in both competitive and recreational athletes [48, 49]. Surgery has been described for the treatment of recalcitrant adductor and rectus abdominis tendinosis [41, 44, 45].

Larson et al. recently published an article looking to evaluate the results of surgical treatment in athletes with associated intra-articular hip pathology and extra-articular sports pubalgia [50]. They followed a series of 37 hips (mean patient age, 25 years) that were diagnosed with both symptomatic athletic pubalgia and symptomatic intra-articular hip joint pathology. Hip arthroscopy was performed in 32 hips (30 cases of femoroacetabular impingement treatment, 1 traumatic labral tear, and 1 borderline dysplasia). Of 16 hips that had athletic pubalgia surgery as the index procedure, 4 (25%) returned to sports without limitations, and 11 (69%) subsequently had hip arthroscopy at a mean of 20 months after pubalgia surgery. Of 8 hips managed initially with hip arthroscopy alone, 4 (50%) returned to sports without limitations, and 3 (43%) had subsequent pubalgia surgery at a mean of 6 months after hip arthroscopy. Thirteen hips had athletic pubalgia surgery and hip arthroscopy at one setting. Concurrent or eventual surgical treatment of both disorders led to improved postoperative outcome scores ($P \leq .05$) and an unrestricted return to sporting activity in 89% of hips (24 of 27). Based upon this study, when patients present with symptoms involving both pubalgia and intra-articular pathology, surgical management of both disorders concurrently or in a staged manner led to improved postoperative outcome scoring and an unrestricted return to sporting activity in 89% of hips [50].

Posterior Compensatory Patterns

Proximal hamstring tendinopathy, previously reported under the name of proximal hamstring syndrome, is proposed to be an overuse injury that expresses itself by lower gluteal pain, especially during sports [51–54]. It has been reported in athletes in various sports, but especially in sprinters and middle- and long-distance runners [52–54]. Abnormal bony morphology within the realm of FAI may be implicated in exacerbating muscle injuries around the pelvis in athletes. Proximal hamstring tendonitis may have a similar association with FAI, although it has not been definitively proven as of yet [45, 48, 49, 55–57]. This compensatory injury pattern is more commonly seen in female patients with a predominant rim impingement morphology. It has been hypothesized that in an attempt to decrease anterior impingement, these patients will develop a compensatory posterior tilt of the pelvis, which leads to chronic hamstring shortening and ultimately predisposing them to chronic hamstring tendinopathy (Fig. 31.5).

As with all muscle injuries, prevention is the key, consisting of preseason stretching and balance and ROM exercises. Treatment of muscle injuries consists of rest, ice, physical therapy, and ROM exercises [45, 48, 49, 55–57]. Surgery has been described for the treatment of recalcitrant proximal hamstring tendonitis [48, 49, 55–57].

Deep gluteal syndrome (DGS), as described by Martin et al. [6], involves pain in the buttock secondary to entrapment of the sciatic nerve by the piriformis muscle, hamstring, obturator internus/gemellus complex, or scar tissue [51, 58–61]. Radicular-like pain may result with rotation of the hip in flexion and knee extended, similar to nerve root pain associated with lumbar disc disease. The sciatic nerve exits through the sciatic notch inferior to the piriformis muscle. Blunt trauma to the buttock with resultant hematoma formation and secondary scarring between the sciatic nerve and short external rotators can result in piriformis syndrome [58].

The sciatic nerve is also in close proximity to the origin of the hamstrings as it passes within the deep gluteal region between the ischial tuberosity and the greater trochanter [59]. In a cadaveric study, Miller et al. [62] described the nerve as located a mean of 1.2 ± 0.2 cm from the most lateral aspect of the ischial tuberosity, and the proximal origin of the hamstrings was found to be intimately related with the inferior gluteal nerve and artery and sciatic nerve. Normally, with hip flexion, the sciatic nerve can stretch and glide and has a proximal excursion of 28.0 mm [63]. With trauma or avulsion of the hamstring, the nerve can become scarred into the hamstring tendons, resulting in DGS [62].

Patients often present with a history of trauma and symptoms of sitting pain (inability to sit for >30 min), radicular pain, and paresthesias of the ipsilateral leg [6, 58]. Physical examination tests advocated for the clinical diagnosis of DGS include passive stretching and active contraction tests [6]. The Laségue sign is pain with straight-leg raise testing (to 90° hip flexion) [64, 65]. The Pace sign is pain and weakness with resisted abduction and external

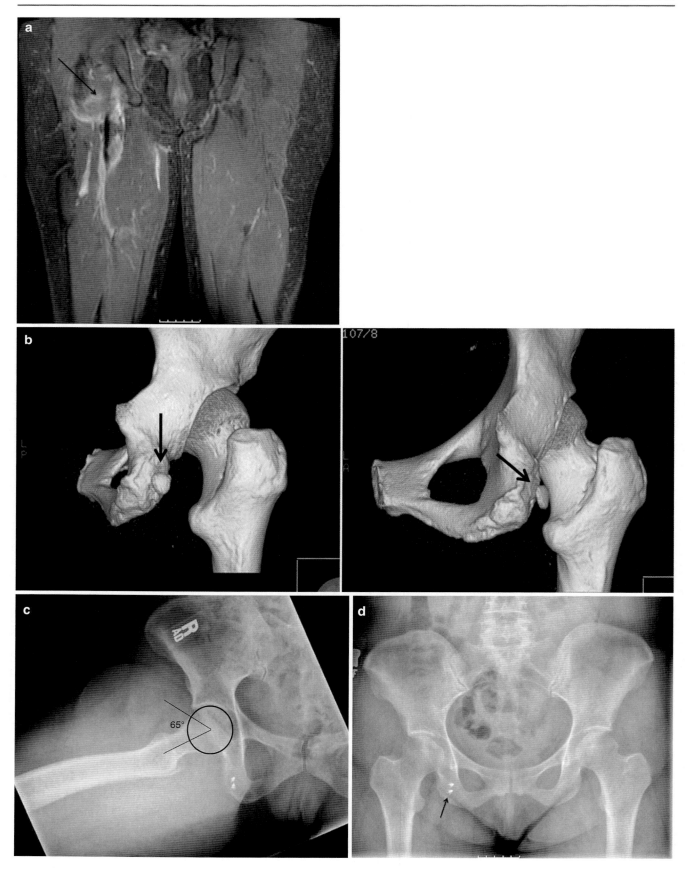

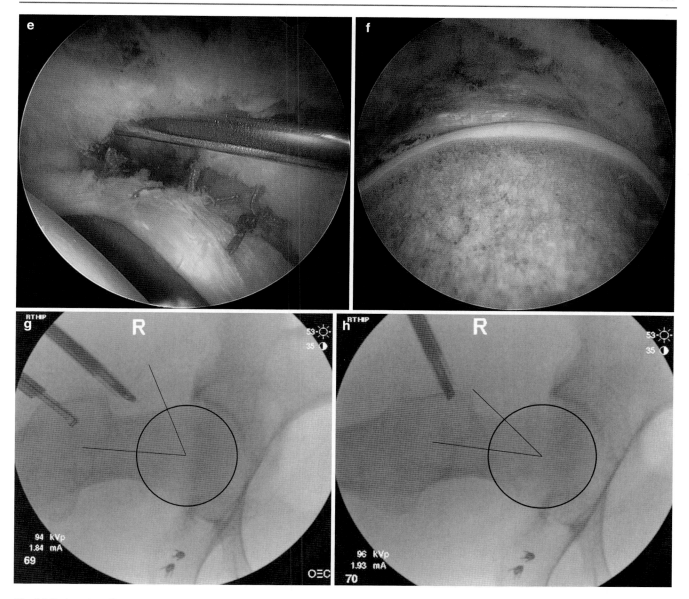

Fig. 31.5 (continued)

rotation of the hip [66]. The Freiberg sign is pain with internal rotation of the extended hip [64, 65]. Martin et al. also postulate that changes in rotational osseous alignment (i.e., decreased femoral anteversion) may affect normal sciatic nerve excursion and may limit the benefits of treatment of DGS [6]. Treatment options include both open and arthroscopic techniques to correct the various entrapment problems [6].

Bony Posterior Compensatory Patterns

SI Joint

The SI joint is a synovial joint surrounded by a thin capsule, and it is stabilized primarily by thick anterior and posterior ligaments. Pain in the SI joint may result from degenerative or inflammatory arthritis, infection, ankylosis, stress fractures,

Fig. 31.5 (**a**) Injury to the proximal hamstring (*arrow*) with associated bony avulsion of the hamstring origin (**b**) (*arrows*) in a female with underlying impingement (**c**). Surgical treatment consisted of staged primary repair of the proximal hamstring avulsion (**d**) (*arrow*), followed by arthroscopic treatment of the underlying FAI with labral refixation (**e**) and femoroplasty (**f–h**)

and either hypermobility or hypomobility [67]. The SI joint is supported by the gluteus maximus and medius, erector spinae, latissimus dorsi, biceps femoris, psoas, piriformis, and oblique and transversus abdominis muscles, and it imparts muscular forces to the pelvic bones [67]. Abnormal motion in the lumbar spine, pubic symphysis, and hip can all lead to increased stress at the SI joint and discomfort. Patients complain of pain near the posterior inferior iliac spine, the buttocks, groin, and occasionally radiating into the thigh. It is important to rule out the lumbar spine as the source of pathology. On examination, palpation of the posterior SI joint may elicit pain. Provocative tests involving rotation of the ipsilateral hip have been described to reproduce symptoms [67, 68] further reinforcing the concept that functional range of motion of the hip beyond the anatomical constraints can lead to increased stresses across the entire hemipelvis and through the SI joint.

Treatment consists of physical therapy focusing on posture, core muscle strength, and range of motion. Oral anti-inflammatory medications and corticosteroid injections may be both diagnostic and therapeutic when other modalities have failed [35]. Arthrodesis of the SI joint has been described in only very select cases of severe joint dysfunction and degeneration [35, 67, 68].

Lumbar Spine

Low back pain in the athlete is common and often difficult to diagnose and treat [68, 69]. Greene et al. concluded athletes with a history of prior low back injuries have a 3–6 times greater risk of sustaining further low back injury relative to other athletes [70]. Additional risk factors for lumbar spine pain in the athlete are decreased range of motion, poor conditioning, excessive or repetitive loading, improper play technique, and abrupt increases in training [69]. Muscle strain is the most common cause of back pain in athletes, but this diagnosis should be made only after other sources have been excluded. When motion of the hemipelvis is limited, increased strain may be placed on the low back to act as a source of motion for the extremity. Stress reactions in the pars interarticularis and posterior facet pain may result and are implicating factors as pain generators [71, 72]. Posterior element pain is commonly reported in sports which require twisting and hyperextension, such as gymnastics, diving, and linemen in football.

On physical examination, pain is exacerbated with hyperextension of the spine. It is important to assess and rule out radicular signs, discogenic pain, spinal deformity, tumor, and infection. Diagnostic imaging should be used in a targeted fashion [22]. Standing radiographs may rule out structural abnormalities, and oblique views allow for assessment of the pars interarticularis. Flexion and extension radiographs evaluate dynamic instability. Cross-sectional imaging, such as CT or MRI, can further delineate bony abnormalities, and

the latter is most useful for evaluation of the soft tissues and edema within the bone.

Treatment of low back pain in athletes is primarily conservative. Relative rest, core strengthening, and the use of lumbar orthosis have been shown to help reduce symptoms. For athletes with persistent pain or with any neurologic symptoms, further workup and evaluation are necessary.

Posterior Hip Subluxation and FAI

The spectrum of posterior hip instability ranges from subluxation to frank dislocation. The most common traumatic mechanism of injury in athletic competition is a fall on a flexed and adducted hip with a posteriorly directed force [45, 73, 74]. Atraumatic and lower energy mechanisms of hip instability have also been described [75–78]. Hip dislocations have been reported in American football, skiing, rugby, gymnastics, jogging, basketball, biking, and soccer [88]. It has been proposed that laxity in capsular tissue or abnormal bony morphology may predispose the athlete to hip instability [1, 74–78].

In the athlete with FAI, functional ROM required in athletic competition is often greater than the limited physiologic motion allowed by the cam and/or pincer lesions. Attempts to increase flexion and internal rotation may result in anterior engagement between the cam lesion and the anterior acetabulum, which results in levering of the femoral head posteriorly. This can lead to failure of the soft tissue and osseous structures, with a subsequent posterior acetabular rim fracture and posterior capsulolabral tear, analogous to a posterior bony Bankart lesion of the shoulder [79] (Fig. 31.6a–c). In the senior author's experience, anterior labral tears have also occurred as part of the spectrum of injury after posterior hip subluxation or dislocation [1, 45]. The proposed mechanism is a labral crush injury at the point where the cam lesion engages the anterior acetabulum and labrum. In certain cases, a posterior hip subluxation or dislocation event may be the first manifestation of occult FAI in competitive athletes [64]. In chronic FAI, particularly with a focal rim lesion creating cephalad retroversion, the anterosuperior labrum is typically degenerated and an associated "contrecoup" pattern of cartilage loss in the posterior capsular-labral junction develops by a distraction force due to the femoral head levering out of the hip socket with continued hip flexion [80, 81]. Increased levering forces during athletic competition could logically thus result in a subluxation episode.

Patients present with painful limitation of hip motion and often discomfort in the hip at rest. A high index of suspicion is critical to avoid missing this injury, which is often misdiagnosed as a muscle strain [1, 45, 73–78]. Posterior subluxation of the hip can be a potentially devastating injury to an athlete, resulting in avascular necrosis, if left unrecognized [82].

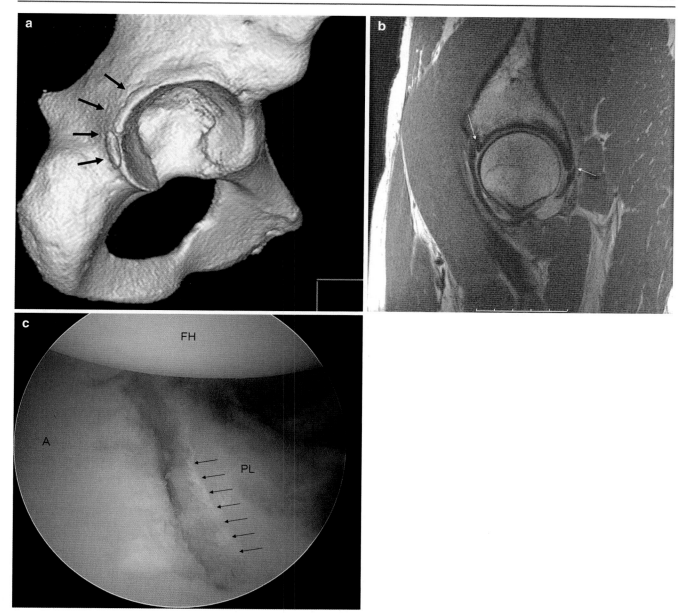

Fig. 31.6 (**a**) 3-D CT scan demonstrating the sequelae of a posterior hip subluxation with an associated bony "Bankart" lesion of the posterior rim of the acetabulum (*arrows*). (**b**) Associated anterior labral tear (*arrows*) associated with underlying anterior FAI leading to premature conflict between the femoral cam lesion and the anterior acetabulum and compensatory posterior subluxation with associated posterior soft tissue and bony injury. (**c**) Intraoperative photo demonstrating the posterior bony "Bankart" injury outlined by the arrows (*PL* posterior labrum, *FH* femoral head, *A* posterior acetabulum)

The classic triad of findings after posterior hip subluxation described in eight American football players has been described as hemarthrosis, iliofemoral ligament disruption, and posterior acetabular lip fracture [73]. Krych et al. reported on a series of 22 athletes presenting with a low energy mechanism of posterior acetabular rim fracture defining a posterior hip instability episode [1]. Eighteen athletes had underlying FAI. The most common pathologic findings observed in their series included a posterior bony Bankart lesion, anterior labral injury, synovitis, chondral injury to the femoral head with loose bodies, and ligamentum teres avulsion. Philippon et al. described the arthroscopic treatment of 14 athletes who sustained a traumatic hip dislocation. Only nine patients had evidence of FAI at the time of arthroscopy. Labral tears, ligamentum teres avulsion, and chondral defects were the most common pathologic findings in their series [74]. Five patients (36%) sustained posterior acetabular rim fractures; however, none required arthroscopic repair. The varying patterns of pathologic findings in these series of patients may be due to differing mechanisms of injury, rates of underlying FAI, as well as differences in MRI and arthroscopy findings.

Lateral Enthesopathy ("Abductor Deficiency")

Mechanical malalignment and intra-articular pathology, such as FAI, may be implicated in lateral enthesopathy or peritrochanteric space disorders. All musculature around the pelvis, including the hip abductor musculature, contributes to the dynamic layer. Chronic overload and compensatory dysfunction of the abductors may lead to chronic trochanteric bursitis, snapping ITB syndrome, and abductor tendon tears. Peritrochanter disorders, including snapping ITB syndrome, trochanteric bursitis, and gluteus medius and minimus tears, have been well documented [83–88]. The peritrochanteric disorders have previously been grouped into the "greater trochanteric pain syndrome" [84, 87, 88]. Static factors which may contribute to chronic overload and lateral enthesopathy include anterior or lateral undercoverage of acetabulum (dysplasia), femoral anteversion, and femoral valgus.

With acetabular dysplasia, a shallow acetabulum results in statically elevated contact pressures, reduced contact area, and instability. While the locally elevated contact pressures may ultimately lead to premature cartilage degeneration and osteoarthritis, this overload may initially manifest with lateral enthesopathy from compensatory dysfunction of the hip abductors.

Increased femoral anteversion may result in either intra-articular or extra-articular symptomatic impingement. Femoral valgus frequently presents in combination with increased femoral anteversion and acetabular dysplasia. Further, as with acetabular dysplasia, increased femoral anteversion and femoral valgus may result in pain from static overload of the anterosuperior head and dome and the anterior capsule and psoas tendon. This overload pattern may also contribute to compensatory dysfunction of the abductor musculature and, consequently, lateral hip pain and the peritrochanteric hip disorders.

A complete discussion on the workup and evaluation of patients with disorders of the peritrochanteric space is included in a separate chapter.

Conclusion

Failure to recognize and address concomitant compensatory injury patterns associated with intra-articular hip pathology can result in continued disability in a subset of patients and athletes. Knowledge of the potential etiology of both intra- and extra-articular hip pain is critical to effectively treating patients who presents with dysfunction of the hip joint, hemipelvis, and surrounding musculature.

References

1. Krych AJ, Byrd TW, Warren RF, Kelly BT. Low energy posterior wall fractures in athletes: evidence of cam induced posterior hip subluxation. Presented at NFL Physicians Society, Indianapolis, Indiana, February 24, 2011.
2. Antolak Jr SJ, Hough DM, Pawlina W, Spinner RJ. Anatomical basis of chronic pelvic pain syndrome: the ischial spine and pudendal nerve entrapment. Med Hypotheses. 2002;59:349–53.
3. Irshad K, Feldman LS, Lavoie C, Lacroix VJ, Mulder DS, Brown RA. Operative management of "hockey groin syndrome": 12 years of experience in National Hockey League players. Surgery. 2001;130:759–64; discussion 64–6.
4. Knockaert DC, D'Heygere FG, Bobbaers HJ. Ilioinguinal nerve entrapment: a little-known cause of iliac fossa pain. Postgrad Med J. 1989;65:632–5.
5. Lacroix VJ, Kinnear DG, Mulder DS, Brown RA. Lower abdominal pain syndrome in national hockey league players: a report of 11 cases. Clin J Sport Med. 1998;8:5–9.
6. Martin HD, Shears SA, Johnson JC, Smathers AM, Palmer IJ. The endoscopic treatment of sciatic nerve entrapment/deep gluteal syndrome. Arthroscopy. 2011;27:172–81.
7. Murata Y, Ogata S, Ikeda Y, Yamagata M. An unusual cause of sciatic pain as a result of the dynamic motion of the obturator internus muscle. Spine J. 2009;9:e16–8.
8. Ziprin P, Williams P, Foster ME. External oblique aponeurosis nerve entrapment as a cause of groin pain in the athlete. Br J Surg. 1999;86:566–8.
9. Armfield DR, Kim DH, Towers JD, Bradley JP, Robertson DD. Sports-related muscle injury in the lower extremity. Clin Sports Med. 2006;25:803–42.
10. Hasselman CT, Best TM, Hughes Ct, Martinez S, Garrett Jr WE. An explanation for various rectus femoris strain injuries using previously undescribed muscle architecture. Am J Sports Med. 1995;23:493–9.
11. Gamradt SC, Brophy RH, Barnes R, Warren RF, Thomas Byrd JW, Kelly BT. Nonoperative treatment for proximal avulsion of the rectus femoris in professional American football. Am J Sports Med. 2009;37:1370–4.
12. Ouellette H, Thomas BJ, Nelson E, Torriani M. MR imaging of rectus femoris origin injuries. Skeletal Radiol. 2006;35:665–72.
13. Frank JB, Jarit GJ, Bravman JT, Rosen JE. Lower extremity injuries in the skeletally immature athlete. J Am Acad Orthop Surg. 2007;15:356–66.
14. Heyworth BE, Voos JE, Metzl JD. Hip injuries in the adolescent athlete. Pediatr Ann. 2007;36:713–8.
15. Metzmaker JN, Pappas AM. Avulsion fractures of the pelvis. Am J Sports Med. 1985;13:349–58.
16. Pan H, Kawanabe K, Akiyama H, Goto K, Onishi E, Nakamura T. Operative treatment of hip impingement caused by hypertrophy of the anterior inferior iliac spine. J Bone Joint Surg Br. 2008;90:677–9.
17. Waters PM, Millis MB. Hip and pelvic injuries in the young athlete. Clin Sports Med. 1988;7:513–26.
18. Brophy RH, Wright RW, Powell JW, Matava MJ. Injuries to kickers in American football: the National Football League experience. Am J Sports Med. 2010;38:1166–73.
19. Hsu JC, Fischer DA, Wright RW. Proximal rectus femoris avulsions in national football league kickers: a report of 2 cases. Am J Sports Med. 2005;33:1085–7.
20. Rajasekhar C, Kumar KS, Bhamra MS. Avulsion fractures of the anterior inferior iliac spine: the case for surgical intervention. Int Orthop. 2001;24:364–5.
21. Allen WC, Cope R. Coxa saltans: the snapping hip revisited. J Am Acad Orthop Surg. 1995;3:303–8.
22. Delp SL, Hess WE, Hungerford DS, Jones LC. Variation of rotation moment arms with hip flexion. J Biomech. 1999;32:493–501.

23. Domb BG, Shindle MK, McArthur B, Voos JE, Magennis E, Kelly BT. Iliopsoas impingement: a newly identified cause of labral pathology in the hip. HSS J. 2011;7:1–6.

24. Heyworth BE, MacArthur BA, Kelly BT. Anterior hip muscle injuries. In: Guanche CA, editor. Hip and pelvis injuries in sports medicine. Philadelphia: Lippincott Williams & Wilkins; 2009. p. 192–9.

25. Lachiewicz PF, Kauk JR. Anterior iliopsoas impingement and tendinitis after total hip arthroplasty. J Am Acad Orthop Surg. 2009;17:337–44.

26. Ilizaliturri Jr VM, Camacho-Galindo J. Endoscopic treatment of snapping hips, iliotibial band, and iliopsoas tendon. Sports Med Arthrosc. 2010;18:120–7.

27. Byrd JW. Evaluation and management of the snapping iliopsoas tendon. Instr Course Lect. 2006;55:347–55.

28. Anderson SA, Keene JS. Results of arthroscopic iliopsoas tendon release in competitive and recreational athletes. Am J Sports Med. 2008;36:2363–71.

29. Hetsroni I, Magennis E, Kelly BT. The anterior inferior iliac spine: morphological classification in people with hip impingement. Arthroscopy. 2011. [In Review].

30. Lamontagne M, Kennedy MJ, Beaule PE. The effect of cam FAI on hip and pelvic motion during maximum squat. Clin Orthop Relat Res. 2009;467:645–50.

31. Kubiak-Langer M, Tannast M, Murphy SB, Siebenrock KA, Langlotz F. Range of motion in anterior femoroacetabular impingement. Clin Orthop Relat Res. 2007;458:117–24.

32. Wyss TF, Clark JM, Weishaupt D, Notzli HP. Correlation between internal rotation and bony anatomy in the hip. Clin Orthop Relat Res. 2007;460:152–8.

33. Paajanen H, Hermunen H, Karonen J. Pubic magnetic resonance imaging findings in surgically and conservatively treated athletes with osteitis pubis compared to asymptomatic athletes during heavy training. Am J Sports Med. 2008;36:117–21.

34. Radic R, Annear P. Use of pubic symphysis curettage for treatment-resistant osteitis pubis in athletes. Am J Sports Med. 2008;36:122–8.

35. Tibor LM, Sekiya JK. Differential diagnosis of pain around the hip joint. Arthroscopy. 2008;24:1407–21.

36. Verrall GM, Slavotinek JP, Barnes PG, Esterman A, Oakeshott RD, Spriggins AJ. Hip joint range of motion restriction precedes athletic chronic groin injury. Aust J Sci Med Sport. 2007;10:463–6.

37. Verrall GM, Hamilton IA, Slavotinek JP, et al. Hip joint range of motion reduction in sports-related chronic groin injury diagnosed as pubic bone stress injury. Aust J Sci Med Sport. 2005;8:77–84.

38. Williams JG. Limitation of hip joint movement as a factor in traumatic osteitis pubis. Br J Sports Med. 1978;12:129–33.

39. Swan Jr KG, Wolcott M. The athletic hernia: a systematic review. Clin Orthop Relat Res. 2007;455:78–87.

40. Farber AJ, Wilckens JH. Sports hernia: diagnosis and therapeutic approach. J Am Acad Orthop Surg. 2007;15:507–14.

41. Meyers WC, Foley DP, Garrett WE, Lohnes JH, Mandlebaum BR. Management of severe lower abdominal or inguinal pain in high-performance athletes. PAIN (Performing Athletes with Abdominal or Inguinal Neuromuscular Pain Study Group). Am J Sports Med. 2000;28:2–8.

42. Brannigan AE, Kerin MJ, McEntee GP. Gilmore's groin repair in athletes. J Orthop Sports Phys Ther. 2000;30:329–32.

43. Kennedy MJ, Lamontagne M, Beaule PE. Femoroacetabular impingement alters hip and pelvic biomechanics during gait Walking biomechanics of FAI. Gait Posture. 2009;30:41–4.

44. Meyers WC, McKechnie A, Philippon MJ, Horner MA, Zoga AC, Devon ON. Experience with "sports hernia" spanning two decades. Ann Surg. 2008;248:656–65.

45. Feeley BT, Powell JW, Muller MS, Barnes RP, Warren RF, Kelly BT. Hip injuries and labral tears in the national football league. Am J Sports Med. 2008;36:2187–95.

46. Caudill P, Nyland J, Smith C, Yerasimides J, Lach J. Sports hernias: a systematic literature review. Br J Sports Med. 2008;42:954–64.

47. Nelson EN, Kassarjian A, Palmer WE. MR imaging of sports-related groin pain. Magn Reson Imaging Clin N Am. 2005;13:727–42.

48. Schilders E, Bismil Q, Robinson P, O'Connor PJ, Gibbon WW, Talbot JC. Adductor-related groin pain in competitive athletes. Role of adductor enthesis, magnetic resonance imaging, and entheseal pubic cleft injections. J Bone Joint Surg Am. 2007;89:2173–8.

49. Schilders E, Talbot JC, Robinson P, Dimitrakopoulou A, Gibbon WW, Bismil Q. Adductor-related groin pain in recreational athletes: role of the adductor enthesis, magnetic resonance imaging, and entheseal pubic cleft injections. J Bone Joint Surg Am. 2009;91:2455–60.

50. Larson CM, Pierce BR, Giveans MR. Treatment of athletes with symptomatic intra-articular hip pathology and athletic pubalgia/sports hernia: a case series. Arthroscopy. 2011;27:768–75.

51. Puranen J, Orava S. The hamstring syndrome. A new diagnosis of gluteal sciatic pain. Am J Sports Med. 1988;16:517–21.

52. Migliorini S, Merlo M. The hamstring syndrome in endurance athletes. Br J Sports Med. 2011;45:363.

53. Orava S. Hamstring syndrome. Oper Tech Sports Med. 1997;5:143–9.

54. Fredericson M, Moore W, Guillet M, Beaulieu C. High hamstring tendinopathy in runners: meeting the challenges of diagnosis, treatment, and rehabilitation. Phys Sportsmed. 2005;33:32–43.

55. Schick DM, Meeuwisse WH. Injury rates and profiles in female ice hockey players. Am J Sports Med. 2003;31:47–52.

56. Nicholas SJ, Tyler TF. Adductor muscle strains in sport. Sports Med. 2002;32:339–44.

57. Akermark C, Johansson C. Tenotomy of the adductor longus tendon in the treatment of chronic groin pain in athletes. Am J Sports Med. 1992;20:640–3.

58. Benson ER, Schutzer SF. Posttraumatic piriformis syndrome: diagnosis and results of operative treatment. J Bone Joint Surg Am. 1999;81:941–9.

59. Clemente C. Gray's anatomy: anatomy of the human body. 13th ed. Baltimore: Williams and Wilkins; 1985.

60. Cox JM, Bakkum BW. Possible generators of retrotrochanteric gluteal and thigh pain: the gemelli-obturator internus complex. J Manipulative Physiol Ther. 2005;28:534–8.

61. Meknas K, Christensen A, Johansen O. The internal obturator muscle may cause sciatic pain. Pain. 2003;104:375–80.

62. Miller SL, Gill J, Webb GR. The proximal origin of the hamstrings and surrounding anatomy encountered during repair. A cadaveric study. J Bone Joint Surg Am. 2007;89:44–8.

63. Coppieters MW, Alshami AM, Babri AS, Souvlis T, Kippers V, Hodges PW. Strain and excursion of the sciatic, tibial, and plantar nerves during a modified straight leg raising test. J Orthop Res. 2006;24:1883–9.

64. Freiberg AH. Sciatic pain and its relief by operations on muscle and fascia. Arch Surg. 1937;34:337–50.

65. Freiberg AH, Vinke TH. Sciatica and the sacroiliac joint. J Bone Joint Surg Am. 1934;16:126–36.

66. Pace JB, Nagle D. Piriform syndrome. West J Med. 1976;124:435–9.

67. Dreyfuss P, Dreyer SJ, Cole A, Mayo K. Sacroiliac joint pain. J Am Acad Orthop Surg. 2004;12:255–65.

68. van der Wurff P, Hagmeijer RH, Meyne W. Clinical tests of the sacroiliac joint. A systematic methodological review. Part 1: reliability. Man Ther. 2000;5:30–6.

69. Lawrence JP, Greene HS, Grauer JN. Back pain in athletes. J Am Acad Orthop Surg. 2006;14:726–35.

70. Greene HS, Cholewicki J, Galloway MT, Nguyen CV, Radebold A. A history of low back injury is a risk factor for recurrent back injuries in varsity athletes. Am J Sports Med. 2001;29:795–800.

71. Sairyo K, Katoh S, Sasa T, et al. Athletes with unilateral spondylolysis are at risk of stress fracture at the contralateral pedicle and pars interarticularis: a clinical and biomechanical study. Am J Sports Med. 2005;33:583–90.

72. Miller SF, Congeni J, Swanson K. Long-term functional and anatomical follow-up of early detected spondylolysis in young athletes. Am J Sports Med. 2004;32:928–33.

73. Moorman 3rd CT, Warren RF, Hershman EB, et al. Traumatic posterior hip subluxation in American football. J Bone Joint Surg Am. 2003;85-A:1190–6.

74. Philippon MJ, Kuppersmith DA, Wolff AB, Briggs KK. Arthroscopic findings following traumatic hip dislocation in 14 professional athletes. Arthroscopy. 2009;25:169–74.

75. Shindle MK, Voos JE, Heyworth BE, et al. Hip arthroscopy in the athletic patient: current techniques and spectrum of disease. J Bone Joint Surg Am. 2007;89 Suppl 3:29–43.

76. Weber M, Ganz R. Recurrent traumatic dislocation of the hip: report of a case and review of the literature. J Orthop Trauma. 1997;11:382–5.

77. Anderson K, Strickland SM, Warren R. Hip and groin injuries in athletes. Am J Sports Med. 2001;29:521–33.

78. Pallia CS, Scott RE, Chao DJ. Traumatic hip dislocation in athletes. Curr Sports Med Rep. 2002;1:338–45.

79. Bankart A. The pathology and treatment of recurrent dislocation of the shoulder joint. J Bone Joint Surg Br. 1938;26:23–9.

80. Zebala LP, Schoenecker PL, Clohisy JC. Anterior femoroacetabular impingement: a diverse disease with evolving treatment options. Iowa Orthop J. 2007;27:71–81.

81. Pfirrmann CW, Mengiardi B, Dora C, Kalberer F, Zanetti M, Hodler J. Cam and pincer femoroacetabular impingement: characteristic MR arthrographic findings in 50 patients. Radiology. 2006;240:778–85.

82. Cooper DE, Warren RF, Barnes R. Traumatic subluxation of the hip resulting in aseptic necrosis and chondrolysis in a professional football player. Am J Sports Med. 1991;19:322–4.

83. Brooker Jr AF. The surgical approach to refractory trochanteric bursitis. Johns Hopkins Med J. 1979;145:98–100.

84. Bunker TD, Esler CN, Leach WJ. Rotator-cuff tear of the hip. J Bone Joint Surg Br. 1997;79:618–20.

85. Collee G, Dijkmans BA, Vandenbroucke JP, Cats A. Greater trochanteric pain syndrome (trochanteric bursitis) in low back pain. Scand J Rheumatol. 1991;20:262–6.

86. Kagan A. Rotator cuff tears of the hip. Clin Orthop Relat Res. 1999;368:135–40.

87. Karpinski MR, Piggott H. Greater trochanteric pain syndrome. A report of 15 cases. J Bone Joint Surg Br. 1985;67:762–3.

88. Tortolani PJ, Carbone JJ, Quartararo LG. Greater trochanteric pain syndrome in patients referred to orthopedic spine specialists. Spine J. 2002;2:251–4.

Complications of Hip Arthroscopy

32

Richard C. Mather III, Avinish Reddy, and Shane J. Nho

Hip arthroscopy is a relatively safe procedure with complications rates reported by several authors around 1.5% [1–4]. As with any surgical procedure, there are potential complications related to bleeding, deep venous thrombosis, infection, and neurovascular injury. There are a number of complications related to hip arthroscopy that have not been reported in any other joint due to issues related to joint distraction, proximity to the abdomen, and treatment of hip-specific pathology. Most of the reported complications involve the use of traction and fluid management. However, the most frequent, but underreported, complications likely result from iatrogenic cartilage injury and over- or undertreatment of the underlying pathology. For example, inadequate resection of a CAM or pincer lesion for femoroacetabular impingement (FAI) may result in persistent pain or revision surgery, while over-resection may cause subtle instability. As our understanding and ability to treat hip pathology have expanded, the rate of complications has not changed, but the types of complications have differed. In the early phases of hip arthroscopy, the complications were related to neurapraxias related to excessive traction time and limited to iatrogenic injury within the central compartment. Hip arthroscopy for FAI has also

Table 32.1 Complications of hip arthroscopy

General
Infection
Bleeding
Wound hematoma
Deep venous thrombosis
Specific to hip arthroscopy
Iatrogenic articular cartilage trauma
Instrument breakage
Heterotopic ossification
Traction
Dysesthesia/hypesthesia of pudendal and lateral cutaneous femoral nerves
Scrotal necrosis
Erectile dysfunction
Fluid management
Abdominal compartment syndrome
Intra-abdominal or retroperitoneal fluid extravasation
Over-/underresection of FAI
Avascular necrosis
Femoral neck fractures
Hip instability/dislocation
Incomplete acetabular and femoral osteoplasty

introduced complications that were not previously encountered (Table 32.1). The goal of this chapter is to review potential complications related to hip arthroscopy and discuss strategies for avoiding them.

General Complications

Certain complications occur with any extremity surgery, such as deep venous thrombosis, bleeding, and infection, but the rates of these complications are very low in hip arthroscopy. Bushnell et al. [5]. reported a 0% incidence in 5,500 cases. Other authors have reported similar rates, but the actual incidence is not known. Routine medical prophylaxis for deep venous thrombosis may be unnecessary, and treatment currently

R.C. Mather III, M.D.
Department of Orthopaedic Surgery,
Duke University Medical Center,
DUMC 2887, Durham, NC 27701, USA
e-mail: chad.mather@gmail.com

A. Reddy, B.S.
Department of Orthopedic Surgery,
Rush University Medical Center,
1611 West Harrison Street Suite 300,
Chicago, IL 60612, USA
e-mail: avinish.reddy@gmail.com

S.J. Nho, M.D., M.S. (✉)
Department of Orthopedic Surgery,
Rush University Medical Center, Midwest Orthopaedics at Rush,
1611 W. Harrison St., Suite 300,
Chicago, IL 60612, USA
e-mail: snho@rushortho.com

J.W.T. Byrd (ed.), *Operative Hip Arthroscopy*,
DOI 10.1007/978-1-4419-7925-4_32, © Springer Science+Business Media New York 2013

follows standards for knee arthroscopy. However, there are no published papers on the rate of deep venous thrombosis or pulmonary embolus after hip arthroscopy, but consideration of each patient's risk factors is necessary and may warrant more postoperative prophylaxis. Intraoperative use of sequential compression devices for all patients may be considered, but no evidence exists regarding its use.

Deep wound infections are rare and were only reported in one patient in a single case series. Clark and Villar [2], in a series of 1,054 hip arthroscopies, reported two hematomas and two portal bleedings. Postoperative hematoma and superficial wound drainage may be higher in the hip than for arthroscopy of other joints. The deep nature of the hip joint and the arthroscopic portals through muscular layers may predispose to this phenomenon, but the overall numbers remain low.

Complications Specific to Hip Arthroscopy

Traction

Traction-related injuries account for the majority of hip arthroscopy complications reported in the literature, and most of these are neurapraxias from prolonged traction time. The pudendal nerve is most frequently cited, followed by the sciatic nerve. Byrd et al. [1]., in a literature review and correspondence from surgeons who perform hip arthroscopy around the world, reported 13 of 20 complications to be nerve injuries, with six pudendal, four sciatic, two lateral femoral cutaneous (LFC), one femoral. Only one of these did not recover, with later evidence suggesting a laceration to the lateral femoral cutaneous nerve. Clark and Villar [2] reported 4 of 15 complications to be neurapraxias, with three related to the sciatic nerve and one femoral nerve.

While nerve injuries account for the large majority of traction-related complications, other complications have also been reported from prolonged leg traction. Byrd et al. [1]. reported one case of scrotal necrosis in their literature review and correspondence from other surgeons of 1,491 hip arthroscopies. Clarke and Villar [2] reported one case of a vaginal laceration that resolved without further treatment. Sexual dysfunction and erectile dysfunction (ED) may also occur with prolonged use of traction. The incidence of ED in patients undergoing femoral fracture fixation using traction is reported to be as high as 40%, but there are no reports of ED in the hip arthroscopy literature which may be, in part, due to a younger patient population [6]. Most of these cases resolved spontaneously and are believed to result from pudendal nerve compression.

Minimizing these complications involves using the least magnitude of traction force required for adequate distraction as well as limiting time of hip distraction. The magnitude of this force is estimated to be between 300 and 900 N [6, 7].

Furthermore, several authors have expressed concern that femoral traction displaces the neurovascular structures, with the lateral femoral cutaneous nerve at greatest risk under traction [7]. Elsaidi and colleagues [2] found in a cadaver study that traction did decrease the distance between the anterior portal and the LFC nerve by only .22 mm, virtually unchanged. However, both the femoral and sciatic nerves were found to be safer under traction. The safe distance between the anterior portal and femoral nerve actually increased by 6.4 mm with 23 kg of traction, while the distance of the sciatic nerve from the posterior portal increased from 40 to 43 mm. While iatrogenic damage to the capsule, labrum, and cartilage can occur with direct manipulation, it appears traction does not damage these structures. Elsaidi et al. [7]. applied up to 64 kg of traction and found macroscopic or histological damage to the labrum, ligamentum teres, or capsule.

Several strategies exist to reduce traction-related complications by minimizing magnitude and time under traction. Brumback and others [8] in a prospective study found that the development of pudendal nerve palsy correlated with traction magnitude. Traction time should be limited to less than two continuous hours. If procedures in the central compartment cannot be completed in less than 2 h, traction should be let down for 30 min before resuming the procedure. Second, efforts should be made to minimize the magnitude of traction force. The surgeon should begin by applying traction with fluoroscopy to obtain 10 mm of joint distraction. We prefer to begin with the hip abducted 30° and flexed 15°, and then axial traction can be applied. The hip is brought to neutral abduction and extension to distract the hip joint. Once 10 mm of joint space has been achieved, the hip is brought to abduction and the traction is released. The hip is brought back into neutral abduction and extension, and the hip can be checked again to determine if adequate joint distraction has been accomplished once the suction seal has been released relying on cantilever bending force. If there is no adequate distraction, then incremental hip distraction can be provided until a joint distraction of 10 mm is achieved with the smallest amount of traction force. In addition, the suction seal can be violated prior to hip distraction without increasing traction force. This is accomplished by placing a sterile needle in the hip joint capsule to allow the intra-articular pressure to equalize with atmospheric pressure. Byrd et al. [9]. described a vacuum phenomenon that occurs when the hip is distracted allowing further separation after this pressure is equalized with atmospheric pressure.

Fluid Management

Several authors have reported cases of fluid extravasation within the thigh and around the hip joint as well as the abdomen and retroperitoneum. Byrd et al. [1]. reported three cases in a literature review and correspondence with other surgeons of 1,491 hips. Sampson et al. [4]. reported ten cases out of a series of 1,000 hips. Fluid extravasation accounted for 3 out of 20 complications in the former series and 10 out of 28 complications in the latter series. Clark and Villar [2] did not report any cases of fluid extravasation in their series of 1,054 hip arthroscopies. In most cases, fluid extravasation is self-limiting and resolves without major intervention or without long-term consequences. Less severe cases have been treated with admission for observation and analgesics. However, some cases have had a more severe presentation, termed abdominal compartment syndrome, necessitating invasive treatment and resulting in long-term morbidity or mortality. In 1989, Fietsam et al. [10]. coined the term abdominal compartment syndrome and described that intra-abdominal pressure greater than 20 mmHg can pose significant risk to vital organs as well as lead to respiratory distress. Findings consist of abdominal pain and distension, increased bladder pressure, increased peak inspiratory pressure, and decreased urine outcome. As in extremity compartment syndrome, treatment is emergent exploratory laparotomy and delayed closure.

Bartlett et al. [11]. reported a case of abdominal compartment syndrome after performing hip arthroscopy for loose body removal in a patient with an acetabular fracture. The patient had previously undergone open reduction and internal fixation through an ilioinguinal approach. The fluid extravasation resulted in an intraoperative cardiac event, but the case did not result in a mortality. Many consider acute ipsilateral acetabular fracture a contraindication to hip arthroscopy.

Low core body temperature may be a sign of fluid extravasation. Haupt et al. [12]. reported a case of a 15-year-old girl who underwent a hip arthroscopy for lysis of adhesions after previously undergoing a surgical dislocation for FAI. The case was uneventful except for the anesthesiologist noting a decrease in core body temperature. In the postanesthesia care unit, the patient complained of abdominal distension and discomfort. Abdominal ultrasound revealed 2–3 l of intraperitoneal and retroperitoneal fluid. She recovered uneventfully in the next 24 h, and the authors suggested that a decrease in core body temperature may be a sign of fluid extravasation and requires further investigation immediately upon discovery.

Capsulotomy and/or psoas tenotomy may also place the patient at risk for abdominal fluid extravasation. Owens et al. [13]. reported a case of abdominal compartment syndrome in a 42-year-old service man who underwent elective hip arthroscopy for FAI. Operating time was 95 min, and pump pressure was maintained at 40 mmHg except for 2 min in which the pump pressure was noted to be at 60 mmHg. After the drapes were removed, the patient's abdomen was extremely distended with elevated bladder and peak inspira-

tory pressures. An emergent laparotomy yielded 1,200 mL of serosanguinous fluid, and the retroperitoneum was boggy with fluid tracking along the iliopsoas muscle and iliac vessels. His abdomen was left open and closed on postoperative day 3. Long-term follow-up revealed complete resolution of the hip symptoms but persistent abdominal complaints. The only risk factor reported in this case was the capsulotomy and psoas tenotomy. Since a capsulotomy is performed frequently in hip arthroscopy, management of fluid dynamics and arthroscopy pumps is critical. This complication may be minimized by maintaining low pressure by using a low flow pump system and minimizing operative time. Additionally, abnormal vital signs such as low core body temperature and blood pressure should be communicated to the surgeon, and the abdomen should be palpated periodically during the case to monitor for distention.

Avascular Necrosis

Avascular necrosis is a devastating potential complication of hip arthroscopy. Fortunately, it has not been reported frequently. Sampson et al. [4]. reported one case after hip arthroscopy with labral debridement. Femoral neck osteochondroplasty was not performed in this case; however, the blood supply is theoretically at greatest risk during CAM osteochondroplasty.

The primary blood supply to the femoral neck is through the deep branch of the medial femoral circumflex artery. It enters the hip capsule at the level of the superior gemellus and branches into two to four intracapsular lateral retinacular vessels [14]. Care must be taken not to extend the capsulotomy too posterior and to visualize the lateral synovial folds to avoid injury to the lateral retinacular vessels while performing lateral femoral neck osteoplasty. The medial and lateral synovial folds contain blood vessels to the head and should be used as landmarks for the medial and lateral extent of the CAM resection.

Cartilage Injury

Cartilage injury is probably the most underreported complication, and its significance is not well understood. Sampson et al. [15]. reported three femoral head scuffings, and Clark and Villar [9] only mentioned it without classifying as an actual complication. Steps can be taken to minimize the risk of cartilage damage including (1) applying adequate traction to allow appropriate working space, (2) pointing the bevel of the spinal needle and scope away from the head when entering the joint, and (3) insufflating the joint with air or saline prior to inserting instruments, and (4) instrument exchange should utilize a cannula whenever possible. If the central compartment cannot be distracted at least 10 mm, the procedure should start with entry into the peripheral compartment. For CAM impingement, in particular, femoral neck osteochondroplasty performed at the outset of the case can improve access to the central compartment.

Femoroacetabular Impingement

The incidence of inappropriate resection of CAM and/or pincer lesions likely accounts for the greatest number of complications and indications for revision hip arthroscopy [16, 17]. In open procedures, the entire head and neck are visible and appropriate resection is technically easier. Arthroscopic treatment of FAI does present unique challenges due to visualization and orientation to perform the adequate amount of bone resection. Careful capsulotomies, capsulectomies, and retraction of the capsule may be used along with fluoroscopy to improve the accuracy of resection. A major focus of current research is to help provide parameters for accurate planning, calculating, and executing the appropriate resection.

Phillipon et al. [17]. reported that underresection of the CAM and/or pincer lesion was present in 92% of their revisions. Heyworth et al. [16]. also reported underresection to be the problem in 79% of revisions. However, overresection can also be problematic as femoral neck stress fractures and iatrogenic instability have been reported in overzealous FAI treatment [4, 18].

Underresection

Incomplete reshaping can be avoided by adhering to one primary principle: visualization. Appropriate visualization is attained through imaging studies, both preoperative and intraoperative and careful surgical treatment of the capsule and manipulation of the extremity.

Preoperative planning is a critical first step. Physical exam can help to define the specific symptomatic anatomic regions. For example, pain with isolated abduction should alert the surgeon that the lateral acetabular rim or superior femoral neck is involved. Pain with flexion, adduction, and internal rotation, the impingement test, indicates pathology at the anterior superior acetabular rim and femoral neck. Pain with neutral flexion suggests subspine impingement, and failure to resect the acetabular rim may lead to a clinical failure.

The second part of preoperative planning involves knowledge of plain radiographs and understanding of the 3D morphology (CT or MRI). The amount of bone resected can be estimated by several parameters on plain radiographs. For example, the crossover sign on an AP radiograph highlights both the amount of bone and the extent of resection necessary. Described by Tannast et al. [19], the crossover sign is

defined as the anterior acetabular wall projecting lateral to the posterior wall. However, a focal overcoverage with a proximal crossover sign must be distinguished from true acetabular retroversion with a deficient posterior wall as the latter may not be appropriately treated with arthroscopy.

Visualization intraoperatively involves the judicious use of imaging, capsulotomy and capsulectomy, and hip positioning. Regarding imaging, a true AP of the hip must be obtained so that the rim lesion that was seen in the office can be reproduced. Capsulectomy or capsulotomy facilitates visualization to correlate the 3D CT scan to the arthroscopic visualization of the CAM/pincer lesion. Furthermore, surgical maneuvers such as a T-capsulotomy allow complete visualization of the femoral neck. Repair afterwards should minimize the risk of symptomatic instability. During femoral neck osteoplasty, the hip position can be frequently changed in several planes, flexion–extension and ER–IR, to improve visualization and to correlate with preoperative evaluation.

Overresection

Femoral Neck Fracture

Femoral neck fracture likely occurs from a combination of two factors, excessive resection and excessive early weight bearing. Lateral CAM lesions are especially at risk given the location on the tension side of the femoral neck. Clinically, only one author has reported a femoral neck fracture, with Sampson et al. [4]. reporting one femoral neck fracture in a series of 120 patients with arthroscopic treatment of a CAM deformity. Cadaveric studies suggest that up to 30% of the anterolateral quadrant of the femoral neck can be resected safely [20]. At 30%, the energy required to produce a fracture decreased by 20%. The typical CAM lesion accounts for 15% of the bone volume, so rarely should a resection approach dangerous levels [21, 22]. Additionally, osteochondroplasty of the femoral head–neck junction should be limited to the level of the femoral neck and, therefore, should minimize, if not, eliminate altogether, the risk of femoral neck fractures.

In addition to careful and appropriate CAM resection, femoral neck fractures that can be minimized with a period of protected weight bearing and patient education. Patients who are at risk for this complication include those with osteopenia or osteoporosis, and female athletic triad should be identified before surgery and may need to be kept on a longer period of protected weight bearing.

Instability

Hip joint instability is a lesser understood pathologic entity in general, and understanding and recognition of iatrogenic instability is has not been well characterized. The causes of hip instability after arthroscopy are thought to be multifactorial. The static hip stabilizers are the osseous, labral, and capsuloligamentous structures, and the dynamic stabilizers include the hip girdle musculature and neuromuscular control [23]. Overresection of the acetabular rim may lead to anterior instability, and treatments for this problem may require a periacetabular osteotomy. Preoperative imaging should be performed, and patients with evidence of acetabular dysplasia should not undergo acetabular rim resection. Capsulotomy or capsulectomy may theoretically predispose patients to develop symptomatic anterior instability. The least amount of capsulotomy/capsulectomy that will allow adequate visualization of the lesion should be performed. Care should especially be taken in patients at risk for this complication: young females and dancers. Capsular repair may be performed in patients at high risk.

To date, there are only three reported cases of hip instability after hip joint preservation surgery, these cases are thought to be underreported, and an additional two cases have been mentioned in another article [23–26]. Benali and Katthagen [24] reported on a case of labral resection in the setting of a dysplastic hip (center-edge angle of 23°) that presented 3 months after arthroscopy with hip subluxation. The unstable hip necessitated conversion to a total hip arthroplasty. The authors conclude that the labrum probably has a larger role in stability in dysplastic hips. Ranawat et al. [26]. reported on a patient with a history of bilateral shoulder capsulorrhaphy for multidirectional instability with a hip labral tear who underwent arthroscopic labral repair. Central and peripheral compartment capsulectomies were performed to access the central compartment, and a double-loaded suture anchor repair was performed. Although there was no evidence of an abnormal femoral head–neck junction on preoperative radiographs, a CAM lesion was indentified intraoperatively. The surgeon elected to decompress the CAM lesion to protect the labral repair in order to prevent secondary impingement due to hyperlaxity. In the central compartment, the anterior capsule was repaired. Postoperatively, the patient was instructed to undergo protected weight bearing with crutches and wore a hip orthosis to prevent hip extension and external rotation to protect the repair. At 6 weeks, the orthosis and crutches were discontinued, and the patient was allowed to bear full weight. At 2 months, the patient fell while walking down a flight of stairs and determined to have an anterior hip dislocation that necessitated closed reduction in the emergency room. The patient was initially managed with a hip orthosis and protected weight bearing but eventually underwent revision hip arthroscopy and anterior capsulorrhaphy. Matsuda [23] reported a case in which a patient with FAI underwent arthroscopy acetabular rim trimming, labral resection, and osteochondroplasty of the femoral head–neck junction. In the recovery room, the patient had an anterior hip dislocation that was unable to be concentrically reduced and maintained in a brace. The patient was brought back to the operating room for a mini-open anterior capsulorrhaphy which was able to maintain hip stability.

Heterotopic Ossification

Heterotopic ossification (HO) is known to occur with open hip surgery, but the incidence in hip arthroscopy is less well studied. None of the major case series on hip arthroscopy complications report HO, but Randelli et al. [15]. examined this complication specifically in the setting of NSAID prophylaxis. They report on a group of 300 patients undergoing hip arthroscopy for FAI with 285 hips receiving NSAID prophylaxis and 15 without HO prophylaxis. The overall prevalence of HO as measured by plain radiographs was 1.6%, but all cases occurred in the group NOT receiving prophylaxis. While further prospective study is needed to evaluate the role of HO prophylaxis, early reports suggest HO does occur with hip arthroscopy and prophylaxis may be considered (Fig. 32.1).

Children and Adolescents

Patients under the age of 18 represent a unique population undergoing hip arthroscopy. Indications may be similar as in adults, such as FAI, or different, for example, slipped capital femoral epiphysis and Perthes disease. Children may be at risk for different complications including physeal separation, triradiate cartilage injury, growth arrest, and avascular necrosis.

Nwachukwu et al. [27]. reported a complication rate of 1.8% in a series of 175 patients. All patients had labral tears, 131 had isolated labral tears and another 37 had labral tears with concomitant hip conditions, including FAI (10), coxa saltans interna (7) and externa (4), and acetabular fracture (1), among others. Other indications included Perthes (10), slipped capital femoral epiphysis (1), juvenile rheumatoid arthritis (3), avascular necrosis (1), and hip dysplasia (5). The complications in this cohort were similar to older patients consisting of transient nerve pudendal nerve palsy (2), instrument breakage (1), and suture abscess (1). There were no cases of proximal femoral epiphyseal separation, triradiate cartilage injury, AVN, or growth arrest. Interestingly, 86.7% of the patients in this cohort were female. The authors suggest that activities common to young women may predispose to hip pathology. For example, dance, gymnastics, ballet, and equestrianism require extremes of range of motion, in particular, hip flexion. This study did not report unique complications to females in this study, but surgery for FAI was only performed on 10 patients. In this study, the high proportion of adolescent female athletes suggests complications such as femoral neck fracture may be theoretically higher in this

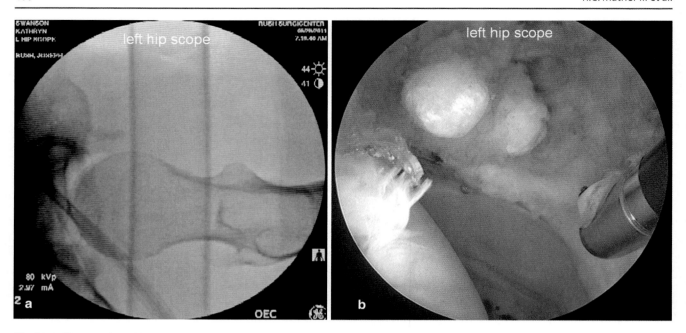

Fig. 32.1 Heterotopic ossification after hip arthroscopy. (**a**) Cross-table lateral view of the hip joint and the appearance of HO in the anterosuperior acetabulum. (**b**) Arthroscopic view of HO within the capsular tissue

group and underlying disorders such as the female athlete triad should be closely monitored.

The Complication: "The Learning Curve"

Hip arthroscopy may have a steep learning curve, and complications differ as surgeon experience increases. Souza et al. [28]. reported on this topic in a series of 194 patients treated over a nine-year period with hip arthroscopy for various indications. Groups of 30 patients were successively examined for complications. The start of this study did mark the beginning of this groups' experience with hip arthroscopy. They reported a 6.1% complication rate with 1% considered major. The two major complications were overresection causing hip dislocation and scrotal necrosis. Other complications were nerve palsies (5 out of 12) of which all recovered and one involved erectile dysfunction, one femoral neck stress fracture due to overresection, and one deep venous thrombosis. In all, 58% were traction-related complications.

This study reported no change in the overall complication rate over time, but rather a change in the type of complications. Vascular complications disappeared over time, and only neurologic complications were observed in the most experienced group. The overwhelming majority of neurologic complications were self-limiting, but the authors did note an increase in major complications including the dislocation and femoral neck stress fracture with the onset of FAI procedures performed by the group.

Conclusions

Hip arthroscopy is a safe and effective means for the treatment of hip pain and dysfunction in the appropriately indicated patient. The rate of complications is thought to be around 1.5% of cases [1–4]. Beyond general surgical complications, many of the complications related to hip arthroscopy can be minimized or avoided altogether. The type of complications has changed as techniques have expanded beyond the central compartment. Whereas the initial complications were related to iatrogenic injury to the cartilage and traction-related dysesthesia around the groin and dorsum of the foot, complications related to the arthroscopic treatment of FAI can be quite devastating and may include abdominal or retroperitoneal fluid extravasation, osteonecrosis, femoral neck fractures, instability, or over-/under-resection of CAM and pincer lesions (Table 32.1). There appears to be a relationship between complications and the number of cases performed. As arthroscopic treatment of disorders in the peritrochanteric space and deep gluteal space expands, there should be a heightened awareness of potential complications that may occur.

References

1. Byrd J. Complications associated with hip arthroscopy. In: Byrd J, editor. Operative Hip arthroscopy. New York: Thieme; 1998. p. 171–6. 70.
2. Clarke MT, Arora A, Villar RN. Hip arthroscopy: complications in 1054 cases. Clin Orthop Relat Res. 2003;406:84–8. doi: 10.1097/01.blo.0000043048.84315.af34.

3. Griffin DR. Complications of arthroscopy of the hip. J Bone Joint Surg Br. 1999;81:604–6. 4.

4. Sampson TG. Complications of hip arthroscopy. Tech Orthop. 2005;20:63–6. 73.

5. Bushnell BD, Anz AW, Bert JM. Venous thromboembolism in lower extremity arthroscopy. Arthroscopy. 2008;24:604–11. doi:10.1016/j.arthro.2007.11.01025. S0749–8063(07)01038–9 [pii].

6. Flierl MA, Stahel PF, Hak DJ, Morgan SJ, Smith WR. Traction table–related complications in orthopaedic surgery. J Am Acad Orthop Surg. 2010;18:668–75. 10.

7. Elsaidi GA, Ruch DS, Schaefer WD, Kuzma K, Smith BP. Complications associated with traction on the hip during arthroscopy. J Bone Joint Surg Br. 2004;86:793–6. 11.

8. Brumback RJ, Ellison TS, Molligan H, Molligan DJ, Mahaffey S, Schmidhauser C. Pudendal nerve palsy complicating intramedullary nailing of the femur. J Bone Joint Surg Am. 1992;74:1450–5. 75.

9. Byrd JW, Chern KY. Traction versus distension for distraction of the joint during hip arthroscopy. Arthroscopy. 1997;13:346–9. 31.

10. Fietsam Jr R, Villalba M, Glover JL, Clark K. Intra-abdominal compartment syndrome as a complication of ruptured abdominal aortic aneurysm repair. Am Surg. 1989;55:396–402. 78.

11. Bartlett CS, DiFelice GS, Buly RL, Quinn TJ, Green DS, Helfet DL. Cardiac arrest as a result of intraabdominal extravasation of fluid during arthroscopic removal of a loose body from the hip joint of a patient with an acetabular fracture. J Orthop Trauma. 1998;12:294–9. 28.

12. Haupt U, Volkle D, Waldherr C, Beck M. Intra- and retroperitoneal irrigation liquid after arthroscopy of the hip joint. Arthroscopy. 2008;24:966–8. doi:10.1016/j.arthro.2007.02.01979. S0749–8063(07)00273–3 [pii].

13. Fowler J, Owens BD. Abdominal compartment syndrome after hip arthroscopy. Arthroscopy. 2010;26:128–30. 1.

14. Glick JM, Sampson TG, Gordon RB, Behr JT, Schmidt E. Hip arthroscopy by the lateral approach. Arthroscopy. 1987;3:4–12. 41.

15. Randelli F, Pierannunzii L, Banci L, Ragone V, Aliprandi A, Buly R. Heterotopic ossifications after arthroscopic management of femoroacetabular impingement: the role of NSAID prophylaxis. J Orthop Traumatol. 2010;11:245–50. doi:10.1007/s10195-010-0121-z82.

16. Heyworth BE, Shindle MK, Voos JE, Rudzki JR, Kelly BT. Radiologic and intraoperative findings in revision hip arthroscopy. Arthroscopy. 2007;23:1295–302. doi:10.1016/j.arthro.2007.09.01543. S0749–8063(07)00961–9 [pii].

17. Philippon MJ, Schenker ML, Briggs KK, Kuppersmith DA, Maxwell RB, Stubbs AJ. Revision hip arthroscopy. Am J Sports Med. 2007;35:1918–21. doi:10.1177/036354650730509752. 0363546507305097 [pii].

18. Ilizaliturri Jr VM. Complications of arthroscopic femoroacetabular impingement treatment: a review. Clin Orthop Relat Res. 2009;467:760–8. 3.

19. Tannast M, Siebenrock KA, Anderson SE. Femoroacetabular impingement: radiographic diagnosis – what the radiologist should know. AJR Am J Roentgenol. 2007;188:1540–52. doi:10.2214/AJR.06.092160. 188/6/1540 [pii].

20. Mardones RM, Gonzalez C, Chen Q, Zobitz M, Kaufman KR, Trousdale RT. Surgical treatment of femoroacetabular impingement: evaluation of the effect of the size of the resection. J Bone Joint Surg Am. 2005;87:273–9. doi:10.2106/JBJS.D.0179348. 87/2/273 [pii].

21. Beck M, Leunig M, Parvizi J, Boutier V, Wyss D, Ganz R. Anterior femoroacetabular impingement: part II. Midterm results of surgical treatment. Clin Orthop Relat Res. 2004;418:67–73.

22. Ilizaliturri Jr VM, Orozco-Rodriguez L, Acosta-Rodriguez E, Camacho-Galindo J. Arthroscopic treatment of cam-type femoroacetabular impingement: preliminary report at 2 years minimum follow-up. J Arthroplasty. 2008;23:226–34. doi:10.1016/j.arth.2007.03.01646. S0883–5403(07)00166–0 [pii].

23. Matsuda DK. Acute iatrogenic dislocation following hip impingement arthroscopic surgery. Arthroscopy. 2009;25:400–4. 55.

24. Benali Y, Katthagen BD. Hip subluxation as a complication of arthroscopic debridement. Arthroscopy. 2009;25:405–7. 54.

25. Ilizaliturri Jr VM. Complications of arthroscopic femoroacetabular impingement treatment: a review. Clin Orthop Relat Res. 2009;467:760–8. 58.

26. Ranawat AS, McClincy M, Sekiya JK. Anterior dislocation of the hip after arthroscopy in a patient with capsular laxity of the hip. A case report. J Bone Joint Surg Am. 2009;91:192–7. 56.

27. Nwachukwu BU, McFeely ED, Nasreddine AY, Krcik JA, Frank J, Kocher MS. Complications of hip arthroscopy in children and adolescents. J Pediatr Orthop. 2011;31:227–31. 9.

28. Souza BG, Dani WS, Honda EK, Ricioli Jr W, Guimarães RP, Ono NK, Polesello GC. Do complications in hip arthroscopy change with experience? Arthroscopy. 2010;26:1053–8. 5.

Rehabilitation of the Hip

33

Erica M. Coplen and Michael L. Voight

Introduction

Over the past decade, hip arthroscopy has gained an increase in popularity. With the advent of hip arthroscopy, there has come an increased recognition of intra-articular hip pathologies and improved techniques for the management of these various pathologies [1–7]. In 2008, more than 30,000 hip arthroscopies were performed, and this number is expected to grow at a rate of 15% over the next 5 years, resulting in more than 70,000 hip arthroscopies performed each year by 2013 [8]. While mechanical problems can often be corrected through surgery, the functional deficits must be corrected through the rehabilitation process. Therefore, the evolution of hip arthroscopy has necessitated a progression in hip rehabilitation to insure optimal postsurgical results. Understanding the process of rehabilitation from preoperative education to the patient's achievement of full function is an integral part of the patient reaching their full potential postsurgery. While it is generally accepted that rehabilitation after hip arthroscopy is vitally important, there is limited evidence-based research to support the rehabilitative guidelines [9–12]. Rehabilitative methodology and techniques commonly employed after minimally invasive surgical techniques for other joints, such as the knee, shoulder, elbow, and ankle, have found application in the management of hip disorders. Understanding and respecting basic principles is always key to obtaining successful outcomes with any technique. As the surgical treatment for hip pain has evolved, the hip rehabilitation process has followed a similar path.

While the rehabilitation protocols following hip arthroscopy continue to evolve, the overall fundamental objective has remained the same: return the patient back to their preinjury level of activity as quickly and as safely as possible with the best possible long-term results. The goal of the rehabilitation plan is to reduce symptoms (modulate pain and inflammation) and improve function (restore mobility, strength, proprioception, and endurance). This is approached through a systematic progression dependent on the patient's status (pathology present) and functional needs. During the assessment process, it is important to determine the patient's level of understanding regarding the pathology, expectations of goals, and the time frame for achieving them. Patient education is the foundation of the rehabilitation plan. The patient must comprehend the related precautions and the recommended progression per their individual situation. Through collaborative consultation with the physician, physical therapist, and patient, reasonable goals and expectations can be formulated for favorable outcomes.

Assessment and Overview

The physician's history, examination, and diagnostic studies determine the patient's diagnosis and prognosis of surgical or nonsurgical treatment. The patient's history and the clinical evaluation assist in determining how the symptoms will respond to treatment. A course of presurgical treatment (prehab) may be indicated in some hip cases to regain neuromotor control and decrease stresses to the joint. An appropriate exercise program can, at times, help restore normal mechanics and minimize joint stresses to facilitate healing. In other circumstances, it can "buy time" when a patient desires and the physician thinks it is beneficial to delay operative intervention. Rehabilitation of a patient preoperatively, when the need for surgery has been confirmed, better prepares patients psychologically and physically for postsurgical recovery.

E.M. Coplen, DPT (✉)
Nashville Sports Medicine Physical Therapy,
2011 Church St, Suite 103, Nashville,
TN 37203, USA
e-mail: erica@nsmoc.com

M.L. Voight, DHSc, PT, OCS, SCS, ATC, FAPTA
School of Physical Therapy, Belmont University,
1900 Belmont Blvd, Nashville,
TN 37212, USA
e-mail: mike.voight@belmont.edu

J.W.T. Byrd (ed.), *Operative Hip Arthroscopy*,
DOI 10.1007/978-1-4419-7925-4_33, © Springer Science+Business Media New York 2013

As direct access and autonomous practice for physical therapists become more prevalent, the rehab provider may have the opportunity to be the initial caregiver for a patient with hip pain. Understanding the hip mechanics and how to properly assess the hip is imperative in deciding whether the severity of the hip dysfunction requires referral back to their orthopedic physician or if the problem can be managed conservatively. Treating a hip patient conservatively can be just as important as treating a patient postoperatively.

The foundation of assessment of a hip dysfunction begins with an understanding of the pathomechanics of the hip and pelvis. Joint dysfunction can manifest as a primary mechanical complaint or secondarily as a compensatory mechanical dysfunction. For example, for a patient with degenerative changes within the joint, the primary disorder is the antalgic gait due to joint pain. The secondary dysfunction may be due to weakness of the gluteus medius presenting as an abductor lurch (Trendelenburg gait) (Fig. 33.1). Disorders of the sacroiliac joint (SI joint) and lumbar spine also become considerations with chronic hip dysfunction because of altered gait and weight-bearing mechanics. Primary problems of symptomatic hip pathology may involve the soft tissue encasing the joint, the surrounding capsule, or the joint structure. The irritation and inflammation of the musculotendinous structures, bursae, or joint capsule can result in concomitant tendinitis, bursitis, or capsulitis. The ligaments of the hip joint are susceptible to acute tearing and chronic degeneration. Within the joint, labral or chondral injury can be responsible for protracted hip symptoms. Femoroacetabular impingement (FAI) has been suggested as playing a role in the development of acetabular labral tears and chondral lesions. FAI is a newly well-recognized indication for arthroscopic hip surgery [13]. Loose bodies and labral lesions are also well-recognized indications for arthroscopic surgery, which tends to produce gratifying results for properly selected patients [3].

Pain-free functional movement necessary to allow participation in sports is composed of many components: posture, ROM, muscle performance, and motor control. Impairments in any of these components can potentially alter required functional movement. The therapeutic plan of care needs to be focused on the patient's functional impairments that are a result and/or cause of pathology. The clinician can then use the traditional parts of the clinical examination to refine and deduce the specific pathoanatomic structures responsible for the functional limitation.

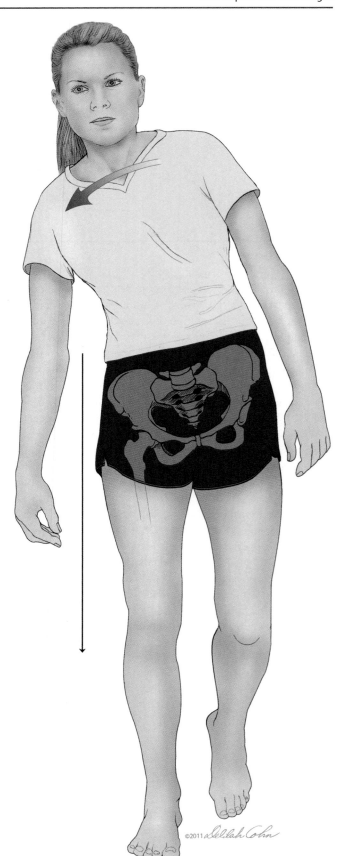

Fig. 33.1 Trendelenburg gait. Abductor lurch may occur as a compensatory mechanism to reduce the forces across the joint. Shifting the torso over the involved hip moves the center of gravity closer to the axis of the hip, shortens the lever arm moment, and reduces compressive joint force. (All rights are retained by Dr. Byrd)

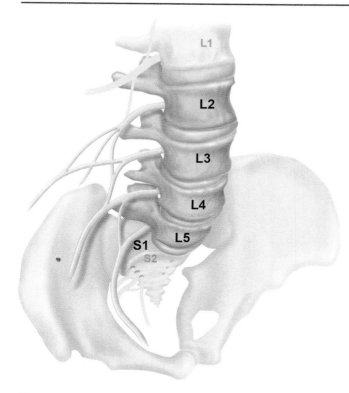

Fig. 33.2 The hip receives innervation predominantly from the L2–S2 nerve roots of the lumbosacral plexus. (All rights are retained by Dr. Byrd)

The clinical presentation of a patient with an acetabular labral tear has shown to be anterior hip or groin pain in greater than 90% of patients. Less often, patients can complain of lateral hip pain or pain deep in the posterior buttock. Data suggests that anterior hip or groin pain is more consistent with an anterior labral tear, whereas buttock pain is more consistent with a posterior labral tear. Mechanical symptoms can include clicking, locking or catching, or giving way, with clicking being the most consistently reported mechanical symptom [14]. The patient can complain of a sharp "catching" pain that is often associated with a popping, and a sensation of locking or giving away of the joint [15, 16]. Patients can have pain in the anterior groin, anterior thigh, buttock, greater trochanter, and medial knee. The reason for the variety in locations of complaints of pain is that the sensory supply to the hip joint is 65% from the obturator nerve; so pain in this area will be referred to the groin and the medial aspect of the knee. Approximately 30% of the sensory distribution is from the femoral nerve, which will refer to the anterior portion of the thigh. The remaining sensory distribution is from a branch of the sciatic nerve; therefore, the pain will be referred to the buttock [19] (Fig. 33.2). In a retrospective study by McCarthy and associates, they reviewed 94 consecutive patients with intractable hip pain who underwent

hip arthroscopy [17]. They found statistically significant associations between the preoperative clinical presentation and arthroscopic operative findings. Acetabular labral tears detected arthroscopically correlated significantly with symptoms of anterior inguinal pain ($r = 1$), painful clicking episodes ($r = 0.809$), transient locking ($r = 0.307$), and giving way ($r = 0.320$). Patients also commonly complain of pain deep in the hip in which they may grasp/cup their lateral hip just above the greater trochanter. This is termed the "C" sign which describes the shape that the hand makes to surround the hip (Fig. 33.3a, b) [4].

History

Taking a thorough history in any patient case can help determine an appropriate tailored rehabilitative program. Understanding the patient's goals preoperatively and/or postoperatively can also help guide the rehab. As there are various disorders that can result in a painful hip, the history may be equally varied as far as onset, duration, and severity of symptoms. For example, acute labral tears associated with an injury have gone undiagnosed for decades, presenting as a chronic disorder. Conversely, patients with a degenerative labral tear may describe the acute onset of symptoms associated with a relatively innocuous episode and gradual progression of symptoms [4]. Many patients with FAI who develop symptoms as adults will often reflect back on the fact that they were never very flexible when they were younger. They commonly complain that they were never able to sit cross-legged on the floor (Fig. 33.4a, b). Common complaints of pain, functional limitations, and impairments are seen among patients that present with hip pain and/or a hip pathology. For example, common functional deficits include pain with prolonged sitting; difficulty donning socks or shoes; inability to squat or sit on low surfaces; and altered gait with a shortened stance phase, protraction of the hip, and decreased hip extension on the involved side. In addition, other common complaints can be loss of ROM, pain with increased stride length during the gait cycle, dyspareunia, and pain with negotiating stairs. Understanding your patient's mechanism of injury, current activity level, and goals for rehab/surgery will help guide your assessment and treatment for the patient.

Physical Examination

The clinical assessment includes observation of gait (Fig. 33.5), assessment of hip ROM and strength, performance of special tests (as referenced in previous chapters), and observation of basic functional transitional movements

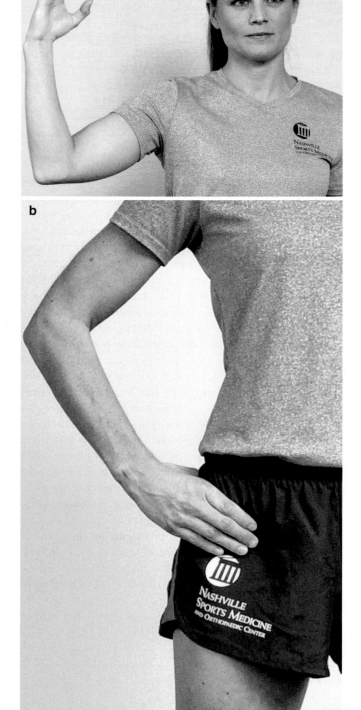

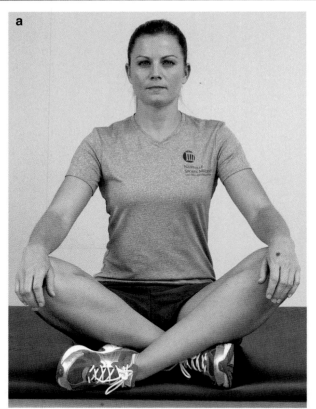

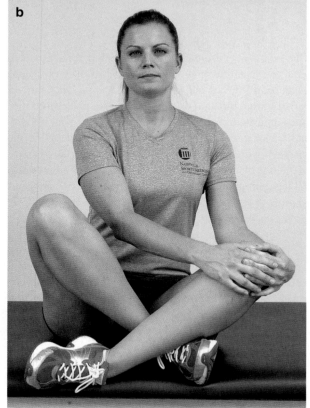

Fig. 33.3 C sign. Patients commonly complain of pain deep in the hip and may grasp/cup their lateral hip just above the greater trochanter. This is termed the "C" sign which describes the shape that the hand (**a**) makes to surround the hip (**b**). (All rights are retained by Dr. Byrd)

Fig. 33.4 (**a**) Normal cross-legged sitting position. (**b**) Patients will commonly demonstrate that they are not able to sit in a cross-legged position due to pain or reduced flexibility. (All rights are retained by Dr. Byrd)

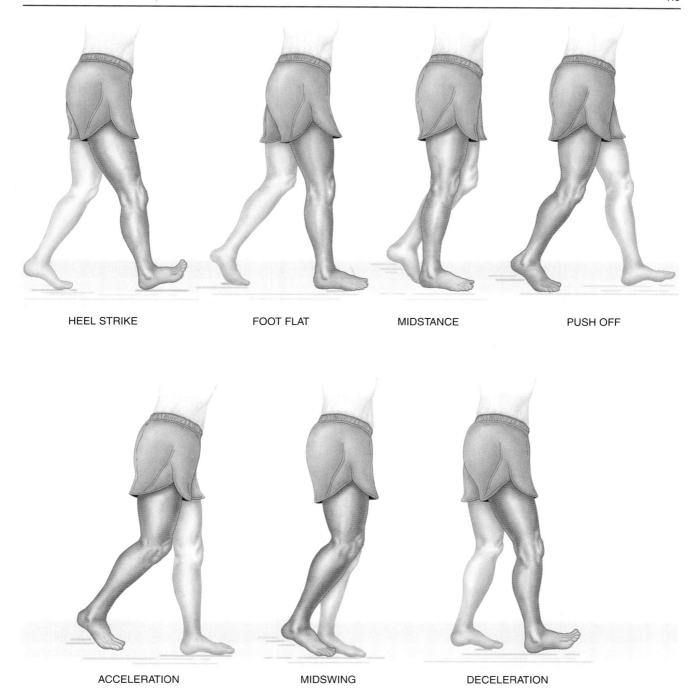

HEEL STRIKE   FOOT FLAT   MIDSTANCE   PUSH OFF

ACCELERATION   MIDSWING   DECELERATION

Fig. 33.5 Gait is continuously assessed throughout the rehab process. Schematic illustrates the normal phases of the gait cycle. (All rights are retained by Dr. Byrd)

such as sit to stand to sit, ascending/descending stairs, and balance activities. This also includes understanding the patient's specific movement patterns and what elicits their painful symptoms. At this time, determining if the patient has involvement of the lumbar spine, pelvis, or sacroiliac joint is important in guiding your physical examination and differential diagnosis. Screening the entire lower extremity chain, including the knees and feet, can be imperative to your evaluation and should be performed during your assessment.

Movement Dysfunction and Assessment

A sport or movement-specific examination is imperative to understanding the contributions of athletic activity to functional limitations or pain. Motion, related to and produced by all the neuromusculoskeletal contributions of the human body, although variable by age remains the prerequisite for function. Traditional rehabilitation approaches used with athletes are often based on identification of inflamed tissues (and subsequent symptomatic treatment of those tissues) rather than on the correction of the mechanical cause of the tissue irritation. The symptom-based approach makes the assumption that the painful tissue is the source of the pain and subsequent dysfunction [18]. Although clinicians are trained to examine both the local area of complaint and the whole patient, typically the sequence of assessment is specific to general, with the examination focused on reproducing the athlete's pain. By looking at specific tissue first, an opportunity is missed to watch the body move as a whole and lost is the overall perspective of what the athlete can functionally achieve. All too often clinicians become too focused on the special tests that serve to confirm a pathologic diagnosis that they fail to refine, qualify, and quantify the functional parameters of the problem at hand. Reversing the sequence of assessment by examining gross movements before looking at component impairments, the therapist may determine where to focus specific assessment. By taking this approach, gross movements may provoke or reveal symptoms in the problem area as well as in other areas. Observing functional movements that the patient is able or unable to perform and those that produce pain may provide a clearer picture of the cause of the problem. One exception to initiating the examination using functional movements is the presence of chemical pain, that is, acute postsurgical or postinjury inflammation. Pain or inflammation of chemical origin is capable of influencing and producing movement dysfunction. Initial treatment emphasis would be directed locally in order to mediate the problem prior to a complete functional examination.

The Selective Functional Movement Assessment

Mobility and stability coexist to create efficient movement in the human body. Mobility and stability are the fundamental building blocks of strength, endurance, speed, power, and agility and therefore of all athletic activities. When these building blocks are decreased, the patient may compensate quality and therefore develop altered biomechanical habits to allow continued performance of an activity. When required movements are changed to accommodate less than optimal musculoskeletal integrity, negative changes and compensations such as altered joint arthrokinematics can occur. Accommodations to altered mobility and stability can produce inefficiency and thus require more energy, resulting in an increased chance of poor performance, pain and likelihood of injury, especially with the years of accumulation of these accommodations combined with the aging changes of the musculoskeletal system.

The Selective Functional Movement Assessment (SFMA) is one way of quantifying the qualitative assessment of functional movement and is not a substitute for the traditional examination process [19]. Rather, the SFMA is the first step in the functional orthopedic examination process, which serves to focus and direct choices made during the remaining portions of the exam, which are pertinent to the functional needs of the older athlete. The SFMA uses functional movement patterns to identify impairments that potentially alter specific functional movements. The approach taken with the SFMA places less emphasis on identifying the source of the symptoms and more on identifying the cause. An example of this assessment scheme is illustrated with a runner that presents with low back pain. Frequently, the symptoms associated with the low back pain are not examined in light of other secondary causes such as hip mobility. Lack of mobility at the hip is compensated for by increased mobility or instability of the spine. The global approach taken by the SFMA would identify the cause of the low back dysfunction.

The functional assessment process emphasizes the analysis of function to restore proper movement of specific physical tasks. Use of movement patterns with the application of specific stresses and overpressure serves to determine if dysfunction and/or pain are elicited. The movement patterns will also reaffirm or redirect the focus of the musculoskeletal problem. Maintaining or restoring proper movement of specific segments is a key to preventing or correcting musculoskeletal pain. The SFMA also identifies where functional exercise may be beneficial and also provides feedback regarding the effectiveness of such exercise. A functional approach to exercise utilizes key specific movements that are common to the patient regardless of the specific sport or activities of daily living they participate in. Exercise that uses repeated movement patterns required for desired function is not only realistic but also practical and time efficient.

The Scoring System for the SFMA

The SFMA uses seven basic movement patterns to rate and rank the two variables of pain and function (Fig. 33.6). The hip is affected by five of these (Video 33.1: http://goo.gl/ZHYvk) (Fig. 33.7). Function comprises mobility and stability. The term *functional* describes any unlimited or unrestricted movement. The term *dysfunctional* describes movements that are limited or restricted in some way, demonstrating a lack of mobility, stability, or symmetry within a given movement pattern. *Painful* denotes a situation where the selective functional movement reproduces symptoms,

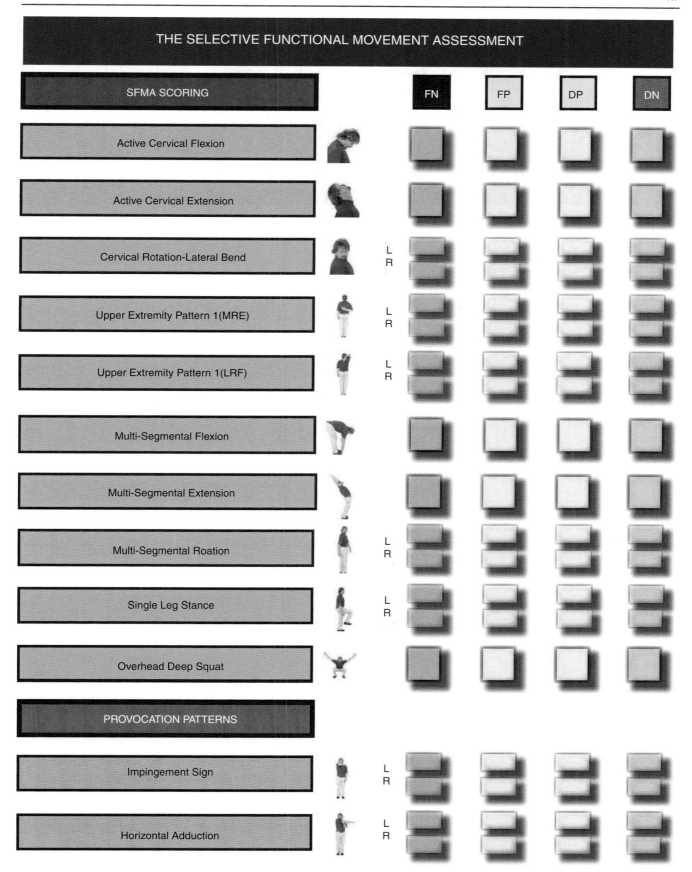

Fig. 33.6 SFMA scoring chart

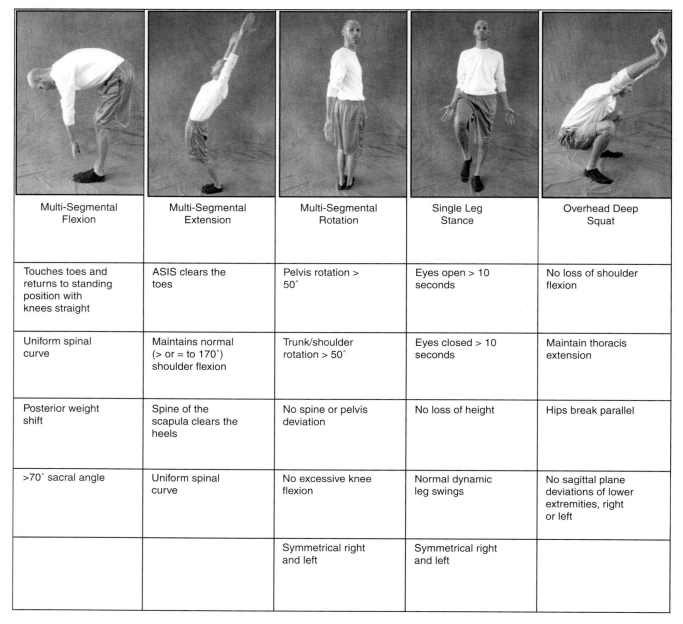

Multi-Segmental Flexion	Multi-Segmental Extension	Multi-Segmental Rotation	Single Leg Stance	Overhead Deep Squat
Touches toes and returns to standing position with knees straight	ASIS clears the toes	Pelvis rotation > 50˚	Eyes open > 10 seconds	No loss of shoulder flexion
Uniform spinal curve	Maintains normal (> or = to 170˚) shoulder flexion	Trunk/shoulder rotation > 50˚	Eyes closed > 10 seconds	Maintain thoracis extension
Posterior weight shift	Spine of the scapula clears the heels	No spine or pelvis deviation	No loss of height	Hips break parallel
>70˚ sacral angle	Uniform spinal curve	No excessive knee flexion	Normal dynamic leg swings	No sagittal plane deviations of lower extremities, right or left
		Symmetrical right and left	Symmetrical right and left	

Fig. 33.7 SFMA movements that affect the hip are shown

increases symptoms, or brings about secondary symptoms that need to be noted. Therefore, each pattern of the SFMA must be scored with one of four possible outcomes.

The seven basic movements or motions that comprise the basic SFMA screen look simple but require good flexibility and control. A patient who is (1) unable to perform a movement correctly, (2) shows a major limitation with one or more of the movement patterns, or (3) demonstrates an obvious difference between the left and right side of the body has exposed a significant finding that may be the key to correcting the problem.

Box 33.1 Functional Assessment (Should Be Done Throughout the Rehab Process, but Official Assessments by the Orthopedic Physician and the Therapist Are Done at 4, 8, 12, and 16 Weeks (Which Coincide with the Phases of Rehab) Unless Otherwise Indicated by the MD)
- Tailor to each pt
- Functional squat (see SMFA assessment)
- Gait

- Job/sport requirements
- Endurance
- Mobility (ROM)
- Strength
- Flexibility

The first five movements examine a combination of upper quarter, lower quarter, and trunk movements. The shoulder and cervical assessments examine upper quarter movement quality. Each movement is graded with a notation of FN, FP, DP, or DN. All responses other than FN are then assessed in greater detail to help refine the movement information and direct the clinical testing. Detailed algorithmic SFMA breakouts are available for each of the movement patterns, but it is beyond the scope of this chapter to describe. Once dysfunction and/or symptoms have been provoked in a functional manner, it is necessary to work backward to more specific assessments of the component parts of the functional movement by using special tests or range of motion comparisons. As the gross functional movement is broken down into component parts, the therapist should examine for consistencies and inconsistencies as well as level of dysfunction for each test as compared to the optimal movement pattern. Provocation of symptoms as well as limitations in movement or the inability to maintain stability during movements should be noted.

Loaded and Unloaded Implications

By performing parts of the test movements in both loaded and unloaded conditions, the clinician can draw conclusions about the interplay between the patient's available mobility and stability. If any of the first five movements are restricted when performed in the loaded position (e.g., limited, and/or in some way painful prior to the end of the ROM), a clue is provided regarding functional movement. For example, if a movement is performed easily (does not provoke symptoms or have any limitation) in an unloaded situation, it would seem logical that the appropriate joint ROM and muscle flexibility exist and therefore a stability problem may be the cause of why the patient cannot perform the movement in a loaded position. In this case, a patient has the requisite available biomechanical ability to go through the necessary ROM to perform the task, but the neurophysiological response needed for stabilization that creates dynamic alignment and postural support is not available when the functional movement is performed.

If the patient is observed to have a limitation, restriction, and pain when unloaded, the patient displays consistent abnormal biomechanical behavior of one or more joints and therefore would require specific clinical assessment of each relevant joint and muscle complex to identify the barriers that restrict movement and that may be responsible for the provocation of pain. Consistent limitation and provocation of symptoms in both the loaded and unloaded conditions may be indicative of a mobility problem [20, 21]. True mobility restrictions often require appropriate manual therapy in conjunction with corrective exercise.

How to Interpret the SFMA

Once the SFMA has been completed, the therapist should be able to do the following: (1) Identify the major sources of dysfunction and movements that are affected. (2) Identify patterns of movement that cause pain where reproduction of pain indicates either mechanical deformation or an inflammatory process affecting the nociceptor in the symptomatic structures. The key follow-up question must be "Which of the functional movements caused the tissue to become painful?" (3) Once the pattern of dysfunction has been identified, the problem is classified as either a mobility or stability dysfunction, determine where intervention should commence. With the SFMA, the choice of treatment is not about alleviating mechanical pain; rather, the SFMA guides the therapist to begin by choosing interventions designed to improve the dysfunctional nonpainful patterns first. This philosophy of intervention does not ignore the source of pain; rather, it takes the approach of removing the mechanical dysfunction that causes the tissues to become symptomatic in the first place.

Conservative Treatment

In some cases, decided by the patient and the surgeon, conservative treatment will be the most desired choice for the patient. The patient may have FAI and/or a labral tear, but some patients are either not ready for surgery or their symptoms may not be affecting their daily functional activities yet. Some may have only had symptoms for a short period of time or only with higher level activities. They may decide to treat their hip conservatively with physical therapy and modification of their current lifestyle before looking to surgery.

The goals of conservative treatment, when the diagnosis is known, focus more on education and comprehensive home exercise programs as compared to the rehabilitative treatment of postoperative patients. Education is imperative in this type of treatment focusing on what activities to avoid (see Box 33.2) that may accelerate their degenerative hip pathology and/or worsen their labral tear. In addition, emphasis is put on teaching the patient what they can do to

---

Box 33.2 Activities to Avoid Long Term

- Deep squats/lunges
- High-impact activities – running, jumping, etc. (articular damage)

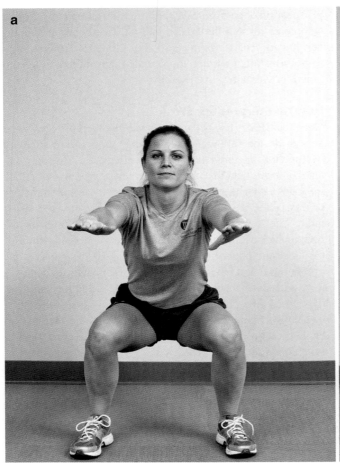

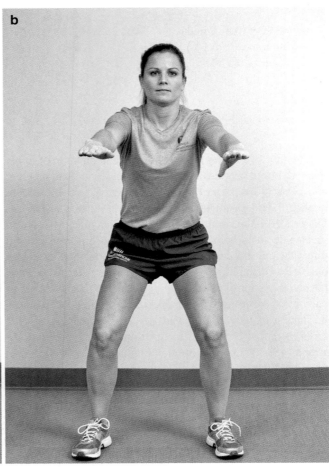

Fig. 33.8 (**a**) Normal squatting position. The depth of the squat may need to be altered postsurgery or if the patient is being treated conservatively for hip pain. (**b**) The patient is instructed to perform the squat no deeper than 45° to decrease the compression on the labrum. (All rights are retained by Dr. Byrd)

decrease the forces on their hip while maintaining or improving their hip strength and function.

Managing or modifying an athlete's training program may be crucial in preventing further irritable forces or damage to the hip. Deep loaded squatting (loaded flexion) >45°, deep lunges, and deep leg press are activities that are avoided if the athlete is trying to avoid surgery or trying to rehab the injured hip (Fig. 33.8a, b). The athlete may benefit from less compressive cardiovascular activities such as swimming and biking to use in between games, practices, etc. In addition, core (lumbopelvic) stabilization may be recommended for the athlete based upon the results of the functional movement assessment (Video 33.2: http://goo.gl/sI4Wm) (Fig. 33.9a–d). Specific findings of your assessment will serve to guide your exercise progression. This in turn will help accentuate a more neutral pelvis which in turn will open up the acetabulum anteriorly and provide some relief of compression in those with pincer FAI.

The focus of the exercise program will be on hip/core strengthening, maintaining full pain-free hip ROM (reduce risk of developing adhesive capsulitis), maintaining/improving flexibility, and helping the patient develop a cardiovascular

routine that will not be detrimental to the hip. Recommendations for cardiovascular exercise are as follows: (in order of least-most compressive for the hip) swimming, biking (no deep hip flexion, may have to adjust seat height), elliptical, walking, and jogging (limit if the patient does not have to perform this activity). If the patient already has a comprehensive workout routine, then the goal will be to help assess their current routine and make changes as needed. The comprehensive programs may be taught in 1–2 visits or over a period of a few weeks to let the patient acclimate to the new program.

Some patients will still respond to manual therapy for temporary symptom relief. Hip mobilizations (described in post-arthroscopic treatment) as well as long axis traction may be tolerated very well. If the patients do respond well, these techniques can easily be taught to a spouse, friend, or family member so they can be performed more often.

During the education process, it is very important to emphasize the importance of compliance with the strengthening program as well as avoiding the activities that worsen their symptoms. If after completing the preliminary phases of a thorough program that is 4–6 weeks in length or if the

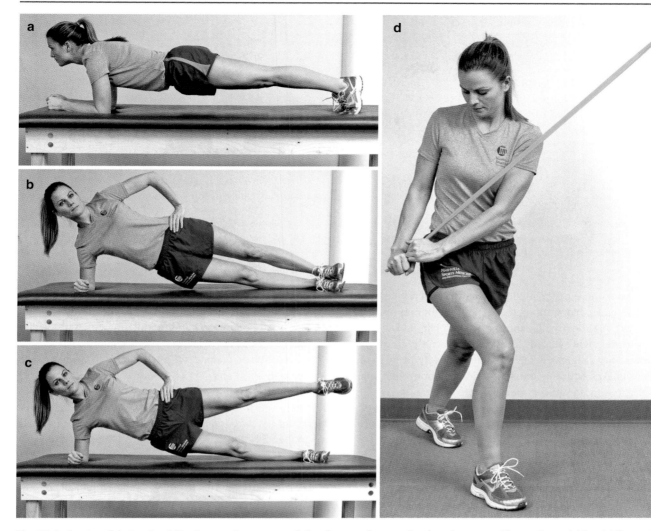

Fig. 33.9 Lumbopelvic (core) stabilization may be recommended to the patient to decrease compression in the hip in someone with a pincer type lesion or in patients who want to get back to higher level functional activities such as running, jumping, or specific sporting activities. (**a**) Forward core planks. (**b**) Side core planks. (**c**) Side plank with leg lift. (**d**) Lunge with shoulder PNF pattern. (All rights are retained by Dr. Byrd)

patient continues to have increasing amounts of pain or does not respond well to conservative treatment, then it will be beneficial to refer the patient back to the orthopedic physician. Failure to respond to a poor conservative treatment program or lack of compliance to an adequate program does not constitute failure of the rehabilitation program.

Treatment/Rehabilitation Progression

From the clinician's subjective and objective assessment and the information provided by the surgeon, specific areas of concern and needs will be identified [4]. To achieve the overall goals for an individual patient, the clinician must assess what instruction, monitoring, and equipment are necessary and must gauge the intensity or aggressiveness of the patient's functional progression. The rehabilitation program must be individualized based upon the evaluation findings of the sur-

geon and the physical therapist and not a strict timeline. The rehabilitation program must be individualized with specific time frames for weight bearing and ROM as determined by the pathology and the specific procedures used for correction (Table 33.1). For example, a patient with significant degenerative changes that undergoes a microfracture will have a slower recovery, dictated primarily by their symptoms and healing precautions. Compliance with the rehabilitation program is vital to allow for optimal soft tissue and bone healing. The rehabilitation program will progress through phases that utilize specific criteria to advance or progress to the next phase. Early in the rehab process (first 1–2 weeks), the exercise prescription is similar for all pathologies while still being mindful of the labral repair ROM restrictions and the microfracture weight-bearing precautions. During phase 1 of the rehab program, the intensity of rehabilitation is very conservative and is accomplished not only by supervision through the first phase but also with the patient performing

Table 33.1 Weight-bearing guidelines

Procedure	WB	Crutches	ROM
Routine arthroscopic procedure (loose body removal, labral debridement, chondroplasty, etc.)	WBAT	5–7 days or when gait is normalized	No limits
Femoroplasty	WBAT	1 month	No limits
Acetabuloplasty	WBAT	2 weeks or until gait is normalized	No limits
Labral repair/refixation	50% BW	1 month	90° of hip flexion; no ER for 4 weeks; week 4–5: increase to 105° hip flexion, ER to 20°; week 5–6: 115–120° of hip flexion, ER: 40° (pain-free); week 6+: Full AROM/PROM (pain-free)
Microfracture	30# PWB	2 months	No limits (emphasize ROM)
Iliopsoas release	WBAT	2 weeks or until gait is normalized	No limits on PROM, limit AROM flexion to allow healing to occur, emphasize passive hip extension to aid in healing process

WB Weight bearing, *ROM* Range of motion, *WBAT* Weight bearing as tolerated, *BW* Body weight, *ER* External rotation, *AROM* Active range of motion, *PROM* Passive range of motion

their home exercise program independently. Progress through this phase is dependent upon the specific pathology that the patient had. A patient with debridement of a labral tear, loose body removal, synovectomy, or otherwise healthy joint may be expected to progress much more aggressively through the protocol phases with the anticipation of regaining full function and return to sports. Because the patient is moving through the protocol at a faster pace, the use of a well-equipped facility is preferred so that the patient has access to rehabilitative tools/equipment that will complement the high level demands of the rehabilitative program. In addition, this higher level patient may require more clinical attention in order to gauge their response to exercise and assure a safe progression. The four phases of rehabilitation include the following: phase 1, mobility and early exercise; phase 2, intermediate exercise and stabilization; phase 3, advanced exercise and neuromuscular control; and phase 4, return to activity.

While pathology-specific protocols have been developed for routine arthroscopic procedures, there are general guidelines that can be applied across four phases of rehabilitation. A sample rehabilitation protocol for routine arthroscopic procedures that require little to no biological healing (loose body removal, labral debridement, synovectomy, ligamentum teres debridement, etc.) has been included as supplemental material with the included DVD. Sample protocols for those arthroscopic procedures that require more extensive biological healing (iliopsoas release, labral repair, femoroplasty, acetabuloplasty, microfracture) have been included in the supplemental material as well.

Postoperative recovery actually begins with the preoperative educational process. This may be a structured prehabilitation program that addresses impairments such as pain, swelling, postural deviations, compensated mobility, muscle length and muscle strength, decreased proprioception, and muscular and cardiovascular endurance. Hip pain may alter lumbopelvic-hip movement, creating patterns which lead to impairments of muscular imbalances and faulty mechanics

[20, 21]. In other cases, a single comprehensive preoperative visit for instruction, explanation, and demonstration of the expected postoperative rehabilitation protocol will suffice. The patient should be aware that their rehabilitative responsibilities such as an understanding of weight-bearing precautions, wound care, and use of assistive devices begin even before leaving the outpatient area. Many of the initial exercises can be performed independently, but the patient should understand the importance of beginning isometric contractions (Video 33.3: http://goo.gl/dY4V5) at the hip and ankle plantarflexion and dorsiflexion pumps (Video 33.4: http://goo.gl/OJX4M) to facilitate lower extremity circulation. Reasonable goals are discussed with the patient depending on the extent of the injury, prior level of function, extent of the surgery, and extent of the damage in the hip.

Initial Visit

The first postoperative visit evaluation (usually day 1 or 2 after surgery) starts when the patient walks through the door. Initiation of treatment begins with normalization of the patient's gait, which involves education about the importance and actual demonstration of proper ambulation (Fig. 33.10). The patient will then start with week 1 exercises that are listed with the supplemental material. These exercises are meant to improve the initial activation of the muscles surrounding the hip/knee as well as decreasing pain, stiffness, and inflammation. The patient should be aware not to "push through" pain as they perform the exercises and as they progress through the rehab program. During this visit, the patient should be educated on their postsurgical restrictions, driving restrictions, sleeping recommendations, and the importance of compliance with their supervised rehab program. For simpler arthroscopic procedures that do not require much biological healing, patients may experience prompt decreased pain and symptoms when existing at a low activity level. This has been

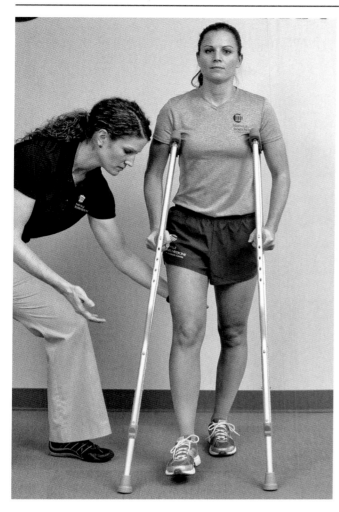

Fig. 33.10 Crutch/gait training is imperative in normalizing the patient's gait and provides better stability as they are ambulating. (All rights are retained by Dr. Byrd)

and inflammation, restore pain-free ROM, prevent muscle inhibition, and normalize gait. The primary constraint during this phase is soft tissue healing and avoiding the negative effects of immobilization [22].

The patient's weight-bearing status can vary depending on the surgeon's findings and procedure performed. If the pathology addressed with the surgical procedure does not require extensive biological healing, then foot-flat weight bearing is allowed as tolerated, and crutches are discontinued within the first week (chondroplasty, debridement, loose body removal, or synovectomy). In those cases where biological healing is required (i.e., microfracture, femoroplasty, acetabuloplasty, and labral repair), the patient may remain on a limited weight-bearing status for up to 8 weeks (see Table 33.1 for details). Although the discomfort associated with arthroscopy might be surprisingly little, due to the combination of capsular penetration with the arthroscopic portals and the traction applied to the capsule during the procedure, there can still be a significant amount of reflex inhibition. This reflex inhibition can lead to limited or poor muscle firing, thereby altering normal patterns of movement [11]. Cold compression devices are often used in the initial stages of rehabilitation to minimize inflammation and reflex inhibition. The gluteus medius muscle is an example of a muscle that commonly exhibits reflex muscle inhibition following hip injury or surgery. In a typical arthroscopic procedure, the anterolateral and posterolateral portals pass through this muscle. Clinically, it is common to see that the patient will have a difficult time regaining muscle tone and appropriate firing of this muscle postsurgery. This is analogous to the effects of an arthroscopic knee surgery on the vastus medialis muscle. Functionally, the gluteus medius muscle is needed to maintain a level pelvis during ambulation. With gluteus medius weakness, a Trendelenburg gait will occur as the contralateral pelvis drops when the limb becomes unsupported in the swing phase of gait. Additionally, due to the short moment arm of the gluteus medius, this muscle causes a large joint compression force when it contracts during the single limb stance phase of gait [23–25]. In a patient with hip articular pathology, it is common to find inhibition of the gluteus medius muscle due to pain [11]. Consequently, assistive devices are helpful to minimize the Trendelenburg pelvis

termed the "honeymoon period" where most patients feel better regardless of their eventual outcome. Early enthusiasm at about 1 month following surgery makes it easy for patients to overdo their activity and results in a flare-up and setback in their recovery. Following more extensive procedures such as correction of FAI, stricter precautions are necessary during the early recovery, and flare-ups are more frequent at around 6–8 weeks as function starts to intensify. A thoughtful rehabilitation strategy can minimize these setbacks, but they are still frequent enough that, by having warned patients of this occurrence, they will have more confidence that it can be corrected and is not a sign of an unsuccessful eventual outcome. See Box 33.3 for how to treat a flare-up if it may occur.

Phase 1: Mobility and Initial Exercise

During the initial phase of rehabilitation, the goals of the program are to protect the repaired tissue, diminish the pain drop and reestablish a normal gait pattern with synchronous muscle activity. The most effective method of neutralizing compressive forces across the hip is to allow the patient to apply the equivalent weight of the leg on the ground [26, 27]. This is especially important with microfracture, protecting the gradually maturing fibrocartilaginous healing response of the articular surface. Maintaining a true non-weight-bearing status requires significant muscle force to suspend the extremity off the ground, thus generating considerable dynamic compression across the joint as a result of muscle contraction [26, 27]. Resting the weight of the lower extremity on the ground neutralizes this dynamic compressive effect of the muscles [26, 27]. The decision on when to discontinue assistive devices is based upon the patient's tolerance to weight bearing and the demonstration of proper firing of the gluteal muscles without a Trendelenburg gait pattern.

Early range of motion (ROM) (Video 33.5: http://goo.gl/yEuQm) is initiated to restore joint motion and decrease the likelihood of adhesions forming about the joint [22]. Joint range of motion is normalized by restoring capsular extensibility. Emphasis with passive range of motion is placed upon internal rotation and flexion to help prevent scarring between the hip joint capsule and the acetabular labrum. Limitation of hip flexion and internal rotation also commonly occurs because of the FAI [12]. Hip extension past neutral is initially restricted due to increased anterior hip forces and excessive stress on the anterior labrum and capsule. Active assisted range of motion exercises are initiated and progressed to active range of motion, gravity-assisted and then to gravity-resisted exercises during the postoperative recovery. Exercises are directed in all planes of hip motion, and the end ranges for motion are determined by the patient's level of discomfort. Stretching is typically pushed only to tolerance, and the patient is educated as to these parameters. Manual mobilization techniques can assist in the reduction of compressive forces across the articular surfaces. This may lessen discomfort and over time enhance cartilage healing [28]. Regaining full functional pain-free ROM is critical in preventing concurrent compensatory patterns with the lower back, SI joint, etc. Small accessory oscillation movements stimulate joint mechanoreceptors assisting in pain modulation while at the same time help to maintain capsular mobility. Graded mobilization with flexion and adduction movement or internal rotation is gently implemented with the moderately painful joint [12]. Stationary bicycling with minimal to no resistance is an excellent adjunct to the range of motion program and should be done daily.

Hip Mobilizations

Distraction techniques (longitudinal movement) (Video 33.6: http://goo.gl/uu0Bf) are most useful when hip movements are painful and also following compressive exercises

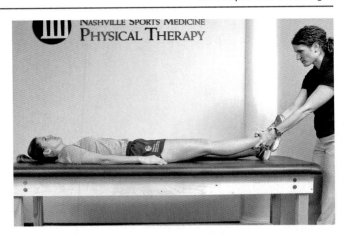

Fig. 33.11 Longitudinal hip distraction. Distraction techniques (longitudinal movement) are most useful when hip movements are painful and also following compressive exercises. (All rights are retained by Dr. Byrd)

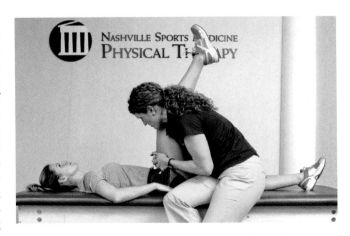

Fig. 33.12 Inferior/caudal glide mobilization. This technique can be performed in varying degrees of flexion. During this mobilization, some longitudinal distraction is performed to decrease compression as the hip is brought into more flexion and the inferior glide is performed. (All rights are retained by Dr. Byrd)

(Fig. 33.11). Oscillatory longitudinal movements are produced by pulling gently on the lower extremity down the long axis of the femur which can be performed in varying degrees of flexion. In addition, capsular stretching can be made more specific with three-dimensional mobilization by rotating the femur into the restrictive barrier and performing an inferior or caudal glide (Fig. 33.12). During the inferior glide mobilization (Video 33.7: http://goo.gl/3vgY7), it is key that some longitudinal distraction is provided to prevent increased force on the labrum rather than actually mobilizing the joint within the capsule. This mobilization can be done in all quadrants of hip flexion and is imperative to regaining full functional pain-free mobility. Changing the hand position to be more medial or lateral is all that has to be done to achieve this goal. To improve internal and external rotation movement, rotational mobilizations can be performed with support under the knees of the patient. A bolster may be used to

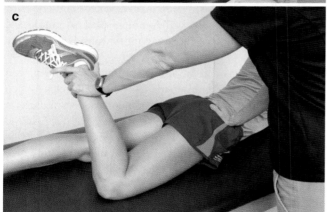

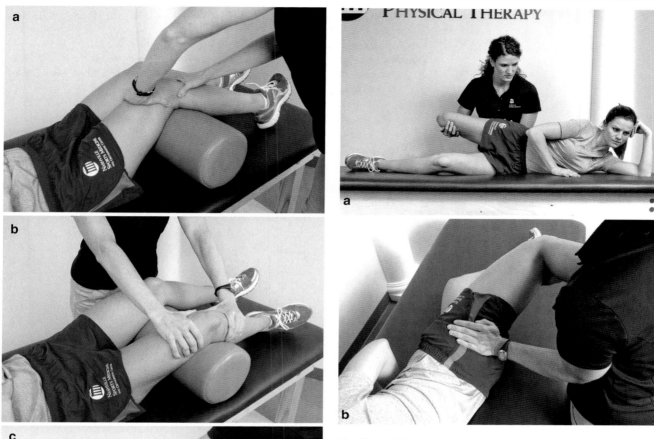

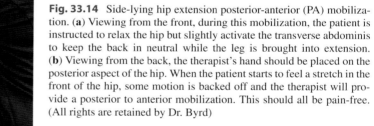

Fig. 33.14 Side-lying hip extension posterior-anterior (PA) mobilization. (**a**) Viewing from the front, during this mobilization, the patient is instructed to relax the hip but slightly activate the transverse abdominis to keep the back in neutral while the leg is brought into extension. (**b**) Viewing from the back, the therapist's hand should be placed on the posterior aspect of the hip. When the patient starts to feel a stretch in the front of the hip, some motion is backed off and the therapist will provide a posterior to anterior mobilization. This should all be pain-free. (All rights are retained by Dr. Byrd)

Fig. 33.13 (**a**) Internal rotation mobilizations. (**a**) bolster is used to prop the hip up into approximately 30° to allow the capsule to be on slack. This will help relax the patient as the mobilization is performed. (**b**) External rotation mobilizations. (**c**) Prone internal/external stretch. The patient's pelvis should be stabilized while the hip is stretched into internal or external rotation. A contract-relax method can also be utilized in this position. (All rights are retained by Dr. Byrd)

put the hip into about 30° of hip flexion which allows the capsule to be on slack (Fig. 33.13a, b). Rotational mobilizations (Video 33.8: http://goo.gl/KZNNK) into each end range direction can be started during week 3–4 of the initial phase of rehab unless the patient has ROM restrictions. Working into small amplitude end range rotational mobilizations are

well tolerated by postoperative patients and may be started during week 4 and on. If patients continue to have ROM limitations long term, then it is important that mobilizations be taught to someone who is available to perform them on the patient on a more consistent basis. Another option for those who have limitations in IR/ER is to have the patient in prone and perform IR/ER stretching at 90° of knee flexion. The patient is to initiate the motion after an outside force (therapist) stabilizes the pelvis with one hand, then the other hand either pushes or pulls the hip into more internal or external rotation as tolerated by the patient (perform 3–5 reps of 10 s). The prone position can be useful to perform a contract-relax method for increased IR/ER (Fig. 33.13c). Limitations in anterior hip mobility can be seen in the terminal stance phase of gait and can be addressed with the side-lying hip extension posterior-anterior mobilization (Fig. 33.14a). The patient begins side-lying on the nonoperative side, and the leg is passively brought into extension,

Table 33.2 Single leg squat criterion

Criterion	To be rated "good"
Overall impression across five trials	
Ability to maintain balance	Patient does not lose balance
Perturbations of the person	Movement is performed smoothly
Depth of the squat	The squat is performed to at least 60° knee flexion
Speed of the squat	Squat is performed at a rate of 1 per s
Trunk posture	
Trunk/thoracic lateral deviation	No trunk/thoracic lateral deviation
Trunk/thoracic rotation	No trunk/thoracic rotation
Trunk/thoracic lateral flexion	No trunk/thoracic lateral flexion
Trunk/thoracic forward flexion	No trunk/thoracic forward flexion
The pelvis "in space"	
Pelvic lateral deviation	No pelvic lateral deviation
Pelvic rotation	No pelvic rotation
Pelvic tilt	No pelvic tilt
Hip joint	
Hip adduction	No hip adduction
Hip "femoral" internal rotation	No hip "femoral" internal rotation
Knee joint	
Apparent knee valgus	No apparent knee valgus
Knee position relative to foot position	Center of knee remains over the center of the foot

keeping the lumbar spine in neutral. The hip is brought back far enough to feel a stretch in the anterior hip, but no pain should be felt. Some extension motion is then released, and a posterior-anterior mobilization is performed with the heel of the hand placed in the posterior hip area (Fig. 33.14b). Small oscillatory motions (10–15) are made by the therapist utilizing their own core, and then the leg is brought back to neutral. This can be repeated as tolerated. Oscillatory movements in a compression mode, stopping short of the pain position, can be helpful especially for patients with pain in weight bearing. The posterior-anterior mobilization can also be used as an accessory movement at the limit of physiological range when a goal of treatment is to increase the range of motion of the joint. The presence of a capsular pattern of the hip as described by Cyriax is often found secondary to the postoperative effusion [28]. Characteristic of that pattern is a gross limitation of flexion, abduction, and internal rotation with minimal loss of extension and external rotation [17, 28]. Regardless of the pattern of restriction, every attempt must be made to restore full capsular mobility and all physiological range of motions. In cases with painful restricted motion, the clinician must carefully assess the end feel to motion and physical status of the joint in order to determine whether mobilization techniques are a viable treatment option.

A key postoperative goal is the restoration of dynamic hip stability. The prevention of muscle inhibition can be achieved through early muscle-toning exercises (Video 33.9: http://goo.gl/jRBPZ) which are performed within the first week after surgery. Progression is dependent on the patient's tolerance but should not be overly aggressive. Exercise selection should be based upon evidence related to the specific muscles

recruited while at the same time maintain all surgical precautions with regard to forces on the healing tissues. Isometric exercises are the simplest and least likely to aggravate underlying joint symptoms [29]. These include isometric sets for the gluteals, quadriceps, hamstrings, adductor and abductor muscle groups, and lower abdominals [29]. Additionally, isometric contraction of the antagonistic muscle group may inhibit spasms and promote pain relief.

Specific emphasis in the strengthening program is placed upon isolating and strengthening the gluteal muscles (Video 33.10: http://goo.gl/nwldn). The gluteus medius muscle is one of the key stabilizers of the hip during gait [25]. Initial assessment of isolated gluteal muscle weakness can best be accomplished with standardized manual muscle testing procedures in the side-lying and prone positions. The dynamic quality of single leg support as a part of the kinetic chain can be assessed functionally with a single leg squat. The single limb squat test requires frontal plane stability of the pelvis and control of the lower limb in both the frontal and transverse plane, both of which require high gluteus medius muscle activation (Table 33.2 with scoring criterion). The single leg squat test also significantly activates the gluteus maximus muscle. The relationship between hip muscle strength and control of the hip and knee motions during a single leg task has been established [30]. The motion of the single limb squat requires stability of the lumbopelvic region while at the same time providing eccentric control of hip flexion and concentric hip extension.

Weak or fatigued gluteal muscles can result in excessive pelvic rotation and femoral internal rotation. Gluteal isometrics in a neutral pelvic position may decrease

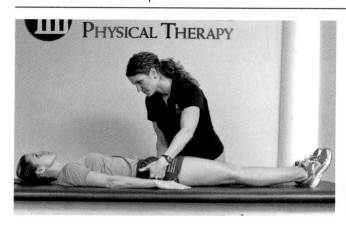

Fig. 33.15 Gluteal isometrics done in a neutral pelvis position may decrease overactivity of the iliopsoas and provide a decrease in anterior hip pain. (All rights are retained by Dr. Byrd)

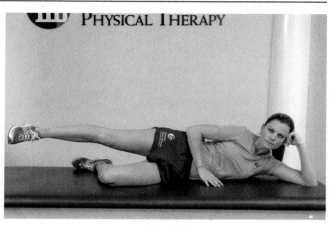

Fig. 33.16 Side-lying hip abduction may be done to aid in strengthening the gluteus medius, but if the patient has concurrent hip flexor irritation, this may need to be done in slight internal rotation. (All rights are retained by Dr. Byrd)

overactivity of the iliopsoas and provide a decrease in anterior hip pain [31–33] (Fig. 33.15). Proper strength and conditioning of these muscles is important due to the influence on the hip, pelvis, and back [34]. A commonly seen substitution pattern for gluteus medius weakness is overactivation of the tensor fascia lata and the iliopsoas with abduction strength testing. Typically, the patient will flex and externally rotate their hip in order to achieve abduction. In order to alleviate this problem, the patient is asked to keep their hip in neutral or in slight extension while lifting their hip into abduction.

It has been established that iliopsoas pain and tenderness can be common during postoperative rehabilitation [12, 35]. The same exercises that are used to strengthen the gluteal muscles may also aggravate an inflamed iliopsoas muscle. Therefore, exercise selection for strengthening the gluteal muscles must also reduce the activation of the iliopsoas muscle 34. Supine hip flexion, side-lying hip abduction with external hip rotation, and the hip clamshell progression have been identified to also activate the iliopsoas muscle considerably and should be avoided with concurrent hip flexor irritation [35] (Figs. 33.16 and 33.17a–f). The clamshell progression (Video 33.11: http://goo.gl/UJIl0) is used to emphasize both internal and external rotations while strengthening the gluteus medius in the neutral position significantly activate the iliopsoas and is safe to use [35]. Other strengthening exercises with low concurrent iliopsoas activation include double to single leg bridging (Video 33.12: http://goo.gl/yIj8q), stool hip rotations, resisted hip extension, side-lying hip abduction with the heel against the wall, prone heel squeezes, and side-lying hip abduction (Video 33.13: http://goo.gl/33OAW) with internal hip rotation [35] (Fig. 33.18a–i). In addition, patients can also start performing a limited arc leg press (Video 33.14: http://goo.gl/ew19Q) and mini-squats (Video 33.15: http://goo.gl/HVnCf) to also work on gluteus maximus. Table 33.3 provides a list of gluteal exercises listed in hierarchy of activation based upon EMG data that was normalized to a maximum volitional isometric contraction (MVIC). Previous research has indicated that muscle activation greater than 50–60% MVIC is considered adequate for muscle strengthening [36].

An aquatic program is often beneficial for allowing early return to exercise and can begin as soon as the portal sites have healed and the sutures have been removed [11]. A pool program will allow for muscle relaxation which allows for earlier joint mobilization and gentle strengthening in a reduced-weight environment. The water buoyancy can provide assistance to movement in all planes and safer resistance with active exercises. Gait activities can be progressed in waist deep water with minimized compression of the surgical site. Once the goals of phase 1 have been met and there is minimal to no pain with the phase 1 exercise program, patients are progressed to the intermediate phase of the rehabilitation program. The patients should have achieved close to full range of motion and accomplished a normalized gait pattern without crutches in order to progress.

Box 33.4 Common Complaints Postsurgery

- Nonpainful popping
- Feeling of stiffness
- Mild swelling (should return to normal within 2 weeks)
- Sharp pains with quick or rotating movement of the hip up to 12 weeks post-op

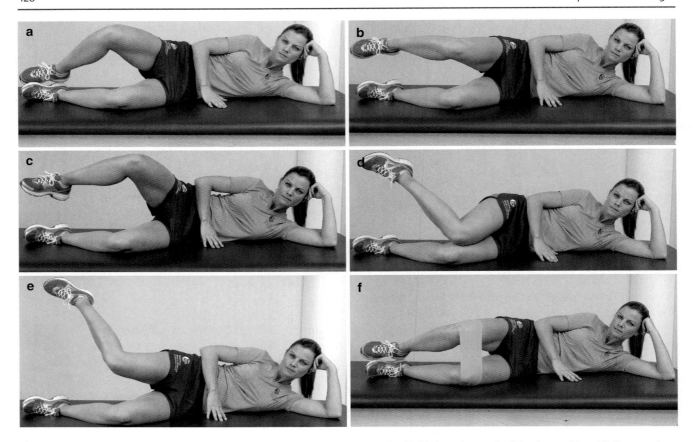

Fig. 33.17 Clamshell progression. (**a**) Classic clamshell. (**b**, **c**) Level 2 clamshell with hip in an isometric abduction position. (**d**) Reverse clamshell. (**e**) Level 2 reverse clamshell. (**f**) Resisted clamshell. (All rights are retained by Dr. Byrd)

Phase 2: Intermediate Exercise and Stabilization

The intermediate phase of rehabilitation typically begins around week 4 and is a progression of the range of motion/stretching (Video 33.16: http://goo.gl/LF0Vi and Video 33.17: http://goo.gl/AJx93) and strengthening exercises (Video 33.18: http://goo.gl/zzSTs) started in phase 1. The range of motion exercises should be continued until full pain-free range of motion is present. Strengthening and stabilization exercises should advance throughout this phase to challenge the patient and correct any muscle weakness or imbalance that was present. Weight-bearing (progressive resistive exercises) resistance exercise (Video 33.19: http://goo.gl/hz5Jh) and resistance to the bicycling program can be added during this phase. Emphasis must be placed upon the elimination of muscle imbalances and motor substitution patterns that occur with tasks of ADL. The most common cause for muscle imbalance is chronic overuse or injury which leads to neuromuscular compromise and an eventual change in the elasticity of the muscle. The neuro-

muscular compromise can manifest by three different mechanisms: (1) *Arthrokinetic Inhibition:* The neuromuscular phenomenon that occurs when a muscle is inhibited by joint dysfunction or the capsule that crosses the joint. Overuse leads to shortening/tightening (not spasm) of postural muscles; disuse leads to a weakening/inhibition of phasic muscles. (2) *Synergistic Dominance:* The neuromuscular phenomenon that occurs when synergists, stabilizers, and neutralizers take over for a weak or inhibited prime mover. (3) *Reciprocal Inhibition:* The neuromuscular phenomenon that occurs when a tight muscle decreases the neural drive to its functional antagonist. This leads to compensation patterns and predictable injury patterns. The most common muscle imbalance seen is tightness of the hip flexors and erector spinae muscles with weakness of the gluteals and abdominal musculature resulting in an anterior pelvic tilt with an increased lumbar lordotic curve. Therefore, core stabilization exercises (Video 33.20: http://goo.gl/FSwdO) are progressed in conjunction with the hip progressive resistive exercise program (Video 33.21: http://goo.gl/SrYh0).

Core stability is an exceedingly important, yet often overlooked, aspect of hip rehabilitation after both injury and surgery, and may be especially critical in optimizing performance and minimizing the risk of reinjury. Core stabilization/strengthening emphasizes training of the trunk musculature to develop better pelvic stability and abdominal control. A simple analogy could be made comparing the core stabilization component after surgery to that of a scapular stabilization program with injury in the upper quarter. Often patients develop the strength, power, and endurance of specific extremity musculature to perform required activities but are deficient in muscular strength of the lumbopelvic-hip complex. The core stabilization system must be checked as part of the assessment and specifically challenged as part of the rehabilitation program [4]. The basic screen involves several basic screening tests. The *Pelvic Tilt Test*

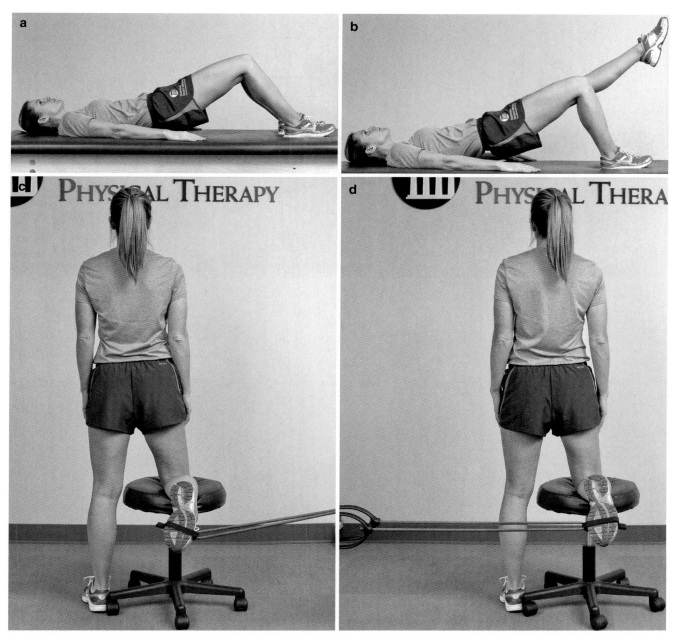

Fig. 33.18 (**a**) Double leg bridge. (**b**) Single leg bridge. (**c**, **d**) Stool hip internal/external rotation. (**e**) Resisted hip extension. (**f**) Side-lying hip abduction with heel against the wall. (**g**) Prone heel squeezes. (**h**) Hip abduction with hip in internally rotated position. (**i**) Mini-squat. (All rights are retained by Dr. Byrd)

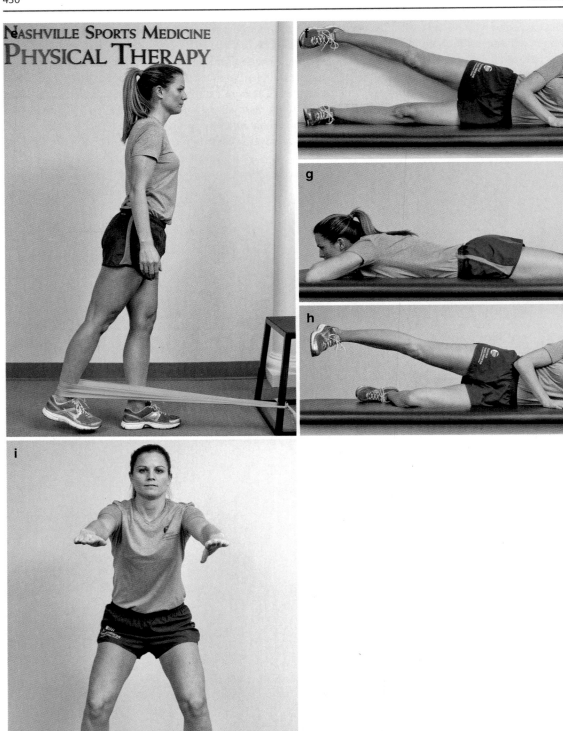

Fig. 33.18 (continued)

Table 33.3 Results: gluteus medius

Exercise	%MVIC gluteus medius
Side plank abduction, DL down	103.11
Side plank abduction, DL up	88.82
Single limb squat	82.26
Clamshell (hip clam) 4	76.88
Front plank	75.13
Clamshell (hip clam) 3	67.63
Side-lying abduction	62.91
Clamshell (hip clam) 2	62.45
Lateral step-up	59.87
Skater squat	59.84
Pelvic drop	58.43
Hip circumduction, stable	57.39
Dynamic leg swing	57.30
Single limb dead lift	56.08
Single limb bridge, stable	54.99
Forward step-up	54.62
Single limb bridge, unstable	47.29
Clamshell (hip clam) 1	47.23
Quadruped hip ext, DOM	46.67
Gluteal squeeze	43.72
Hip circumduction, unstable	37.88
Quadruped hip ext, non-DOM	22.03

– especially the gluteal muscles. This test will highlight any inhibition or weakness in the gluteus maximus due to over-recruitment of the synergistic muscles, like the hamstrings and lower back. If the pelvis on the unsupported side drops or the support leg shakes, this indicates instability in the gluteal muscles on the support side. If the support leg hamstrings or lower back start to cramp, this also indicates inhibition of the gluteals and recruitment of synergistic muscles – LOOK FOR CRAMPING. The most common reason for a failed test is a deactivation of the gluteals. The patient is used to recruiting the hamstrings and lower back for hip extension, so when asked to go into a bridge position those muscles go into hyperactivity. Next, when the leg is extended, this position should normally be easy for the gluteals to support, but if the gluteals are inhibited, cramping of the synergistic muscles will usually occur. Weakness in the abdominals, legs, and gluteals can also show a positive test. The patient will not show signs of cramping, but instead they will say the test is not easy or that one leg is easier than the other. An integrated functional unit of an effective core stabilization system plus a strong lumbopelvic-hip musculature complex is important for efficient weight distribution, absorption, and transfer of compressive forces [36].

(Video 33.22: http://goo.gl/JKuUU) is a great test for overall mobility of the hips and the lumbar spine and the patient's ability to control the position of their pelvic posture. This test examines the ability to mobilize and control the movement of the pelvis linking the lower body with the upper body. The test begins with having the patient tilt their pelvis forward and backwards. Begin by having the patient create an arch in their back (rolling pelvis forward) and then flattening their lower back (rolling their pelvis backward). Observe for both the motion available and the smoothness or nature of the movement. The quality of the movement indicates the frequency of use on a day-to-day basis. The *Pelvic Rotation Test* (Video 33.23: http://goo.gl/x7TDY) checks the patient's ability to rotate their lower body independently from their upper body. This movement requires good mobility of the spine, hips and pelvis, and simultaneous stability of the trunk. Look for smooth turns to the right and left with no choppiness or lateral movement (no lateral movement of the pelvis). This test requires the use of hip rotators and oblique abdominals to rotate the pelvis. The *Torso Rotation Test* (Video 33.24: http://goo.gl/z8gvu) checks the patient's ability to rotate their upper body independently from their lower body. This movement requires good mobility of the trunk and simultaneous stability of the hips and pelvis. Look for any movement of the hips or extension/side bending of the thoracic spine vs. rotation. (There should be no motion below the waistline.) The *Bridge with Leg Extension Test* (Video 33.25: http://goo.gl/tIwqq) is a great test for stability in the pelvis, lumbar spine, and core

Phase 3: Advanced Exercise and Neuromotor Control

Proprioceptive deficits routinely occur in conjunction with articular injuries [18]. The acetabular labrum contains free nerve endings and sensory organs [11, 25]. It is believed that these free nerve endings contribute in nociceptive and proprioceptive mechanisms [18]. The acetabular labrum also improves the stability of the hip joint by maintaining a negative intra-articular pressure [37]. With injury to the labrum, this negative pressure is lost and stability of the hip is adversely affected. This inhibits normal motor response and decreases neuromuscular stabilization of the joint. The aim of proprioceptive retraining is to restore these deficits and assist in reestablishing neuromotor control. The elements necessary for reestablishing neuromuscular control are proprioception, dynamic joint stability, reactive neuromuscular control, and functional motor pathways [18]. Joint positioning tasks performed early in the rehabilitative process can enhance proprioceptive and kinesthetic awareness. More advanced proprioceptive neuromuscular techniques incorporated in functional patterns of movement or modified ranges may be acceptable transition exercises, depending on the symptoms and status of the hip (Fig. 33.19a–c).

Dynamic stabilization exercises encourage muscular co-contractions to balance joint forces. Closed chain methods allow progressive weight-bearing transference to the lower

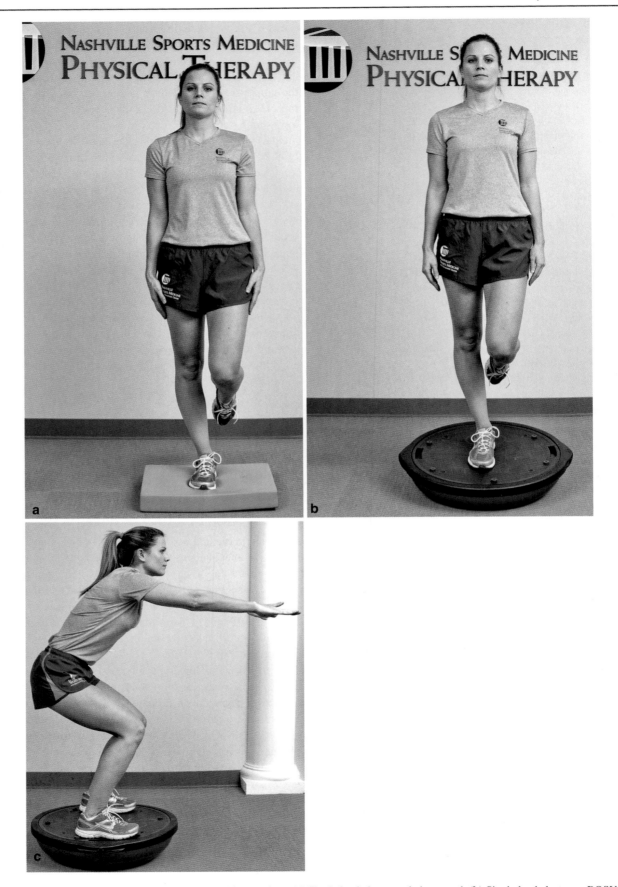

Fig. 33.19 Advanced proprioceptive neuromuscular hip exercises. (**a**) Single leg balance on balance pad. (**b**) Single leg balance on BOSU ball. (**c**) Mini-squats on BOSU ball. (All rights are retained by Dr. Byrd)

extremity in a manner that lessens the shear and translational forces across the joint surface [18]. This begins with simple static balance maneuvers, starting with full stance, and evolving to single limb stance, with and without visual input. Progression is then made to a combination of balance and strength activities. Bilateral heel raises (Video 33.26: http://goo.gl/svEd1) and mini-squats (Video 33.27: http://goo.gl/KEFsI) are progressed to unilateral heel raises and mini-squats (Video 33.28: http://goo.gl/9zpNw). More advanced closed kinetic exercises such as partial squats, lunges (Video 33.29: http://goo.gl/WHcdw), and dynamic weight shifts are encouraged initially in the pool. Low force, slow speed, and controlled activities may be transitioned to high progressive force, fast speed, and uncontrolled activities if the joint allows without becoming overstressed. For example, balance devices (Video 33.30: http://goo.gl/Y4DPu), mini-trampolines, and unlimited creative upper extremity activities while balancing can further challenge the neuromuscular system (Fig. 33.20a–m). Emphasis in the balance and functional training program (Video 33.31: http://goo.gl/X77M2) should be focused upon core stabilization and proper recruitment of the gluteus medius muscle group.

Static stabilization, transitional stabilization, and dynamic stabilization are phases of progression from closed chain loading and unloading, to conscious controlled motion with high joint tolerance, and ultimately to unconscious control and loading of the joint. Thus, depending on the patient's tolerance, the exercise program may progress from slow to fast, simple to complex, stable to unstable, low force to high force, and general to specific [18].

Phase 4: Return to Activity

The ultimate time frame for return to function depends upon the type of hip pathology present and the specific demands of the patient's anticipated activities.

Functional exercises simulating the patient's daily activities or sport-specific programs must be individualized to meet the patient's goals. Each patient or athlete's reassessment and phase 4 rehab program will need to be tailored to their specific demands of their sport or activity. It is beyond the scope of this chapter to include individualized programs for each sport for phase 4 rehab and specific functional tests. Functional tests are used at this time to assess the readiness of the patient to return to unrestricted activity (Fig. 33.21).

> **Box 33.5 Timeline of Cardio**
> - Bike (day 3–1 week post-op depending on procedure)
> - Elliptical (4–5 weeks post-op or 8–9 weeks for microfracture)
> - Walking program (week 8)
> - Jogging (start assessment at week 10–12 depending on type of surgery and extent of bone work)
> - Sprinting (week 14+)

> **Box 33.6 Checklist for Return to Play a Specific Sport**
> - Can perform all required activities to participate in a game without compensation or pain
> - Full functional ROM/strength
> - May need to communicate with athlete's trainer/coach to discuss return to play
> - Educate athlete on the importance of maintaining full strength/ROM, flexibility, and activities to avoid long term

These may include a functional squat test, a functional single leg step-down test, running/sprinting assessments, cutting/lateral movements, and sport-specific tests. These must be kept within the constraints dictated by the type of hip pathology that has been addressed. Improving quality of life is certainly a goal of arthroscopic procedures but must be kept within the framework of a realistic outlook.

For some cases, depending on the extent of pathology and the extent of surgical debridement, the explosive character of compressive forces generated by certain specific physical and sports activities may need to be curtailed or modified with substitutions that the joint can tolerate during healing. In fact, some patients or athletes may need to change the sport position or the sport altogether. Lastly, the clinician must ensure that the patient's expectations and the goals of rehabilitation coincide by emphasizing education for current and future hip management. The patient's compliance with a continued management program should include maintaining muscle balance (strength, flexibility, and proprioception) and improving overall function.

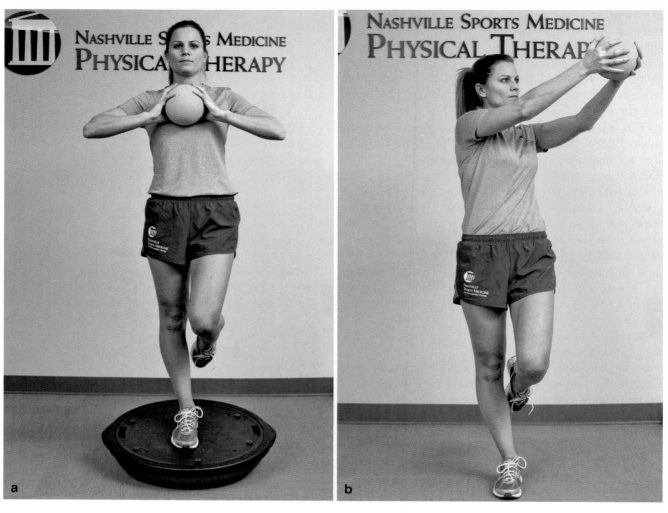

Fig. 33.20 Dynamic stabilization exercises. (**a**) Single leg ball toss on BOSU ball. (**b**) Single leg balance with PNF pattern. (**c–e**) Airplane balance activity. (**f**) Plyobox jumps. (**g**) Jumping mechanics are assessed and corrected during these exercises. (**h**) Forward quick steps on plyobox. (**i**) Lateral quick steps on plyobox. (**j**) Double leg hops on plyobox. (**k**) Double leg hop hurdle drill. (**l**) Single leg hop hurdle drill. (**m**) Double leg lateral hop hurdle drill. (All rights are retained by Dr. Byrd)

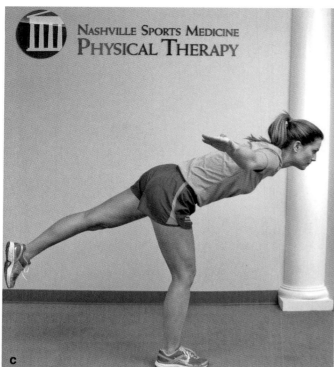

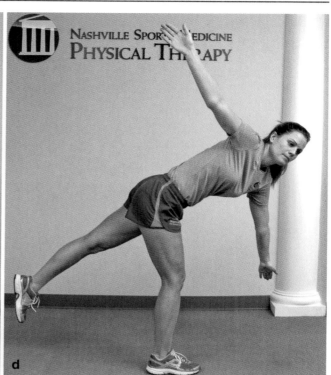

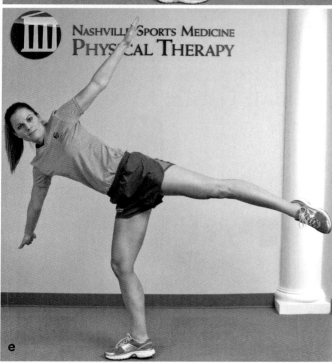

Fig. 33.20   (continued)

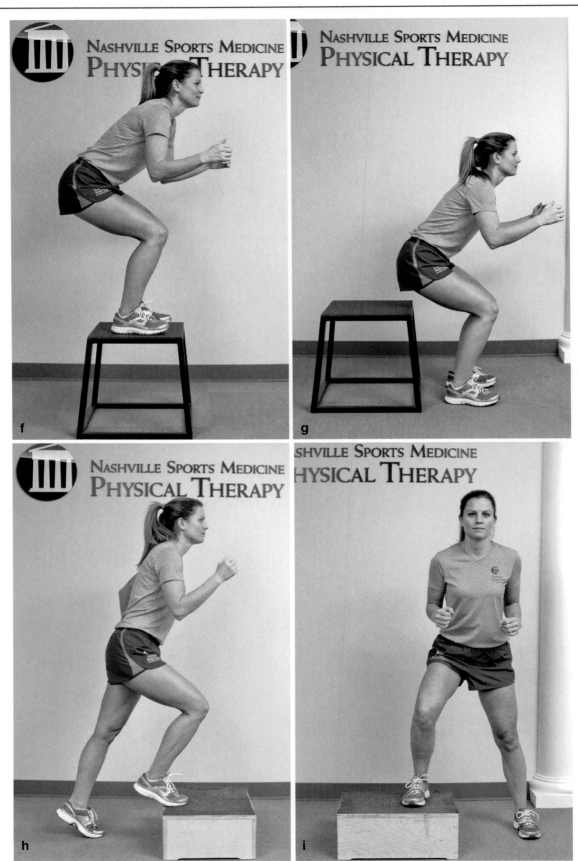

Fig. 33.20 (continued)

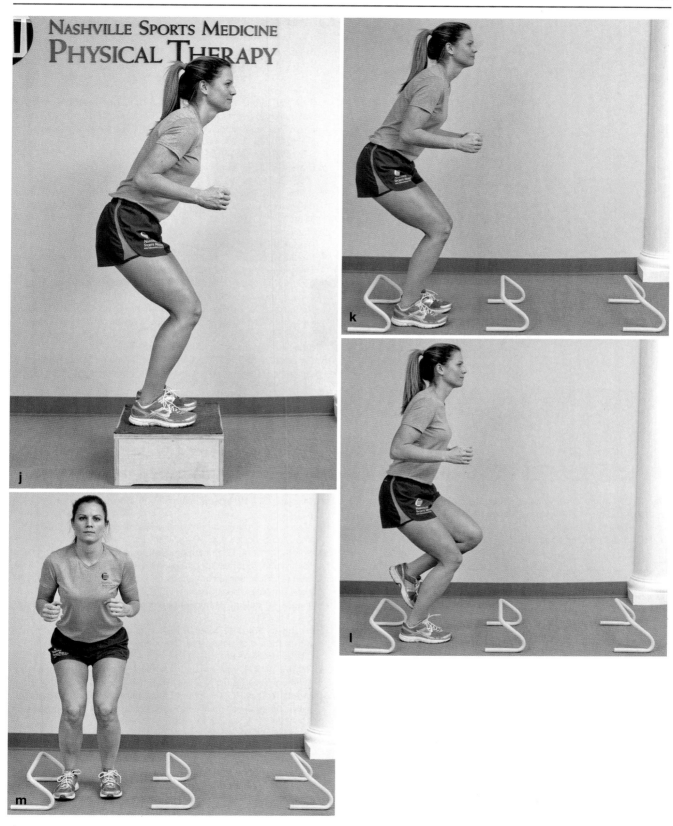

Fig. 33.20 (continued)

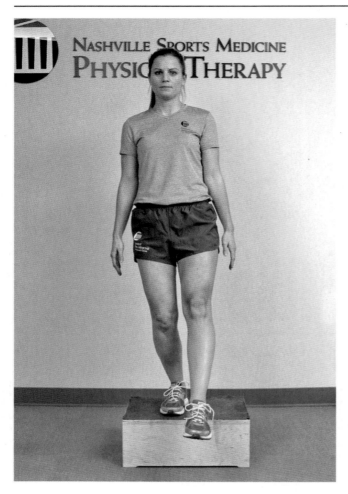

Fig. 33.21 Single limb squat test. The stance leg is assessed for correct knee and hip position during this motion. This test may be helpful when assessing if athletes are ready to go back to their desired sport. (All rights are retained by Dr. Byrd)

Conclusions

The principles of rehabilitation following hip arthroscopy continue to evolve based on expanding knowledge gained both from improved diagnostics and surgical management. The development of effective evidence-based rehabilitation protocols is advancing in conjunction with concepts that protect the integrity of the healing tissues. A common goal of hip rehabilitation should remain focused on the return to pain-free function and long-term restoration of the hip joint. A cornerstone to a successful treatment plan is constant reassessment. Outcome data indicates that this goal is being met, but further data will be required to completely validate the long-term success [38].

References

1. Boyd KT, Peirce NS, Batt ME. Common hip injuries in sport. Sports Med. 1997;24:273–80.
2. Byrd JWT. Hip arthroscopy utilizing the supine position. Arthroscopy. 1994;10(3):275–80.
3. Byrd JW. Labral lesions: an elusive source of hip pain case reports and literature review. Arthroscopy. 1996;12:603–12.
4. Byrd JW. Examination of the hip: history and physical examination. NAJSPT. 2007;2:231–40.
5. Byrd JW. Hip arthroscopy in the athlete. NAJSPT. 2007;2:217–30.
6. Byrd JW. Hip arthroscopy in athletes. Op Tech Sports Med. 2005;13:24–36.
7. Kelley BT, Riley JW, Philippon MJ. Hip arthroscopy: current indications, treatment options, and management issues. Am J Sports Med. 2003;31:1020–37.
8. US markets for arthroscopy devices 2009. Report by Millennium Research Group (MRG). 2009.
9. Enseki K, Martin R, Draovitch P, et al. The hip joint: arthroscopic procedures and postoperative rehabilitation. JOSPT. 2006;36:516–25.
10. Griffin KM, Henry CO, Byrd JWT. Rehabilitation after hip arthroscopy. J Sport Rehabil. 2000;9:77–88.
11. Robinson TK, Griffin KM. Rehabilitation. In: Byrd JWT, editor. Operative hip arthroscopy. New York: Springer; 2004. p. 236–51.
12. Stalzer S, Wahoff M, Scanlon M. Rehabilitation following hip arthroscopy. Clin Sports Med. 2006;25:337–57.
13. Enseki KR, Martin R, Kelly BT. Rehabilitation after arthroscopic decompression for femoroacetabular impingement. Clin Sports Med. 2010;29:247–55.
14. Lewis Cara L, Sahrmann Shirley A. Acetabular labral tears. Phys Ther. 2006;86:110–21.
15. McCarthy JC, Busconi B. The role of hip arthroscopy in the diagnosis and treatment of hip disease. Orthopedics. 1995;18:753–6.
16. Farjo LA, Glick JM, Sampson TG. Hip arthroscopy for acetabular labrum tears. Arthroscopy. 1999;15:132–7.
17. Hase T, Ueo T. Acetabular labral tear: arthroscopic diagnosis and treatment. Arthroscopy. 1999;15:138–41.
18. Maitland GD. Peripheral manipulation. Boston: Butterworth; 1977. p. 207–29.
19. Magee DJ. Orthopedic physical assessment. 3rd ed. Philadelphia: WB Saunders; 1997. p. 20–6.
20. Voight M, Cook G. Impaired neuromuscular control: reactive neuromuscular training. In: Voight M, Hoogenboom B, Prentice W, editors. Musculoskeletal interventions-techniques for therapeutic exercise. New York: McGraw-Hill; 2007. p. 181–212.
21. Voight M. Selective functional movement assessment. Nashville: NASMI; 2002.
22. Austin A, Souza R, Meer J, Powers C. Identification of abnormal hip motion associated with acetabular labral pathology. JOSPT. 2008;38:558–65.
23. Sahrmann S. Diagnosis and treatment of movement impairment syndromes. St Louis: Mosby; 2002. p. 1–50.
24. Dehne E, Tory R. Treatment of joint injuries by immediate mobilization based upon spinal adaptation concept. Clin Orthop. 1971;77:218–32.
25. Anderson FC, Pandy MG. Individual muscle contribution to support in walking. Gait Posture. 2003;17:159–69.
26. Crowninsheild RD, Johnston RC, Andrews JG, et al. A biomechanical investigation of the human hip. J Biomech. 1978;11:75–85.

27. Tackson SJ, Krebs DE, Harris BA. Acetabular pressures during hip arthritis exercises. Arthritis Care Res. 1997;10:308–19.
28. McCarthy J, Day B, Busconi B. Hip arthroscopy: applications and technique. J Am Acad Orthop Surg. 1995;3:115–22.
29. Ekstrom R, Donatelli R, Carp K. Electromyographic analysis of core trunk, hip, and thigh muscles during 9 rehabilitation exercises. JOSPT. 2007;37:754–62.
30. Norkin C, Levangie PK. Joint structure and function: a comprehensive analysis. 2nd ed. Philadelphia: FA Davis; 1992. p. 300–32.
31. Crossley KM, Zhang WJ, Schache AG, Bryant A, Cowan SM. Performance on the single-leg squat task indicates hip abductor muscle function. Am J Sports Med. 2011;39:866–73.
32. Zeller BL, McCrory JL, Kibler WB, Uhl TL. Differences in kinematics and EMG activity between men and women during the single leg squat. Am J Sports Med. 2003;31:449–56.
33. Boling MC, Bolga LA, Mattacola CG, Uhl TL, Hosey RG. Outcomes of a weight bearing rehabilitation program for patients diagnosed with patellofemoral pain syndrome. Arch Phys Med Rehabil. 2006;87:1428–35.
34. Mascal CL, Landel R, Powers C. Management of patellofemoral pain targeting the hip, pelvis, and trunk muscle function: 2 case reports. J Orthop Sports Phys Ther. 2003;21:647–60.
35. Nakagawa TH, Muniz TB, Baldon RM. The effect of additional strengthening of hip abductor and internal rotator muscles in patellofemoral pain syndrome: a randomized controlled pilot study. Clin Rehabil. 2008;22:1051–60.
36. Bolga LA, Uhl TL. EMG analysis of hip rehabilitation exercises in a group of healthy subjects. J Orthop Sports Phys Ther. 2005;35:487–94.
37. Philippon MJ, Decker MJ, Giphart JE, et al. Rehabilitation exercise progression for the gluteus medius muscle with consideration for iliopsoas tendinitis. Am J Sports Med. 2011;39(8):1777–85.
38. Byrd JW, Jones K. Hip arthroscopy in athletes: a 10 year follow-up. Am J Sports Med. 2009;27:2140–3.

Perioperative Care

34

Kay S. Jones, Elizabeth A. Potts, and J.W. Thomas Byrd

In hip arthroscopy, the physician places great emphasis on patient selection, the surgical procedure, and the rehabilitation process after surgery. It is also important to provide the necessary perioperative care to the patient during this time of disability and altered functional state. The clinical nurse and physician extender have multifaceted roles and play an integral part in the patient's perioperative experience. This commences even before the decision for surgery is made and continues until recuperation and rehabilitation are complete. Much of the clinical nurse's efforts are spent preparing the patient and the patient's family, which will be referred to as caregivers, for the postoperative period. It is important for the nurse to assure that the expectations of patients and caregivers are reasonable and appropriate and that they are prepared for what is to come. The physician extender can provide physical exam and diagnostic information to the surgeon to help guide the patient through the perioperative process.

The clinical nurse and physician extender provide comprehensive care, education, continuity, and support to patients undergoing hip arthroscopy. They serve as a resource not only for the patients but also for the surgeon, outpatient personnel, physical therapists, and other ancillary agencies. The clinical nurse's role includes consulting and collaborating with others to help increase the effectiveness, efficiency, and safety of the care rendered to the patient. Both the clinical nurse and physician extender play an important role in facilitating communication among members of the health care team.

As health care resources and patient needs become more sophisticated, so must the skills of the person to whom the patients and staff turn for assistance and direction. To function most effectively in these multiple roles, the clinical nurse and physician extender must be knowledgeable of all aspects of hip arthroscopy including anatomy and physical examination of the hip, appropriate diagnostic testing, the surgical procedure and its indications, expected outcomes, possible complications, and the postoperative rehabilitation process. This knowledge enables the nurse to provide the necessary nursing care and enables the physician extender to perform the advanced practice roles of provider, educator, practitioner, consultant, and collaborator.

Preoperative Care

An outpatient surgical setting is routine for many surgical procedures. It is advantageous because it reduces costs and allows patients to recuperate in their own environment. This requires that the patient and caregivers become actively involved in and responsible in the perioperative care [1]. Patient preparation starts with the first visit to the orthopedic office. This visit may be for diagnostic purposes, conservative treatment measures, or for the decision for surgery. It is important to establish an open and trusting relationship with the patient and other caregivers from the first encounter. It is through this special relationship and unique interaction that the foundation for the perioperative course is laid.

It is important to provide continuity of care through direct patient interaction. Both the nurse and physician extender can serve as a resource with whom patients can feel comfortable conversing and asking questions. This is important in helping patients and caregivers manage their anxiety and to provide information regarding diagnoses, testing, surgery, and postoperative recovery.

It takes a comprehensive systematic approach to care for the patient undergoing hip arthroscopy. The providers must demonstrate an aptitude to foresee and discuss care options including potential short-term and long-term consequences. This requires continual assessment, diagnosis, intervention, and evaluation of the patient and the plan of care.

K.S. Jones, MSN, RN (✉) • E.A. Potts, MSN, APN, ACNP-BC
J.W.T. Byrd, M.D.
Nashville Sports Medicine Foundation,
2011 Church St., Suite 100,
Nashville, TN 37203, USA
e-mail: kay@nsmfoundation.org; info@nsmfoundation.org

J.W.T. Byrd (ed.), *Operative Hip Arthroscopy*,
DOI 10.1007/978-1-4419-7925-4_34, © Springer Science+Business Media New York 2013

Patient Health History

To obtain a thorough health history, adequate time must be spent with the patient. This is done on the patient's first visit to the office. This history is a composition of subjective and objective data that will assist in identifying diagnoses and collaborative health problems.

In our opinion, the history is the single most essential element in patient evaluation. The surgeon may use some of the information provided by the clinical nurse specialist or physician extender, but he or she may also ask their own set of questions based on their dialogue with the patient. Nonetheless, this initial history is important for two reasons. First, it provides the patient an opportunity to formulate and organize their thoughts, making the subsequent interaction with the surgeon more time-efficient. Also, just as part of human nature, it is not uncommon to encounter contradictions in the patient's response between the two interviews. This provides an opportunity to establish clarification since the information obtained may have significant influence on the subsequent course of treatment.

Subjective Data

The patient interview is a communication process that focuses on developmental, psychological, sociocultural, and spiritual responses. It is important to be cognizant of the patient's comfort and anxiety levels, age, and current health status. These factors can influence the patient's ability to fully participate in the interview.

The interview process has three phases. During the introductory phase, the nurse or extender and the patient get to know each other. At this time, the patient is given a brief overview of the interview process, and its purpose is explained. The second phase is the working phase, in which the history is obtained. It is important to take cues from the patient, listen, and use critical thinking skills in interpreting and validating the information received from the patient. The final phase of the interview process is the summary phase, in which the information obtained is summarized to ensure accuracy and to validate problems and goals. Possible plans for problem resolution are discussed with the patient during the summary phase [2].

A few specific communication techniques can be employed to facilitate the interview and ensure its efficiency. It is important to ask open-ended questions to obtain patient perceptions. These questions begin with "What," "When," "Where," and "How" and are important because they encourage the patient to use more than a one-word response. Close-ended questions are also important to help obtain facts and elicit specific information. This may help keep the patient from rambling. Offering the patient a list of words to choose from may help obtain specific answers while reducing the

chance that patients will perceive and try to provide an expected answer. For example, in reference to the quality of pain, one might ask, "Is the pain dull, sharp, or stabbing?"

When data is obtained that digresses from normal, further exploration is necessary. These questions are useful: "What alleviates or aggravates the problem?" "How long has it occurred?" "When does it occur?" "Was the onset gradual or sudden?" Throughout the interview, it is important to rephrase the patient's responses to clarify information obtained [2].

There are several key points to remember when interviewing a patient. The first is to avoid being judgmental. This will help put the patient at ease and more inclined to provide specific information. It is important to utilize silence to help patients organize their thoughts. It is also helpful to provide answers to questions as they arise during the interview. Avoid leading questions, rushing the patient, and performing other tasks while taking the history [2]. By employing these principles during the interview, the information obtained is used in developing a plan of care and in providing information necessary for making a diagnosis.

While obtaining the patient's history, one must be aware that many disorders can present as a painful hip, including problems of the lower back as well as visceral disorders and that the patient may describe "hip pain" that actually represents referred symptoms from a different origin. Once the problem has been localized to the hip area, a distinction must be made between intra-articular and extra-articular symptoms.

A few characteristic features may clue the examiner to suspect an intra-articular hip problem. These hallmarks include complaints of anterior, inguinal, or medial thigh pain. Complaints of lateral hip pain or posterior or buttock symptoms are more commonly caused by extra-articular sources such as trochanteric bursitis, abductor muscle injury, or sciatica. A history of catching or popping in the hip may be related to intra-articular pathology but can also occur with disorders outside the joint.

Patients with abnormal intra-articular hip pathology commonly complain of pain in the groin with standing and ambulation. They may relate that they cannot sit for prolonged periods of time and that sitting with the hip in a flexed position is especially uncomfortable. Increased pain may be experienced with weight-bearing activities and when ascending or descending stairs. The patient may report difficulty with putting on socks and shoes or getting in and out of the car. Usually, a correlation is seen between the activity level and the pain perceived.

Objective Data: Physical Examination

After the subjective information has been obtained, the objective aspects of the patient's complaints can be explored. The physician extender or surgeon may obtain this information, but it is important for the clinical nurse to understand the physical assessment process. This is discussed in detail in Chap. 2 and summarized here.

Examination of the patient with a complaint of hip pain is straightforward but inclusive of the lumbar spine and pelvis. Many patients present with a chief complaint of "hip pain" but do not have an intra-articular hip problem. Therefore, the examiner must first consider extra-articular sources that could cause the patient's "hip pain." Once the extra-articular sources are ruled out, intra-articular sources of the patient's pain can be considered.

Some extra-articular disorders may mimic a hip problem and may sometimes coexist with a hip disorder. A common example among athletes is athletic pubalgia ("sports hernia"), which can occur in conjunction with femoroacetabular impingement (FAI). Some patients with early signs of hip disease may also have a component of lumbar spine disease. Patients with chronic hip problems may demonstrate gluteal tenderness to palpation simply as these muscles have been overworked attempting to protect the joint. Snapping of the iliopsoas tendon is incidentally present in up to 10% of a normal active population and could simply be present in conjunction with a joint problem. For every one of these apparent extra-articular problems, there are numerous less obvious disorders of the lumbar spine, pelvis, and viscera that may be the source of symptoms.

Observation of the patient's gait pattern is meaningful. The gait may be antalgic or possibly reveal an abductor lurch, which reduces the forces generated across the hip. The patient may use an assistive device such as a cane or crutches. It is important to note the patient's base of support. While standing, the patient may assume a slightly flexed position of the affected hip. When seated, the patient may slouch to avoid excessive hip flexion or lean to the uninvolved side with the hip in a slightly abducted, externally rotated position.

It is important to inspect the patient's hips and lower extremities for any asymmetry, gross atrophy, spinal malalignment, or pelvic obliquity that may be fixed or associated with a gross leg length discrepancy. Leg lengths can be measured as a routine part of the exam. In some situations, documenting thigh circumference may reflect the chronicity of the problem and may be a rough indicator of the response to therapy. It is also important to document range of motion of the affected hip compared with the unaffected hip.

It is helpful to ask the patient to use one finger to point to the area of most discomfort. This is a useful way of determining the area of maximal involvement. Intra-articular hip pathology typically has a component of anterior hip pain. The patient may also relate a sensation of deep, lateral discomfort or posterior pain, but this is usually in conjunction with a significant anterior component. Often, the patient will demonstrate the C-sign in describing deep hip pain. This sign is characterized by placing the index finger and thumb around the hip, forming a C-shaped pattern over the area of involvement. The index finger rests in the groin area and the thumb rests over the posterior aspect of the trochanter.

Palpation is rarely helpful in determining intra-articular pathology, but it is important in the overall assessment of other sources of pain in the hip region, such as trochanteric bursitis or abductor tendinopathy. The examiner palpates the lumbar spine, sacroiliac joints, ischium, iliac crest, and the lateral hip around the greater trochanter, always comparing the unaffected to the affected side and examining the unaffected hip first.

Range of motion should be assessed and recorded, looking for asymmetry or bilateral anomalies. While reduced rotation often accompanies FAI, excessive mobility may imply dysplasia or capsular laxity. Popping or snapping may be present and can occur from a variety of intra-articular and extra-articular sources which can be indicative of pathology or sometimes just a normal finding. Manual muscle testing is a crude measure of hip function but may elicit symptoms localized to a specific muscle injury. The most specific indicator for hip joint pain is log rolling of the patient's leg. This action moves only the femoral head in relation to the acetabulum and the surrounding capsule. The absence of pain on log rolling does not preclude the hip as the source of symptoms, but the presence of pain with this maneuver greatly raises the suspicion of mechanical joint pathology.

Extreme forceful end ranges of motion may elicit pain with even subtle hip pathology. Maximal flexion with internal rotation is referred to as an "impingement test," but we have found this maneuver to be uncomfortable in association with virtually any intra-articular pathology and not just specific for impingement. The Patrick or FABER (flexion, abduction, external rotation) test has been used to induce symptoms from both the hip and sacroiliac joint. The distinction is usually based on the origin of the pain. An active straight leg raise will often elicit symptoms. This maneuver creates a force of several times body weight across the articular surfaces and actually generates more force than walking.

Objective Data: Diagnostic Testing

Patient history and clinical examination are important tools, but diagnostic testing also plays a large role in the evaluation of hip arthroscopy candidates. This begins with plain radiographs and may include various advanced imaging as discussed in Chap. 3. Beyond the normal clinical assessment, the best indicator of true joint pathology is pronounced temporary pain relief from an intra-articular injection of anesthetic. We have reported that positive anesthetic relief of hip pain has been found to be indicative of abnormal intra-articular pathology with 90% accuracy [3]. Traditionally, fluoroscopy has been used for this type of injection, which is not readily available in most orthopedic offices.

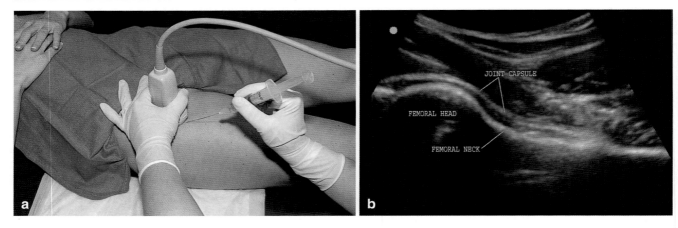

Fig. 34.1 (**a**) Visualization of the hip is performed by placing the transducer firmly over the area of the femoral head/neck junction in long axis and slightly oblique. A slight oblique angle to the transducer allows a more lateral entry site for the needle into the joint and increases the distance between the needle and the femoral neurovascular structures

anterior to the hip. The skin has been sterilely prepped and sterile gel is used. Prior to the injection, a scan should be performed to visualize the location of the neurovascular bundle. (**b**) Ultrasound image of anterior hip joint with probe positioned over femoral head/neck junction as described above. (All rights are retained by Dr. Byrd)

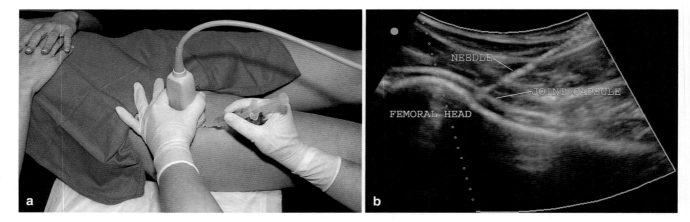

Fig. 34.2 (**a**) The needle is inserted in plane with the transducer which allows visualization of the needle throughout the course of its advancement to the capsule. (**b**) The needle can be seen entering the joint capsule at the base of the femoral head. (All rights are retained by Dr. Byrd)

Ultrasonography

There have been substantial technological advancements in ultrasonography since the second edition of this textbook. It is now available in an office setting with numerous diagnostic and interventional roles applicable to surgeons and physician extenders.

Intra-articular hip injections for diagnostic and therapeutic purposes can be reliably performed under ultrasound guidance (Video 34.1: http://goo.gl/F5kEs) (Figs. 34.1, 34.2, 34.3, and 34.4). We have found the technique to be very reproducible. Perhaps most importantly, our patients have uniformly found that the experience of an in-office ultrasound injection of the joint is a much gentler experience than one performed under fluoroscopy. This is especially compounded by the convenience when the patient does not have to travel

to a hospital or imaging center for fluoroscopy. The clinical advantage is substantial, as a real-time assessment of the patient's pre- and postinjection pain level is readily obtained. Sometimes this may necessitate specific functional activities on the part of the patient in order to make this determination.

Ultrasound is much more than just an injection tool. It can be used to look for an effusion which, historically, has been one of the most reliable positive indicators of hip pathology. Extra-articular structures can be assessed including the iliopsoas tendon (Video 34.2: http://goo.gl/e0SRr), (Video 34.3: http://goo.gl/VNefU) (Figs. 34.5, 34.6, 34.7, and 34.8), abductor tears (Figs. 34.9, and 34.10), (Video 34.4: http://goo.gl/7Aod1) and the piriformis (Video 34.5: http://goo.gl/FOSiu) (Figs. 34.11, 34.12, 34.13, and 34.14), among others. Diagnostic and therapeutic injections of these areas can be

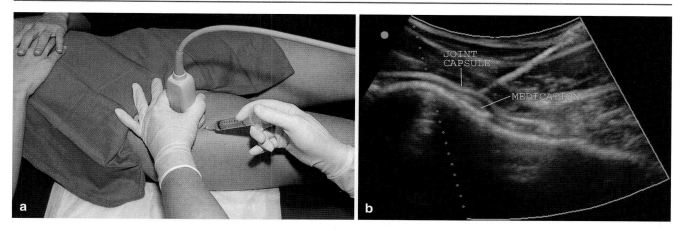

Fig. 34.3 (a) The transducer remains in the same plane throughout the injection. (b) The medication can be visualized entering the joint capsule. (All rights are retained by Dr. Byrd)

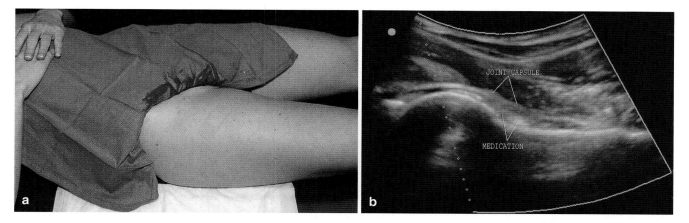

Fig. 34.4 (a) After completing the injection process, the syringe is removed and a small bandage is applied. (b) The medication can be visualized in the joint capsule. (All rights are retained by Dr. Byrd)

performed with reliable localization for corticosteroids or platelet-rich plasma for select conditions.

Ultrasound also offers the ability for dynamic examination of numerous soft tissue structures, including muscles and tendons, ligaments, and neurovascular structures. There is much ongoing work in this area evaluating the contribution of these numerous structures as causes of pain and dysfunction in the hip region.

Postoperative Care

By the time the patient arrives in the operating suite, the educational process should be complete and the patient prepared to handle the events that will follow. As discussed earlier, this educational process is best accomplished before the patient arrives at the hospital. Three salient features are important in the postoperative care of the patient: pain control, wound care, and activity level. It is important that these

are understood by the patient and the caregivers. These concepts may be difficult to comprehend preoperatively but should be discussed.

It is helpful to have written postoperative instructions for the patient and caregiver (Appendix). This will reiterate much of the information that has been verbalized preoperatively and immediately postoperatively. Providing written discharge instructions will help increase retention and understanding of the information provided [4]. The 1994 study by Oberle et al. [5] showed that timing of preoperative teaching is critical to retention and patient satisfaction. Approximately 25% of the patients in the study reported being given little or no information about their surgery even through nurses had provided information during the perioperative period. This report suggests that patients and their caregivers do not always hear and understand the information being conveyed. Written postoperative discharge instructions can serve as a reference once the patient has returned home.

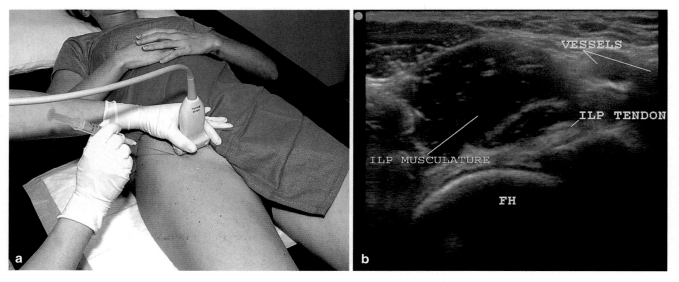

Fig. 34.5 (**a**) Visualization of the iliopsoas is performed with the transducer placed over the area of the iliopsoas in short axis. (**b**) Short axis ultrasound image illustrates visualization of the iliopsoas (*ILP*) tendon, musculature, blood vessels, and femoral head (*FH*). (All rights are retained by Dr. Byrd)

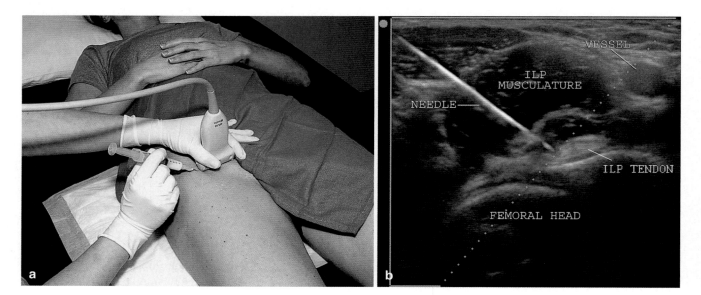

Fig. 34.6 (**a**) The needle is inserted in plane with the transducer to allow visualization of the needle during the injection. The tip of the needle should be placed just lateral to the tendon and into the anterior recess of the bursa. (**b**) Ultrasound image depicts position of needle in relation to the iliopsoas tendon. (All rights are retained by Dr. Byrd)

Pain Control

Postoperative pain is one of the greatest fears patients have about surgery and is often poorly addressed by physicians [6]. Pain control should be discussed preoperatively to allay patient apprehension. Patients should expect postoperative pain and/or discomfort. The pain experienced is typically the worst in the recovery room. Once the acute postsurgical pain is controlled, many patients are surprised at the low intensity of pain they actually experience. Patients describe postoperative pain as a burning ache in the hip, but the severity depends on the pathology addressed. For example, a patient with loose bodies may find that the postoperative pain is less than the discomfort experienced preoperatively. Conversely, a patient undergoing bony work for impingement may experience considerably more discomfort immediately after surgery.

Educating patients about postoperative pain is an important step in the preoperative discussion. The patient should

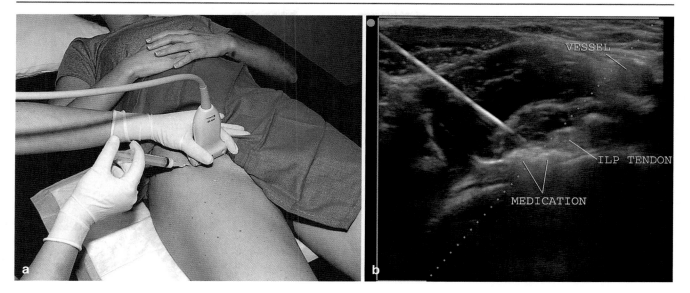

Fig. 34.7 (**a**) The medication is injected. (**b**) The medication is visualized entering the anterior recess of the iliopsoas bursa. (All rights are retained by Dr. Byrd)

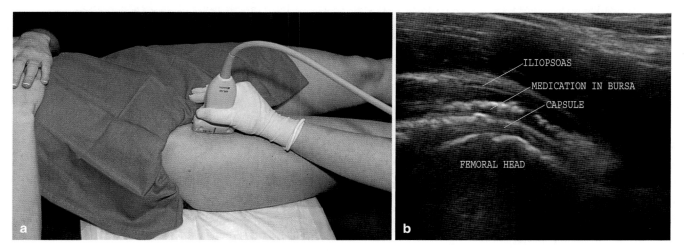

Fig. 34.8 (**a**) After the injection, placing the transducer over the iliopsoas in long axis will allow visualization of the medication in the bursa between the joint capsule and the iliopsoas musculature. (**b**) Long axis ultrasound image after injection of medication into the bursa. The image shows clearly defined layers indicating the femoral head, joint capsule, bursa, and the iliopsoas musculature. (All rights are retained by Dr. Byrd)

know to expect pain from instrumentation of the joint and any bony work performed as well as muscular soreness in the operative leg that is often noted after the acute surgical pain has abated. This muscular soreness can be caused by manipulation of the hip, traction forces applied during the procedure, and the use of the perineal post. The typical description is overall soreness around the hip and many patients report feeling like they have ridden a horse and have soreness in the saddle area. Ankle soreness in the operative leg is also a common complaint and is related to the traction boot. It is reassuring for the patient to know that these various aches normally resolve in 5–7 days. The amount of dis-

comfort is variable, but we generally find the greatest pain control issues in conjunction with extensive bony work to the acetabulum and concomitant labral refixation. The peak of pain usually subsides within 8–10 h. Adequate pain control is one criterion for discharge from the recovery room. Occasionally, some patients may not achieve adequate control with oral analgesics. For these circumstances, patients may be well suited for a regional block performed by the anesthesia service. We do not use these routinely for all patients, but all patients are assessed in the recovery area and, if initial pain control is problematic, a regional block can be chosen.

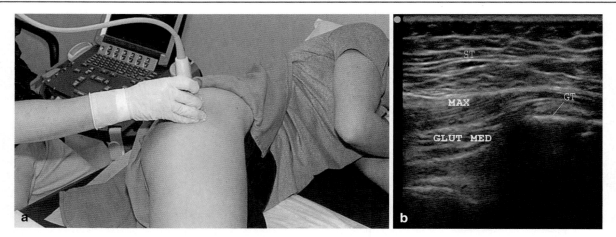

Fig. 34.9 (a) The peritrochanteric region is scanned over the lateral hip. The location of the transducer will vary depending on the location of the pathology and desired injection site. (b) Ultrasound image shows the subcutaneous tissues (*ST*), gluteus maximus (*MAX*), gluteus medius (*GLUT MED*), and the greater trochanter (*GT*). (All rights are retained by Dr. Byrd)

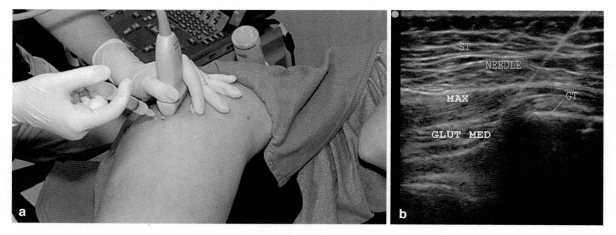

Fig. 34.10 (a) The needle is placed in plane with the transducer to allow visualization of the needle throughout the procedure. Visualization of the needle ensures that the medication is injected into the desired location. (b) Ultrasound image demonstrates the needle entering the tissue of the gluteus medius as it nears its insertion on the greater trochanter. (All rights are retained by Dr. Byrd)

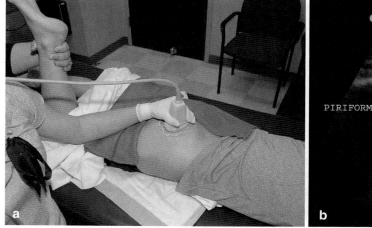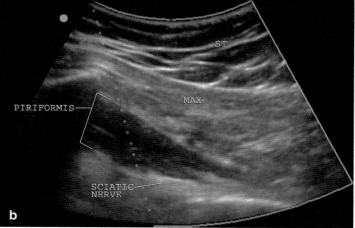

Fig. 34.11 (a) Inspection of the piriformis is performed with the patient prone and the transducer placed firmly over the piriformis in long axis. With the knee flexed, an assistant can internally and externally rotate the leg allowing visualization of the piriformis in motion throughout the subgluteal space. (b) This long axis ultrasound image depicts the relationship between the subcutaneous tissue (*ST*), gluteus maximus (*MAX*), piriformis, and sciatic nerve. (All rights are retained by Dr. Byrd)

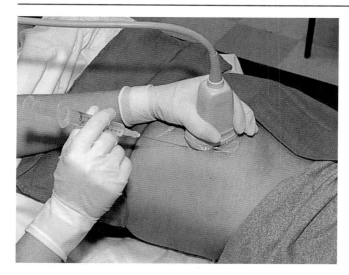

Fig. 34.12 The needle is placed in plane with the transducer. This allows the needle to be visualized throughout its advancement to the piriformis, avoiding the sciatic nerve. (All rights are retained by Dr. Byrd)

A lateral femoral cutaneous nerve block or fascia iliacus compartment block is most commonly used. These types of regional nerve blocks are preferred because they give mostly sensory nerve anesthesia with very little motor nerve anesthesia. Occasionally, these blocks do not provide the patient with adequate pain control so a femoral nerve block is used. One caution about femoral blocks is that there is concomitant motor inhibition of the quadriceps. Patients must be educated regarding the potential for falls and should be instructed on strict protected weight bearing until they regain full motor function.

Narcotics or oral centrally acting medications, such as oxycodone 5 mg with acetaminophen 325 mg, are prescribed for pain control. Prescription pain medicine is generally used for the first 5–7 days after surgery. By the end of the first postoperative week, the need for narcotic pain control is more sporadic. Patients should be reminded to take medications with food to prevent gastrointestinal discomfort. They

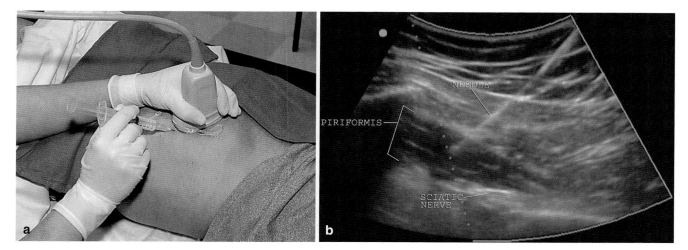

Fig. 34.13 (**a**) The needle is inserted into the musculature of the piriformis avoiding the sciatic nerve. (**b**) The ultrasound image shows the needle entering the piriformis a safe distance from the sciatic nerve. (All rights are retained by Dr. Byrd)

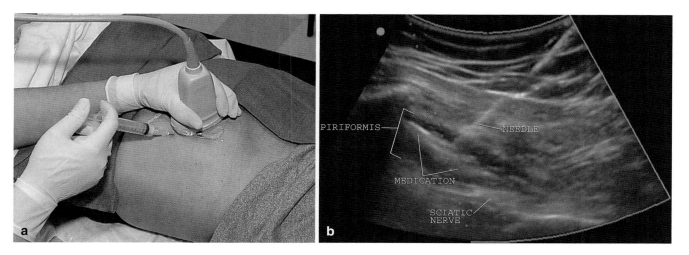

Fig. 34.14 (**a**) The medication is injected. (**b**) The medication is visualized entering the muscle tissue of the piriformis. (All rights are retained by Dr. Byrd)

should also be instructed to refrain from driving or operating heavy machinery while medicated.

With the introduction of impingement surgery, the need to prevent heterotopic ossification must be considered by the surgeon. This is routinely accomplished with nonsteroidal anti-inflammatory drugs. The patient should be educated on the purpose of the drug regime and the importance of their compliance in the prevention of heterotopic ossification. The patient should also be reminded about the potential side effects that can be experienced and to call the surgeon's office if they experience any such effects.

After narcotics are discontinued, alternative nonprescription medications such as acetaminophen, ibuprofen, or other nonsteroidal anti-inflammatories may be useful to ameliorate discomfort. It is important to note that analgesics, possibly narcotics, may be needed when physical therapy is initiated or when performing exercises. Some patients may experience prolonged discomfort or more intense pain. The reasons for this should be explored by the clinician.

The use of ice (cryotherapy) has several beneficial effects for tissues that have been injured, whether from trauma or surgery. When ice is applied immediately after surgery, the body attempts to preserve core heat by constricting superficial cutaneous vessels, causing decreased capillary permeability and hemorrhaging. This therapeutically alters the physiologic response of the tissues to injury by reducing inflammation, swelling, and pain [7].

Ice is most effective when used immediately after surgery. The ice bag can first be applied by the recovery room nurse. The patient should be instructed to apply ice for 15–20 min every 3 h for the first 24 h and even for 2–3 days after surgery if it helps alleviate discomfort. There are several different cold therapy devices available that are effective to help control pain. They are convenient in that they often cycle through the cooling process and are designed to maintain a constant cool temperature over the joint. Patients who use cold compression therapy devices rave over the difference that they make compared to traditional ice packs.

Cryotherapy is not without hazards. Cold should not be used for longer than 30 min with conventional methods (ice bags/packs) due to the potential for freezing the skin. This could result in frostnip or frostbite. Nerve palsies can result from the application of cold to an extremity for longer than 30 min, or when cold is improperly applied to vulnerable areas [8].

Contraindications to cryotherapy include patients recovering from an epidural infusion or spinal/nerve block. Ice should not be used until full sensation has returned in both lower extremities. Cryotherapy should not be used at all in the patient with a suspected neuropathy, such as with diabetes or on patients with a true hypersensitivity or allergy to cold [8].

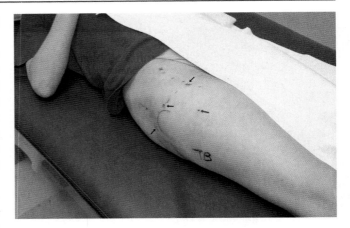

Fig. 34.15 A first postoperative day wound site following correction of FAI including acetabuloplasty with labral refixation and femoroplasty. The three standard portals (*black arrows*) were used for access to the central compartment. A distal puncture wound (*green arrow*) was used for percutaneous anchor placement, and an accessory proximal portal (*gray arrow*) aided in access to the periphery and femoroplasty. (All rights are retained by Dr. Byrd)

Wound Care

A bulky dressing is applied to the surgical site. This dressing is left in place until the first postoperative day, allowing time for extravasated fluid from surgery to be absorbed into the dressing. Usually, this has subsided enough to remove the dressing within the first 24 h. The patient should be reassured that it is normal for the dressing to feel wet from the irrigation fluid and that it may be blood-tinged.

The patient should be aware that the surgeon will make several arthroscopy portals. Each of these portals is typically about 1 cm but could be larger and will be closed with sutures. Patients, and even allied health professionals, are often surprised at the anatomic location of the portals. They envision them being located more cephalad (Fig. 34.15).

The portals are cleaned daily with hydrogen peroxide and water. A small adhesive bandage can then be placed over each portal site until the sutures are removed. The patient may shower on the first postoperative day, taking care to keep water from running directly over the portals. If the portals show signs of adequate healing, the sutures may be removed approximately 7 days postoperatively and Steri-Strips applied.

It takes approximately 10–14 days for the portals to heal completely. During this time, showering is allowed, but the patient should avoid submersing the operative hip in a bathtub, hot tub, or swimming pool.

It is important to educate patients regarding the signs and symptoms of infection. They should be advised to contact the nurse if they develop any redness or drainage at the portal sites or if they develop a high fever.

Activity Level

The activity level prescribed after hip arthroscopy is variable, depending on the pathology found at the time of surgery and the surgeon's preference. Assistive devices, usually crutches, are used at least until the gait pattern is normalized and limp resolved, which can take 5–7 days. At a minimum, patients are encouraged to use their assistive devices until they have been seen by the physical therapist or return to the surgeon's office. More complex procedures such as correction of FAI, labral repair or refixation, microfracture or capsular stabilizations may require a more protracted period of protected weight bearing ranging from 4 to 8 weeks. The specifics of this must be directed by the surgeon and can be implemented by the clinical nurse and physician extender.

The patient will be most comfortable immediately after surgery in a reclining or sitting position. The most comfortable sleeping positions are usually supine or on the nonoperative side with a pillow between the legs. Sleeping on the operative side has no known adverse effects, but this is usually not comfortable for several weeks postoperatively.

Patients need to be reminded that it is easy for them to overdo in the first few days after surgery and should be encouraged to limit their activities. Once they feel like being up and around, daily activities can be performed to tolerance, but they should be respectful of any discomfort felt in the hip. Oftentimes, for simpler procedures, patients experience a "honeymoon" phase for the first 3–4 weeks postoperatively. During this time, the patient experiences pronounced pain relief compared to their preoperative status. They do need to be reminded that they have just had hip surgery and need to pace themselves accordingly. Often, the patients are not back to regular activities of daily living, and when they do return to their normal level of functioning, they will experience pain and soreness. When this does happen, the patient often gets discouraged or thinks that the surgical procedure was not successful. The nurse can explain to them that it really takes a month to get over the actual surgical procedure. After that initial month, it can take 3–4 months before they may actually appreciate the benefits of the surgery.

For more complex procedures such as FAI, it is not uncommon for patients to spontaneously experience a setback at around 8–10 weeks postoperatively. The etiology is not always clear, but it is probably a combination of the patient starting to do more and the joint experiencing forces for the first time since surgery. This requires attention on behalf of the patients to assure them that this is not necessarily a worrisome sign but may obligate some alteration in the rehab strategy to accommodate their discomfort and perhaps a brief course of anti-inflammatory medication. It is best to warn patients preoperatively about this occasional occurrence. Thus, they will have more confidence in your explanation and encouragement that things will be okay when this occurs postoperatively.

Fatigue is one of the biggest considerations after surgery [4]. This can be related to several factors including the anesthetic, analgesics, pain, or sleep disruption. The nurse should inform the patient that this will generally dissipate after postoperative day 3 but can last as long as several weeks.

Physical therapy is usually initiated 1–2 days after surgery. The rehabilitation program for the postoperative patient is individualized to the pathology and the procedure performed. The primary focus of the rehabilitation process is to reduce discomfort and improve function. A successful result after surgery is often dependent on a properly constructed rehabilitation program. This is an important concept to be relayed to the patient because there may often be a reluctance to go to physical therapy. When the hip hurts, the idea of "exercise" may not be appealing to the patient.

The most frequently asked question regarding activity is "When can I drive?" General guidelines include the following two parameters: the patient must have discontinued the use of narcotic analgesics and have regained adequate leg control to operate the accelerator and brake pedals or clutch. Right hip arthroscopy often delays the resumption of driving. Restrictions for up to a month may be necessary for complex procedures, especially with labral repair in the driving leg.

It is important for the clinical nurse and physician extender to remember several things pertinent to the postoperative recuperation. Patients want and need to hear that they are doing well and are on schedule in their recovery. Patients are often impatient and may expect to recover more quickly than they actually do. Rarely will a patient tell you that their recovery was quicker than they had anticipated. Many prefer to have guidelines by which to gauge their progress. They want to know how other patients normally respond under the same circumstances [5]. Patients and their caregivers may have selective hearing or may forget to read postoperative instructions; therefore, frequent contact by telephone is one of the keys to the successful recovery of the hip arthroscopy patient [9]. The frequent contact between the clinical nurse and the patient and/or their caregivers can have a positive effect on patient satisfaction and also provides a mechanism for feedback [4].

Conclusions

Appropriate patient selection and education, skillful implementation of the surgical procedure, and a properly constructed rehabilitation program are all important factors in the success of hip arthroscopy. Of equal importance, the patient's expectations must be properly matched with the results anticipated by the surgeon. The clinical nurse and physician extender play a crucial role in assuring the integration of these factors, all of which are critical to an optimal outcome.

The role of the clinical nurse is an integral part of the perioperative experience. While the patient is carefully guided through surgery and the rehabilitation process, the nurse monitors expectations to assure the most likely degree of overall patient satisfaction. The clinical nurse's perspective, attained through direct patient assessment and interaction, can help to define coexistent conditions or circumstances that could potentially influence the success of arthroscopy.

Physician extenders facilitate all aspects of patient care but also provide a useful additional diagnostic and therapeutic resource for surgeons. The history and physical examination direct most patient care, but adjunct imaging such as office ultrasonography greatly enhances both diagnosis and treatment while leaving the surgeon free to steer all aspects of the patient's care.

Success is also dependent on patients' ability not only to understand what is happening but also to be an active participant in their perioperative care. The focus on ambulatory outpatient surgery allows more efficient utilization of resources but places more responsibility on patients and caregivers. Patients undergoing arthroscopic surgery of the hip must be equipped to handle their postoperative course. This is best accomplished with detailed education and nursing care, beginning preoperatively.

An optimal outcome is dependent on coordination of the perioperative care, from preoperative assessment through postoperative rehabilitation. The clinical nurse and physician extender help facilitate the patient's smooth transition through this experience and serve as a vital resource for other members of the health care team. The nurse and extender are educators, practitioners, consultants, and collaborators. By serving in this multifaceted role, they ensure appropriate and efficient utilization of resources through close patient follow-up and timely response to changes in the clinical circumstance. This allows the other members of the health care team, whether it is as the patient, caregiver, surgeon, operating room personnel, or physical therapist, to better fulfill their respective roles.

Appendix: Postoperative Instructions

J.W. Thomas Byrd

Arthroscopic Surgery of the Hip

The following information is designed to answer some of the frequently asked questions regarding what to expect and what to do after arthroscopic surgery. These are general guidelines, if you have any questions or concerns, please give us a call.

Dressing and Wound Care – During arthroscopic surgery, the joint is irrigated with water. There will typically be 3 to 5 small incisions closed with sutures. Your hip will be covered with a bulky dressing. Water may gradually leak through these incisions, saturating the bandage. This blood-tinged drainage may persist for 24–36 h. If it has not significantly decreased by this time, please call our office.

The bandage may be removed the day after surgery. The incisions should be cleaned with hydrogen peroxide then covered with band-aids. As soon as the incisions are dry, you may leave them uncovered. Do not use ointments such as Neosporin on the incisions. You may shower the day after surgery, but avoid water running directly over the incisions. The incisions should not be soaked under water (e.g., bathtub, hot tub, swimming pool, etc.). The sutures should be removed 7–10 days after surgery.

If the incisions show any signs of infection, please contact our office. Specifically, if there is increased redness, persistent drainage, if you have fever, or if the pain does not progressively decrease, you should call the office.

ICE – During the first 48 h, ice can be helpful to decrease pain and swelling and is especially important during the first 24 h. Ice bags/packs should never be applied directly to the skin. They should be wrapped in a towel and applied for 15 min at a time every 2–3 h. If the skin becomes very cold or burns, discontinue the ice application immediately. If you are using the Game Ready system, please use the program outlined at the time of your instruction on how to use the machine.

Ambulation and Movement – Unless you have been otherwise instructed, you will be allowed to bear as much weight on your leg as is comfortable immediately after surgery. Crutches should be used and are necessary to help decrease discomfort and to protect your hip while walking after surgery. If there is any question about how much weight to place on your leg or how long to be on crutches, please call our office.

Your level of discomfort will most often be your best guide in determining how much activity is allowed. Remember that it is very easy to overdo in the first few days after surgery and any increase in pain or swelling usually indicates that you need to decrease your activities. Please be careful on slippery surfaces, steps, or anywhere you might fall and injure yourself.

Medications – You will be given a prescription for pain medication. You may also be given a prescription for an anti-inflammatory medication that you will need to take twice a day for 3 weeks. It is very important that you start this medication the night of your surgery and that you take this medication for the full 3 weeks. If there is any problem with you tolerating this medication, please call and let the nurse know. If you have any known drug allergies, check with the nurse prior to taking any medication.

Some medications do have side effects. If you have any difficulty with itching, nausea, or other side effects, discontinue the medication immediately and call our office. Pain medication often causes drowsiness and we advise that you do not drive, operate machinery, or make important decisions while taking medication.

Please note that we are unable to call in prescriptions for narcotics (pain pills) after office hours. If you need a refill, please call early in the day or before the weekend so the nurses can take care of that for you.

If you are able to take aspirin, you should take one aspirin (325 mg) twice daily for two weeks following your surgery. Aspirin serves as a mild blood thinner and may decrease the chance of blood clots forming in the leg. Although this is uncommon, it can be a difficult problem. It is best to take one in the morning and one in the evening and to avoid taking them on an empty stomach. If you are under the age of 16 or have any unusual medical problems, please check with the nurse about whether you should take aspirin.

Exercise/Physical Therapy – Physical therapy usually begins within a few days after your surgery. The therapist will outline an exercise program specific to your type of surgery. The purpose of physical therapy is to help you regain the use of your hip in a safe and progressive fashion. If you have any questions regarding your exercise program, please contact the physical therapist. If you are unaware of when or where your therapy is, please call the nurse and she can help you determine this.

First Post-Operative Visit – Your first post-operative appointment will be within one week of your surgery. The findings at surgery, long-term prognosis, and plans for rehabilitation will be discussed at this appointment. If you are unsure of when your first post-op visit with Dr. Byrd is, please call the office and someone will help get one scheduled.

Communications – If you are having any problems, contact us right away. If it is after office hours, the answering service will contact the nurse or doctor on call.

Remember, if your pain increases, check for signs of infection (redness, fever, etc.), decrease your activities, use ice, and take your pain medication as prescribed. If the pain persists, or if there are signs of infection, call our office (615) 284–5800.

References

1. Sutherland E. Day surgery: all in a day's work. Nurs Times. 1991;87(11):26–30.
2. Weber J. Nurses' handbook of health assessment. Philadelphia: J.B. Lippincott; 1988. p. 1–7.
3. Byrd JWT, Jones KS. Diagnostic accuracy of clinical assessment. MRI, gadolinium MRI, and intraarticular injection in hip arthroscopy patients. Am J Sports Med. 2004;32(7):1668–74.
4. Dougherty J. Same-day surgery: the nurse's role. Orthop Nurs. 1996;15(4):15–8.
5. Oberle K, Allen M, Lynkowski P. Follow-up of same day surgery patients. AORN J. 1994;59(5):1016–25.
6. Stephenson ME. Discharge criteria in day surgery. J Adv Nurs. 1990;15(5):601–13.
7. Knight KL. Cryotherapy. Am Fam Physician. 1990;23(3):141–4.
8. McDowell JH, McFarland EG, Nalli BJ. Cryotherapy in the orthopaedic patient. Orthop Nurs. 1994;13(5):21–30.
9. Burden N. Telephone follow-up of ambulatory surgery patients following discharge is a nursing responsibility. J Post Anesth Nurs. 1992;7(4):256–61.

Acetabuloplasty

This protocol should be used as a guideline for progression and should be tailored to the needs of the individual patient.

- **Weight bearing as tolerated, use crutches to normalize gait.**
  - · Crutches are usually discontinued at 5-7 days, once gait is normalized.

- **Strict impact precautions unnecessary, but functional progression may still be protracted because of severity of associated damage.**
  - · May still need to be delayed for 12 weeks to minimize exacerbation of symptoms.

- **Always use pharmacologic prophylaxis against heterotopic ossification (unless contraindicated.)**
  - · Quiz patient
  - · Must initiate and maintain immediately postop

PHASE 1:	WEEK 1

Initial Exercise *(Weeks 1-3)*

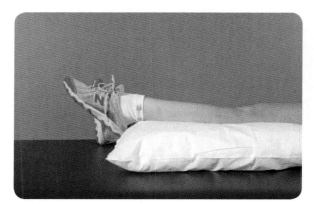

Ankle pump

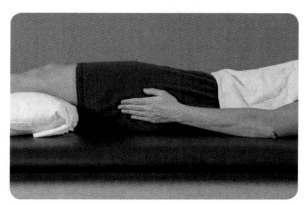

Glut sets

J.W.T. Byrd (ed.), *Operative Hip Arthroscopy*,
DOI 10.1007/978-1-4419-7925-4, © Springer Science+Business Media New York 2013

Initial Exercises *(Weeks 1-3)*

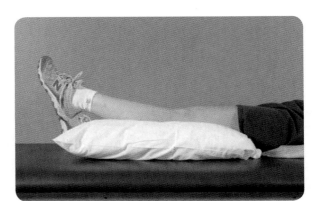

Quad sets

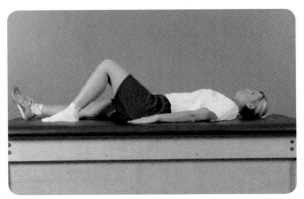

Heel slides, active-assisted range of motion

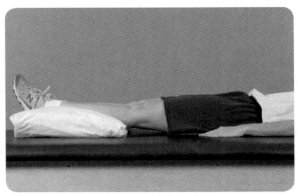

Hamstring sets

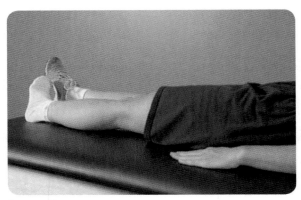

Log rolling

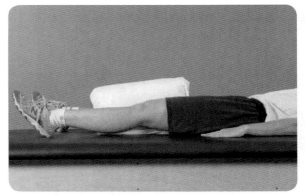

Adductor isometrics

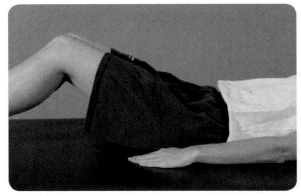

Pelvic tilt

PHASE 1:   WEEK 1
Initial Exercises *(Weeks 1-3)*

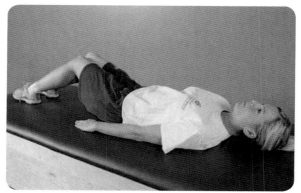

Trunk rotation

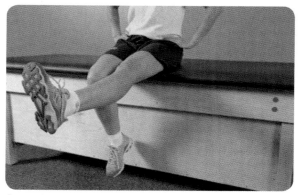

Seated knee extensions

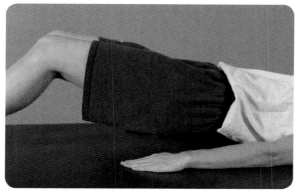

Double leg bridges

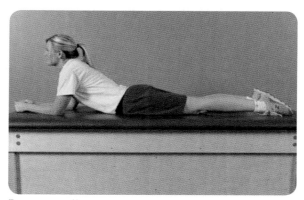

Prone on elbows

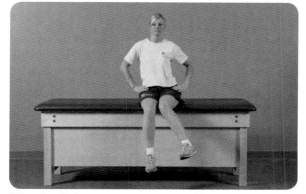

Weight shifts – sitting, supported, anterior/
posterior, lateral

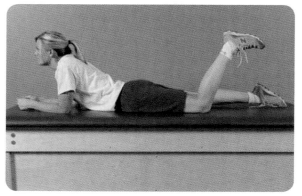

Prone knee flexion

PHASE 1:
Initial Exercises (Weeks 1-3)

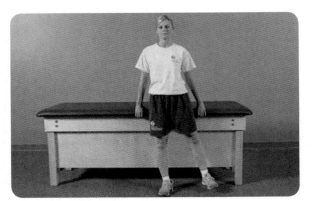

Standing abduction without resistance

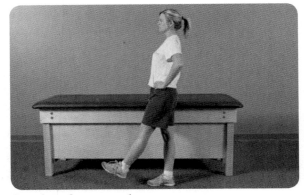

Standing flexion without resistance

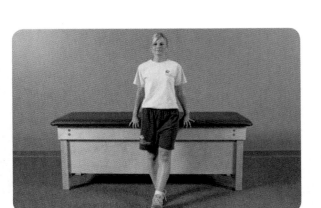

Standing adduction without resistance

Other Exercises Week 1

• Seated heel lifts

• Standard stationary bike without resistance at 3 days post-op (10 min. if tolerated)

• Upper body ergometer, upper body strengthening

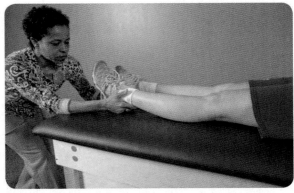

Pain dominant hip mobilization – grades I, II

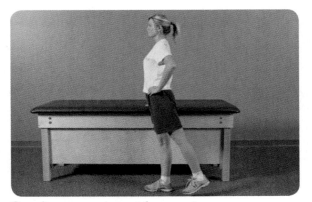

Standing extension without resistance

In Addition to Previous Exercises *(Weeks 1-3)*

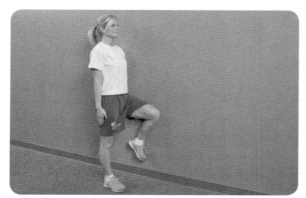

Abduction isometrics

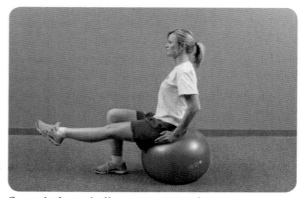

Seated physioball progression – knee extension

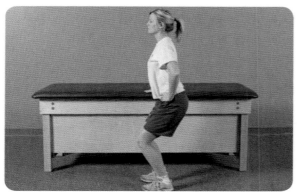

¼ Mini squats

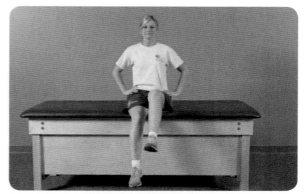

Hip flexion, IR/ER in pain-free range

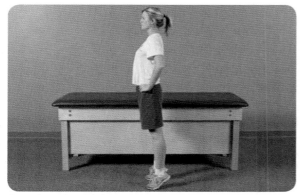

Standing heel lifts

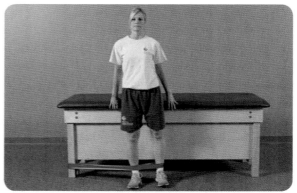

Theraband resistance on affected side – Abduction (start very low resistance)

PHASE 1:   WEEK 2
In Addition to Previous Exercises *(Weeks 1-3)*

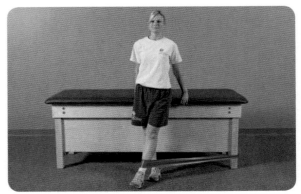

Theraband resistance on affected side – Adduction (start very low resistance)

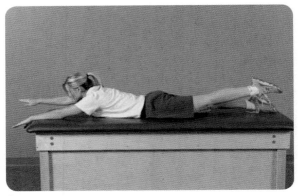

Superman

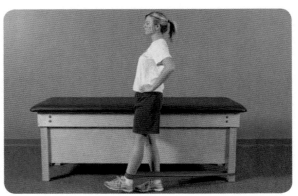

Theraband resistance on affected side – Flexion (start very low resistance)

Other Exercises Week 2

- Wall mini-squats

- Physioball mini-squats with cocontraction

- Pool exercises (water walking, range of motion, march steps, lateral steps, backward walking, mini-squats, heel raises, hamstring and hip flexor stretches)

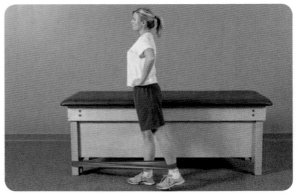

Theraband resistance on affected side – Extension (start very low resistance)

In Addition to Previous Exercises *(Weeks 1-3)*

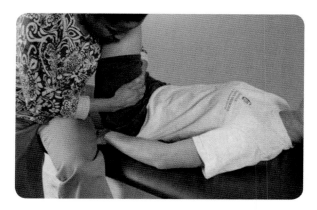

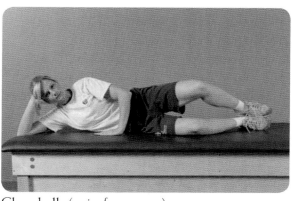

Clamshells (pain-free range)

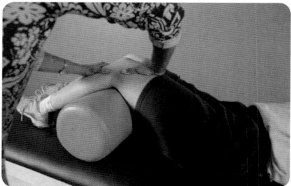

Stiffness dominant hip mobilization – grades III, IV

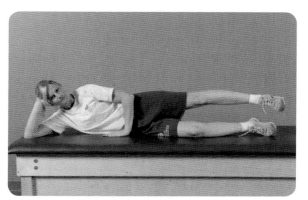

Leg raise – Abduction

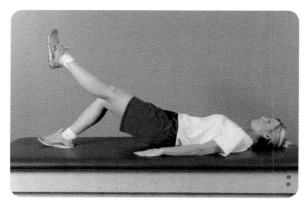

Double leg bridges to single leg bridges

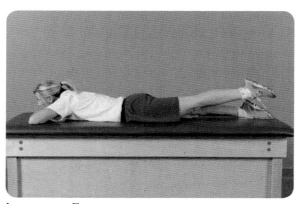

Leg raise – Extension

PHASE 1:   WEEK 3
In Addition to Previous Exercises *(Weeks 1-3)*

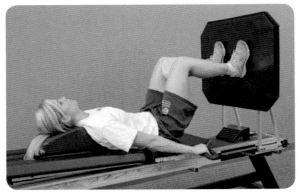

Shuttle leg press 90 degree hip flexion with co-contraction of adductors

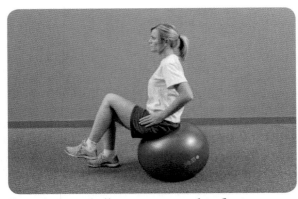

Seated physioball progression – hip flexion

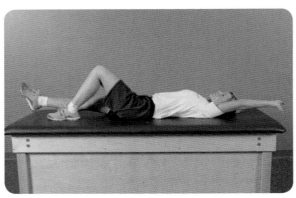

Dead bug

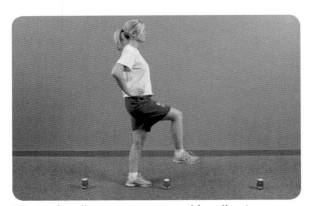

Forward walking over cups and hurdles (pause on affected limb), add ball toss while walking

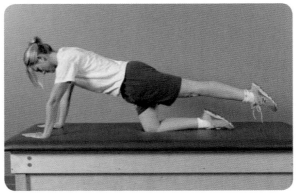

Quadriped 4 point support, progress 3 point support, progress 2 point

Other Exercises Week 3

- Continue stationary bike with minimal resistance – 5 min. increase daily

- Active range of motion with gradual end range stretch within tolerance

- Leg raise – Adduction

- Single leg sports cord leg press (long sitting) limiting hip flexion

PHASE 1:   WEEK 3
In Addition to Previous Exercises (Weeks 1-3)

Goals of Phase 1

☐ Restore range of motion

☐ Diminish pain and inflammation

☐ Prevent muscular inhibition

☐ Normalize gait

Criteria for progression to Phase 2

☐ Minimal pain with phase 1 exercises

☐ Minimal range of motion limitations

☐ Normalized gait without crutches

PHASE 2:   WEEKS 4-5
Intermediate Exercises (Weeks 4-6)

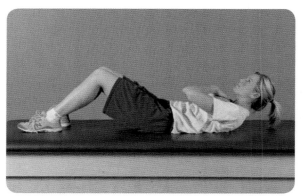

Crunches

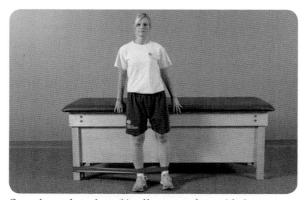

Standing theraband/pulley weight – Abduction

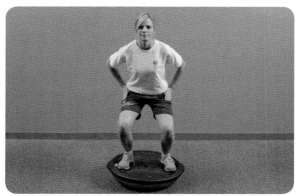

Bosu squats

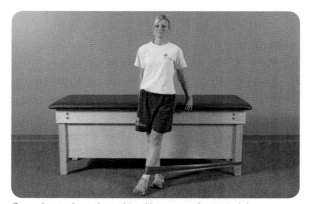

Standing theraband/pulley weight – Adduction

Intermediate Exercises *(Weeks 4-6)*

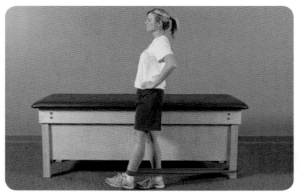

Standing theraband/pulley weight – Flexion

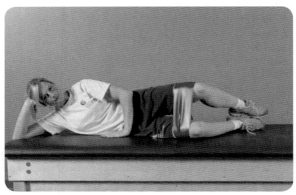

Clamshells with theraband

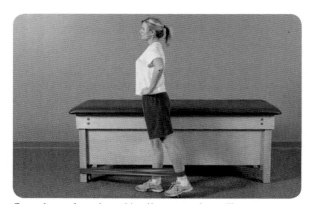

Standing theraband/pulley weight – Extension

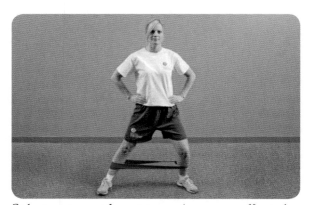

Sidestepping with resistance (pause on affected limb), sports cord walking forward and backward (pause on affected limb)

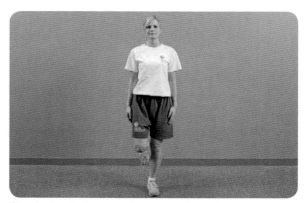

Single leg balance – firm to soft surface

Other Exercises Weeks 4-5

- Gradually increase resistance with stationary bike

- Initiate elliptical machine

- Pool water exercises – flutterkick swimming, 4 way hip with water weights, step-ups

Intermediate Exercises *(Weeks 4-6)*

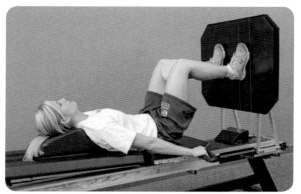

Leg press (gradually increasing weight)

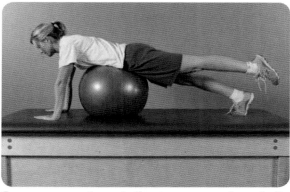

Superman on physioball – 2 point on physioball

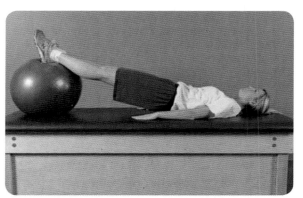

Physioball hamstring exercises – hip lift, bent knee hip lift, curls, balance

Other Exercises Week 6

- Single leg balance – firm to soft surface with external perturbation (ball catch, sports specific/simulated ex.)

- Knee extensions, hamstring curls

Goals of Phase 2

☐ Restore pain-free range of motion

☐ Initiate proprioception exercises

☐ Progressively increase muscle strength and endurance

Criteria for progression to Phase 3

☐ Minimum pain with phase 2 exercises

☐ Single leg stance with level pelvis

Advanced Exercises (Weeks 7-8)

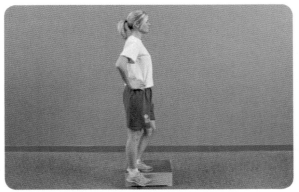

Step-ups with eccentric lowering

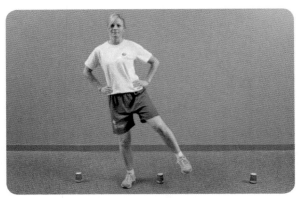

Side steps over cups/hurdles (with ball toss and external sports cord resistance), increase speed

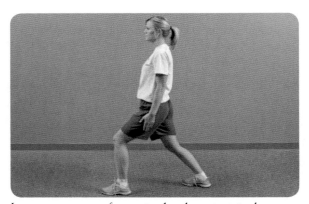

Lunges progress from single plane to tri-planar, add medicine balls for resistance and rotation

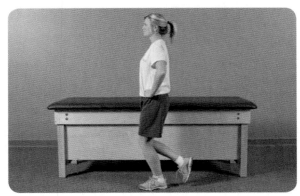

Single leg body weight squats, increase external resistance, stand on soft surface

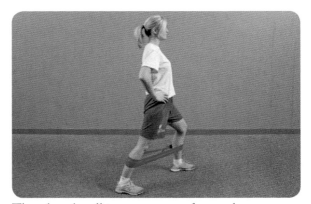

Theraband walking patterns – forward, sidestepping, carioca, monster steps, backward, ½ circles forward/backward – 25 yds. Start band at knee height and progress to ankle height

Other Exercises Weeks 7-8

• Full squats

• Single stability ball bridges

Goals for Phase 3

☐ Restoration of muscular endurance/strength

☐ Restoration of cardiovascular endurance

☐ Optimize neuromuscular control/balance/proprioception

PHASE 3:   WEEKS 7-8
Advanced Exercises *(Weeks 7-8)*

Criteria for Progression to Phase 4

☐ Single leg mini-squat with level pelvis

☐ Cardiovascular fitness equal to preinjury level

☐ Demonstration of initial agility drills with proper body mechanics

PHASE 4:   WEEKS 9-11
Sports specific training rehab clinic based progression

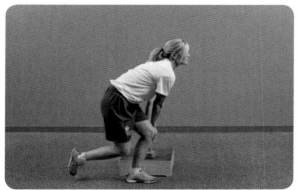

Single leg pick-ups, add soft surface

Other Exercises Weeks 9-11

• All phase 3 exercises

• Pool running (progress from chest deep to waist deep), treadmill jogging

• Step drills, quick feet step-ups (4-6 inch box) forward, lateral, carioca

• Plyometrics, double leg and single leg shuttle jumps

• Theraband walking patterns 1 rep of six exercises x 50yds, progress to band at knee height and ankle height

PHASE 4:   WEEKS 12 & BEYOND
Sports specific training rehab clinic based progression

Other Exercises Weeks 12 & Beyond

• Running progression

• Sport specific drills

• Traditional weight training

Criteria for full return to competition

☐ Full range of motion

☐ Hip strength equal to uninvolved side, single leg pick-up with level pelvis

☐ Ability to perform sport-specific drills at full speed without pain

☐ Completion of functional sports test

Femoroplasty

This protocol should be used as a guideline for progression and should be tailored to the needs of the individual patient.

- **Allowed full weight bearing, but use crutches for four weeks.**
  - Avoids risk of fracture through area of recontoured head/neck junction.
  - Protects against unexpected inordinate torsional or twisting forces, while muscle strength and response are regained.
  - Bony strength mostly unchanged at four weeks, but muscular function can protect the joint.

- **Vigorous impact loading avoided for 12 weeks.**
  - Allows for bone remodeling/healing.

- **Aggressive functional progression delayed until 12 weeks.**
  - Then progressed to tolerance.

- **Resumption of full activities anticipated at 4-6 months.**
  - Variable as dictated by hip symptoms.

- **Always use pharmacologic prophylaxis against heterotopic ossification (unless contraindicated.)**
  - Quiz patient
  - Must initiate and maintain immediately postop

PHASE 1:   WEEK 1
Initial Exercises *(Weeks 1-3)*

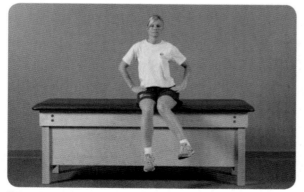

Weight shifts – sitting, supported, anterior/ posterior, lateral

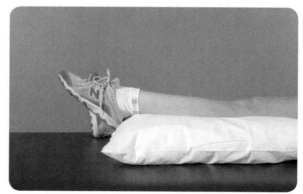

Ankle pumps

Initial Exercises *(Weeks 1-3)*

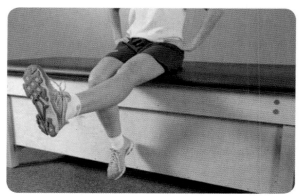

Seated knee extensions

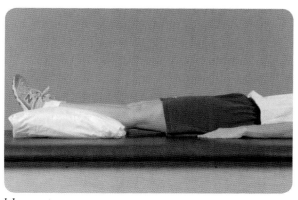

Hamstring sets

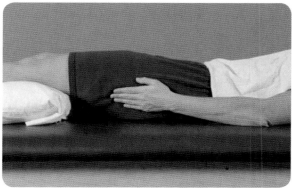

Glut sets

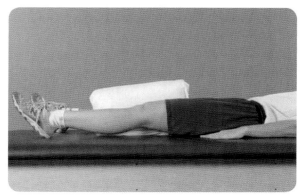

Adductor isometrics

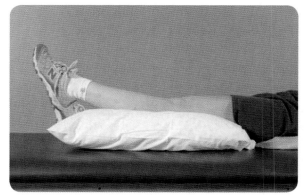

Quad sets

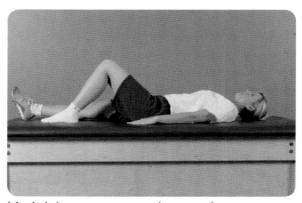

Heel slides, active-assisted range of motion

PHASE 1:
Initial Exercises *(Weeks 1-3)*

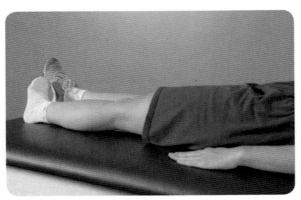

Log rolling

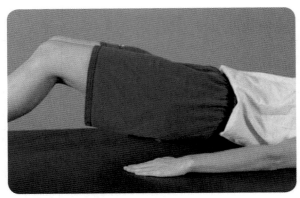

Double leg bridges

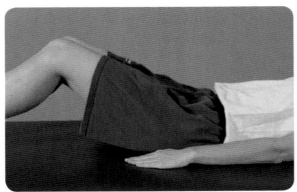

Pelvic tilt

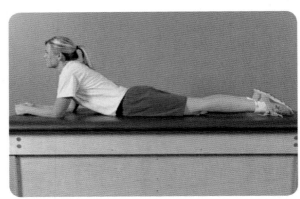

Prone on elbows

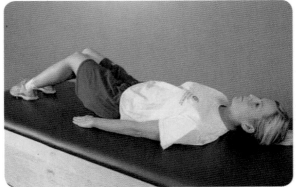

Trunk rotation

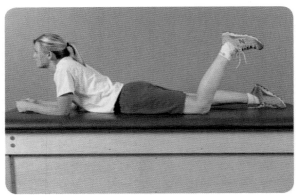

Prone knee flexion

Initial Exercises *(Weeks 1-3)*

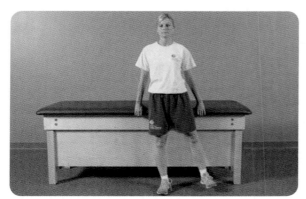

Standing abduction without resistance

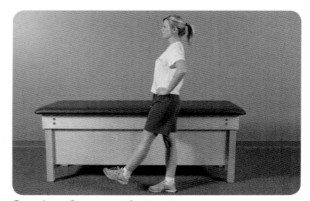

Standing flexion without resistance

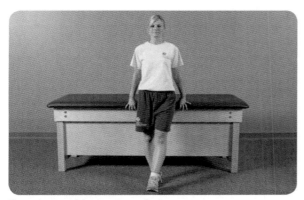

Standing adduction without resistance

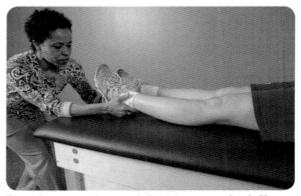

Pain dominant hip mobilization – grades I, II

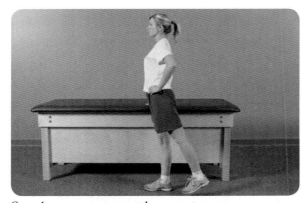

Standing extension without resistance

Other Exercises Week 1

- Standard stationary bike without resistance at 3 days post-op (10 min. if tolerated)

- Upper body ergometer, upper body strengthening

PHASE 1:   WEEK 2
In Addition to Previous Exercises *(Weeks 1-3)*

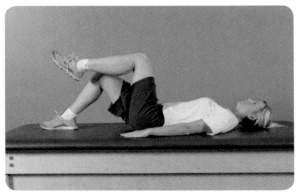

Supine marching, modified dead bug

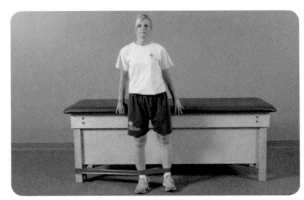

Theraband resistance on affected side –
Abduction (start very low resistance)

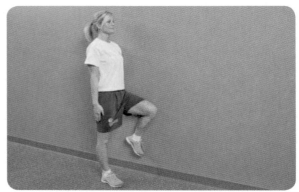

Abduction isometrics

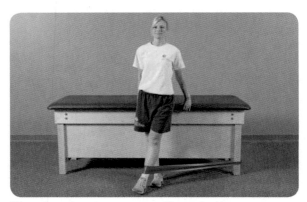

Theraband resistance on affected side –
Adduction (start very low resistance)

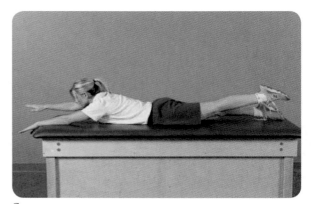

Superman

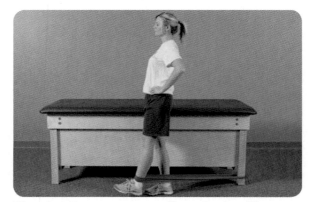

Theraband resistance on affected side – Flexion
(start very low resistance)

PHASE 1:   WEEK 2
In Addition to Previous Exercises *(Weeks 1-3)*

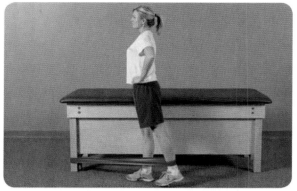

Theraband resistance on affected side –
Extension (start very low resistance)

Other Exercises Week 2

- Pool exercises (water walking, range of motion, march steps, lateral steps, backward walking, mini-squats, heel raises, hamstring and hip flexor stretches)

PHASE 1:   WEEK 3
In Addition to Previous Exercises *(Weeks 1-3)*

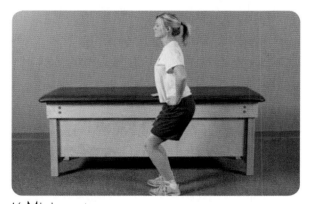

¼ Mini squats

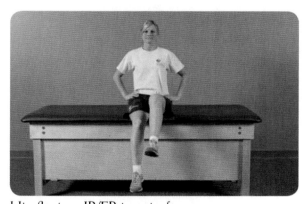

Hip flexion, IR/ER in pain-free range

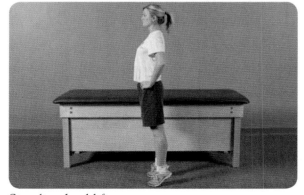

Standing heel lifts

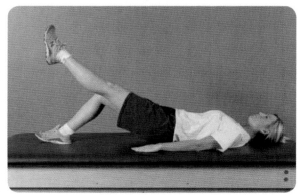

Double leg bridges to single leg bridges

PHASE 1:   WEEK 3
In Addition to Previous Exercises *(Weeks 1-3)*

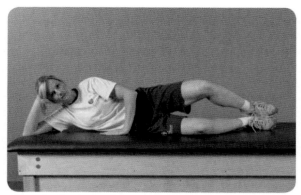

Clamshells (pain-free range)

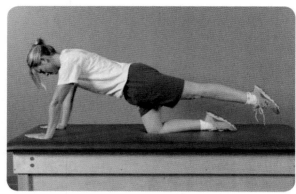

Quadriped 4 point support, progress 3 point support, progress 2 point

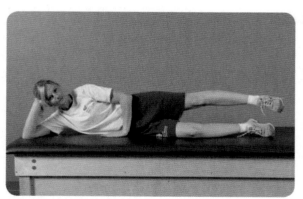

Leg raise – Abduction

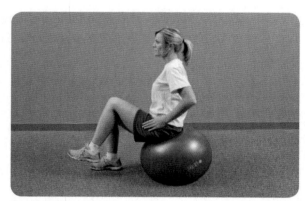

Seated physioball progression – hip flexion

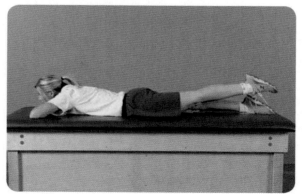

Leg raise – Extension

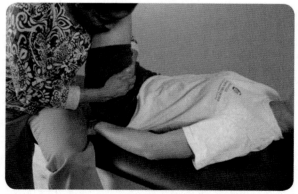

Hip mobilization – inferior glides in flexion

PHASE 1:
In Addition to Previous Exercises *(Weeks 1-3)*

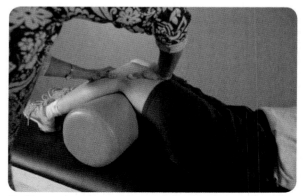

Stiffness dominant hip mobilization – grades III, IV

Goals of Phase 1

☐ Restore range of motion

☐ Diminish pain and inflammation

☐ Prevent muscular inhibition

☐ Normalize gait

Criteria for progression to Phase 2

☐ Minimal pain with phase 1 exercises

☐ Minimal range of motion limitations

☐ Normalized gait without crutches

Other Exercises Week 3

• Wall mini-squats

• Physioball mini-squats with cocontraction

• Leg raise – Adduction

• Kneeling hip flexor stretch (short of pain)

• Active range of motion with gradual end range stretch within tolerance

PHASE 2:
Intermediate Exercises *(Weeks 4-6)*

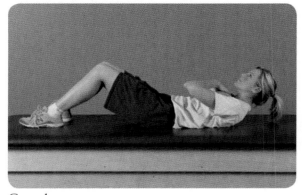

Crunches

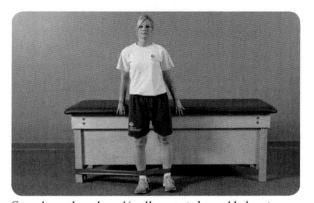

Standing theraband/pulley weight – Abduction

Intermediate Exercises *(Weeks 4-6)*

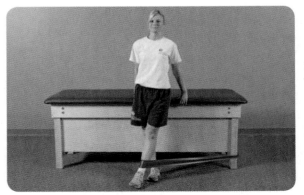

Standing theraband/pulley weight – Adduction

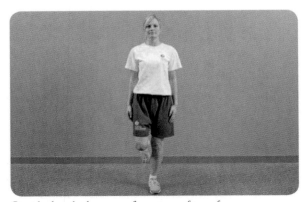

Single leg balance – firm to soft surface

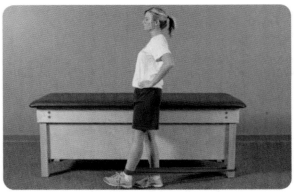

Standing theraband/pulley weight – Flexion

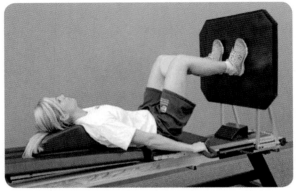

Shuttle leg press 90 degree hip flexion with co-contraction of adductors

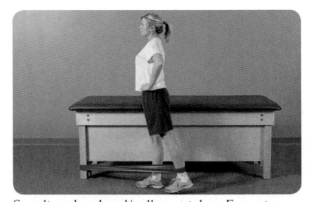

Standing theraband/pulley weight – Extension

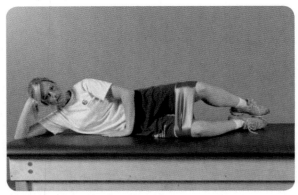

Clamshells with theraband

PHASE 2:   WEEKS 4-5
Intermediate Exercises *(Weeks 4-6)*

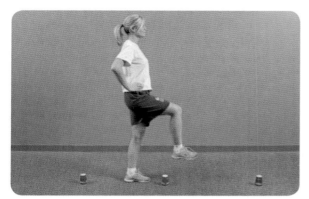

Forward walking over cups and hurdles (pause on affected limb), add ball toss while walking

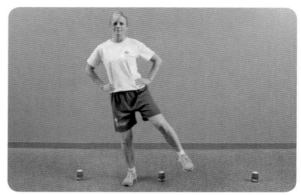

Lateral walking over cups and hurdles (pause on affected limb), add ball toss while walking

Other Exercises Weeks 4-5

- Wean off crutches after 4 weeks
- Gradually increase resistance with stationary bike
- Single leg sports cord leg press (long sitting) limiting hip flexion
- Pool water exercises – flutterkick swimming, 4 way hip with water weights, step-ups
- Initiate elliptical machine

PHASE 2:   WEEK 6
Intermediate Exercises *(Weeks 4-6)*

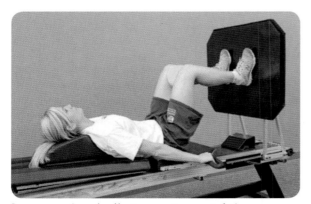

Leg press (gradually increasing weight)

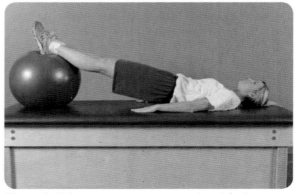

Physioball hamstring exercises – hip lift, bent knee hip lift, curls, balance

PHASE 2: WEEK 6

Intermediate Exercises *(Weeks 4-6)*

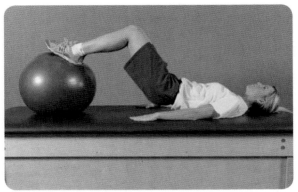

Superman on physioball – 2 point on physioball

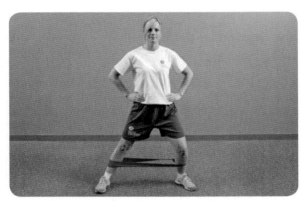

Sidestepping with resistance (pause on affected limb), sports cord walking forward and backward (pause on affected limb)

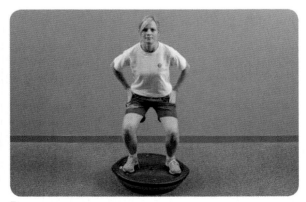

Bosu squats

Other Exercises Week 6

- Single leg balance – firm to soft surface with external perturbation (ball catch, sports specific/simulated ex.)

- Knee extensions, hamstring curls

Goals of Phase 2

☐ Restore pain-free range of motion

☐ Initiate proprioception exercises

☐ Progressively increase muscle strength and endurance

Criteria for progression to Phase 3

☐ Minimum pain with phase 2 exercises

☐ Single leg stance with level pelvis

PHASE 3:
WEEKS 7-8

Advanced Exercises *(Weeks 7-8)*

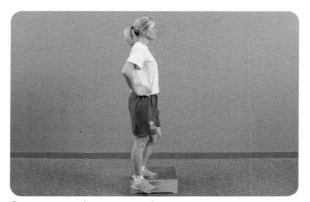

Step-ups with eccentric lowering

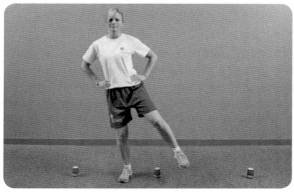

Side steps over cups/hurdles (with ball toss and external sports cord resistance), increase speed

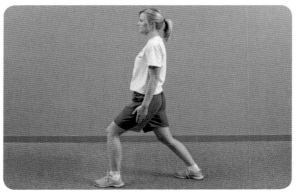

Lunges progress from single plane to tri-planar, add medicine balls for resistance and rotation

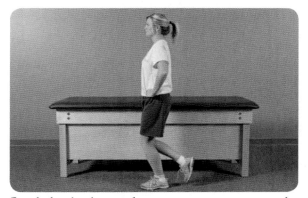

Single leg body weight squats, increase external resistance, stand on soft surface

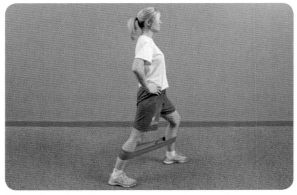

Theraband walking patterns – forward, sidestepping, carioca, monster steps, backward, ½ circles forward/backward – 25 yds. Start band at knee height and progress to ankle height

Other Exercises Weeks 7-8

- Full squats
- Single stability ball bridges

Goals for Phase 3

☐ Restoration of muscular endurance/strength

☐ Restoration of cardiovascular endurance

☐ Optimize neuromuscular control/balance/ proprioception

PHASE 3:   WEEKS 7-8
Advanced Exercises *(Weeks 7-8)*

Criteria for Progression to Phase 4

☐ Single leg mini-squat with level pelvis

☐ Cardiovascular fitness equal to preinjury level

☐ Demonstration of initial agility drills with proper body mechanics

PHASE 4:   WEEKS 9-11
Sports specific training rehab clinic based progression

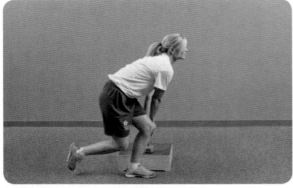

Single leg pick-ups, add soft surface

Other Exercises Weeks 9-11

• All phase 3 exercises

• Pool running (progress from chest deep to waist deep), treadmill jogging

• Step drills, quick feet step-ups (4-6 inch box) forward, lateral, carioca

• Plyometrics, double leg and single leg shuttle jumps

• Theraband walking patterns 1 rep of six exercises x 50yds, progress to band at knee height and ankle height

PHASE 4:   WEEKS 12 & BEYOND
Sports specific training on field or court

Other Exercises Weeks 12 & Beyond

• Running progression

• Sport specific drills

• Traditional weight training

Criteria for full return to competition

☐ Full range of motion

☐ Hip strength equal to uninvolved side, single leg pick-up with level pelvis

☐ Ability to perform sport-specific drills at full speed without pain

☐ Completion of functional sports test

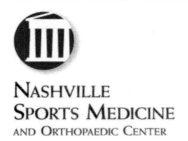

J. W. Thomas Byrd, M.D.

2011 Church Street
Suite 100
Nashville, TN 37203
615-284-5800
fax 615-284-5819

Hip Luxation Protocol
(Stable Posterior Acetabular Fracture)

- Initial xrays, CT scan & MRI (high-resolution!)
    - Stable fracture pattern without obvious major intraarticular damage, then candidate for conservative treatment

- Crutches, partial WB 4 weeks
    - Minimize risk of fracture displacement
    - Slight loading stimulates healing process
    - At 4 weeks fracture should be "sticky"

- 4 weeks
    - Limited CT scan
        - Check for signs of displacement
    - Alignment good & painfree, then transition off crutches
    - Follow-up MRI
        - Check for resolution of soft tissue edema
        - Check for early signs of subchondral femoral edema (bone bruise) indicative of FH impaction injury
            - May necessitate more conservative approach because of uncertain prognostic significance

- 4-6 weeks, avoid loading of flexed hip

- Functional progression at 6 weeks, if pain-free

- Return to unrestricted activities 8-10 weeks, if pain-free

- F/U xrays at 1, 2, 3 & 6 months

- F/U MRI 3 & 6 months
    - Assess for early signs of AVN
    - Assess for progression/resolution of subchondral edema, if present

- F/U CT scan, if needed due to symptoms
    - Bony bridging of fracture often partial / incomplete
    - May develop asymptomatic fibrous union

Iliopsoas Release

This protocol should be used as a guideline for progression and should be tailored to the needs of the individual patient.

- **Weight bearing as tolerated – use crutches to normalize gait.**
  - May be needed for 2-4 weeks

- **Gentle emphasis on passive extension exercises.**

- **Aggressive hip flexion strengthening delayed 6 weeks.**

- **Functional progression as tolerated.**

- **Resumption of full activities allowed as tolerated after 3 months.**

- **Always use pharmacologic prophylaxis against heterotopic ossification (unless contraindicated).**
  - Quiz patient
  - Must initiate and maintain immediately postop

PHASE 1:   WEEK 1
Initial Exercise *(Weeks 1-3)*

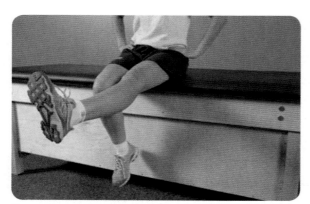

Seated knee extensions

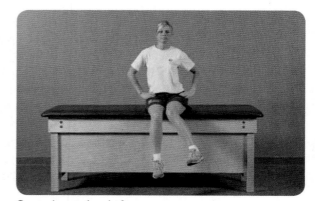

Seated weight shifts

PHASE 1:   WEEK 1
Initial Exercises *(Weeks 1-3)*

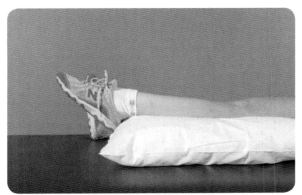

Ankle pumps

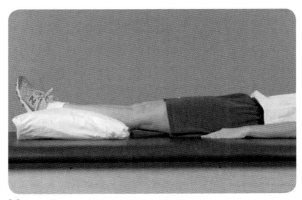

Hamstring sets

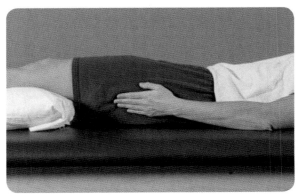

Glut sets

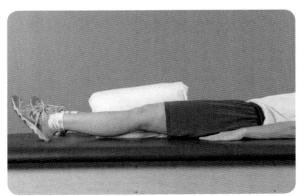

Adductor isometrics

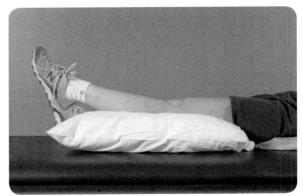

Quad sets

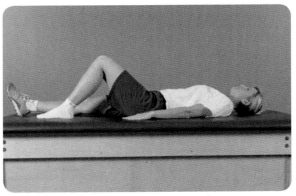

Heel slides, active-assisted range of motion

Initial Exercises *(Weeks 1-3)*

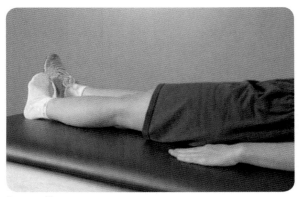

Log rolling

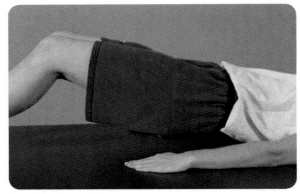

Double leg bridges

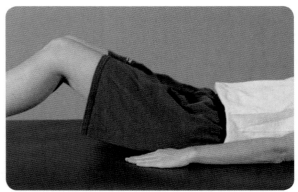

Pelvic tilt

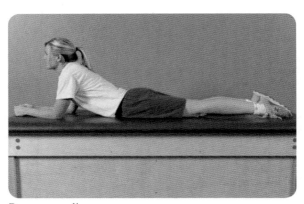

Prone on elbows

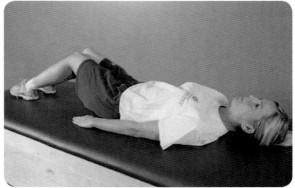

Trunk rotation

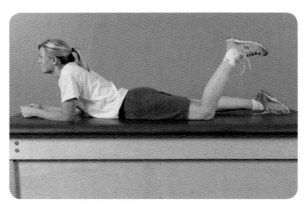

Prone knee flexion

Initial Exercises (Weeks 1-3)

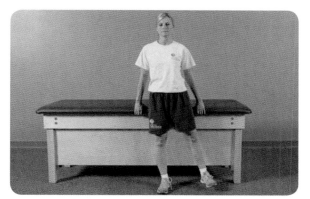

Standing abduction without resistance

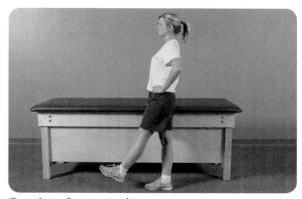

Standing flexion without resistance

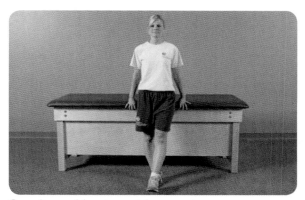

Standing adduction without resistance

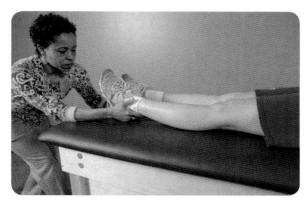

Pain dominant hip mobilization – grades I, II

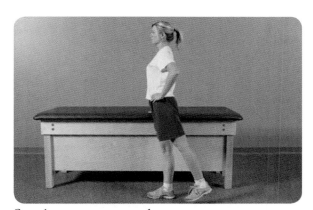

Standing extension without resistance

Other Exercises Week 1

- Standard stationary bike without resistance at 3 days post-op (10 min. if tolerated)

- Upper body ergometer, upper body strengthening

PHASE 1:   WEEK 2
In Addition to Previous Exercises *(Weeks 1-3)*

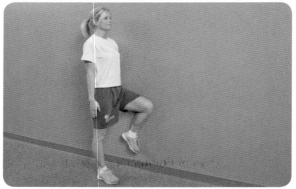

Abduction isometrics

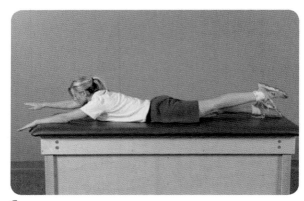

Superman

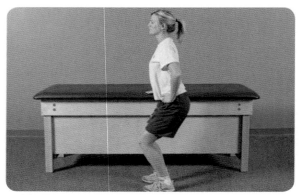

¼ Mini squats

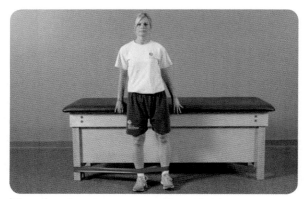

Theraband resistance on affected side –
Abduction (start very low resistance)

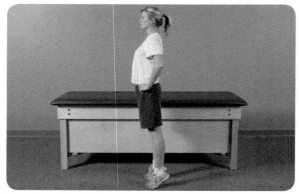

Standing heel lifts

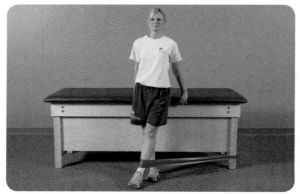

Theraband resistance on affected side –
Adduction (start very low resistance)

PHASE 1:   WEEK 2
In Addition to Previous Exercises (Weeks 1-3)

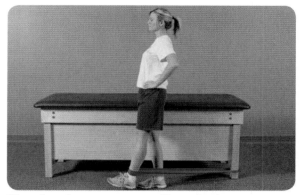

Theraband resistance on affected side – Flexion (start very low resistance) ONLY IF TOLERATED

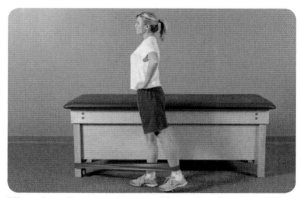

Theraband resistance on affected side – Extension (start very low resistance)

Other Exercises Week 2

- Wall mini-squats
- Physioball mini-squats with cocontraction
- Pool exercises (water walking, range of motion, march steps, lateral steps, backward walking, mini-squats, heel raises, hamstring and hip flexor stretches)

PHASE 1:   WEEK 3
In Addition to Previous Exercises (Weeks 1-3)

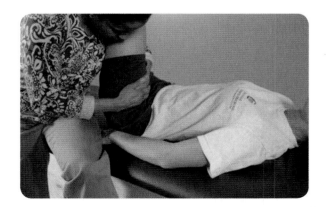

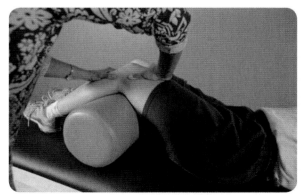

Stiffness dominant hip mobilization – grades III, IV

PHASE 1:   WEEK 3
In Addition to Previous Exercises *(Weeks 1-3)*

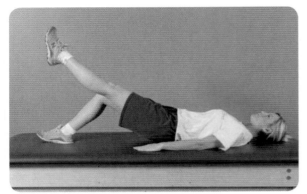

Double leg bridges to single leg bridges

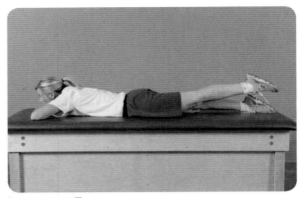

Leg raise – Extension

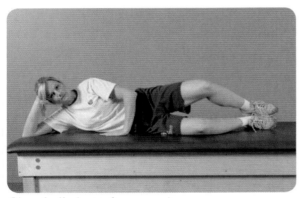

Clamshells (pain-free range)

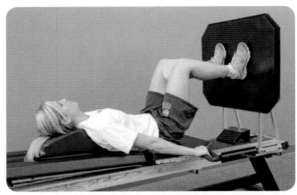

Shuttle leg press 90 degree hip flexion with co-contraction of adductors

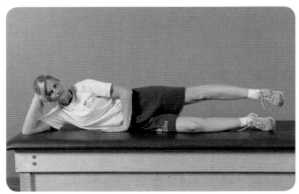

Leg raise – Abduction

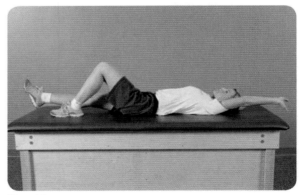

Dead bug

In Addition to Previous Exercises *(Weeks 1-3)*

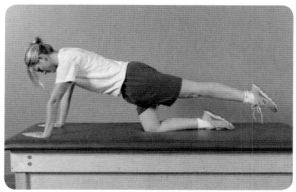

Quadriped 4 point support, progress 3 point support, progress 2 point

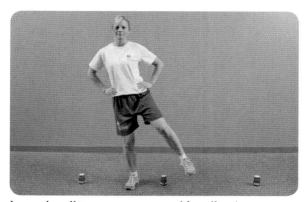

Lateral walking over cups and hurdles (pause on affected limb), add ball toss while walking

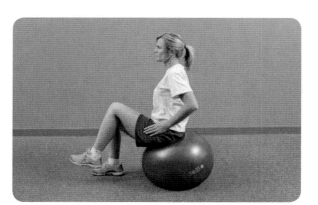

Seated physioball progression – hip flexion

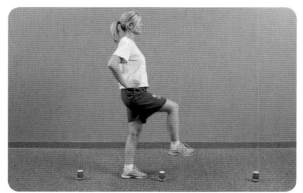

Forward walking over cups and hurdles (pause on affected limb), add ball toss while walking

Other Exercises Week 3

- Continue stationary bike with minimal resistance – 5 min. increase daily
- Active range of motion with gradual end range stretch within tolerance
- Leg raise – Adduction
- Single leg sports cord leg press (long sitting) limiting hip flexion

Goals of Phase 1

☐ Restore range of motion
☐ Diminish pain and inflammation
☐ Prevent muscular inhibition
☐ Normalize gait

Criteria for progression to Phase 2

☐ Minimal pain with phase 1 exercises
☐ Minimal range of motion limitations
☐ Normalized gait without crutches

PHASE 2:   WEEKS 4-5
Intermediate Exercises *(Weeks 4-6)*

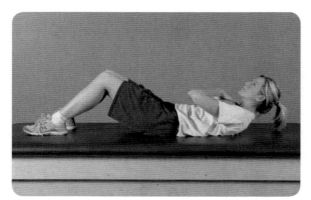

Crunches

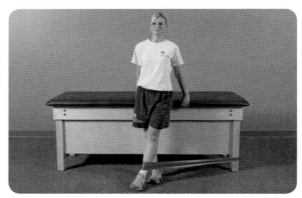

Standing theraband/pulley weight – Adduction

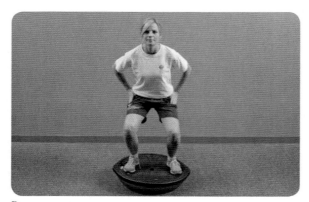

Bosu squats

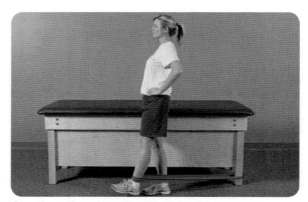

Standing theraband/pulley weight – Flexion

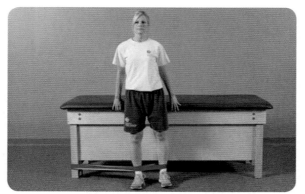

Standing theraband/pulley weight – Abduction

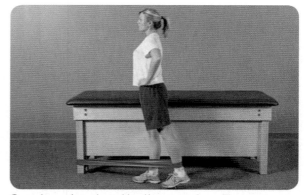

Standing theraband/pulley weight – Extension

PHASE 1: WEEKS 4-5
Intermediate Exercises *(Weeks 4-6)*

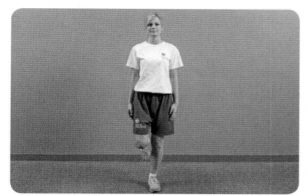

Single leg balance – firm to soft surface

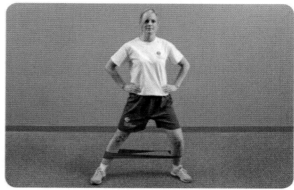

Sidestepping with resistance (pause on affected limb), sports cord walking forward and backward (pause on affected limb)

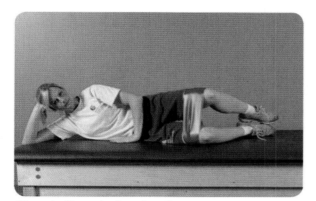

Clamshells with theraband

Other Exercises Weeks 4-5

- Gradually increase resistance with stationary bike

- Initiate elliptical machine

- Pool water exercises – flutterkick swimming, 4 way hip with water weights, step-ups

PHASE 1: WEEK 6
Intermediate Exercises *(Weeks 4-6)*

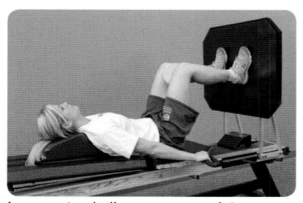

Leg press (gradually increasing weight)

PHASE 1:   WEEK 6
Intermediate Exercises (*Weeks 4-6*)

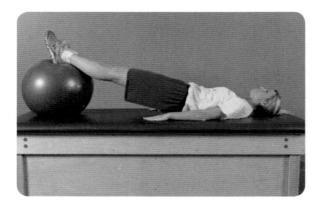

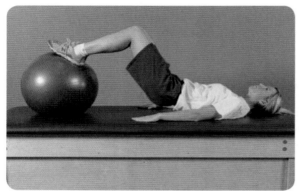

Physioball hamstring exercises – hip lift, bent knee hip lift, curls, balance

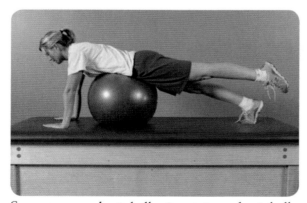

Superman on physioball – 2 point on physioball

Other Exercises Week 6

• Single leg balance – firm to soft surface with external perturbation (ball catch, sports specific/simulated ex.)

• Knee extensions, hamstring curls

Goals of Phase 2

☐ Restore pain-free range of motion

☐ Initiate proprioception exercises

☐ Progressively increase muscle strength and endurance

Criteria for progression to Phase 3

☐ Minimum pain with phase 2 exercises

☐ Single leg stance with level pelvis

PHASE 3:
Advanced Exercises *(Weeks 7-8)*

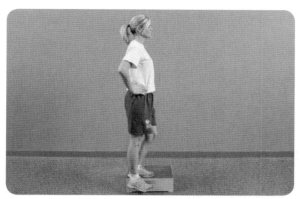

Step-ups with eccentric lowering

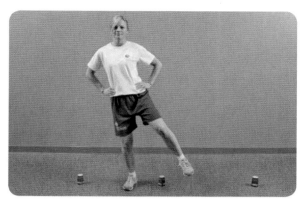

Side steps over cups/hurdles (with ball toss and external sports cord resistance), increase speed

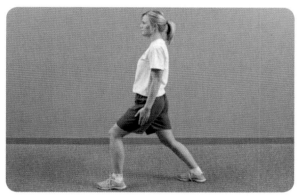

Lunges progress from single plane to tri-planar, add medicine balls for resistance and rotation

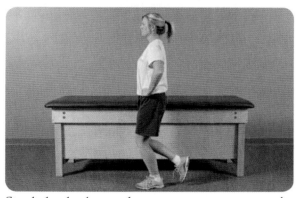

Single leg body weight squats, increase external resistance, stand on soft surface

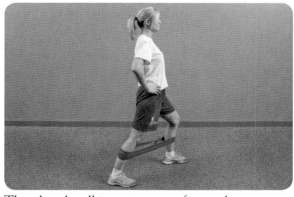

Theraband walking patterns – forward, sidestepping, carioca, monster steps, backward, ½ circles forward/backward – 25 yds. Start band at knee height and progress to ankle height

Other Exercises Weeks 7-8

• Full squats

• Single stability ball bridges

Goals for Phase 3

☐ Restoration of muscular endurance/strength

☐ Restoration of cardiovascular endurance

☐ Optimize neuromuscular control/balance/ proprioception

PHASE 3:   WEEKS 7-8
Advanced Exercises *(Weeks 7-8)*

Criteria for Progression to Phase 4

☐ Single leg mini-squat with level pelvis

☐ Cardiovascular fitness equal to preinjury level

☐ Demonstration of initial agility drills with proper body mechanics

PHASE 4:   WEEKS 9-11
Sports specific training rehab clinic based progression

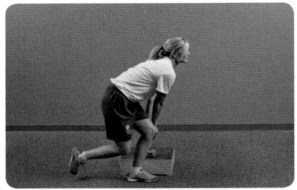

Single leg pick-ups, add soft surface

Other Exercises Weeks 9-11

• All phase 3 exercises

• Pool running (progress from chest deep to waist deep), treadmill jogging

• Step drills, quick feet step-ups (4-6 inch box) forward, lateral, carioca

• Plyometrics, double leg and single leg shuttle jumps

• Theraband walking patterns 1 rep of six exercises x 50yds, progress to band at knee height and ankle height

PHASE 4:   WEEKS 12 & BEYOND
Sports specific training on field or court

Other Exercises Weeks 12 & Beyond

• Running progression

• Sport specific drills

• Traditional weight training

Criteria for full return to competition

☐ Full range of motion

☐ Hip strength equal to uninvolved side, single leg pick-up with level pelvis

☐ Ability to perform sport-specific drills at full speed without pain

☐ Completion of functional sports test

Labral Repair

This protocol should be used as a guideline for progression and should be tailored to the needs of the individual patient.

- **Partial weight bearing (50%) four weeks.**

- **Encourage, but limit hip flexion to 90 degrees.**
  - Flexion inhibits adhesions within anterior capsule.
  - Flexion beyond 90 degrees starts to stress the repair site.

- **Avoid external rotation!**
  - 6 weeks
  - External rotation stresses anterior labrum.
  - Especially cautious in bed (bolster with pillow).

PHASE 1:   WEEK 1
Initial Exercises *(Weeks 1-3)*

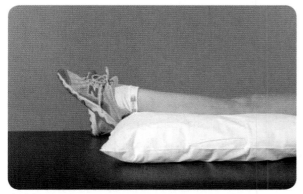

Ankle pumps

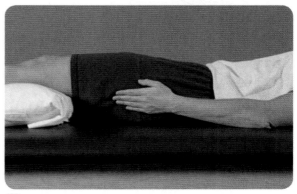

Glut sets

Initial Exercises *(Weeks 1-3)*

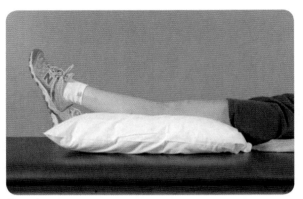

Quad sets

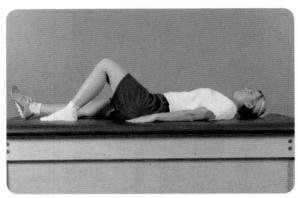

Heel slides, active-assisted range of motion

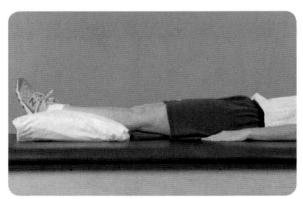

Hamstring sets

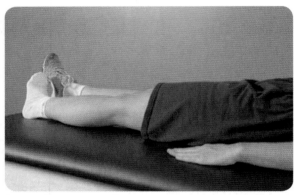

Log rolling internal rotation

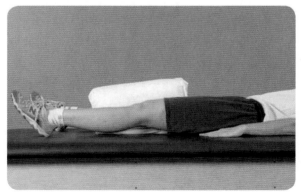

Adductor isometrics

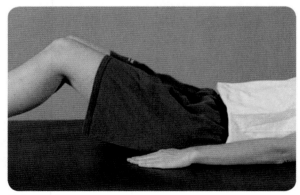

Pelvic tilt

PHASE 1:
Initial Exercises (Weeks 1-3)

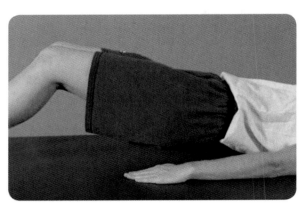

Double leg bridges

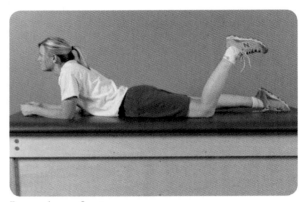

Prone knee flexion

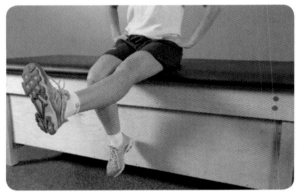

Seated knee extensions

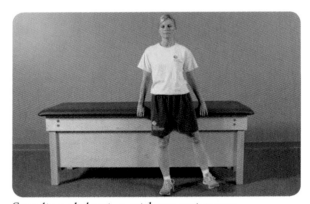

Standing abduction without resistance

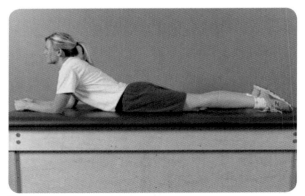

Prone on elbows

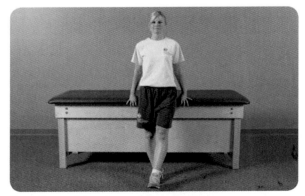

Standing adduction without resistance

PHASE **1**:   WEEK **1**
Initial Exercises *(Weeks 1-3)*

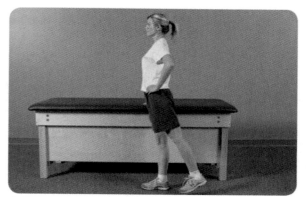

Standing extension without resistance

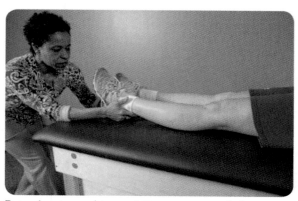

Pain dominant hip mobilization – grade I

Other Exercises Week 1

• Upper body ergometer, upper body strengthening

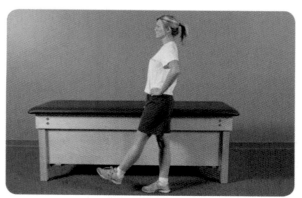

Standing flexion without resistance

PHASE **1**:   WEEK **2**
In Addition to Previous Exercises *(Weeks 1-3)*

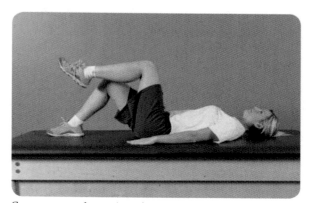

Supine marching (90 degrees)

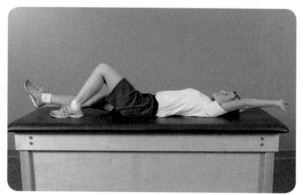

Modified deadbug (90 degrees)

PHASE 1:
Initial Exercises *(Weeks 1-3)*

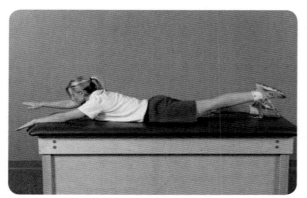

Superman

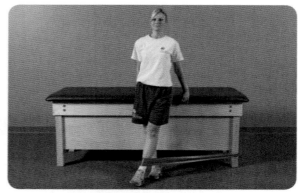

Theraband resistance on affected side –
Adduction (start very low resistance)

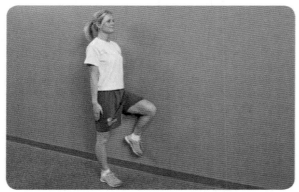

Abduction isometrics

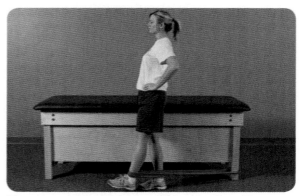

Theraband resistance on affected side – Flexion
(start very low resistance)

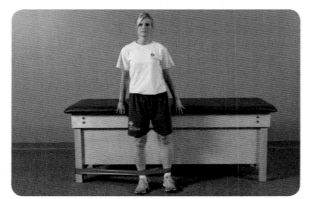

Theraband resistance on affected side –
Abduction (start very low resistance)

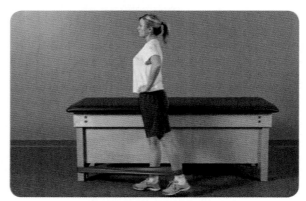

Theraband resistance on affected side –
Extension (start very low resistance)

PHASE 1:   WEEK 2
Initial Exercises *(Weeks 1-3)*

Other Exercises Week 2

- Standard stationary bike without resistance (10 min. if tolerated; no more than 90 degrees of hip flexion)

- Pool exercises (water walking, range of motion, march steps, lateral steps, backward walking, mini-squats, heel raises, hamstring and hip flexor stretches)

PHASE 1:   WEEK 3
Initial Exercise *(Weeks 1-3)*

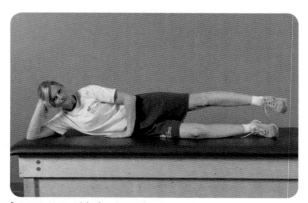

Leg raise – Abduction

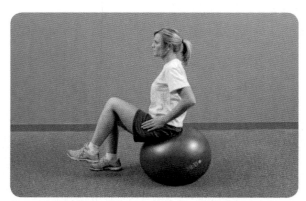

Seated physioball progression – hip flexion to 90 degrees

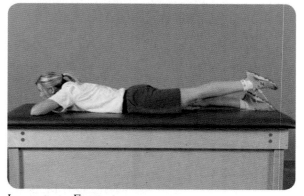

Leg raise – Extension

Goals of Phase 1

- ☐ Protect integrity of repaired labrum
- ☐ Restore range of motion within restrictions
- ☐ Diminish pain and inflammation
- ☐ Prevent muscular inhibition
- ☐ Normalize gait using two crutches (50% weight bearing)

Other Exercises Week 3

- Active range of motion with gradual end range stretch within tolerance
- Leg raise – Adduction

Criteria for progression to Phase 2

- ☐ Minimal pain with phase 1 exercises
- ☐ 90 degrees of pain-free flexion
- ☐ Minimal range of motion limitations with internal rotation, extension and abduction
- ☐ Normalized heel to toe gait with two crutches (50% weight bearing)

PHASE 2: WEEKS 4-5
Intermediate Exercises *(Weeks 4-6)*

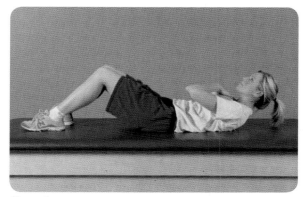

Crunches

Other Exercises Weeks 4 and 5

- Gradually increase resistance with stationary bike

- Front and side standing weight shifts

- Pool water exercises – flutterkick swimming, 4 way hip with water weights, step-ups

PHASE 2: WEEK 6
Intermediate Exercises *(Weeks 4-6)*

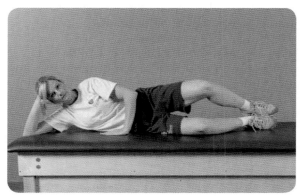

Clamshells

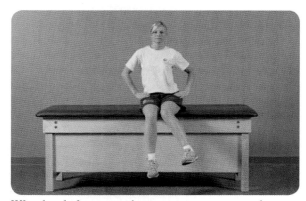

Weight shifts – standing, sitting, supported, anterior/posterior, laterals, physioball

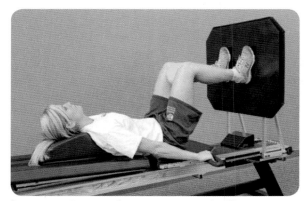

Leg press (minimal resistance, gradually increasing resistance to patient tolerance)

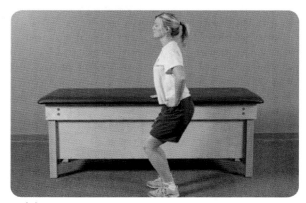

¼ Mini squats

PHASE 2:

Intermediate Exercises *(Weeks 4-6)*

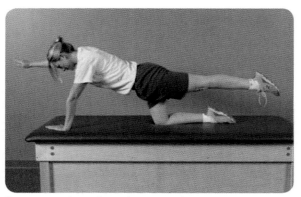

Superman (quadriped position)

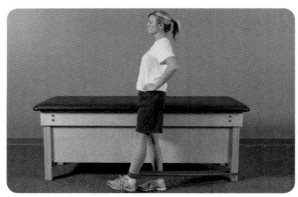

Standing theraband – Flexion

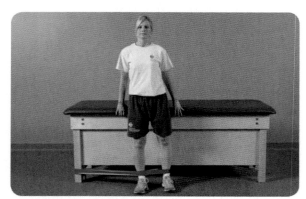

Standing theraband – Abduction

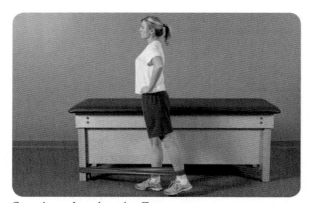

Standing theraband – Extension

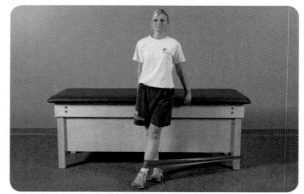

Standing theraband – Adduction

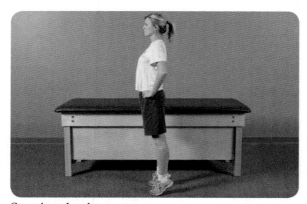

Standing heel raises

PHASE 2:   WEEK 6
Intermediate Exercises *(Weeks 4-6)*

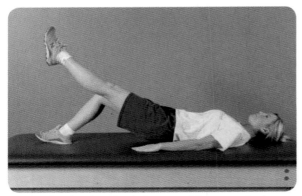

Single leg bridges/stabilization/alternate kickouts

Other Exercises Week 6

- Gradually wean off crutches if no gait deviations

- Passive range of motion (gradually incorporate gentle external rotation and flexion sort of pain; limit to 20 degrees of ER and 105 degrees of flexion)

- Wall mini-squats

- Physioball mini-squats with cocontraction

- Elliptical machine

Goals of Phase 2

☐ Protect integrity of repaired tissue

☐ Increase range of motion

☐ Normalize gait with no crutches

☐ Progressively increase muscle strength

Criteria for progression to Phase 3

☐ 105 degrees of flexion; 20 degrees of external rotation

☐ Pain-free/normal gait pattern

☐ Hip flexion strength >60% of the uninvolved side

☐ Hip adduction, extension, internal and external rotation strength >70% of the uninvolved side

PHASE 3:   WEEK 7
Advanced Exercises *(Weeks 7-8)*

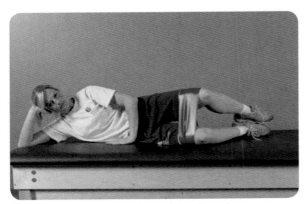

Clamshells with resistive tubing/band

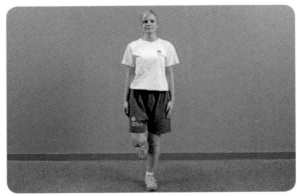

Single leg balance – firm to soft surface with external perturbation (ball catch, sports specific/simulated ex.)

PHASE 3:
Advanced Exercises *(Weeks 7-8)*

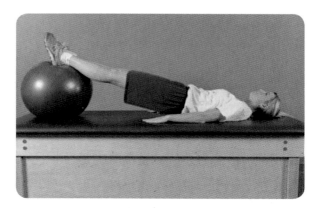

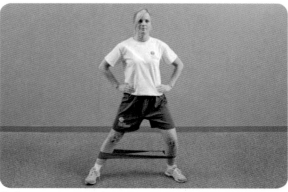

Side stepping with resistance (pause on affected limb), sports cord walking forward and backward (pause on affected limb)

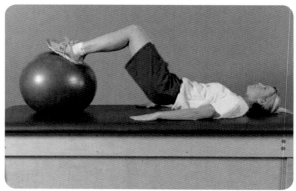

Physioball hamstring ex. – hip lift, bent knee hip lift, curls, balance

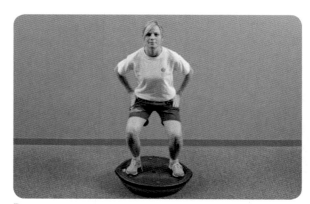

Bosu squats

Other Exercises Week 7

• Restore full passive range of motion

• Knee extensions, hamstring curls

PHASE 3:
Advanced Exercises (*Weeks* 7-8)

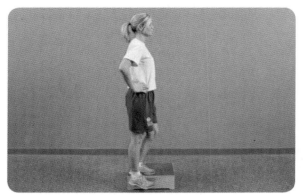

Step-ups with eccentric lowering

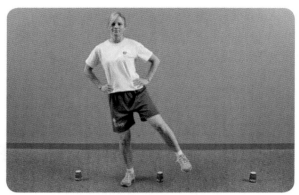

Side steps over cups/hurdles (with ball toss and external sports cord resistance), increase speed

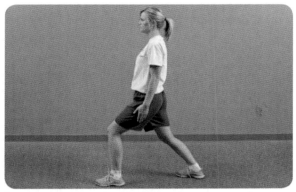

Lunges progress from single plane to tri-planar, add medicine balls for resistance and rotation

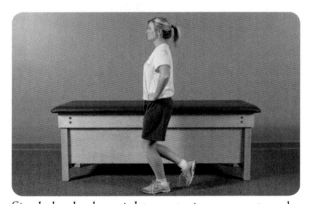

Single leg body weight squats, increase external resistance, stand on soft surface

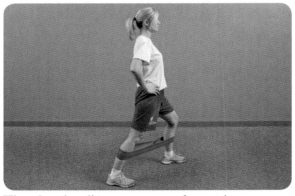

Theraband walking patterns – forward, sidestepping, carioca, monster steps, backward, ½ circles forward/backward – 25 yds. Start band at knee height and progress to ankle height

Other Exercises Week 8

- Full squats
- Single stability ball bridges

Goals for Phase 3

☐ Restoration of muscular endurance/strength

☐ Restoration of cardiovascular endurance

☐ Optimize neuromuscular control/balance/ proprioception

PHASE 3:   WEEK 8
Advanced Exercises *(Weeks 7-8)*

Criteria for Progression to Phase 4

- ☐ Hip flexion strength >70% of the uninvolved side
- ☐ Hip adduction, abduction, extension, internal and external rotation >80% of the uninvolved side

- ☐ Cardiovascular fitness equal to preinjury level
- ☐ Demonstration of initial agility drills with proper body mechanics

PHASE 4:   WEEKS 9-11
Sports specific training rehab clinic based progression

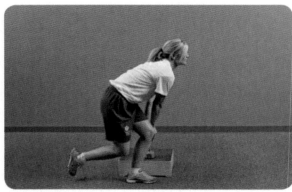

Single leg pick-ups, add soft surface

Other Exercises Weeks 9-11

- All phase 3 exercises
- Pool running (progress from chest deep to waist deep), treadmill jogging
- Step drills, quick feet step-ups (4-6 inch box) forward, lateral, carioca
- Plyometrics, double leg and single leg shuttle jumps
- Theraband walking patterns 1 rep of six exercises x 50yds, progress to band at knee height and ankle height
- Sports specific training on field or court

PHASE 4:   WEEKS 12 & BEYOND
Sports specific training on field or court

Other Exercises Weeks 12 & Beyond

- Running progression
- Sport specific drills
- Traditional weight training

Criteria for full return to competition

- ☐ Full range of motion
- ☐ Hip strength equal to uninvolved side, single leg pick-up with level pelvis
- ☐ Ability to perform sport-specific drills at full speed without pain
- ☐ Completion of functional sports test

Microfracture

This protocol should be used as a guideline for progression and should be tailored to the needs of the individual patient.

- **Strict protective weight bearing status for two months (8-9 weeks).**
  - Allow to place weight of leg on ground (neutralizes joint reaction forces).

- **Emphasis on range of motion.**
  - Active assisted motion for home program.

- **Pool program to initiate functional exercises in reduced weight environment.**

- **Emphasis on cycling for range of motion without resistance (as long as this is tolerated by the individual).**

- **At 2 months, transition to full weight bearing (transition variable).**
  - Some transition immediately to full weight bearing status.
  - Some require transition to 1 crutch or continued support for distances, which may be needed for 1-2 weeks.

- **Minimum three months before progression of functional activities as tolerated.**

PHASE 1:   WEEK 1
Initial Exercises *(Weeks 1-3)*

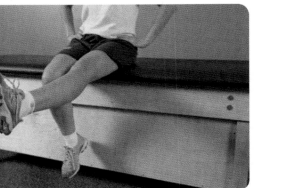

Seated knee extensions

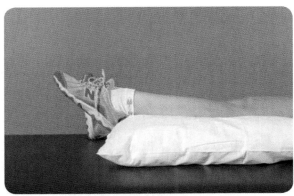

Ankle pumps

Initial Exercises *(Weeks 1-3)*

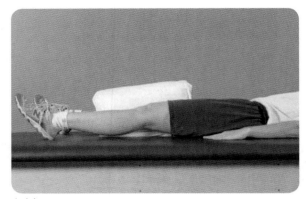

Glut sets

Adductor isometrics

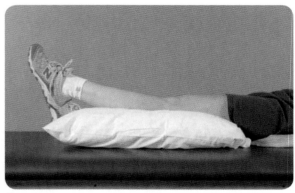

Quad sets

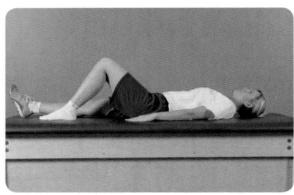

Heel slides, active-assisted range of motion

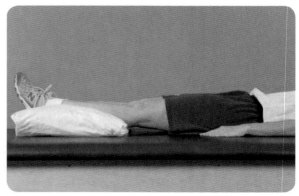

Hamstring sets

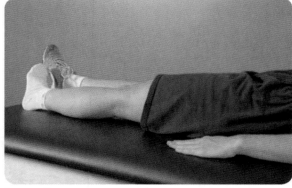

Log rolling

PHASE 1: WEEK **1**

Initial Exercises *(Weeks 1-3)*

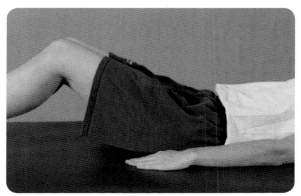

Pelvic tilt

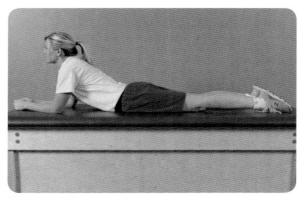

Prone on elbows

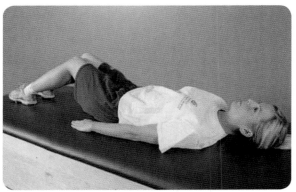

Trunk rotation

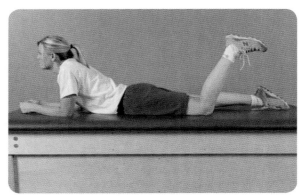

Prone knee flexion

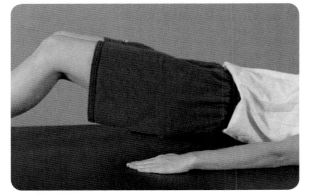

Double leg bridges

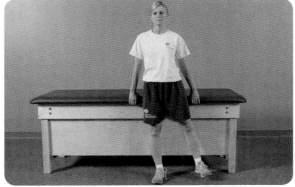

Standing abduction without resistance

PHASE 1:   WEEK 1
Initial Exercises (*Weeks 1-3*)

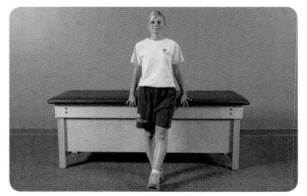

Standing adduction without resistance

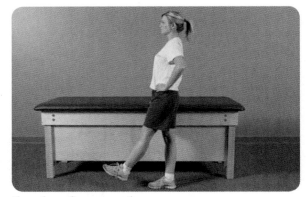

Standing flexion without resistance

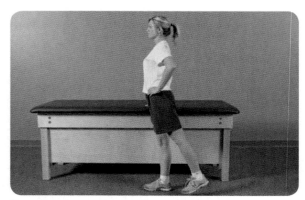

Standing extension without resistance

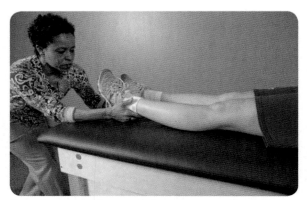

Pain dominant hip mobilization – grades I, II

Other Exercises Week 1

• Upper body ergometer, upper body strengthening

Initial Exercises *(Weeks 1–3)*

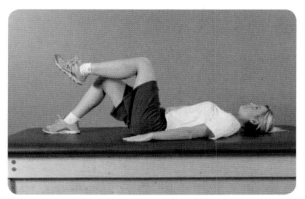

Supine marching, modified dead bug

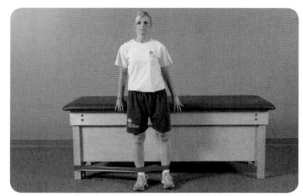

Theraband resistance on affected side –
Abduction (start very low resistance)

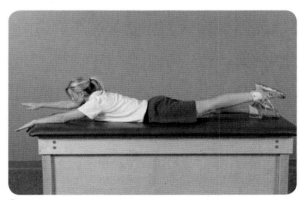

Superman

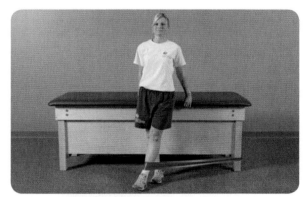

Theraband resistance on affected side –
Adduction (start very low resistance)

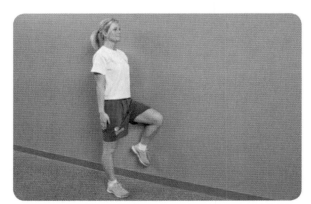

Abduction isometrics

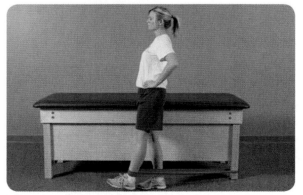

Theraband resistance on affected side – Flexion
(start very low resistance)

PHASE 1:   WEEK 2
Initial Exercises *(Weeks 1-3)*

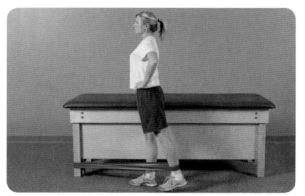

Theraband resistance on affected side –
Extension (start very low resistance)

Other Exercises Week 2

- Standard stationary bike without resistance at 3 days post-op (10 min. if tolerated)
- Pool exercises (water walking, range of motion, march steps, lateral steps, backward walking, mini-squats, heel raises, hamstring and hip flexor stretches)

PHASE 1:   WEEK 3
Initial Exercises *(Weeks 1-3)*

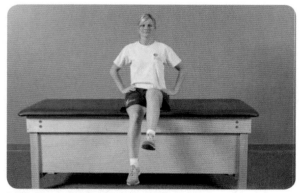

Hip flexion, IR/ER in pain-free range

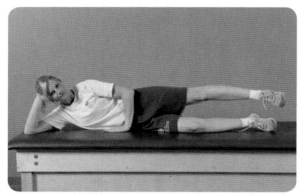

Leg raise – Abduction

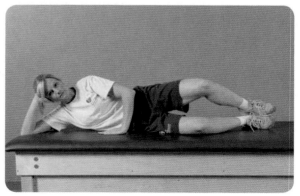

Clamshells

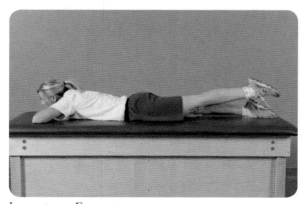

Leg raise – Extension

PHASE 1:
Initial Exercises (Weeks 1-3)

WEEK 3

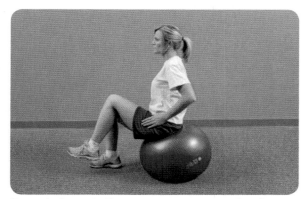

Seated physioball progression – active hip/knee

Other Exercises Week 3

- Active range of motion with gradual end range stretch within tolerance
- Leg raise – Adduction

Goals of Phase 1

- ☐ Protect integrity of healing microfracture
- ☐ Restore range of motion within patient tolerance
- ☐ Diminish pain and inflammation
- ☐ Prevent muscular inhibition
- ☐ Normalize gait using two crutches with strict protective weight bearing of no more than the weight of the leg

Criteria for progression to Phase 2

- ☐ Minimal pain with phase 1 exercises
- ☐ Minimal range of motion limitations
- ☐ Demonstrates restircted weight bearing during gait

PHASE 2:
Intermediate Exercises (Weeks 4-6)

WEEKS 4-6

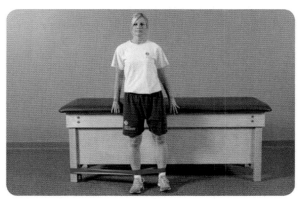

Theraband resistance on affected side –
Abduction (start very low resistance)

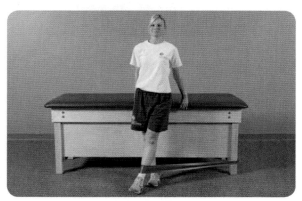

Theraband resistance on affected side –
Adduction (start very low resistance)

PHASE 2:   WEEKS 4-6
Intermediate Exercises *(Weeks 4-6)*

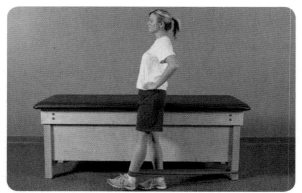

Theraband resistance on affected side – Flexion
(start very low resistance)

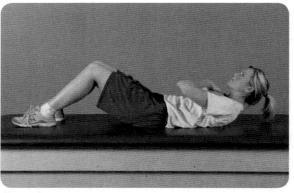

Crunches

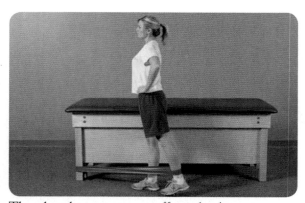

Theraband resistance on affected side –
Extension (start very low resistance)

Other Exercises Weeks 4-6

- Initiate elliptical machine
- Pool water exercises – flutterkick swimming, 4
  way hip with water weights, step-ups

Goals of Phase 2

☐ Protect integrity of healing tissue

☐ Restore pain-free range of motion

☐ Progressively increase muscle strength and
  endurance

☐ Continue to respect weight bearing
  precautions

Criteria for progression to Phase 3

☐ Minimum pain with phase 2 exercises

PHASE 3:   **WEEK 7**
Advanced Exercises *(Weeks 7-10)*

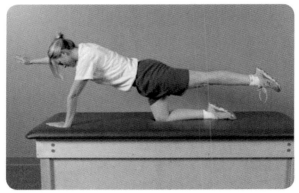

Superman (quadriped position)

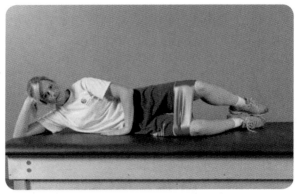

Clamshells with resistive tubing/band

Other Exercises Week 7

- Standing theraband/pulley flexion, adduction, abductio and extenion or multi-hip

- Pool water exercises – flutterkick swimming, 4 way hip with water weights, step-ups

PHASE 3:   **WEEK 8**
Advanced Exercises *(Weeks 7-10)*

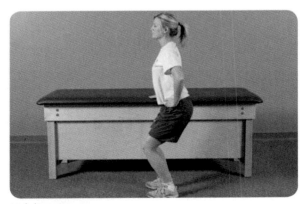

¼ Mini squats

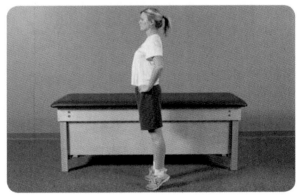

Standing heel lifts

PHASE 3:   WEEK 8
Advanced Exercises (*Weeks 7-10*)

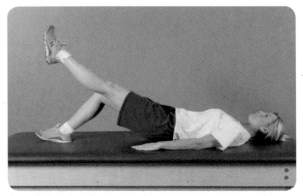

Single leg bridges/stabilization/alternate kickouts

Other Exercises Week 8

- Gradually wean off crutches
- Wall mini-squats
- Physioball mini-squats with cocontraction
- Leg Press (minimal resistance, gradually increasing resistance to patient tolerance)

PHASE 3:   WEEK 9
Advanced Exercises (*Weeks 7-10*)

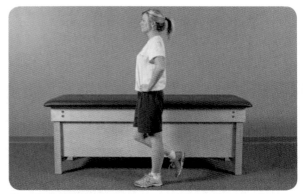

Single leg balance – firm to soft surface with external perturbation (ball catch, sports specific/simulated ex.)

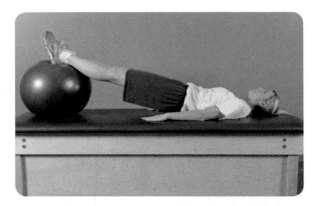

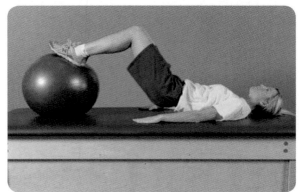

Physioball hamstring exercises – hip lift, bent knee hip lift, curls, balance

PHASE 3:
Advanced Exercises (Weeks 7-10)

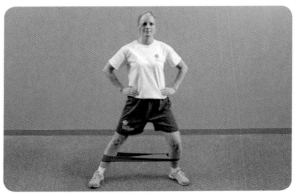

Sidestepping with resistance (pause on affected limb), sports cord walking forward and backward (pause on affected limb)

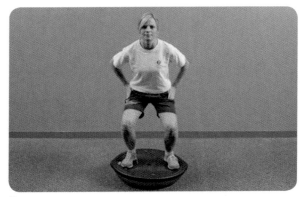

Bosu squats

Other Exercises Week 9

• Knee extensions, hamstring curls

• Single stability ball bridges

PHASE 3:
Advanced Exercises (Weeks 7-10)

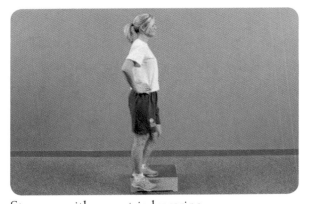

Step-ups with eccentric lowering

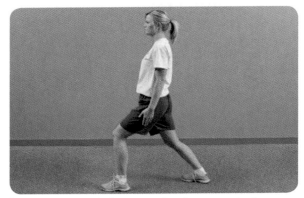

Lunges progress from single plane to tri-planar lunges, add medicine balls for resistance and rotation

PHASE 3:   WEEK 10
Advanced Exercises *(Weeks 7-10)*

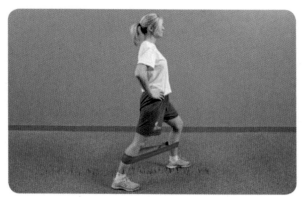

Theraband walking patterns – forward, sidestepping, carioca, monster steps, backward, ½ circles forward/backward – 25 yds. Start band at knee height and progress to ankle height

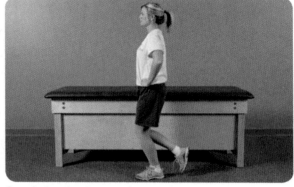

Single leg body weight squats, increase external resistance, stand on soft surface

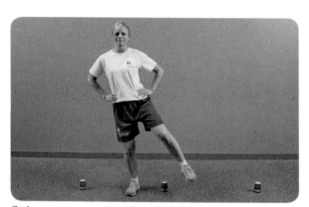

Side steps over cups/hurdles (with ball toss and external sports cord resistance), increase speed

Goals for Phase 3

☐ Restoration of muscular endurance/strength

☐ Restoration of cardiovascular endurance

☐ Optimize neuromuscular control/balance/ proprioception

Criteria for Progression to Phase 4

☐ Single leg mini-squat with level pelvis

☐ Cardiovascular fitness equal to preinjury level

☐ Demonstration of initial agility drills with proper body mechanics

PHASE 4:   WEEKS 11-13
Sports specific training rehab clinic based progression

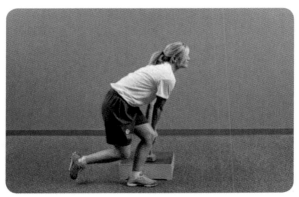

Single leg pick-ups, add soft surface

Other Exercises Weeks 11-13

- All phase 3 exercises

- Pool running (progress from chest deep to waist deep), treadmill jogging

- Step drills, quick feet step-ups (4-6 inch box) forward, lateral, carioca

- Plyometrics, double leg and single leg shuttle jumps

- Theraband walking patterns 1 rep of six exercises x 50yds, progress to band at knee height and ankle height

FINAL PHASE: WEEKS 14 & BEYOND
Sports specific training on field or court

Other Exercises Weeks 14 & beyond

☐ Running progression
☐ Sport specific drills
☐ Traditional weight training

Criteria for full return to competition

☐ Full range of motion
☐ Hip strength equal to uninvolved side, single leg pick-up with level pelvis
☐ Ability to perform sport-specific drills at full speed without pain
☐ Completion of functional sports test

Routine Arthroscopic Procedure

(Loose body removal, labral debridement, chondroplasty, synovectomy, ligamentum teres debridement)

This protocol should be used as a guideline for progression and should be tailored to the needs of the individual patient.

- **Weight bearing as tolerated – use crutches to normalize gait.**
  - Crutches are usually discontinued at 5-7 days, once gait is normalized

- **Initiate supervised physical therapy, postop day 1 or 2.**

- **Isometrics, co-contractions, closed chain exercises.**

- **Initiate stationary bike as symptoms allow.**
  - Seat raised to avoid uncomfortable hip flexion.
  - Low resistance with the emphasis on fluid range of motion.

- **Pool program initiated when sutures removed and portals healed.**
  (approximately 10 days; sutures removed at 1 week)

- **Rehab deliberate for the first 2-3 months, then initiate functional progression as symptoms allow.**
  - (2 vs. 3 months dictated by nature of pathology).
  - 2 months: loose fragment, simple labral tears, ruptured ligamentum teres.
  - 3 months: tenuous preserved labrum (i.e. thermal treatment for stabilization); or extensive articular damage.

- **"Honeymoon period"**
  - At 1 month most patients feel like they are doing better than they really are (regardless of eventual outcome).
  - Probably due to expectations of surgery being more disabling.
  - Risk of overdoing it!
  - Delaying functional progression based on tolerance to 2-3 months more reliable with less risk of setback.
  - Functional progression more liberal for athletes with close supervision.

PHASE 1: WEEK 1
Initial Exercises *(Weeks 1-3)*

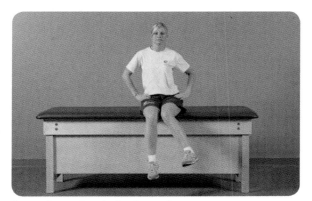

Seated weight shifts, lateral

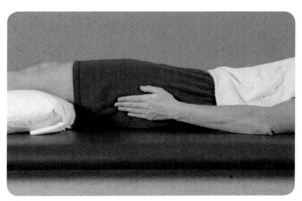

Glut sets

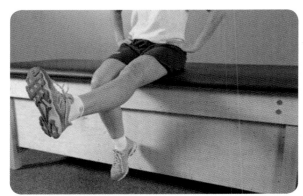

Seated knee extensions

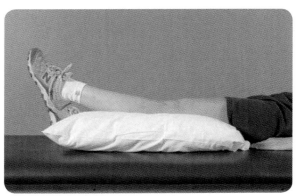

Quad sets

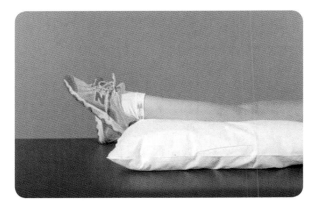

Ankle pumps

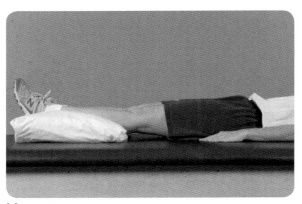

Hamstring sets

Initial Exercises *(Weeks 1-3)*

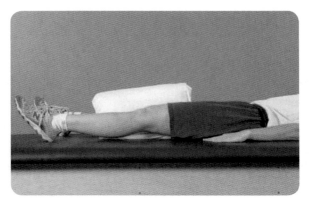

Adductor isometrics

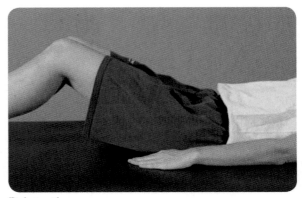

Pelvic tilt

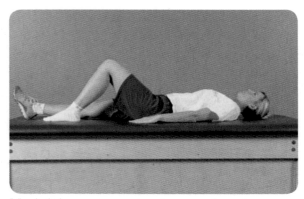

Heel slides, active-assisted range of motion

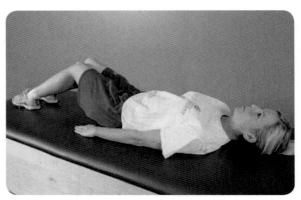

Trunk rotation

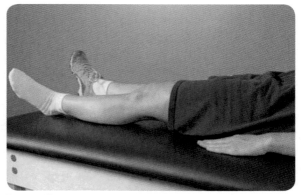

Log rolling

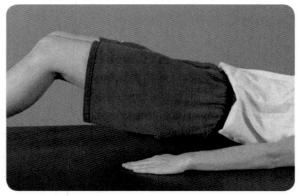

Double leg bridges

PHASE 1:
Initial Exercises *(Weeks 1-3)*

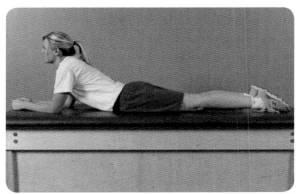

Prone on elbows

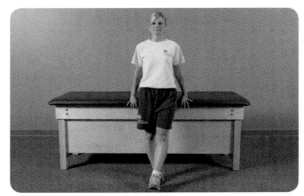

Standing adduction without resistance

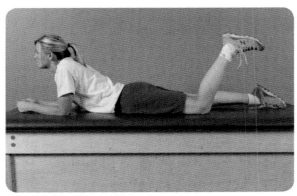

Prone knee flexion

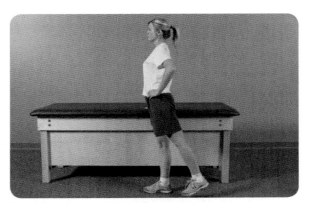

Standing extension without resistance

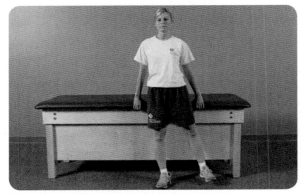

Standing abduction without resistance

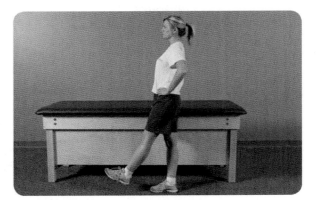

Standing flexion without resistance

PHASE 1:   WEEK 1
Initial Exercises *(Weeks 1-3)*

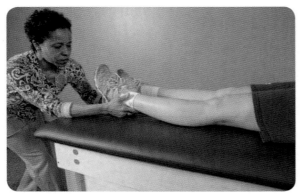

Pain dominant hip mobilization – grades I, II

Other Exercises Week 1

- Standard stationary bike without resistance at 3 days post-op (10 min. if tolerated)

- Upper body ergometer, upper body strengthening

PHASE 1:   WEEK 2
In Addition to Previous Exercises *(Weeks 1-3)*

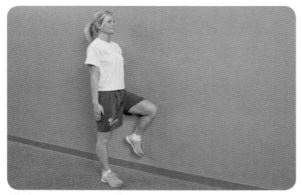

Abduction isometrics

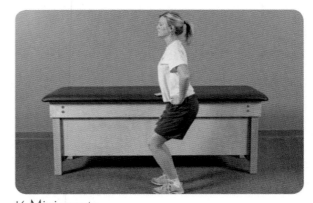

¼ Mini squats

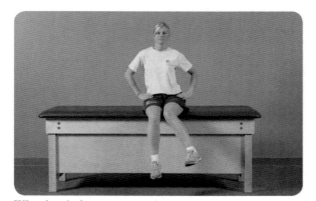

Weight shifts – anterior/posterior

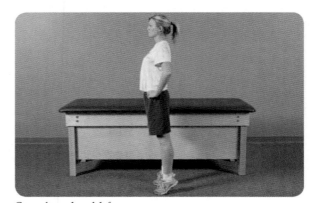

Standing heel lifts

PHASE 1:
WEEK 3

In Addition to Previous Exercises *(Weeks 1-3)*

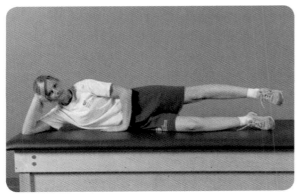

Leg raise – Abduction

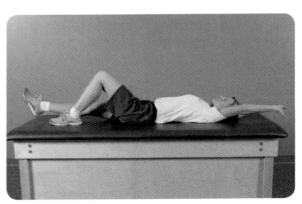

Dead bug

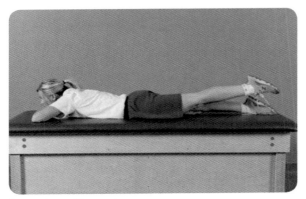

Leg raise – Extension

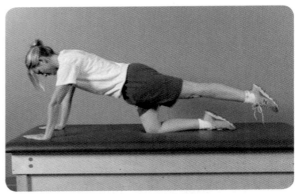

Quadriped 4 point support, progress 3 point support, progress 2 point

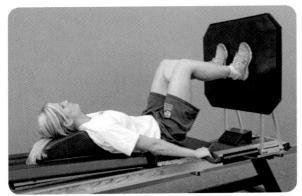

Shuttle leg press 90 degree hip flexion with co-contraction of adductors

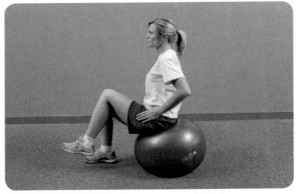

Seated physioball progression – hip flexion

PHASE 1:   WEEK 3
In Addition to Previous Exercises *(Weeks 1-3)*

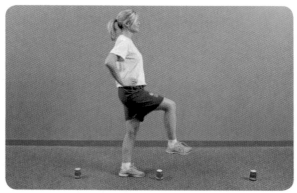

Forward walking over cups and hurdles (pause on affected limb), add ball toss while walking

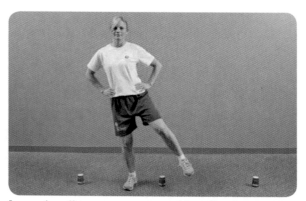

Lateral walking over cups and hurdles (pause on affected limb), add ball toss while walking

Other Exercises Week 3

- Continue stationary bike with minimal resistance – 5 min. increase daily

- Active range of motion with gradual end range stretch within tolerance

- Leg raise – Adduction

- Single leg sports cord leg press (long sitting) limiting hip flexion

Goals of Phase 1

☐ Restore range of motion

☐ Diminish pain and inflammation

☐ Prevent muscular inhibition

☐ Normalize gait

Criteria for progression to Phase 2

☐ Minimal pain with phase 1 exercises

☐ Minimal range of motion limitations

☐ Normalized gait without crutches

PHASE 2:
Intermediate Exercises *(Weeks 4-6)*

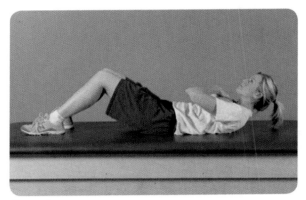

Crunches

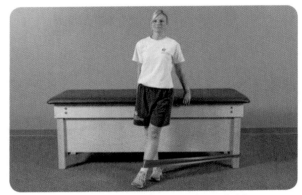

Standing theraband/pulley weight – Adduction

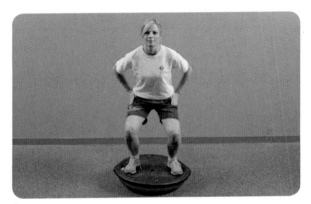

Bosu squats

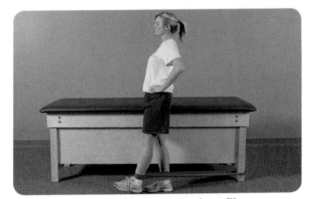

Standing theraband/pulley weight – Flexion

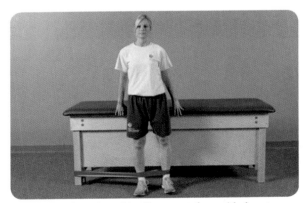

Standing theraband/pulley weight – Abduction

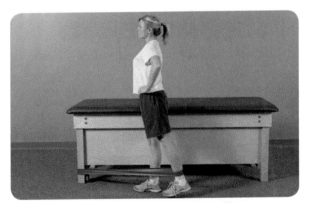

Standing theraband/pulley weight – Extension

PHASE 2:   WEEKS 4-5
Intermediate Exercises *(Weeks 4-6)*

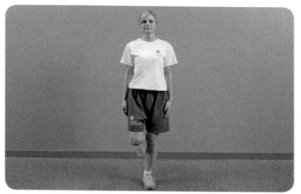

Single leg balance – firm to soft surface

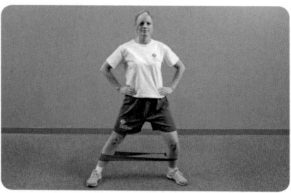

Sidestepping with resistance (pause on affected limb), sports cord walking forward and backward (pause on affected limb)

Other Exercises Weeks 4-5

- Gradually increase resistance with stationary bike

- Initiate elliptical machine

- Pool water exercises – flutterkick swimming, 4 way hip with water weights, step-ups

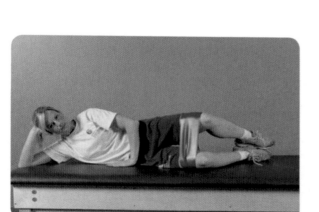

Clamshells with theraband

PHASE 2:   WEEK 6
Intermediate Exercises *(Week 6)*

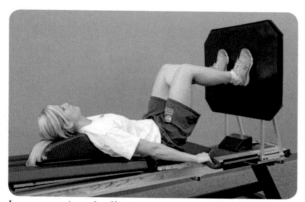

Leg press (gradually increasing weight)

PHASE 2:   WEEK 6
Intermediate Exercises *(Week 6)*

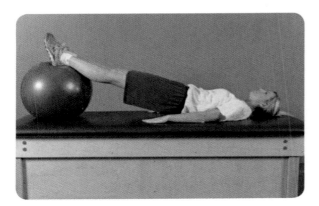

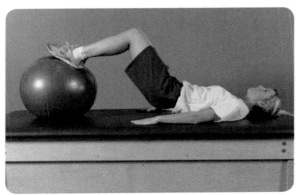

Physioball hamstring exercises – hip lift, bent knee hip lift, curls, balance

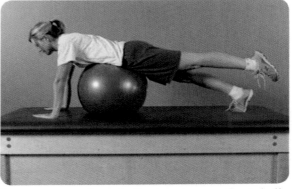

Superman on physioball – 2 point on physioball

Other Exercises Week 6

• Single leg balance – firm to soft surface with external perturbation (ball catch, sports specific/simulated ex.)

• Knee extensions, hamstring curls

Goals of Phase 2

☐ Restore pain-free range of motion

☐ Initiate proprioception exercises

☐ Progressively increase muscle strength and endurance

Criteria for progression to Phase 3

☐ Minimum pain with phase 2 exercises

☐ Single leg stance with level pelvis

Advanced Exercises (*Weeks 7-8*)

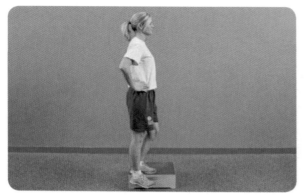

Step-ups with eccentric lowering

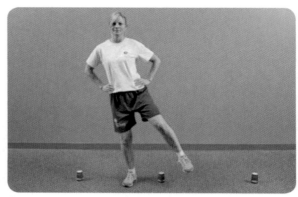

Side steps over cups/hurdles (with ball toss and external sports cord resistance), increase speed

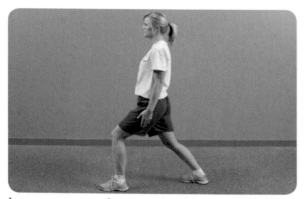

Lunges progress from single plane to tri-planar, add medicine balls for resistance and rotation

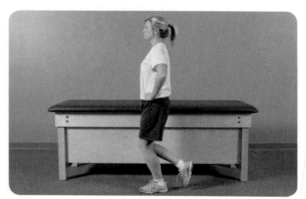

Single leg body weight squats, increase external resistance, stand on soft surface

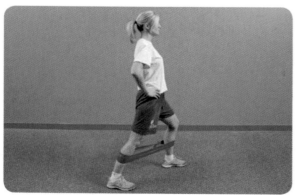

Theraband walking patterns – forward, sidestepping, carioca, monster steps, backward, ½ circles forward/backward – 25yds. Start band at knee height and progress to ankle height

Other Exercises Weeks 7-8

• Full squats

• Single stability ball bridges

Goals for Phase 3

☐ Restoration of muscular endurance/strength

☐ Restoration of cardiovascular endurance

☐ Optimize neuromuscular control/balance/proprioception

PHASE 3:   WEEKS 7-8
Advanced Exercises *(Weeks 7-8)*

Criteria for Progression to Phase 4

☐ Single leg mini-squat with level pelvis

☐ Cardiovascular fitness equal to preinjury level

☐ Demonstration of initial agility drills with proper body mechanics

PHASE 4:   WEEKS 9-11
Sports specific training rehab clinic based progression

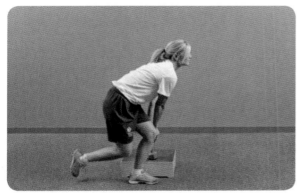

Single leg pick-ups, add soft surface

Other Exercises Weeks 9-11

• All phase 3 exercises

• Pool running (progress from chest deep to waist deep), treadmill jogging

• Step drills, quick feet step-ups (4-6 inch box) forward, lateral, carioca

• Plyometrics, double leg and single leg shuttle jumps

• Theraband walking patterns 1 rep of six exercises x 50yds, progress to band at knee height and ankle height

FINAL PHASE: WEEKS 12 & BEYOND
Sports specific training rehab clinic based progression

Other Exercises Weeks 12 & Beyond

• Running progression

• Sport specific drills

• Traditional weight training

Criteria for full return to competition

☐ Full range of motion

☐ Hip strength equal to uninvolved side, single leg pick-up with level pelvis

☐ Ability to perform sport-specific drills at full speed without pain

☐ Completion of functional sports test

Acetabuloplasty Exercises

Page	Exercise	Link to video demonstration
P. 455	Ankle pump	http://goo.gl/1KTvU
	Glut sets	http://goo.gl/sx4Ze
P. 456	Quad sets	http://goo.gl/NKRg6
	Heel slides, active-assisted range of motion	http://goo.gl/2zYZ2
	Hamstring sets	http://goo.gl/cPku0
	Log rolling	http://goo.gl/GJHvs
	Adductor isometrics	http://goo.gl/ZmlWZ
	Pelvic tilt	http://goo.gl/8rHkO
P. 457	Trunk rotation	http://goo.gl/nO9ob
	Seated knee extensions	http://goo.gl/HOSmk
	Double leg bridges	http://goo.gl/GrbI0
	Prone on elbows	http://goo.gl/Cb7OJ
	Weight shifts - sitting, supported, anterior/posterior, lateral	http://goo.gl/QF6un
	Prone knee flexion	http://goo.gl/OdaSb
P. 458	Standing abduction without resistance	http://goo.gl/xvSH2
	Standing flexion without resistance	http://goo.gl/y0HjG
	Standing adduction without resistance	http://goo.gl/Qt9MN
	Standing extension without resistance	http://goo.gl/WVYwP
	Pain dominant hip mobilization, grades I, II	http://goo.gl/pJ1OY
P. 459	Abduction isometrics	http://goo.gl/k2zB3
	Seated physioball progression - knee extension	http://goo.gl/Qj0b2
	1/4 mini squats	http://goo.gl/xiTd4
	Hip flexion, IR/ER in pain-free range	http://goo.gl/h7Ktd
	Standing heel lifts	http://goo.gl/TbHu0
	Theraband resistance on affected side - abduction (start very low resistance)	http://goo.gl/skh1u
P. 460	Theraband resistance on affected side - adduction (start very low resistance)	http://goo.gl/zWFGC
	Superman	http://goo.gl/U0CBw
	Theraband resistance on affected side - flexion (start very low resistance)	http://goo.gl/IshHg
	Theraband resistance on affected side - extension (start very low resistance)	http://goo.gl/NvZnN
P. 461	Stiffness dominant hip mobilization - grades III, IV	http://goo.gl/MQEFE
	Stiffness dominant hip mobilization - grades III, IV	http://goo.gl/GAWJz
	Clamshells (pain-free range)	http://goo.gl/mBydg
	Leg raise - Abduction	http://goo.gl/BfKa8
	Leg raise - Extension	http://goo.gl/yjNad
	Double leg bridges to single leg bridges	http://goo.gl/6Iuk8
P. 462	Shuttle leg press 90 degree hip flexion with co-contraction of adductors	http://goo.gl/BCpCe
	Seated physioball progression - hip flexion	http://goo.gl/rwov6
	Dead bug	http://goo.gl/KzAVu
	Forward walking over cups and hurdles (pause on affected limb), add ball toss while walking	http://goo.gl/LxCsl
	Quadriped 4 point support, progress 3 point support, progress 2 point	http://goo.gl/WeS8g
P. 463	Crunches	http://goo.gl/2jcQx
	Standing theraband/pulley weight - Abduction	http://goo.gl/P1J9h
	Bosu squats	http://goo.gl/m5mFL
	Standing theraband/pulley weight - Adduction	http://goo.gl/mUOHd
P. 464	Standing theraband/pulley weight - Flexion	http://goo.gl/IshHg
	Clamshells with theraband	http://goo.gl/RxWsS
	Standing theraband/pulley weight - Extension	http://goo.gl/cpxNY
	Sidestepping with resistance (pause on affected limb), sports cord walking forward and backward (pause on affected limb)	http://goo.gl/5ylq3
	Single leg balance - firm to soft surface	http://goo.gl/7YV8S
P. 465	Leg press (gradually increasing weight)	http://goo.gl/BCpCe
	Superman on physioball - 2 point on physioball	http://goo.gl/ThWMa
	Physioball hamstring exercises - hip lift, bent knee hip lift, curls, balance	http://goo.gl/kLYq5

P. 466	Step-ups with eccentric lowering	http://goo.gl/TaaDa
	Side steps over cups/hurdles (with ball toss and external sports cord resistance), increase speed	http://goo.gl/pv6ci
	Lunges pogress from single plane to tri-planar, add medicine balls for resistance and rotation	http://goo.gl/syM2y
	Single leg body weight squats, increase external resistance, stand on soft surface	http://goo.gl/JXYV7
	Theraband walking patterns	http://goo.gl/g7XQG
P. 467	Single leg pick-ups, add soft surface	http://goo.gl/eiVQL

Femoroplasty Exercises

Page	Exercise	Link to video demonstration
P. 468	Weight shifts - sitting, supported, anterior/posterior, lateral	http://goo.gl/osBPR
	Ankle pumps	http://goo.gl/GaA2R
P. 469	Seated knee extensions	http://goo.gl/Otgh7
	Hamstring sets	http://goo.gl/DHONr
	Glut sets	http://goo.gl/XSMYP
	Adductor isometrics	http://goo.gl/xDXeC
	Quad sets	http://goo.gl/28hCV
	Heel slides, active-assisted range of motion	http://goo.gl/JUcgU
P. 470	Log rolling	http://goo.gl/1OczB
	Double leg bridges	http://goo.gl/Fl9Yh
	Pelvic tilt	http://goo.gl/Fl9Yh
	Prone on elbows	http://goo.gl/LlC83
	Trunk rotation	http://goo.gl/nO9ob
	Prone knee flexion	http://goo.gl/dJEgn
P. 471	Standing abduction without resistance	http://goo.gl/WDm5n
	Standing flexion without resistance	http://goo.gl/ZoPKO
	Standing adduction without resistance	http://goo.gl/Yjq9S
	Pain dominant hip mobilization, grades I, II	http://goo.gl/pJ1OY
	Standing extension without resistance	http://goo.gl/nzb00
P. 472	Supine marching, modified dead bug	http://goo.gl/RB505
	Theraband resistance on affected side - abduction (start very low resistance)	http://goo.gl/IlCPc
	Abduction isometrics	http://goo.gl/rw3x7
	Theraband resistance on affected side - adduction (start very low redsistance)	http://goo.gl/lYNtO
	Superman	http://goo.gl/Sf4kc
	Theraband resistance on affected side - flexion (start very low resistance)	http://goo.gl/IshHg
P. 473	Theraband resistance on affected side - extension (start very low resistance)	http://goo.gl/NvZnN
	1/4 mini squats	http://goo.gl/Ap5Pd
	Hip flexion, IR/ER in pain-free range	http://goo.gl/wdnUS
	Standing heel lifts	http://goo.gl/ZO6Yb
	Double leg bridges to single leg bridges	http://goo.gl/3k6zE
P. 474	Clamshells (pain-free range)	http://goo.gl/uckKA
	Quadriped 4 point support, progress 3 point support, progress 2 point	http://goo.gl/vWgWT
	Leg raise - Abduction	http://goo.gl/Bwzed
	Seated physioball progression - hip flexion	http://goo.gl/0WPPj
	Leg raise - Extension	http://goo.gl/yjNad
	Hip mobilization - inferior glides in flexion	http://goo.gl/MQEFE
P. 475	Stiffness dominant hip mobilization - grades III, IV	http://goo.gl/HRrZV
	Crunches	http://goo.gl/VZ3qT
	Standing theraband/pulley weight - Abduction	http://goo.gl/E5CPE
P. 476	Standing theraband/pulley weight - Adduction	http://goo.gl/KleNf
	Single leg balance - firm to soft surface	http://goo.gl/ni9hg
	Standing theraband/pulley weight - Flexion	http://goo.gl/NeflL
	Shuttle leg press 90 degree hip flexion with co-contraction of adductors	http://goo.gl/BCpCe
	Standing theraband/pulley weight - Extension	http://goo.gl/hQylz
	Clamshells with theraband	http://goo.gl/Jgsb6
P. 477	Forward walking over cups and hurdles (pause on affected limb, add ball toss while walking	http://goo.gl/VNF4i
	Lateral walking over cups and hurdles (pause on affected limb), add ball toss while walking	http://goo.gl/kvdW6
	Leg press (gradually increasing weight)	http://goo.gl/BCpCe
	Physioball hamstring exercises - hip lift, bent knee hip lift, curls, balance	http://goo.gl/sMdX3
P. 478	Superman on physioball - 2 point on physioball	http://goo.gl/Gom9f
	Sidestepping with resistance (pause on affected limb), sports cord walking forward and backward (pause on affected limb)	http://goo.gl/5ylq3
	Bosu squats	http://goo.gl/WAU49

P. 479	Step-ups with eccentric lowering	http://goo.gl/BUHvx
	Side steps over cups/hurdles (with ball toss and external sports cord resistance), increase speed	http://goo.gl/LZ2U1
	Lunges progress from single plane to tri-planar, add medicine balls for resistance and rotation	http://goo.gl/V4S0T
	Single leg body weight squats, incerase external resistance, stand on soft surface	http://goo.gl/NzbKh
	Theraband walking patterns	http://goo.gl/3ovrA
P. 480	Single leg pick-ups, add soft surface	http://goo.gl/RzSrr

Iliopsoas Release Exercises

Page	Exercise	Link to video demonstration
P. 482	Seated knee extensions	http://goo.gl/BY5ec
	Seated weight shifts	http://goo.gl/LkxoY
P. 483	Ankle pumps	http://goo.gl/ZgqKk
	Hamstring sets	http://goo.gl/oB8PN
	Glut sets	http://goo.gl/Eiq9M
	Adductor isometrics	http://goo.gl/gE9UF
	Quad sets	http://goo.gl/cJcBG
	Heel slides, active-assisted range of motion	http://goo.gl/txSao
P. 484	Log rolling	http://goo.gl/nAOjL
	Double leg bridges	http://goo.gl/417CV
	Pelvic tilt	http://goo.gl/417CV
	Prone on elbows	http://goo.gl/LlC83
	Trunk rotation	http://goo.gl/nO9ob
	Prone knee flexion	http://goo.gl/Iz4kH
P. 485	Standing abduction without resistance	http://goo.gl/0IrpB
	Standing flexion without resistance	http://goo.gl/QbtFl
	Standing adduction without resistance	http://goo.gl/eyU9i
	Pain dominant hip mobilization, grades I, II	http://goo.gl/pJ1OY
	Standing extension without resistance	http://goo.gl/nzb00
P. 486	Abduction isometrics	http://goo.gl/rw3x7
	Superman	http://goo.gl/CspFC
	1/4 mini squats	http://goo.gl/3mf4I
	Theraband resistance on affected side - abduction (start very low resistance)	http://goo.gl/E5CPE
	Standing heel lifts	http://goo.gl/TUekm
	Theraband resistance on affected side - adduction (start very low resistance)	http://goo.gl/lYNtO
P. 487	Theraband resistance on affected side - flexion (start very low resistance) ONLY IF TOLERATED	http://goo.gl/IshHg
	Theraband resistance on affected side - extension (start very low resistance)	http://goo.gl/NvZnN
	Stiffness dominant hip mobilization (left photo)	http://goo.gl/MQEFE
	Stiffness dominant hip mobilization (right photo)	http://goo.gl/Br94X
P. 488	Double leg bridges to single leg bridges	http://goo.gl/Xng3v
	Leg raise - Extension	http://goo.gl/yjNad
	Clamshells (pain-free range)	http://goo.gl/uckKA
	Shuttle leg press 90 degree hip flexion with co-contractionof adductors	http://goo.gl/BCpCe
	Leg raise - Abduction	http://goo.gl/dbj0t
	Dead bug	http://goo.gl/Vy5F3
P. 489	Quadriped 4 point support, progress 3 point support, progress 2 point	http://goo.gl/ExPJN
	Lateral walking over cups and hurdles (pause on affected limb), add ball toss while walking	http://goo.gl/FiYvY
	Seated physioball progression - hip flexion	http://goo.gl/rwov6
	Forward walking over cups and hurdles (pause on affected limb), add ball toss while walking	http://goo.gl/1Ps3O
P. 490	Crunches	http://goo.gl/Vq467
	Standing theraband/pulley weight - Adduction	http://goo.gl/lYNtO
	Bosu squats	http://goo.gl/WAU49
	Standing theraband/pulley weight - Flexion	http://goo.gl/IshHg
	Standing theraband/pulley weight - Abduction	http://goo.gl/E5CPE
	Standing theraband/pulley weight - Extension	http://goo.gl/NvZnN
P. 491	Single leg balance - firm to soft surface	http://goo.gl/ni9hg
	Sidestepping with resistance (pause on affected limb), sports cord walking forward and backward (pause on affected limb)	http://goo.gl/H7Thn
	Clamshells with theraband	http://goo.gl/Jgsb6
	Leg press (gradually increasing weight)	http://goo.gl/BCpCe

Labral Repair Exercises

Page	Exercise	Link to video demonstration
P. 495	Ankle pumps	http://goo.gl/ZgqKk
	Glut sets	http://goo.gl/Eiq9M
P. 496	Quad sets	http://goo.gl/cJcBG
	Heel slides, active-assisted range of motion	http://goo.gl/txSao
	Hamstring sets	http://goo.gl/oB8PN
	Log rolling internal rotation	http://goo.gl/nAOjL
	Adductor isometrics	http://goo.gl/gE9UF
	Pelvic tilt	http://goo.gl/417CV
P. 497	Double leg bridges	http://goo.gl/417CV
	Prone knee flexion	http://goo.gl/Iz4kH
	Seated knee extensions	http://goo.gl/BY5ec
	Standing abduction without resistance	http://goo.gl/0IrpB
	Prone on elbows	http://goo.gl/LlC83
	Standing adduction without resistance	http://goo.gl/eyU9i
P. 498	Standing extension without resistance	http://goo.gl/nzb00
	Pain dominant hip mobilization, grade I	http://goo.gl/pJ1OY
	Standing flexion without resistance	http://goo.gl/QbtFl
	Supine marching (90 degrees)	http://goo.gl/sI4Wm
	Modified deadbug (90 degrees)	http://goo.gl/Vy5F3
P. 499	Superman	http://goo.gl/CspFC
	Theraband resistance on affected side - Adduction (start very low resistance)	http://goo.gl/lYNtO
	Abduction isometrics	http://goo.gl/rw3x7
	Theraband resistance on affected side - Flexion (start very low resistance)	http://goo.gl/IshHg
	Theraband resistance on affected side - Abduction (start very low resistance)	http://goo.gl/E5CPE
	Theraband resistance on affected side - Extension (start very low resistance)	http://goo.gl/NvZnN
P. 500	Leg raise - Abduction	http://goo.gl/dbj0t
	Seated physioball progression - hip flexion to 90 degrees	http://goo.gl/rwov6
	Leg raise - Extension	http://goo.gl/yjNad
P. 501	Crunches	http://goo.gl/Vq467
	Clamshells	http://goo.gl/uckKA
	Weight shifts - standing, sitting, supported, anterior/posterior, laterals, physioball	http://goo.gl/LkxoY
	Leg press (minimal resistance, gradually increasing resistance to patient tolerance)	http://goo.gl/BCpCe
	1/4 mini squats	http://goo.gl/3mf4I
P. 502	Superman (quadriped position)	http://goo.gl/ExPJN
	Standing theraband - Flexion	http://goo.gl/IshHg
	Standing theraband - Abduction	http://goo.gl/E5CPE
	Standing theraband - Extension	http://goo.gl/NvZnN
	Standing theraband - Adduction	http://goo.gl/lYNtO
	Standing heel raises	http://goo.gl/TUekm
P. 503	Single leg bridges/stabilization/alternate kickouts	http://goo.gl/Xng3v
	Clamshells with restrictive tubing/band	http://goo.gl/Jgsb6
	Single leg balance - firm to soft surface with external perturbation (ball catch, sports specific/simulated ex.)	http://goo.gl/ni9hg
P. 504	Physioball hamstring ex. - hip lift, bent knee hip lift, curls, balance (top photo)	http://goo.gl/sMdX3
	Physioball hamstring ex. - hip lift, bent knee hip lift, curls, balance (bottom photo)	http://goo.gl/lcitg
	Side stepping with resistance (pause on affected limb), sports cord walking forward and backward (pause on affected limb)	http://goo.gl/H7Thn
	Bosu squats	http://goo.gl/WAU49
P. 505	Step-ups with eccentric lowering	http://goo.gl/Oho0S
	Side steps over cups/hurdles (with ball toss and external sports cord resistance), increase speed	http://goo.gl/vBLGc
	Lunges progress from single plane to tri-planar, add medicine balls for resistance and rotation	http://goo.gl/syM2y
	Single leg body weight squats, increase external resistance, stand on soft surface	http://goo.gl/NzbKh
	Theraband walking patterns	http://goo.gl/3ovrA
P. 506	Single leg pick-ups, add soft surface	http://goo.gl/RzSrr

Microfracture Exercises

Page	Exercise	Link to video demonstration
P. 507	Seated knee extensions	http://goo.gl/BY5ec
	Ankle pumps	http://goo.gl/QcQ3L
P. 508	Glut sets	http://goo.gl/pr1AM
	Adductor isometrics	http://goo.gl/gE9UF
	Quad sets	http://goo.gl/cJcBG
	Heel slides, active-assisted range of motion	http://goo.gl/txSao
	Hamstring sets	http://goo.gl/oB8PN
	Log rolling	http://goo.gl/nAOjL
P. 509	Pelvic tilt	http://goo.gl/Fl9Yh
	Prone on elbows	http://goo.gl/LlC83
	Trunk rotation	http://goo.gl/nO9ob
	Prone knee flexion	http://goo.gl/Iz4kH
	Double leg bridges	http://goo.gl/Fl9Yh
	Standing abduction without resistance	http://goo.gl/WDm5n
P. 510	Standing adduction without resistance	http://goo.gl/Yjq9S
	Standing flexion without resistance	http://goo.gl/ZoPKO
	Standing extension without resistance	http://goo.gl/nzb00
	Pain dominant hip mobilization, grades I, II	http://goo.gl/pJ1OY
P. 511	Supine marching, modified dead bug	http://goo.gl/Vy5F3
	Theraband resistance on affected side - Abduction (start very low resistance)	http://goo.gl/E5CPE
	Superman	http://goo.gl/CspFC
	Theraband resistance on affected side - Adduction (start very low resistance)	http://goo.gl/lYNtO
	Abduction isometrics	http://goo.gl/rw3x7
	Theraband resistance on affected side - Flexion (start very low resistance)	http://goo.gl/IshHg
P. 512	Theraband resistance on affected side - Extension (start very low resistance)	http://goo.gl/NvZnN
	Hip flexion, IR/ER in pain-free range	http://goo.gl/wdnUS
	Leg raise - Abduction	http://goo.gl/dbj0t
	Clamshells	http://goo.gl/uckKA
	Leg raise - Extension	http://goo.gl/yjNad
P. 513	Seated physioball progression - active hip/knee	http://goo.gl/rwov6
	Theraband resistance on affected side - Abduction (start very low resistance)	http://goo.gl/E5CPE
	Theraband resistance on affected side - Adduction (start very low resistance)	http://goo.gl/lYNtO
P. 514	Theraband resistance on affected side - Flexion (start very low resistance)	http://goo.gl/IshHg
	Crunches	http://goo.gl/Vq467
	Theraband resistance on affected side - Extension (start very low resistance)	http://goo.gl/NvZnN
P. 515	Superman (quadriped position)	http://goo.gl/ExPJN
	Clamshells with resistive tubing/band	http://goo.gl/Jgsb6
	1/4 mini squats	http://goo.gl/3mf4I
	Standing heel lifts	http://goo.gl/TUekm
P. 516	Single leg bridges/stabilization/alternate kickouts	http://goo.gl/Xng3v
	Single leg balance - firm to soft surface with external perturbation (ball catch, sports specific/ simulated ex.)	http://goo.gl/ni9hg
	Physioball hamstring exercises - hip lift, bent knee hip lift, curls, balance (top photo)	http://goo.gl/sMdX3
	Physioball hamstring exercises - hip lift, bent knee hip lift, curls, balance (bottom photo)	http://goo.gl/lcitg
P. 517	Sidestepping with resistance (pause on affected limb), sports cord walking forward and backward (pause on affected limb)	http://goo.gl/H7Thn
	Bosu squats	http://goo.gl/WAU49
	Step-ups with eccentric lowering	http://goo.gl/Oho0S
	Lunges progress from single plane to tri-planar lunges, add medicine balls for resistance and rotation	http://goo.gl/syM2y
P. 518	Theraband walking patterns	http://goo.gl/3ovrA
	Single leg body weight squats, increase external ressistance, stand on soft surface	http://goo.gl/NzbKh
	Side steps over cups/hurdles (with ball toss and external sports cord resistance), increase speed	http://goo.gl/vBLGc
P. 519	Single leg pick-ups, add soft surface	http://goo.gl/RzSrr

Routine Arthroscopic Procedure Exercises

Page	Exercise	Link to video demonstration
P. 521	Seated weight shifts, lateral	http://goo.gl/LkxoY
	Glut sets	http://goo.gl/pr1AM
	Seated knee extensions	http://goo.gl/BY5ec
	Quad sets	http://goo.gl/cJcBG
	Ankle pumps	http://goo.gl/QcQ3L
	Hamstring sets	http://goo.gl/oB8PN
P. 522	Adductor isometrics	http://goo.gl/gE9UF
	Pelvic tilt	http://goo.gl/Fl9Yh
	Heel slides, active-assisted range of motion	http://goo.gl/txSao
	Trunk rotation	http://goo.gl/nO9ob
	Log rolling	http://goo.gl/nAOjL
	Double leg bridges	http://goo.gl/Fl9Yh
P. 523	Prone on elbows	http://goo.gl/LlC83
	Standing adduction without resistance	http://goo.gl/Yjq9S
	Prone knee flexion	http://goo.gl/Iz4kH
	Standing extension without resistance	http://goo.gl/nzb00
	Standing abduction without resistance	http://goo.gl/WDm5n
	Standing flexion without resistance	http://goo.gl/ZoPKO
P. 524	Pain dominant hip mobilization - grades I, II	http://goo.gl/pJ1OY
	Abduction isometrics	http://goo.gl/rw3x7
	1/4 mini squats	http://goo.gl/3mf4I
	Weight shifts - anterior/posterior	http://goo.gl/kdRPI
	Standing heel lifts	http://goo.gl/TUekm
P. 525	Hip flexion, IR/ER in pain-free range	http://goo.gl/wdnUS
	Theraband resistance on affected side - Flexion (start very low resistance)	http://goo.gl/IshHg
	Theraband resistance on affected side - Abduction (start very low resistance)	http://goo.gl/E5CPE
	Theraband resistance on affected side - Extension (start very low resistance)	http://goo.gl/NvZnN
	Theraband resistance on affected side - Adduction (start very low resistance)	http://goo.gl/lYNtO
	Superman	http://goo.gl/CspFC
P. 526	Stiffness dominant hip mobilization, grades III, IV (top photo)	http://goo.gl/MQEFE
	Stiffness dominant hip mobilization, grades III, IV (bottom photo)	http://goo.gl/Br94X
	Double leg bridges to single leg bridges	http://goo.gl/Xng3v
	Clamshells (pain-free range)	http://goo.gl/uckKA
P. 527	Leg raise - Abduction	http://goo.gl/dbj0t
	Dead bug	http://goo.gl/Vy5F3
	Leg raise - Extension	http://goo.gl/yjNad
	Quadriped 4 point support, progress 3 point support, progress 2 point	http://goo.gl/SsafD
	Shuttle leg press 90 degree hip flexion with co-contraction of adductors	http://goo.gl/BCpCe
	Seated physioball progression - hip flexion	http://goo.gl/rwov6
P. 528	Forward walking over cups and hurdles (pause on affected limb), add ball toss while walking	http://goo.gl/1Ps3O
	Lateral walking over cups and hurdles (pause on affected limb), add ball toss while walking	http://goo.gl/vBLGc
P. 529	Crunches	http://goo.gl/Vq467
	Standing theraband/pulley weight - Adduction	http://goo.gl/lYNtO
	Bosu squats	http://goo.gl/WAU49
	Standing theraband/pulley weight - Flexion	http://goo.gl/IshHg
	Standing theraband/pulley weight - Abduction	http://goo.gl/E5CPE
	Standing theraband/pulley weight - Extension	http://goo.gl/NvZnN
P. 530	Single leg balance - firm to soft surface	http://goo.gl/ni9hg
	Side stepping with resistance (pause on affected limb), sports cord walking forward and backward (pause on affected limb)	http://goo.gl/H7Thn
	Clamshells with theraband	http://goo.gl/Jgsb6
	Leg press (gradually increasing weight)	http://goo.gl/BCpCe

Index

J.W.T. Byrd (ed.), *Operative Hip Arthroscopy*,
DOI 10.1007/978-1-4419-7925-4, © Springer Science+Business Media New York 2013